Neuromusculoskeletal Examination and Assessment

A Handbook for therapists

FOURTH EDITION

Edited by

Nicola J Petty DPT MSc FMACP FHEA
Principal Lecturer, School of Health Professions, University of Brighton, UK

Foreword by

Dr Alison Rushton EdD MSc Grad Dip Phys Dip TP mILT FMACP

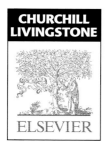

CHURCHILL
LIVINGSTONE

ELSEVIER

Edinburgh   London   New York   Oxford   Philadelphia   St Louis   Sydney   Toronto   2011

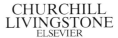

CHURCHILL
LIVINGSTONE
ELSEVIER

© 2013 Elsevier Ltd. All rights reserved.

No part of this publication may be reproduced or transmitted in any form or by any means, electronic or mechanical, including photocopying, recording, or any information storage and retrieval system, without permission in writing from the publisher. Details on how to seek permission, further information about the Publisher's permissions policies and our arrangements with organizations such as the Copyright Clearance Center and the Copyright Licensing Agency, can be found at our website: http://www.elsevier.com/permissions.

This book and the individual contributions contained in it are protected under copyright by the Publisher (other than as may be noted herein).

First edition 1997
Second edition 2001
Third edition 2006
Fourth edition 2013

ISBN 978-0-7020-55041
Formerly 978-0-7020-2990-5

British Library Cataloguing in Publication Data
A catalogue record for this book is available from the British Library

Library of Congress Cataloging in Publication Data
A catalog record for this book is available from the Library of Congress

Notices
Knowledge and best practice in this field are constantly changing. As new research and experience broaden our understanding, changes in research methods, professional practices, or medical treatment may become necessary.

Practitioners and researchers must always rely on their own experience and knowledge in evaluating and using any information, methods, compounds, or experiments described herein. In using such information or methods they should be mindful of their own safety and the safety of others, including parties for whom they have a professional responsibility.

With respect to any drug or pharmaceutical products identified, readers are advised to check the most current information provided (i) on procedures featured or (ii) by the manufacturer of each product to be administered, to verify the recommended dose or formula, the method and duration of administration, and contraindications. It is the responsibility of practitioners, relying on their own experience and knowledge of their patients, to make diagnoses, to determine dosages and the best treatment for each individual patient, and to take all appropriate safety precautions.

To the fullest extent of the law, neither the Publisher nor the authors, contributors, or editors assume any liability for any injury and/or damage to persons or property as a matter of products liability, negligence or otherwise, or from any use or operation of any methods, products, instructions, or ideas contained in the material herein.

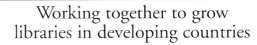
Printed in China

369 0226240

DATE DUE

30A|19			

N⯀ ⯀ation

A I

Demco, Inc. 38-293

Commissioning Editor: Rita Demetriou-Swanwick
Development Editor: Nicola Lally
Project Manager: K Anand Kumar and Deepthi Unni
Designer: Kirsteen Wright
Illustration Manager: Merlyn Harvey
Illustrator: Antbits

Dedication

In memory of Geoff Maitland, visionary pioneer of musculoskeletal physiotherapy

Contents

List of contributors

Kieran Barnard MSc BSc(Hons) MCSP MMACP
Extended Scope Physiotherapist, West Sussex Primary Care Trust, Horsham, UK

Linda Exelby BSc(Physio) GradDipManTher FMACP
Senior Lecturer, School of Health and Emergency Professions, University of Hertfordshire and Clinical Specialist, Pinehill Hospital, UK

Laura Finucane MSc BSc(Hons) MCSP MMACP HPC Reg
Consultant Musculoskeletal Physiotherapist, Physiotherapy Department, East Surrey Hospital, Redhill, UK

Roger Kerry MSc FMACP
Associate Professor, Division of Physiotherapy Education, University of Nottingham, UK

Chris Mercer MSc MCSP MMACP PGCert(Clin Ed)
Consultant Physiotherapist, Western Sussex Hospitals NHS Trust, West Sussex, UK

Chris Murphy MSc MCSP MMACP PGCert
PhysioUK, Epsom, Surrey, UK

Nicola J Petty DPT MSc FMACP FHEA
Principal Lecturer, School of Health Professions, University of Brighton, Eastbourne, UK

Colette Ridehalgh MSc BSc(Hons) MMACP
Senior Lecturer, School of Health Professions, University of Brighton, Eastbourne, UK

Dionne Ryder MSc MMACP FHEA
Senior Lecturer, School of Health and Emergency Professions, University of Hertfordshire, UK

Foreword from the first edition

The authors are to be congratulated on being able to put together the work of a number of clinical manipulative therapists, some of whom have dealt with manual therapy as a whole while others have concentrated on specific aspects of manipulative physiotherapy.

The standard of the whole field has grown almost out of recognition over the last 50 years. Latterly this coming together has been largely due to Gwen Jull's 'prove it or lose it' approach. Another significant factor has been the improved communication of a shrinking world; this has brought together the different approaches to the basis, teaching and performance of manipulative physiotherapy.

In our profession knowledge, skills and opportunities have increased substantially. It is wonderful to see these two authors, Nikki Petty and Ann Moore, making such an excellent job of putting together the contributions of all the familiar names into one volume. The coming generation needs to continue this trend; it won't all happen quickly but this start is excellent. The text is appropriate for the undergraduate, postgraduate and the practising therapist who is not fully aware of the diversity of concepts within manipulative physiotherapy.

G.D. Maitland

Foreword from the third edition

Do we need textbooks with lengthy, detailed and precise descriptions of clinical examination and assessment? Is it worthwhile for a clinician/academic to spend countless hours putting together a text that will, in part, contain information that will no longer be the latest information available by the time it goes to press? Perhaps you think that I should not be posing these questions in the foreword of a textbook, and that this is the time for praise of the author? Let me assure you that this will come later, now let me deal with the questions.

Learning is a life event without space and time limitations, and with no single 'right' way. Different learning processes work for different individuals; however, most of us require a structure to enable the first steps to take place. We must all start somewhere, and if we are lucky enough to have a wide-based structure as our springboard it gives us a solid foundation upon which to build the rest of our lives' work experience. For example, take undergraduate students with no concept of the process of clinical reasoning; they can easily understand why they have to learn the structure of the body, the workings and pathological patterns of those structures. To arrive at what has gone wrong in specific clinical presentations and to formulate a management programme tailored to the patient's individual situation and needs, the students are required to incorporate many areas of knowledge combined with their own life experience. 'Fortune favours the prepared mind', yes, but not in order to limit what information we take on board, instead to be discerning, critical and questioning to an appropriate degree. Without the knowledge of how to technically examine, why we perform these tests specifically and how to interpret them, the clinician would be lost.

This textbook provides the way forward. The detail with which the examinations are described and the possible interpretation for a wide variety of findings will be invaluable for any student of manual therapy at under- or post-graduate level. It is gratifying to see that the author allows for variation in body size and shape, both of the therapist and the patient, in her suggestions of manual examination. This textbook has a greater global approach than many of its predecessors (as indicated in its title) and is successful in reflecting the multifaceted approach taken by contemporary expert clinicians. It is for these reasons that the answer to my first question has to be yes.

In the last 15 years the UK has seen an explosive growth in manual therapy-related research. In some countries research in this area was prolific much earlier, and in some they are just starting. The emerging information from these studies is increasingly easier to access via the internet and, therefore, available to a far greater number of practitioners than ever before. This gives us no excuse for not being well informed and up to date. For the student the situation is different. The nature of being at the beginning of the learning process means that it is not always possible to know which questions to ask to get the most informed answer. Questions arising from clinical examination may not be answered by the most recent studies. Some of the information most frequently used by clinicians is patterns of referred pain. The definitive texts in this area were published following research in the 1940s and 1950s. Ergo it is necessary for the student to utilise information from a multitude of sources, produced by professionals from a variety of areas relevant to manual therapy and at different time periods in the development of this clinical field.

This textbook provides information for the beginning of the learning process and beyond. It utilizes up-to-date information combined with previous studies, providing that broad base essential for the 'probing' and critical clinician. The text takes the student through a logical sequence of questioning, examination and assessment, providing an open-minded approach to the diagnosis. It sets out possible management pathways and encourages further exploration and learning by providing ample references for each chapter. Again, the answer to the second question has to be yes.

Nikki Petty is to be congratulated on this mammoth task and clinicians of the future will thank her for her dedication and commitment to detail and be grateful for the ease with which she initiated their learning.

Agneta Lando,
August 2005

Foreword

It is difficult to write a foreword for a text that is now in its fourth edition as the necessity for a further edition speaks for itself. I therefore turn to quotations from Albert Einstein (1879 – 1955) for assistance:

"A man (or woman) should look for what is, and not for what he (she) thinks should be".

"Any intelligent fool can make things bigger and more complex. . . It takes a touch of genius - and a lot of courage to move in the opposite direction".

As well as being a great physicist, Einstein is also acknowledged as an excellent theorist and philosopher and was a leading intellectual of the modern world. His quotes serve to illustrate the distinctiveness of this text. Firstly, that it focuses us to examine (patient history and physical testing) and assess (clinical reasoning) a patient with an open mind free of bias, using the clinical evidence from the patient interpreted in the context of our knowledge. Secondly, that it makes the many components of a complex process of patient examination and assessment as clear as possible. Our effectiveness of practice within the speciality of neuromusculoskeletal is dependent upon an accurate and reasoned analysis of an individual patient's presentation. Owing to the complexities of the process, we require a framework to enable our learning and development to achieve proficiency and effectiveness in examination and assessment. By making all components of the process as clear and logical as possible, this text therefore provides a valuable and structured framework for learning and development.

The complexity of the process of examination and assessment is illustrated by the International Federation of Orthopaedic Manipulative Physical Therapists (IFOMPT), through its definition of educational standards in neuromusculoskeletal practice:

". . . practice in Orthopaedic Manipulative Therapy (OMT, neuromusculoskeletal) is informed by a complex integration of research evidence, the patient's preferences and the patient's individual clinical presentation. . ."

"The application of OMT is based on a comprehensive assessment of the patient's neuromusculoskeletal system and of the patient's functional abilities. This examination serves to define the presenting dysfunction(s) in the articular, muscular, nervous and other relevant systems; and how these relate to any disability or functional limitation as described by the World Health Organisation's International Classification of Functioning, Disability and Health. Equally, the examination aims to distinguish those conditions that are indications or contraindications to OMT Physical Therapy and / or demand special precautions, as well as those where anatomical anomalies or pathological processes limit or direct the use of OMT procedures".

(IFOMPT Standards Document, 2008)

In this edition, Nicola Petty takes an editorial role and has invited experienced clinicians and academics to review and write each chapter. All contributors are members of the Manipulation Association of Chartered Physiotherapists (MACP) that is the UK's Member Organisation of IFOMPT, and collectively, their considerable clinical experience ensures application of the content to practice situations, for example through case studies in the new assessment chapter. This provides challenge to our existing level of practice to ensure learning and development, and most importantly the stimulus for wider reading. The reference lists at the end of each chapter enable us to follow up additional reading to further inform our depth of understanding in key areas.

The first edition was published in 1997. At that time, as remains the case now, the text is unique in synthesising the different approaches to examination and assessment of neuromusculoskeletal dysfunction. The text is constructed and written from an educational perspective to provide a framework for the examination and assessment of a patient without being prescriptive. It facilitates application of the principles to the individual patient within the patient centred and evidence based framework of practice illustrated in the IFOMPT description of practice. The focus of the original edition is maintained, to explore the subjective history, the physical examination and then each of the body's regions in turn, building on the foundations established through the introductory chapters. This contributes to an analysis of the theoretical rationale underpinning examination and assessment principles, questions, tests, and their interpretation. A new chapter focused to the principles of assessment is a valuable addition; strengthening the clinical reasoning components of the process. The photographs throughout each chapter are new, and provide greater clarity to enable our development of sensitivity and specificity of handling in the physical examination.

This updated text continues to strive to present best current practice to assist our development of the processes of examination and assessment. The increased emphasis on the processes of clinical reasoning is timely to develop the framework for learning further. The detailed attention to the many components of the processes of examination and assessment, and the application to key regions of the body, therefore continue to make this text a valuable resource. The analysis and synthesis that this text provides is of unique value for both the development of beginning clinicians and more experienced clinicians who are striving to develop their practice further. The components of the process of examination and assessment are effectively simplified to enable learning and development - although as we all know, the 'whole' is not simpler. . . . . .

"Make everything as simple as possible, but not simpler".

(Albert Einstein, 1879 – 1955)

Alison Rushton

Preface

This new edition has been refreshed in a number of ways. The book has been strengthened by the involvement and contribution of a number of key clinicians and academics who bring specialised knowledge and expertise in the field of neuromusculoskeletal examination and assessment. All contributors are members of the Manipulation Association of Chartered Physiotherapists (MACP) and as such hold a recognised postregistration qualification in neuromusculoskeletal physiotherapy.

A number of years ago, it was planned to merge this book with the companion textbook, entitled *Principles of Neuromusculoskeletal Treatment and Management*. Feedback from users indicated it would be better to keep them separate. However, to enhance the way each book complements the other, new editions of both books have been prepared at the same time; it has been a busy year!

Contributors for this text have worked with chapters from the previous edition of this book. They have updated references, edited the text and created new photographs. A further change is the addition of a new chapter on assessment (moved out from the companion treatment and management textbook). This offers a top-down explanation of the clinical reasoning process and explanation of hypotheses categories derived from clinical examination findings.

A number of people have contributed to this text. Thanks to Caroline Green for acting as model and Jackie Hollowell, the photographer, for Chapters 5–7. Thanks to Matthew Percival for acting as model for Chapter 8. Thanks to Adam Rochford and Anna Milford for acting as model and to Tania Newton for taking the photographs for Chapter 9. Thanks to models Robyn Davies and Rowan Galloway for Chapter 12 and Lisa Mallett and Becca Stone for Chapter 13. Thanks to Lucy Lewin for acting as the model for Chapters 14 and 15. Thanks to proofreader Sally Davenport, models Alan Barbero and Matthew Percival and photographer Jane Simmonds for Chapters 3, 10 and 11.

The skills required of the clinician are therapeutically to come alongside another person and facilitate his or her rehabilitation. When successful, it can bring immense satisfaction and reward; however success is not always easy to achieve with the inherent uncertainty of clinical practice. Each person is a unique blend of physical being, intellect, will, emotion and spirit, living within, and being influenced by, a social and cultural world. Rehabilitation is thus a complex process and requires high levels of clinical expertise. This text aims to provide a comprehensive step-by-step approach to the technical skills involved in the examination and assessment of people with neuromusculoskeletal conditions.

Nicola J Petty
Eastbourne 2010

Introduction

Nicola J Petty

This text aims to provide guidance to the process of examination and assessment of patients with neuromusculoskeletal dysfunction. Examination refers to the subjective questioning and physical testing procedures, while assessment refers to the interpretation of clinical findings by the clinician – often referred to as clinical reasoning.

The text provides a step-by-step approach to the subjective and physical examination of the various regions in the body. The next chapter (Chapter 2) on subjective examination provides a general guide to the way in which questions might be asked as well as the clinical relevance of questions. Chapter 3, on the physical examination, provides a guide to performing the testing procedures and to understand the relevance of the tests. While Chapters 2 and 3 provide a bottom-up approach on how to collect and interpret clinical data from patients, Chapter 4, on assessment, provides a top-down approach to the clinical reasoning process from a variety of hypotheses categories. All subsequent chapters explore the examination and assessment process for specific regions of the body and include: temporomandibular, upper cervical, cervicothoracic, thoracic, shoulder, elbow, wrist/hand, lumbar, pelvis, hip, knee and foot/ankle. There is a deliberate repetition of information from Chapters 2 and 3 into each of the regional chapters to help reinforce the information and avoid excessive page turning. Similarly, within each regional chapter, reference is made to Chapters 2 and 3.

The division of the body into regions is anatomically, biomechanically, functionally and clinically false and contrived. More realistic regions might, for example, be the cervico-thoracic-shoulder region and the lumbo-pelvic-hip region. So, while readers are introduced here to the individual regions, they need to maintain an awareness of the wider regional areas that are clinically and functionally relevant.

A word of warning to the novice clinician who may believe what is shown in this text is the right way to do something. What you see in this text is one way of doing a technique favoured by the particular clinician on the particular model at that time. Furthermore, the ability of the photographer to capture the technique will also have affected how the clinician performed it. Initially, novices have to start somewhere, and may want to replicate the techniques shown. Once novices understand what they are trying to achieve with a technique, then they would be wise to consider alternative ways of carrying out the technique, making adaptations for themselves and for their patients. They can determine whether or not their adapted technique is effective and efficient by asking themselves whether:

- it is easy and comfortable to perform. A technique is easy and comfortable when posture is carefully considered to produce forces easily; the position of the feet, legs, trunk and arms, as well as the position of the patient and plinth height, will all contribute to the ease with which a technique is carried out. When learning, an easy way of checking whether a technique is easy to do is to prolong your position and force applied much longer than it needs to be, and see whether it continues to feel easy. If it becomes tiring small alterations may be needed.
- comfortable for the student model or patient. While learning, it can be helpful for models to imagine they are a patient in pain, so they raise the

standard of comfort required and then provide honest and constructive feedback to their partner.

- achieves what it intends to achieve. A technique achieves what it intends to achieve when it is comfortable, accurate, specific, controlled, appropriate and handling is sensitively adapted to the tissue response. Whenever a technique is being carried out, it is helpful, to ask whether you think you are achieving what you are intending to achieve, and if not, then change your technique. This is not just for novices as they learn techniques; normal everyday clinical practice requires clinicians to adapt their examination procedures to individual patients.

For those learning these examination procedures for the first time, here are some tips on how you might improve your handling:

- Practise, practise and practise! There is no substitute for plenty of good-quality practice.
- When practising, split the task into bite-sized chunks, building up into a whole. For example, practise hand holds, then application of force, then the hand hold and force on different individuals, then the communication needed with your model, then everything all together on different individuals.
- Imagine what is happening to the tissues when you are carrying out an examination procedure.
- Tell your model very specifically what you want in terms of feedback; model feedback needs to be honest and constructive.

- Verbalise out loud to your model what you are doing.
- When you do a technique, evaluate it and predict the feedback you will receive from your model, so you learn to become independent of your model's feedback.
- Act as a model and feel what is happening.
- Act as an observer: if you can see a good technique and feel a good technique then this can help you to perform a good technique.
- Use a video recorder to observe yourself.
- Imagine yourself doing the examination procedures in your mind in any spare moments.

It is perhaps worth mentioning at the outset that the clinician examining patients with neuromusculoskeletal dysfunction may not be able to identify a particular pathological process. In some patients it may be possible – for example, the clinician may suspect a meniscal tear in the knee, or a lateral ligament sprain of the ankle. However, in other patients, when one integrates current knowledge of pain mechanisms, and considers these effects on the presenting symptoms, the goal of identifying exact pathology is clouded. When the detailed analysis of movement dysfunction is considered in conjunction with psychosocial factors, the clinician is then in a position to establish a reasoned treatment and management strategy. The reader is referred to the companion text for further information on the principles of treatment and management of patients with neuromusculoskeletal dysfunction (Petty 2011).

Reference

Petty, N.J., 2011. Principles of neuromusculoskeletal treatment and management, a guide for therapists, second ed. Elsevier, Edinburgh.

Subjective examination

2

Dionne Ryder

CHAPTER CONTENTS

Introduction

This chapter and Chapter 3 cover the general principles and procedures for examination of the neuromusculoskeletal system. This chapter is concerned with the subjective examination, during which information is gathered from the patient and from other sources such as their medical notes, while Chapter 3 covers the objective or physical examination. This examination system provides a framework that can be adapted to fulfil the examination requirements for people with neuromusculoskeletal problems in various clinical settings.

Clinical reasoning within health and disability

In order to understand fully a patient's problems the clinician must consider all factors capable of having an impact on a person's health (Figure 2.1) (World Health Organization 2001).

Throughout the subjective examination the clinician looks for cues to identify possible sources of a patient's symptoms and the existence of psychosocial factors so that appropriate management options relevant to that individual patient can be selected.

The process of clinical reasoning will help to determine whether these factors are relevant to an individual patient's presenting problem and so whether they must be considered in the physical assessment. Clinical reasoning has been defined as:

> a process in which the clinician, interacting with significant others (client, caregivers, health care team members), structures meaning, goals and health management strategies based on clinical data, client choices, and professional judgment and knowledge
>
> Higgs & Jones (2000, p. 11).

Research has demonstrated that a number of clinical reasoning models are used by therapists and these can be broadly divided into those with a more cognitive/thinking process such as hypotheticodeductive reasoning (Rivett & Higgs 1997) or

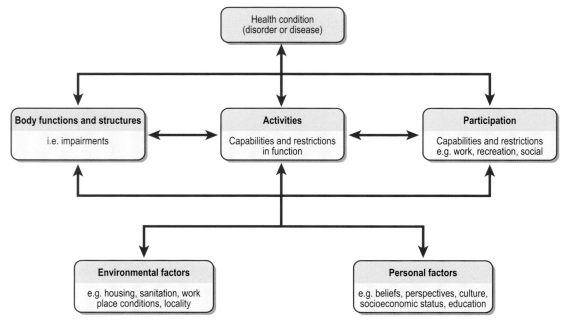

Figure 2.1 • Framework of health and disability. World Health Organisation 2001 International classification of functioning, disability and health. World Health Organisation, Geneva. http://www.who.int/classifications/icf/en/

pattern recognition (Barrows & Feltovich 1987) and those utilising more interactive processes such as narrative or collaborative reasoning (Jones 1995; Edwards et al. 2004, 2006; Jones & Rivett 2004; Jones et al. 2008).

Figure 2.2 presents the patient-centred collaborative model of reasoning. This model brings together both cognitive and interactive processes, recognising that these are intrinsically linked and are central to understanding the complexity of the mind–body interaction. To provide a framework to assist in the organisation of knowledge and reasoning throughout the subjective and physical examination, hypothesis categories have been proposed (Jones & Rivett 2004) which reflect the framework of health and disability (World Health Organization 2001) (Box 2.1).

The subjective examination step by step

The accuracy of the information gained in the subjective examination depends to a large extent on the quality of the communication between the clinician and patient. The clinician should speak slowly and deliberately, keep questions short and ask only one question at a time (Maitland et al. 2005). For further

details, readers are directed to an excellent chapter on interviewing skills by Maitland et al. (2005).

The usefulness of the information gained in the subjective examination depends to a large extent on the clinician using clinical reasoning skills to ask pertinent questions. This chapter aims to give this background in regard to the questions asked, so that clinicians are able to question effectively and obtain a wealth of useful information on which to base the physical examination.

This chapter outlines a very detailed subjective examination, which will not be required for every patient. Not every question will need to be asked to the same depth – the clinician must tailor the examination to the patient. An illuminating text on the theoretical concepts underlying the subjective and physical examination can be found in Refshauge & Gass (2004).

The most important findings in the subjective examination are highlighted with asterisks (*) for easy reference and can be used at subsequent treatment sessions to evaluate the effects of treatment intervention.

The aim of the subjective examination is to obtain sufficient information about the patient's symptoms so as to be able to plan an efficient, effective and safe physical examination. A summary of the subjective examination is shown in Table 2.1.

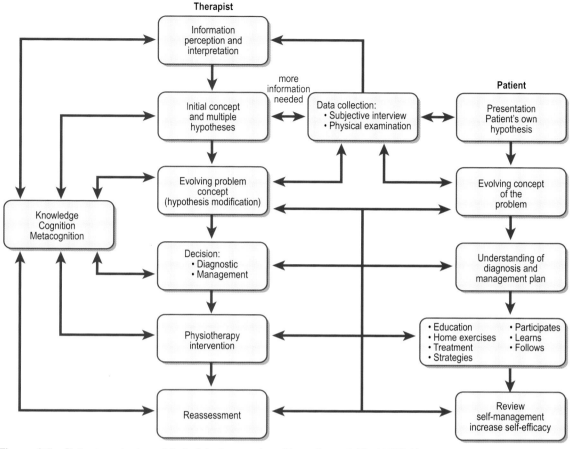

Figure 2.2 • Patient-centred model of clinical reasoning. (From Jones & Rivett 2004.)

Body chart

A body chart (Figure 2.3) is a useful and quick way of recording and communicating information about the area and type of symptoms the patient is experiencing. Its completion early on in the examination ensures that the clinician has an appreciation of the type and extent of the patient's symptoms, thereby facilitating more focused questioning and allowing more experienced clinicians to use pattern recognition reasoning.

Area of current symptoms

The exact area of the symptoms can be mapped out. Although the most common symptom allied to neuromusculoskeletal dysfunction is pain, it must not be assumed to be the only presenting symptom. A clear demarcation between areas of pain, paraesthesia, stiffness or weakness will distinguish symptoms and the clinician can then establish their relationship to each other (see Figures 2.12 and 2.13 in Appendix 2.2).

The area of the symptoms does not always identify the structure at fault, since symptoms can be felt in one area but emanate from a distant area; for example, pain felt in the elbow may be locally produced or may be due to pathology in the cervical spine. When the manifestation of symptoms is distant to the pathological tissue, this is known as referred pain. The more central the lesion, the more extensive is the possible area of referral; for example, the zygapophyseal joints in the lumbar spine can refer symptoms to the foot (Mooney & Robertson 1976), the hip joint classically refers symptoms as far as the knee, whereas the joints of the foot tend to produce local symptoms.

Although the exact mechanism is still unknown, several theories have been proposed in an effort to

Box 2.1

Subjective and physical examination hypotheses categories (Jones & Rivett 2004)

- **Activity capability/restriction**: what activities the patient is able and unable to do, e.g. walking, lifting, sitting
- **Participant capability/restriction**: the patient's ability/inability to be involved in life situations, i.e. work, family and leisure activities
- **Patients' perspectives on their experience**: an important category in its own right as it must be acknowledged that patients' perceptions will have a significant impact on their presentation and response to treatment
- **Pathobiological mechanisms**: the state of the structures or tissues thought to be producing the patient's symptoms in relation to tissue pathology, ongoing tissue damage, the stage of the healing process and the pain mechanisms involved
- **Physical impairments and associated structure/tissue sources**: the target tissue from where symptoms may be coming, in conjunction with the resulting impairment. Sole identification of specific tissues is often difficult and management directed to the resulting impairment whilst hypothesising the pathological processes involved is most effective
- **Contributing factors to the development and maintenance of the problem**: these may be environmental, psychosocial, behavioural, physical or heredity factors. Environmental factors may include a patient's work station or work environment, home and

car. Psychosocial factors may include the patient's belief that pain or exercise is 'bad', or misunderstanding the nature of the problem. Behavioural factors may include what patients do at work or at home, their choice of activities, such as they may lead a very sedentary lifestyle. Physical contributing factors include elements such as reduced range of movement and muscle weakness. Heredity factors play a part in the development of some musculoskeletal conditions, such as ankylosing spondylitis and osteoarthritis (Solomon et al. 2001)

- **Precautions/contraindications to physical examination, treatment and management**: this includes the severity and irritability of the patient's symptoms, response to special questions and the underlying nature of the problem
- **Management strategy and treatment plan**
- **Prognosis**: this can be affected by factors such as the stage and extent of the injury as well as the patient's expectation, personality and lifestyle. Psychosocial (yellow flags) risk factors, patient's perceived stress at work (blue flags) and work conditions, including employment and sickness policy as well as type and amount of work (black flags), are considered to influence the outcome of treatment strongly. Orange flags indicate mental health disorders which will need to be managed by a mental health professional (Main & Spanswick 2000; Jones & Rivett 2004)

Table 2.1 Summary of subjective examination

Area of examination	Information gained
Body chart	Type and area of current symptoms, depth, quality, intensity, abnormal sensation, relationship of symptoms
Behaviour of symptoms	Aggravating factors, easing factors, severity and irritability of the condition, 24-hour behaviour, daily activities, stage of the condition
Special questions	General health, drugs, steroids, anticoagulants, recent unexplained weight loss, rheumatoid arthritis, spinal cord or cauda equina symptoms, dizziness, recent radiographs
History of present condition	History of each symptomatic area – how and when it started, how it has changed
Past medical history	Relevant medical history, previous attacks, effect of previous treatment
Social and family history	Age and gender, home and work situation, dependants and leisure activities

explain the complex phenomenon of referred pain, as identified in Figure 2.4. These include:

- the convergence projection theory, in which it is suggested that separate peripheral sensory nerves

converge on to one cell in the dorsal horn of the spinal cord

- the axon reflex model, in which it is suggested that axons in peripheral sensory nerves innervating

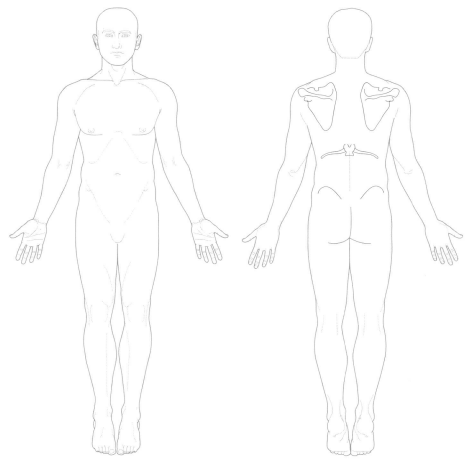

Figure 2.3 • Body chart. (Redrawn from Grieve 1991, with permission.)

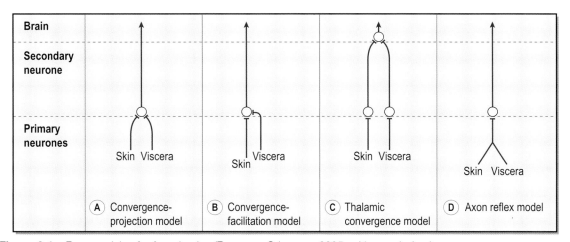

Figure 2.4 • Four models of referred pain. (From van Griensven 2005, with permission.)

different structures share the same cell body in the dorsal root ganglion prior to converging in the dorsal horn

- the convergence facilitation theory, in which it is proposed that visceral input causes central sensitisation so that normal somatic input is perceived as pain in the dorsal horn
- the thalamic convergence theory, in which it is suggested that summation of peripheral inputs occurs in the thalamus rather than at spinal cord level.

The areas of referred symptoms from the viscera are shown in Figure 2.5 (Lindsay et al. 1997). Pain is most likely to be referred to tissues innervated by the same segments as pain is 'projected' from the viscera to the area supplied by corresponding somatic afferent fibres (Figure 2.6). In addition the uterus is capable of referring symptoms to the T10–L2 and S2–S5 regions (van Cranenburgh 1989). Symptoms referred from the viscera can sometimes be distinguished from those originating in the neuromusculoskeletal system, as the symptoms are not usually aggravated by activity or relieved by rest, but this is not always the case (Appendix 2.3). The clinician needs to be aware that symptoms can be referred from the spine to the periphery, from the periphery to other peripheral regions or more centrally, from the viscera to the spine, or from the spine to the viscera.

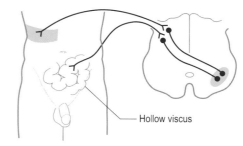

Figure 2.6 • A mechanism of referred pain from the viscera. (From Lindsay et al. 1997, with permission.)

Using the body chart the clinician ascertains which is the worst symptom (if more than one area). This can help to focus the examination to the most important areas and may help to prioritise treatment.

In addition, the patient is asked where s/he feels the symptoms are coming from: 'If you had to put your finger on one spot where you feel it is coming from, where would you put it?' When the patient is able to do this, it can help to pinpoint the source of the symptoms. Care is needed, however, as it may simply be an area of pain referral.

Areas relevant to the region being examined

All other relevant areas are checked for the presence of any symptoms and any unaffected areas are marked with ticks (✓) on the body chart. It is important to

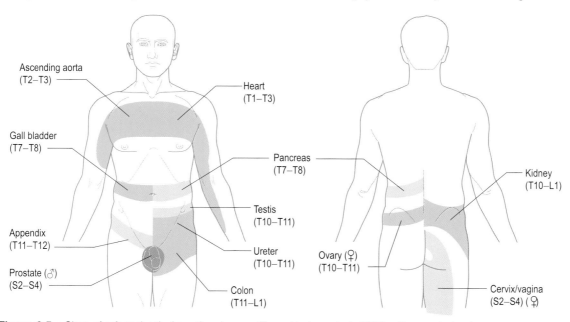

Figure 2.5 • Sites of referred pain from the viscera. (From Lindsay et al. 1997, with permission.)

remember that the patient may describe only the worst symptom, not thinking that it is important to mention an area of slight discomfort, although this may be highly relevant to the understanding of the patient's condition. The cervical and thoracic spinal segments can, for example, give rise to referred symptoms in the upper limb; and the lumbar spine and sacroiliac joints can give rise to referred symptoms in the lower limb. Quite frequently, patients can present with classical signs and symptoms of a peripheral condition such as tennis elbow, but on examination the symptoms are found to emanate from the cervical spine, which is confirmed when palpation or other diagnostic tests of the spine either relieve or aggravate the symptoms.

Pain: the most common presenting symptom

The International Association for the Study of Pain (IASP) defines pain as:

> An unpleasant sensory and emotional experience associated with actual or potential tissue damage, or described in terms of such damage
> (Available online at: http://www.iasp-pain.org).

Pain is complex: it may be widespread or focal and may follow either an anatomical or a non-anatomical distribution. It is important that clinicians recognise that pain is a subjective phenomenon and is different for each individual as it includes many dimensions, as shown in Figure 2.7. It is therefore difficult to estimate the extent of another's psychological and emotional experience of pain. Patients may demonstrate signs of illness behaviour, also called non-organic signs, in the way they report symptoms of pain and record them on a body chart. For an overview of illness behaviours, see Box 2.2.

The clinician should apply the criteria for illness behaviour with care and be aware of the following (Waddell 2004):

- You need to examine the patient fully.
- Avoid observer bias.
- Isolated behavioural symptoms mean nothing; only multiple findings are relevant.
- Illness behaviour does not explain the cause of the patient's pain, nor does it suggest that the patient has no 'real' pain.
- Illness behaviour does not mean that there is no physical disease; most patients have both a physical problem and a degree of illness behaviour.
- Illness behaviour is not in itself a diagnosis.
- Illness behaviour does not mean that the patient is faking or malingering.

One group of patients who may be unjustly labelled as having predominantly psychological problems are those with joint hypermobility syndrome (JHS). They may present with widespread diffuse pain, whilst also reporting a range of symptoms such as

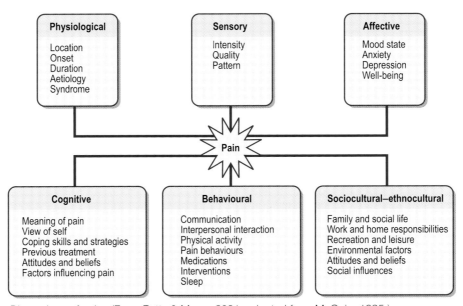

Figure 2.7 • Dimensions of pain. (From Petty & Moore 2001, adapted from McGuire 1995.)

Box 2.2

Illness behaviours (Keefe & Block 1982; Waddell 2004)

- Pain drawing
- Pain adjectives and description
- Non-anatomical or behavioural descriptions of symptoms
- Non-organic or behavioural signs
- Overt pain behaviours:
  - Guarding – abnormally stiff, interrupted or rigid movement while moving from one position to another
  - Bracing – a stationary position in which a fully extended limb supports and maintains an abnormal distribution of weight

- Rubbing – any contact between hand and back, i.e. touching, rubbing or holding the painful area
- Grimacing – obvious facial expression of pain that may include furrowed brow, narrowed eyes, tightened lips, corners of mouth pulled back and clenched teeth
- Sighing – obvious exaggerated exhalation of air, usually accompanied by the shoulders first rising and then falling; the cheeks may be expanded first
- Use of walking aids
- Down time
- Help with personal care

---

clunking, clicking, stiffness and tiredness (Simmonds & Keer 2007). If JHS is suspected there are five simple questions that can help to subjectively identify this syndrome (Hakim & Grahame 2003):

1. Can you now (or could you ever) place your hands flat on the floor without bending your knees?
2. Can you now (or could you ever) bend your thumb to touch your forearm?
3. As a child, did you amuse your friends by contorting your body into strange shapes or could you do the splits?
4. As a child or teenager, did your kneecap or shoulder dislocate on more than one occasion?
5. Do you consider yourself 'double-jointed'?

Quality of the pain

The clinician asks the patient: 'How would you describe your pain?' The quality of the pain may give a clue as to the anatomical structure at fault (Table 2.2), although care must be taken because it can be misleading (Dalton & Jull 1989; Austen 1991). The adjective the patient uses to describe the pain may be of an emotional nature, such as torturous, miserable or terrifying, which may suggest that a behavioural component is playing a role in this patient's problem. Alternatively physical descriptions of pain such as burning, sharp, stabbing can assist identification of the pain mechanism producing the patient's pain. This, along with the location and behaviour of symptoms, may assist in determining the structures at fault. An understanding of the

Table 2.2 Type of pain thought to be produced by various structures (Newham & Mills 1999; Magee 2006)

Structure	Pain
Bone	Deep, nagging, dull
Muscle	Dull ache
Nerve root	Sharp, shooting
Nerve	Sharp, bright, lightning-like
Sympathetic nerve	Burning, pressure-like, stinging, aching
Vascular	Throbbing, diffuse

neurobiological mechanisms responsible for pain has led to the development of treatment approaches specifically targeting certain pain mechanisms (Woolf 2004). The mechanism of pain production can be broadly categorised into nociceptive, peripheral neurogenic, central sensitisation, autonomic and affective. The characteristics for each mechanism are given in Box 2.3.

Intensity of pain

The intensity of pain can be measured by the use of a descriptive, numerical or visual analogue rating scale (Hinnant 1994). These are outlined in Figure 2.8. To complete the descriptive and numerical rating scales, the patient is asked to indicate the description or number which best describes the intensity of their pain. For the visual analogue scale (VAS), the patient is asked to mark on a

Box 2.3

Characteristics of pain mechanisms (Fields 1995; Gifford 1996; Doubell et al. 2002)

Nociceptive pain

Pain arising from all innervated tissues which can be further subdivided into mechanical, inflammatory and ischaemic causes.

Characterised by:

Mechanical	Inflammatory	Ischaemic
Localised intermittent pain	Constant/ varying pain	Usually intermittent
Predictable consistent response, e.g. to stretch, compression or movement	Worsened rapidly by movement	Predictable pattern – aggravated by sustained postures and/or repetitive activities
No pain on waking but pain on rising	Latent pain	
	Night pain and pain on waking	
	High irritability and severity	
Usually mild to moderate severity	Movements limited by pain	Eased by change of position or by cessation of a repetitive activity
Responds to simple painkillers	Responds to non-steroidal anti-inflammatory drugs (NSAIDs)	

Peripheral neurogenic pain

Pain arising from a peripheral nerve axon, due to damage or pathology to the axons / nerve fibres themselves in the peripheral nervous system.

Characterised by:

- Anatomical distribution, i.e. along a spinal segment or peripheral/cranial nerve pathway/course
- Burning, sharp, shooting, electric shock-like
- Allodynia (pain provoked by stimuli that are normally innocuous), dysaesthesia (heightened or diminished skin sensation), paraesthesia (abnormal sensation), possibly a mixture of these
- Provoked by nerve stretch, compression or palpation
- Possible associated sensory loss, muscle weakness and autonomic changes
- Poor response to simple painkillers and anti-inflammatories
- Response to passive treatment varies

Central sensitisation

Pain initiated or caused by a primary lesion or dysfunction in the central nervous system.

Characterised by:

- Widespread, non-anatomical distribution
- Hyperalgesia (increased sensitivity to pain), allodynia evident
- Inconsistent response to stimuli and tests
- Patients have difficulty in locating and describing their pain
- Pain seems to have 'a mind of its own'
- Simple analgesics are ineffective
- Unpredictable or failed response to passive treatments

Autonomic

The autonomic nervous system has an indirect impact on pain systems through the release of chemicals, i.e. adrenaline affecting capillary response and indirectly cortisol levels via the adrenal medulla, blocking inflammation. Although this is beneficial to the body immediately following injury, if this stress response is maintained over a period of time cortisol may reduce the availability of amino acids for the repair of soft tissues, resulting in poor tissue healing (Gifford & Thacker 2002; van Griensven 2005). Recognition of autonomic system arousal is important so it can be explained to the patient and initial management aimed towards a reduction of the cortisol levels using relaxation techniques and exercise.

Characterised by:

- Symptoms often develop following trauma
- Hyperaesthesia (heightened perception to touch), hyperalgesia and allodynia
- Pain often described as burning, deep, crawling, unusual type of pain
- Pain often comes on by itself, with varying different activities and at varying different times, is eased by itself and is not consistent. Often described by the patient as 'having a mind of its own'
- Patient overprotective of the affected limb
- Associated alterations in circulation and sweat production identified by skin colour changes and distal oedema
- Trophic changes such as excessive hair growth and a decline in skin quality
- Sensory deficits – sock and glove distribution
- Weakness tremor

Affective

The affective component of pain is related to thought processes, e.g. fear, anxiety and mood, which are powerful enough to maintain a pain state (Price 2000). Butler & Moseley (2003) refer to these as 'thought viruses'. Their text *Explain Pain* provides a very useful resource for both clinicians and patients as it explains the basis of pain using simple analogies and powerful images that may help patients modify their thought processes. Depression can either be a consequence of or predate the current pain state and there are numerous screening tools available to assess its impact formally, e.g. Distress Risk Assessment Method (DRAM) (Main et al. 1992). As a starting point to identify whether further screening or referral on to a mental health professional is indicated, Aroll et al. (2003) identified two questions that had reasonable sensitivity and specificity in detecting depression:

- During the past month have you often been bothered by feeling down, depressed or hopeless?
- During the past month have you often been bothered by little interest or pleasure in doing things?

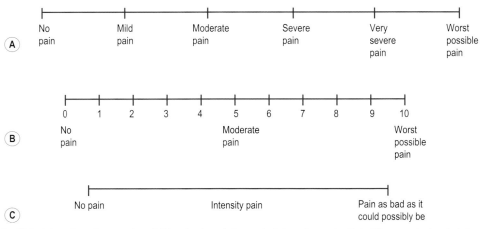

Figure 2.8 • Pain intensity rating scales. A Simple descriptive pain intensity scale. B 1–10 numerical pain intensity scale. C Visual analogue scale. (From Hinnant 1994. © Williams and Wilkins.)

10-cm line the point that best represents the intensity of their pain, where 0 denotes 'no pain' and 10 denotes 'pain as bad as it could possibly be'. The distance of the mark from the left end of the line is measured in millimetres and then becomes a numerical value, which can be recorded. The Present Pain Intensity, which is part of the McGill Pain Questionnaire (Melzack & Wall 1996), measures intensity of pain by asking patients to choose the word listed below that best describes the intensity of their pain now, at its worst and at its least:

- mild
- discomforting
- distressing
- horrible
- excruciating.

For comparison, patients are also asked to score their worst ever toothache, headache and stomachache. Only the descriptors are shown to patients, to ensure that they do not choose a numerical value to match their pain. The numbers are strictly for recording purposes only.

It is important to realise that the various pain scales are not interchangeable. Someone who marks their pain at 80 mm on the VAS will not necessarily give the pain a description of 8 out of 10 on the Numerical Scale, or a Present Pain Intensity of 4. A score can only be compared with another score on the same scale. The intensity of pain score can be repeated several times a day or during a period of treatment, thereby developing a pain diary. This can then be used to construct a pain profile from which the behaviour of pain, or the effectiveness of a treatment for pain, can be judged. There is however recognition that a focus on functional goals rather than on pain can be more important in managing patients with chronic problems (Harding & Williams 1995).

Depth of pain

The clinician asks: 'Is the pain deep down or is it on the surface?' The depth of pain may give some indication as to the structure at fault but, like quality, this can be misleading (Austen 1991). Muscles are thought to produce deep pain (Mense 1993), whilst joints tend to refer superficially (Mooney & Robertson 1976).

Abnormal sensation

Areas of abnormal sensation are mapped out on the body chart and include paraesthesia (abnormal sensation), anaesthesia (complete loss of sensation), hypoaesthesia (reduced touch sensation), hyperaesthesia (heightened perception to touch), allodynia (pain provoked by stimuli that are normally innocuous), analgesia (absence of appreciation of pain), hypoalgesia (reduced appreciation of pain) and hyperalgesia (increased sensitivity to pain). Paraesthesia includes sensations of tingling, pins and needles, swelling of a limb, tight bands tied around part of the body and water trickling over the skin.

The sensory changes listed above can be generated anywhere along a peripheral or cranial nerve, including the nerve root. A common cause for more sensory changes is ischaemia of the nerve, e.g. when part of the brachial plexus is compressed by a cervical rib or when a median nerve compression results in carpal tunnel syndrome. Knowledge of the cutaneous distribution of nerve roots (dermatomes), brachial and lumbosacral plexuses and peripheral nerves enables the clinician to distinguish the sensory loss resulting from a root lesion from that resulting from a peripheral nerve lesion. The cutaneous nerve distribution and dermatome areas are shown in Chapter 3.

Symptoms may also have their origin in the central nervous system. A spinal cord lesion or stroke, for example, can cause a variety of sensory changes and long-term pain can sensitise or modify structures like the dorsal horn.

Constant or intermittent symptoms

The word 'constant' is used here to mean symptoms that are felt unremittingly for 24 hours a day; any relief of symptoms even for a few minutes would mean that the symptoms were intermittent. The frequency of intermittent symptoms is important as there may be wide variations, from symptoms being felt once a month to once an hour. Specific details are useful at this stage so that progress can be clearly monitored at subsequent treatment sessions. Constant pain that does not vary is characteristic of serious pathology, e.g. malignancy. Constant pain that varies in intensity may be suggestive of inflammatory or infective processes or may occur following trauma due to chemical irritation. Intermittent pain is suggestive of a mechanical disturbance such that forces sufficient to stimulate free nerve endings are producing pain that stops when the force is removed (McKenzie 1981).

Relationship of symptoms

The question of the relationship of symptomatic areas to each other is very important as it helps to establish links between symptoms and gives clues as to the structure(s) at fault. For example, if posterior leg pain is felt when back pain is made worse, then it suggests that the leg pain and the back pain are being produced by the same structure. If, on the other hand, the symptoms occur separately, so that the patient can have back pain without leg pain and leg pain without back pain, then different structures would be thought to be producing these two symptoms.

This completes the information that can be documented on the body chart. An example of a completed body chart is shown in Figures 2.12 and 2.13 in Appendix 2.2.

Behaviour of symptoms

Information about the behaviour of symptoms provides a valuable contribution to the subjective assessment of the patient. It is used to hypothesise the structure(s) at fault, to give an indication of functional impairments and to allow the therapist to come to a decision on the severity (S), irritability (I) and nature (N) of the condition. This gives valuable information as to the ease or difficulty that the clinician may have in reproducing the patient's symptom(s), and therefore an indication of the required vigour and/or extent of the physical examination.

Aggravating and easing factors

Aggravating and easing factors are used in the first instance to establish an indication of the severity and irritability of the problem, and in the generation of possible hypotheses as to the cause. The behaviour of symptoms can be further assessed by indepth questioning as described below.

Aggravating factors. These are movements or postures that produce or increase the patient's symptoms. The exact movement or posture and the time it takes to bring on the symptoms (or make them worse) need to be established and indicate how irritable the condition is and so how difficult or easy it may be to reproduce the patient's symptoms in the physical examination. For example, symptoms that are felt after 2 hours of hard physical exercise may well be harder to reproduce than symptoms provoked by one single movement such as elbow flexion. The clinician must analyse in detail the aggravating movement or posture in order to hypothesise what structures are being stressed and thereby causing the symptoms.

Aggravating factors are determined for each symptomatic area. The effect of aggravating one symptom on the other symptoms is established, as this helps to confirm the relationship between the symptoms. If different symptoms are aggravated by the same position or movement, it suggests that the symptoms are being produced by the same source or structure(s).

To assist with the clinical reasoning process the clinician can ask the patient about theoretically known aggravating factors for structures that could be hypothesised as a source of the symptoms, e.g. squatting and going up and down stairs for suspected hip and knee problems, and lifting the head to look upwards for cervical spine problems. A list of common aggravating factors for each joint as well as for muscle and neurological tissue can be found in Table 2.3. Some worked examples can be found in Appendix 2.2.

The clinician asks how the symptoms affect function, e.g. sitting, standing, lying, bending, walking, running, walking on uneven ground, walking up and down stairs, washing, driving, lifting and digging, work, sport and leisure activities. For any sporting activities note details of the training regimen. The clinician finds out whether the patient is left- or right-handed/footed as there may be increased stress on the dominant side.

Table 2.3 Common aggravating factors – for each region or structure, examples of various functional activities and a basic analysis of the activity are given

	Functional activity	Analysis of the activity
Temporomandibular joint	Yawning	Depression of mandible
	Chewing	Elevation/depression of mandible
	Talking	Elevation/depression of mandible
Headaches	Stress, eye strain, noise, excessive eating, drinking, smoking, inadequate ventilation, odours	
Cervical spine	Reversing the car	Rotation
	Sitting reading/writing	Sustained flexion
Thoracic spine	Reversing the car	Rotation
	Deep breath	Extension
Shoulder	Tucking shirt in	Hand behind back
	Fastening bra	Hand behind back
	Lying on shoulder	Joint compression
	Reaching up	Flexion
Elbow	Eating	Flexion/extension
	Carrying	Distraction
	Gripping	Flexion/extension
	Leaning on elbow	Compression
Forearm	Turning key in a lock	Pronation/supination
Wrist/hand	Typing/writing	Sustained extension
	Gripping	Extension
	Power gripping	Extension
	Power gripping with twist	Ulnar deviation and pronation/supination
	Turning a key	Thumb adduction with supination
	Leaning on hand	Compression
Lumbar spine	Sitting	Flexion
	Standing/walking	Extension
	Lifting/stooping	Flexion
Sacroiliac joint	Standing on one leg	Ipsilateral upward shear, contralateral downward shear
	Turning over in bed	Nutation/counternutation of sacrum
	Getting out of bed	Nutation/counternutation of sacrum
	Walking	Nutation/counternutation of sacrum

(Continued)

Table 2.3 Common aggravating factors – for each region or structure, examples of various functional activities and a basic analysis of the activity are given—cont'd

	Functional activity	Analysis of the activity
Hip	Squat Walking Side-lying with painful hip uppermost Stairs	Flexion Flexion/extension Adduction and medial rotation Flexion/extension
Knee	Squat Walking Stairs	Flexion Flexion/extension Flexion/extension
Foot and ankle	Walking Running	Dorsiflexion/plantarflexion, inversion/eversion Dorsiflexion/plantarflexion, inversion/eversion
Muscular tissue		Contraction of muscle Passive stretch of muscle
Nervous tissue		Passive stretch or compression of nervous tissue

Detailed information on each of the above activities is useful in order to help determine the structure(s) at fault and identify functional restrictions. This information can be used to determine the aims of treatment and any advice that may be required. The most notable functional restrictions are highlighted on the patient's clinical records with asterisks (*), explored in the physical examination, and reassessed at subsequent treatment sessions to evaluate treatment intervention.

The clinician must identify whether patients have changed or abandoned activities in response to their symptoms. For example, short-term reduction or avoidance of some activities can be an effective strategy to overcome an injury, and is known as adaptive, but avoiding most activities over a longer period of time is recognised as maladaptive, and may lead to a decline in function and possible chronicity. Maladaptive coping strategies can easily contribute to and perpetuate the patient's problem and compromise treatment (Harding & Williams 1995; Shorland 1998). Coping strategies include:

- Activity avoidance – disuse, lack of fitness, strength and flexibility. May also lead to withdrawal from leisure activities and interfere with work.
- Underactivity/overactivity cycles (activity avoidance on days with pain, very active on days with less pain). Reduced activity tolerance due to disuse on 'bad' days leads to tissue overload on

'good' days. Over time there may be a gradual increase in pain and decrease in activity.

- Long-term use of medication which may lead to side-effects such as constipation, indigestion, drowsiness. This may interfere with general function and hinder recovery, as well as perhaps causing the patient to become drug-dependent.
- Visiting a range of therapists and specialists in the pursuit of a diagnosis or cure (Butler & Moseley 2003).
- The patient is not willing to take control, not willing to apply adaptive coping strategies.

Easing factors. These are movements or positions that ease the patient's symptoms. As with the aggravating factors, the exact movement or posture and the time it takes to ease the symptoms are established. This indicates how difficult or easy it may be to relieve the patient's symptoms in the physical examination and, more importantly, in treatment, and gives an indication of irritability. Symptoms that are readily eased may respond to treatment more quickly than symptoms that are not readily eased. The clinician analyses in detail the easing movement or posture in order to hypothesise which structures are causing the symptoms.

Again, easing factors are determined for each symptomatic area. The effect of the easing of one symptom on the other symptoms is established as this helps to confirm the relationship between symptoms.

If different symptomatic areas ease with the same position or movement, it suggests that the symptoms are being produced by the same source or structure.

The clinician asks the patient about theoretically known easing factors for structures that could be a source of their symptoms; for instance, crook-lying for a painful lumbar spine may ease pain by reducing intradiscal pressure (Nachemson 1992) as well as reducing the forces produced by muscle activity (Jull 1986). However, if patients feel that they can only manage the pain by lying down regularly for long periods this may indicate possible illness behaviour which, if not recognised and managed, can be an indicator of a poor prognostic outcome.

Severity and irritability of symptoms

The severity and irritability of symptoms must be determined in order to identify patients who will not be able to tolerate a full physical examination and also to establish guidelines concerning the vigour of the examination strategy. Generally, the tests carried out in the physical examination require the patient to move and sustain positions that provoke symptoms. Sometimes the intensity of the provoked symptoms is too great for these positions to be sustained, i.e. the patient's symptoms are severe. At other times, the symptoms gradually increase with each movement tested until eventually they may become intolerable to the patient and the examination may have to be stopped until the symptoms subside; in this case the patient's symptoms are said to be irritable. The clinician must know before starting the physical examination whether the patient's symptoms are severe and/or irritable so that an appropriate examination is carried out in a way that avoids unnecessary exacerbation of the patient's symptoms.

Severity of the symptoms. The severity of the symptoms is the degree to which symptoms restrict movement and/or function and is related to the intensity of the symptoms. If a movement at a certain point in range provokes pain and this pain is so intense that the movement must be ceased immediately, then the symptoms are defined as severe. If the symptoms are severe then the patient will not be able to tolerate structures being tested more extensively, e.g. overpressures, and movements must be performed just short of, or just up to, the first point of pain. If the intensity is such that the patient is able to maintain or increase a movement that provokes the symptoms, then the symptoms are not considered to be severe and in this case overpressures can be performed.

In order to determine the severity of the condition, the clinician chooses an aggravating movement and, when examining a patient with symptoms emanating from the cervical spine, for example, asks: 'When you turn your head around to the left and you get your neck pain (or you get more pain), can you stay in that position or do you have to bring your head back straight away because the pain is too severe?' If the patient is able to stay in the position, the symptoms are considered non-severe; if the patient is unable to maintain the position, the symptoms are deemed to be severe.

Irritability of the symptoms. The irritability of the symptoms is the degree to which symptoms increase and reduce with provocation. Asking questions about the same aggravating movement as for severity, the clinician finds out how long it takes for the provoked symptom to ease. When a movement is performed and pain, for example, is produced (or increased) and continues to be present for a period of time, then the symptom is considered to be irritable. Anything more than a few seconds would require a pause between testing procedures, to allow symptoms to return to their resting level. If the symptom disappears as soon as the movement is stopped, then the symptom is considered to be non-irritable.

Using the same example as above, the clinician might ask: 'When you turn your head around to the left and feel the sharp pain and then immediately turn your head back, does that sharp pain ease immediately or does it take a while to go?' The clinician needs to make sure that the patient has understood by asking: 'You mean that sharp pain, that extra pain that was felt at the end of the movement, takes 10 minutes to go?' If the pain eases immediately, the symptoms are considered to be non-irritable and all movements can be examined. If the symptoms take a few minutes to disappear then the symptoms are irritable and the patient may not be able to tolerate all movements as the symptoms may gradually get worse. The clinician may choose to carry out movements just to the onset of symptom provocation, reduce the number of movements carried out and allow a pause for the symptoms to settle after each movement. Alternatively, the clinician may choose to carry out all movements just short of the onset of symptom provocation, so that all movements can be carried out and no pauses are needed.

Occasionally, latent irritability may occur where a movement or position may induce symptoms that are delayed by some minutes and often continue for a considerable length of time. Careful management is required with these patients to avoid unnecessary exacerbation of their symptoms.

A patient's condition may be non-severe but irritable or it may be severe but non-irritable or both severe and irritable.

Twenty-four-hour behaviour of symptoms

Night symptoms. The following information is gathered from the patient:

- Does the patient have difficulty getting to sleep because of the symptom(s)? Lying may in some way alter the stress on the structure(s) at fault and provoke or ease symptoms. For example, weight-bearing joints such as the spine, sacroiliac joints, hips, knees and ankles have reduced compressive forces in lying compared with upright postures.
- Which positions are most comfortable and uncomfortable for the patient? The clinician can then analyse these positions to help confirm the possible structures at fault.
- How many and what type of pillows are used by the patient? How are they placed? For example, foam pillows are often uncomfortable for patients with cervical spine symptoms because their size and non-malleability create highly flexed or highly side-flexed sleeping positions.
- Does the patient use a firm or soft mattress, and has it recently been changed? Alteration in sleeping posture caused by a new mattress is sometimes sufficient to provoke spinal symptoms.
- Is the patient woken by symptoms, and, if so, which symptoms and are they associated with movement, e.g. turning over in bed?
- To what extent do the symptoms disturb the patient at night?
  - ○ How many times in any one night is the patient woken?
  - ○ How many nights in the past week was the patient woken?
  - ○ What does the patient do when woken? For example, can the patient reposition him- or herself or does s/he have to get up?
  - ○ Can the patient get back to sleep?
  - ○ How long does it take to get back to sleep?
- It is useful to be as specific as possible as this information can then be used at subsequent attendances to determine the effect of treatment on the condition.

Morning symptoms. What are the patient's symptoms like in the morning immediately on waking before movement and also after getting up? Prolonged morning pain and stiffness that improves minimally with movement suggests an inflammatory process (Magee 2006). Minimal or absent pain with stiffness in the morning is associated with degenerative conditions such as osteoarthrosis (Huskisson et al. 1979).

Evening symptoms. The patient's symptoms at the beginning of the day are compared with those through to the end of the day. Symptoms may depend upon the patient's daily activity levels. Pain that is aggravated by movement and eased by rest generally indicates a mechanical problem of the neuro musculoskeletal system (Corrigan & Maitland 1994). Pain that increases with activity may be due to repeated mechanical stress, an inflammatory process or a degenerative process (Jull 1986). Ischaemic pain is eased with activity. If pain is worse in the evening when the person has been at work all day compared with when off work, it would be important to explore the activities involved at work to identify what may be aggravating the symptoms.

Stage of the condition

Knowing whether the symptoms are getting better, getting worse or remaining static gives an indication of the stage of the condition and helps the clinician to determine the time for recovery. Symptoms that are deteriorating will tend to take longer to respond to treatment than symptoms that are resolving.

Special questions

The clinician needs to determine the nature of the patient's condition, differentiating between benign neuromusculoskeletal conditions that are suitable for manual therapy and systemic, neoplastic or other non-neuromusculoskeletal conditions, which are not suitable for treatment. It is important that the clinician realises that serious conditions may masquerade as neuromusculoskeletal conditions. This is discussed at length by Grieve (1994a) and a published paper by the same author (Grieve 1994b) is reproduced in Appendix 2.3 of this chapter. A number of questions are asked to enable the clinician to establish the nature of the patient's condition and to identify any precautions or absolute contraindications to further examination and application of treatment techniques. Table 2.4 identifies the precautions to neuromusculoskeletal examination and treatment. Further

Table 2.4 Precautions to spinal and peripheral passive joint mobilisations and nerve mobilisations

Aspects of subjective examination	Subjective information	Possible cause/implication for examination and/or treatment
Body chart	Constant unremitting pain	Malignancy, systemic, inflammatory cause
	Symptoms in the upper limb below the acromion or symptoms in the lower limb below the gluteal crease	Nerve root compression. Carry out appropriate neurological integrity tests in physical examination
	Widespread sensory changes and/or weakness in upper or lower limb	Compression on more than one nerve root, metabolic (e.g. diabetes, vitamin B_{12}), systemic (e.g. rheumatoid arthritis)
Aggravating factors	Symptoms severe and/or irritable	Care in treatment to avoid unnecessary provocation or exacerbation
Special questions	Feeling unwell	Systemic or metabolic disease
	General health: – history of malignant disease, in remission – active malignant disease if associated with present symptoms – active malignant disease not associated with present symptoms – hysterectomy	Not relevant Contraindicates neuromusculoskeletal treatment, may do gentle maintenance exercises Not relevant Increased risk of osteoporosis
	Recent unexplained weight loss	Malignancy, systemic
	Diagnosis of bone disease (e.g. osteoporosis, Paget's brittle bone)	Bone may be abnormal and/or weakened Avoid strong direct force to bone, especially the ribs
	Diagnosis of rheumatoid arthritis or other inflammatory joint disease	Avoid accessory and physiological movements to upper cervical spine and care with other joints
	Diagnosis of infective arthritis	In active stage immobilisation is treatment of choice
	Diagnosis of spondylolysis or spondylolisthesis	Avoid strong direct pressure to the subluxed vertebral level
	Systemic steroids	Osteoporosis, poor skin condition requires careful handling, avoid tape
	Anticoagulant therapy	Increased time for blood to clot. Soft tissues may bruise easily
	Human immunodeficiency virus (HIV)	Check medication and possible side-effects
	Pregnancy	Ligament laxity, may want to avoid strong forces
	Diabetes	Delayed healing, peripheral neuropathies
	Bilateral hand/feet pins and needles and/or numbness	Spinal cord compression, peripheral neuropathy
	Difficulty walking	Spinal cord compression, peripheral neuropathy, upper motor neurone lesion
	Disturbance of bladder and/or bowel function	Cauda equina syndrome

(Continued)

Table 2.4 Precautions to spinal and peripheral passive joint mobilisations and nerve mobilisations—cont'd

Aspects of subjective examination	Subjective information	Possible cause/implication for examination and/or treatment
	Perineum (saddle)	Cauda equina syndrome
	Anaesthesia/paraesthesia	
	For patients with cervicothoracic symptoms: dizziness, altered vision, nausea, ataxia, drop attacks, altered facial sensation, difficulty speaking, difficulty swallowing, sympathoplegia, hemianaesthesia, hemiplegia	Cervical artery dysfunction, upper cervical instability, disease of the inner ear
	Heart or respiratory disease	May preclude some treatment positions
	Oral contraception	Increased possibility of thrombosis – may avoid strong techniques to cervical spine
	History of smoking	Circulatory problems – increased possibility of thrombosis
Recent history	Trauma	Possible undetected fracture, e.g. scaphoid

information can be obtained from textbooks, for example Goodman & Boisonnault (1998) and Greenhalgh & Selfe (2006).

For all patients, the following information is gathered.

General health. Ascertain the general health of the patient, as poor general health can be suggestive of various systemic disease processes. The clinician asks about any feelings of general malaise or fatigue, fever, nausea or vomiting, stress, anxiety or depression. Feeling unwell or tired is common with systemic, metabolic or neoplastic disease (O'Connor & Currier 1992), whereas malaise, lassitude and depression are often associated with rheumatoid arthritis (Dickson & Wright 1984) and tuberculosis (TB) (Greenhalgh & Selfe 2006).

Weight loss. Has the patient noticed any recent weight loss? This may be due to the patient feeling unwell, perhaps with nausea and vomiting, especially if pain is severe. If there is no explanation for rapid weight loss, it may be indicative of malignancy or systemic diseases such as TB and the clinician should urgently contact the patient's medical practitioner to raise these concerns.

Cancer. It is important to ask specifically about a history of cancer both personally and also a family history of the disease (Greenhalgh & Selfe 2006). For the presence of malignant disease which is in remission, there are no precautions to examination or treatment. If, on the other hand, there is active malignancy, then the primary aim of the day 1 examination will be to clarify whether the presenting symptoms are being caused by the malignancy or whether there is a separate neuromusculoskeletal disorder. If the symptoms are thought to be associated with the malignancy then this may contraindicate most neuromusculoskeletal treatment techniques, although gentle maintenance exercises may be given.

Tuberculosis. With the incidence of TB on the rise, particularly in deprived socioeconomic groups (Bhatti et al. 1995), asking patients about exposure to TB is relevant. A previous history should be noted as TB can remain dormant. Greenhalgh & Selfe (2006) suggest that patients presenting with both systemic illness and low-back pain should raise concerns.

Human immunodeficiency virus (HIV). In cases of HIV infection a combination of several factors, including age, immunosuppression, nutritional status and chronicity, can contribute to the development of distal peripheral nerve dysfunction (Tagliati et al. 1999).

Inflammatory arthritis. Has the patient ever been diagnosed as having rheumatoid arthritis (RA) or reactive arthritis such as ankylosing spondylitis? The clinician also needs to find out if a member of the patient's family has ever been diagnosed as having this disease, as it is hereditary and the patient may be presenting with the first signs. Manual treatment of the cervical spine is avoided in patients with RA and other joints are not treated with manual therapy during the acute inflammatory stage of the disease (Grieve 1991). Common symptoms of RA are red swollen joints, pain that is worst in the morning and systemic symptoms (Huskisson et al. 1979).

Cardiovascular disease. Does the patient have a history of cardiovascular disease, e.g. angina, previous myocardial infarction, stroke? If the patient has a pacemaker fitted then s/he will need to be treated away from pulse shortwave diathermy equipment.

Respiratory disease. Does the patient have any condition which affects breathing? If so, how is it managed? This is important to establish as there may be implications for patient positioning during assessment. For instance the patient may be unable to lie supine or prone due to breathlessness.

Epilepsy. Is the patient epileptic? What type of seizures does s/he have and when was the last seizure?

Thyroid disease. Does the patient have a history of thyroid disease? How well is it managed? Thyroid dysfunction is associated with a higher incidence of neuromusculoskeletal conditions such as adhesive capsulitis, Dupuytren's contracture, trigger finger and carpal tunnel syndrome (Cakir et al. 2003).

Diabetes mellitus. Has the patient been diagnosed as having diabetes? How long since diagnosis? How is the diabetes managed? How well controlled is the condition? Healing of tissues is likely to be slower in the presence of this disease (Brem & Tomic-Canic 2007). Also distal sensory loss is indicative of a peripheral neuropathy, an associated symptom of diabetes.

Osteoporosis. As the age of the population rises, so does the incidence of osteoporosis. Clinicians should be aware of the factors likely to increase risk of osteoporosis such as postmenopause, smoking, poor diet and limited exercise (Siris et al. 2001). Patients who present with a history of fractures following falls should be considered at risk. Have they been investigated with a dual-energy X-ray absorptiometry scan? If so, when and what was the result?

Neurological symptoms. Has the patient experienced any neural tissue symptoms such as tingling, pins and needles, pain weakness or hypersensitivity? Consider whether symptoms are likely to be central, spinal or peripheral in origin. Are these symptoms unilateral or bilateral? For spinal conditions, the following information is acquired:

- Has the patient experienced symptoms of spinal cord compression (i.e. compression of the spinal cord that runs from the foramen magnum to L1)? Positive spinal cord symptoms are bilateral tingling in hands or feet and/or disturbance of gait due to disturbance of the sensory and motor pathways of the spinal cord. This can occur at any spinal level but most commonly occurs in the cervical spine (Adams & Logue 1971), causing cervical myelopathy. Recent onset of spinal cord compression may require a prompt referral to a medical practitioner. These symptoms can be further tested in the physical examination by carrying out neurological integrity tests, including the plantar response.

- Has the patient experienced symptoms of cauda equina compression (compression below L1) such as saddle (perineum) anaesthesia/paraesthesia and bladder or bowel sphincter disturbance (loss of control, retention, hesitancy, urgency or a sense of incomplete evacuation) (Grieve 1991)? These symptoms may be due to interference of S3 and S4 nerve roots (Grieve 1981). Prompt surgical intervention is required to prevent permanent sphincter paralysis.

Cervical artery dysfunction. For symptoms emanating from the cervical spine, the clinician should ask about symptoms that may be caused by cervical artery dysfunction. Symptoms include: dizziness (most commonly), altered vision (including diplopia), nausea, ataxia, 'drop attacks', altered facial sensation, difficulty speaking, difficulty swallowing, sympathoplegia, hemianaesthesia and hemiplegia (Bogduk 1994). If present, the clinician determines the aggravating and easing factors in the usual way. For further information the reader is directed to Chapter 7 and to Kerry & Taylor (2006) and Kerry et al. (2008). These symptoms can also be due to upper cervical instability and diseases of the inner ear.

Drug therapy. In this area, there are three relevant questions.

1. Has the patient been on long-term medication/steroids? High doses of corticosteroids for a long period of time can weaken the skin and cause osteoporosis. In this case, the patient requires careful handling and avoidance of the use of tape

so that the skin is not damaged. Owing to the raised likelihood of osteoporosis, strong direct forces to the bones may be inadvisable. Long-term use of medication may lead to side-effects such as constipation, indigestion and drowsiness as well as perhaps causing the patient to become drug-dependent. This may interfere with their general function and hinder their recovery.

2. Has the patient been taking anticoagulants? If so, care is needed in the physical examination in order to avoid trauma to tissues and consequent bleeding.

3. Has drug therapy been prescribed for the patient's neuromusculoskeletal problem or is the patient self-medicating with over-the-counter preparations? This can give useful information about the pathological process and may affect treatment. For example, the strength of any painkillers may indicate the intensity of the patient's pain. A neurogenic or central pain component does not tend to respond to simple analgesic or anti-inflammatory drugs. Care may be needed if the patient attends for assessment/treatment soon after taking painkillers as the pain may be temporarily masked and assessment/treatment may cause exacerbation of the patient's condition. In addition, the clinician needs to be aware of any side-effects of the drugs taken. The clinician must continue to monitor medication use throughout treatment.

Radiographs, medical imaging and tests. Has the patient been X-rayed or had any other medical tests? Radiographs are useful to diagnose fractures, arthritis and serious bone pathology such as infection, osteo-porosis or tumour and to determine the extent of the injury following trauma. Radiographs can provide useful additional information but the findings must be correlated with the patient's clinical presentation. This is particularly true for spinal radiographs, which may reveal the normal age-related degenerative changes of the spine that do not necessarily correlate with the patient's symptoms. For this reason, routine spinal radiographs are no longer considered necessary for non-traumatic spinal pain (Clinical Standards Advisory Report 1994). Other imaging techniques include computed tomography, magnetic resonance imaging, myelography, discography, bone scans and arthrography. The results of these tests can help to determine the nature of the patient's condition.

Further details of these tests and their diagnostic value can be found in Refshauge & Gass (2004). In addition has the patient had any other investigations such as blood tests? Erythrocyte sedimentation rate and C-reactive protein blood tests are commonly used to detect inflammation seen in certain types of arthritis, tissue injury, muscular and connective tissue disorders.

History of the present condition (HPC)

For each symptomatic area, the clinician should ascertain:

- how long the symptom has been present
- whether there was a sudden or slow onset of the symptom
- whether there was a known or unknown cause that provoked the onset of the symptom, i.e. trauma or change in lifestyle that may have triggered symptoms
- if the patient has sought any treatment already and, if so, to what effect
- whether the patient feels the symptoms are getting better, worse or staying the same.

These questions give information about the nature of the problem, the possible pathological processes involved and whether trauma was a feature in the production of symptoms.

- To confirm the relationship of symptoms, the clinician asks when each symptom began in relation to others. If, for example, anterior knee joint pain started 3 weeks ago and increased 2 days ago when anterior calf pain developed, it would suggest that the knee and calf pain are associated and that the same structures may well be at fault. If there was no change in the knee pain when the calf pain began, the symptoms may not be related and different structures may be producing the two pain areas.

- History of any previous attacks, e.g. the number of episodes, when they occurred, the cause, the duration of the episodes and whether the patient fully recovered between episodes. If there have been no previous attacks, has the patient had any episodes of stiffness which may have been a precursor to the development of pain?

- Has the patient had treatment previously? If so, what was the outcome of any past treatments for the same or a similar problem? Past treatment records, if available, may then be obtained for further information. It may well be the case that a previously successful treatment modality will be successful again, but greater efforts may be needed to prevent a recurrence. Physical, psychological or social factors may need to be examined in more detail as they may be responsible for the recurrence of the problem.

Past medical history (PMH)

The following information is obtained from the patient and/or medical notes:

- Details of any medical history such as major or long-standing illnesses, accidents or surgery that are relevant to the patient's condition.

Social history (SH)

Social history that is relevant to the onset and progression of the patient's problem is recorded. This includes the patient's perspectives, experience and expectations, age, employment, home situation and details of any leisure activities. In order to treat appropriately, it is important that the condition is managed within the context of the patient's social and work environment.

The following factors are considered to predict poor treatment outcome in patients with low-back pain (Waddell 2004):

- belief that back pain is harmful or potentially severely disabling
- fear avoidance behaviours and reduced activity levels
- tendency to low mood and withdrawal from social interaction
- expectation that passive treatment will help, rather than active treatment.

The clinician may therefore ask the following types of questions to elucidate these psychosocial risk factors, or 'yellow flags' (Waddell 2004):

- Have you had time off work in the past with back pain?
- What do you understand to be the cause of your back pain?

- What are you expecting will help you?
- How is your employer/co-workers/family responding to your back pain?
- What are you doing to cope with your back pain?
- Do you think you will return to work? When?

Readers are referred to Waddell's text for further information on psychosocial risk factors for patients with low-back pain. While these factors have been identified for low-back pain, it seems reasonable to suggest that they would be useful for patients with cervical and thoracic spine pain, as well as pain in the periphery.

Family history (FH)

The clinician should ask about any relevant family history that may indicate a patient's predisposition for the development of a condition. An understanding of a family history may also help to explain a patient's perceptions of the problem.

Expectations and goals

In order to understand a patient's expectation of therapy, it is helpful at the outset to identify the patient's hopes and expectations of treatment and management. This can reveal a great deal about the patient's perceptions and beliefs about the condition and offers the clinician an opportunity for a collaborative consensual approach to treatment as well as appropriate education for the patient from the outset.

Plan of the physical examination

When all this information has been collected, the subjective examination is complete. It is useful at this stage for the clinician to reconfirm briefly with patients their understanding of their main complaint, and to offer them the opportunity to add anything that they may not have had the opportunity to raise so far, before explaining to them the purpose and plan for the physical examination. For ease of reference, highlight with asterisks (*) important subjective findings and particularly one or more functional restrictions. These can then be re-examined at subsequent treatment sessions to evaluate treatment intervention.

A summary of this first part of the patient examination can be found in Figure 2.9.

In order to plan the physical examination, the hypotheses generated from the subjective examination should be tested (Figure 2.10).

- Are there any precautions and/or contraindications to elements of the physical examination that need to be explored further, such as neurological involvement, recent fracture, trauma, steroid therapy or rheumatoid arthritis? There may also be contraindications to further examination and treatment, e.g. symptoms of cord compression.

- Clinically reasoning throughout the subjective examination using distribution of symptoms, pain mechanisms described, behaviour of symptoms, as well as the history of onset, the clinician must decide on structures that could be the cause of the patient's symptoms. The clinician should have a prioritised list of working hypotheses based on the most likely causes of the patient's symptoms. These may include the structures underneath the symptomatic area, e.g. joints, muscles, nerves and fascia, as well as the regions referring into the area. These possible referring regions will need to be examined as a possible cause of symptoms, e.g. cervical spine, thoracic spine, shoulder and wrist and hand. In complex cases it is not always possible to examine fully at the first attendance and so, using clinical reasoning skills, the clinician will need to prioritise and justify what 'must' be examined in the first assessment session, and what 'should' or 'could' be followed up at subsequent sessions.

- What are the pain mechanisms driving the patient's symptoms and what impact will this information have on an understanding of the problem and subsequent management decisions? For example, pain associated with repetitive activities may indicate inflammatory or neurogenic nociception. This would indicate an early assessment of activities and advice to the patient to pace activities. The patient's acceptance and willingness to be an active participant in management will depend on his or her perspective and subsequent behavioural response to the symptoms. If patients are demonstrating fear avoidance behaviours then the clinician's ability to explain and teach them about their condition will be pivotal to achieving a successful outcome.

- Once the clinician has decided on the tests to include in the physical examination the next consideration should be how the physical tests should be carried out? Are symptoms severe and/or irritable? Will it be easy or hard to reproduce each symptom? If symptoms are severe, physical tests may be carried out to just before the onset of symptom production or just to the onset of symptom production; further stressing of tissues, e.g. overpressures, will not be carried out, as the patient would be unable to tolerate this. If symptoms are irritable, physical tests may be examined to just before symptom production or just to the onset of provocation with fewer physical tests being examined to allow for rest periods between tests. Alternatively will it be necessary to use combined movements, or repetitive movements, in order to reproduce the patient's symptoms?

A planning form for the physical examination, such as the one shown in Appendix 2.1, can be useful for clinicians, to help guide them through the often complex clinical reasoning process (Figure 2.11).

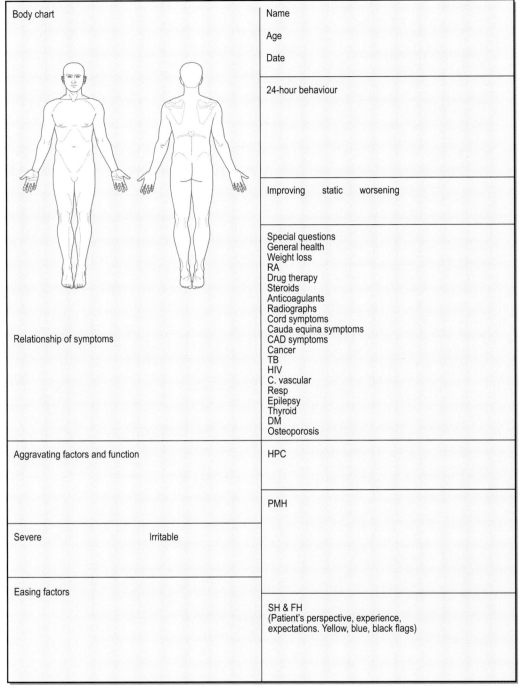

Body chart	Name
	Age
	Date

Figure 2.9 • Subjective examination chart. RA, rheumatoid arthritis; CAD, cervical artery dysfunction; HPC, history of the present condition; PMH, past medical history; SH, social history; FH, family history, DM, diabetes mellitus.

The chart contains the following labelled sections:

- Body chart
- Name
- Age
- Date
- 24-hour behaviour
- Improving   static   worsening
- Relationship of symptoms
- Special questions
  - General health
  - Weight loss
  - RA
  - Drug therapy
  - Steroids
  - Anticoagulants
  - Radiographs
  - Cord symptoms
  - Cauda equina symptoms
  - CAD symptoms
  - Cancer
  - TB
  - HIV
  - C. vascular
  - Resp
  - Epilepsy
  - Thyroid
  - DM
  - Osteoporosis
- Aggravating factors and function
- HPC
- PMH
- Severe   Irritable
- Easing factors
- SH & FH
  (Patient's perspective, experience, expectations. Yellow, blue, black flags)

	Symptom	Symptom	Symptom	Symptom
Is it severe?				
Is it irritable?				
Will you move: – short of production? – point of onset/increase in resting symptoms? – partial reproduction? – total reproduction?				
How will you reproduce symptom: – repeat? – alter speed? – combine? – sustain? – other? (state)				
Are there any precautions or contraindications? Yes No State				
What other factors contributing to the patient's symptom(s) need to be examined?				

Figure 2.10 • Basic physical examination planning form.

APPENDIX 2.1 AN INDEPTH CLINICAL REASONING FORM

1.1 Source of symptoms

Symptomatic area	Structures under area	Structures which can refer to area	Supporting evidence

1.2 What is the mechanism of each symptom?
Explain from information from the subjective and physical examination findings

	Symptom	Symptom	Symptom	Symptom
Subjective				
Physical				

Figure 2.11 • Clinical reasoning form.

(Continued)

1.3 Following the physical examination, what is your clinical diagnosis?

2. Contributing factors

2.1 What factors need to be examined/explored in the physical examination?

2.2 How will you address each contributing factor?

3. Precautions and contraindications

3.1 Are any symptoms severe?   Yes   No
     Which symptoms, and explain why

3.2 Are any symptoms irritable?   Yes   No
     Which symptoms, and explain why

Figure 2.11—cont'd

(Continued)

APPENDIX 2.1 cont'd

3.3 How much of each symptom are you prepared to provoke in the physical examination?

Symptom	Short of P1	Point of onset or increase in resting symptoms	Partial reproduction	Total reproduction

3.4 Will a neurological examination be necessary in the physical?

        Yes   No   Explain why

3.5 Following the subjective examination, are there any precautions or contraindications?

        Yes   No   Explain why

4. Management

4.1 What tests will you do in the physical and what are the expected findings?

Physical tests	Expected findings

Figure 2.11—cont'd

(Continued)

4.2   Were there any unexpected findings from the physical? Explain
4.3   What will be your subjective and physical reassessment asterisks?
4.4   What is your first choice of treatment (be exact) and explain why?
4.5   What do you expect the response to be over the next 24 hours following the 1st visit? Explain
4.6   How do you think you will treat and manage the patient at the 2nd visit, if the patient returns: Same Better Worse
4.7   What advice and education will you give the patient?

Figure 2.11—cont'd

(Continued)

APPENDIX 2.1 cont'd

4.8 What needs to be examined on the 2nd and 3rd visits?

2nd visit	3rd visit

5. Prognosis

5.1 List the positive and negative factors (from both the subjective and physical examination findings) in considering the patient's prognosis

	Positive	Negative
Subjective		
Physical		

5.2 Overall, is the patient's condition:
   improving   worsening   static

5.3 What is your overall prognosis for this patient? Be specific

Figure 2.11—cont'd

(Continued)

6. After 3rd attendance

6.1 Has your understanding of the patient's problem changed from your interpretations made following the initial subjective and physical examination? If so, explain

6.2 On reflection, were there any clues that you initially missed, misinterpreted, under- or over-weighted? If so, explain

7. After discharge

7.1 Has your understanding of the patient's problem changed from your interpretations made following the 3rd attendance? If so, explain how

7.2 What have you learnt from the management of this patient which will be helpful to you in the future?

APPENDIX 2.2 CASE SCENARIOS

The main aim of the examination/assessment is to determine the structures at fault, and this process begins at the outset of the subjective examination with the body chart and behaviour of symptoms. Two examples of the clinical reasoning process during the first part of the subjective examination are given below.

PATIENT A

The symptoms are depicted in the body chart in Figure 2.12.

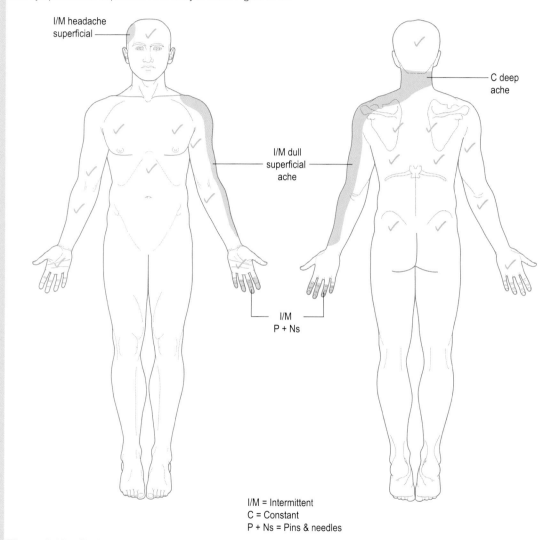

I/M headache superficial

C deep ache

I/M dull superficial ache

I/M P + Ns

I/M = Intermittent
C = Constant
P + Ns = Pins & needles

Figure 2.12 • Body chart patient A.

The relationship of the symptoms is as follows. The left and right cervical spine pains come and go together; they appear to be a single area of pain. When the cervical pain worsens, the headache becomes apparent, but the cervical pain can be present without the headache. The headache cannot be present without the cervical pain. The left arm pain and paraesthesia in the left hand always come and go together, and these symptoms can be present without any neck pain or headache.

This suggests that one structure is producing the left and right neck pain, another structure is producing the arm pain and paraesthesia in the hand and, possibly, a third structure is producing the headache.

(Continued)

The information gathered so far from the body chart suggests various structures giving rise to each symptom and these are listed in Table 2.5. The clinician then uses the behaviour of symptoms to localise further which structures may be at fault.

Table 2.5 Structures suspected to be a source of the symptoms

Symptom	Structure
Left cervical spine pain	Cervical spine*
Right cervical spine pain	Cervical spine
Right headache	Cervical spine Spine and cerebral dura mater
Left arm pain	Cervical spine Neural tissue Individual joints – shoulder, elbow and wrist Individual muscles around shoulder, elbow, wrist and hand
Paraesthesia in left hand	Cervical spine Neural tissue Entrapment of brachial plexus around first rib Entrapment of nerve at wrist

*Note that, because of the complex anatomy of the spine and the fact that most structures are pain-sensitive, it is very difficult to isolate specific structures in the spine at this stage in the examination. For the purposes of this part of the examination, the region is therefore dealt with as one structure.

Behaviour of symptoms

Aggravating factors. The clinician asks the effect on symptoms of specific aggravating movements and positions for each structure suspected to be a source of symptoms. Table 2.6 illustrates the possible responses of symptoms to aggravating factors.

Table 2.6 Possible aggravating factors for each of the symptoms

Symptoms	Extension (includes first rib)	Rotation	Sustained flexion	Depression of shoulder girdle	Carrying loads	Hand behind back	Flexion/extension	Flexion/extension
Cervical spine pain	+	+	+	−	+	−	−	−
Right headache	−	−	+	−	−	−	−	−
Left arm pain	−	−	−	+	+	−	−	−
Pins and needles in left hand	−	−	−	+	+	−	−	−

+, reproduction of symptoms; −, no production of symptoms.

(Continued)

APPENDIX 2.2 cont'd

The logical interpretation of the information on aggravating factors would be that the cervical spine is producing the left and right cervical spine pain and the headache. Abnormal neurodynamics are producing the left arm pain and paraesthesia in the left hand, since the aggravating positions put the nervous system under tension.

Easing factors. The relationship of symptoms and the structures at fault may be further confirmed by establishing the easing factors. The patient may find, for example, that keeping the cervical spine still eases the neck pain, that the headaches are eased by avoiding extreme neck positions, and that the left arm pain and pins and needles in the fingers of the left hand are eased by supporting the left arm with the shoulder girdle elevated. This information would confirm the findings from the body chart and aggravating factors.

Patient B

The symptoms are depicted in the body chart in Figure 2.13.

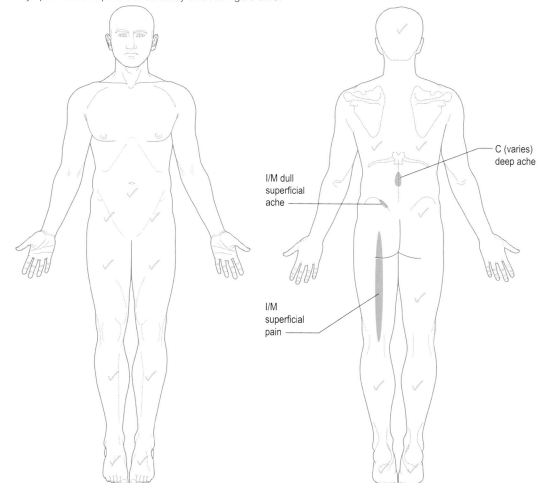

Figure 2.13 • Body chart patient B.

The relationship of symptoms is as follows. When the lumbar spine pain gets worse (it is constant but varies in intensity), there is no change in any of the other pains. The buttock and thigh pains come and go together. The iliac crest pain, buttock and posterior thigh pain come on separately; the patient can have the iliac crest pain without the buttock and thigh pain, and similarly the buttock and thigh pain can come on without the iliac crest pain.

(Continued)

Since none of the symptoms seem to be associated, this would suggest that there are three different structures at fault, each causing one of the three areas of pain.

The information gathered so far from the body chart suggests that various structures are giving rise to each symptom; these are listed in Table 2.7 The clinician then uses the behaviour of symptoms to localise further which structures are at fault.

Table 2.7 Structures suspected to be a source of the symptoms

Symptom	Structure
Central low-back pain	Lumbar spine
Left iliac crest pain	Lumbar spine Sacroiliac joint
Left buttock and thigh pain	Lumbar spine Sacroiliac joint Nervous tissue Muscles

Behaviour of symptoms

Aggravating factors. The clinician asks the effect on symptoms of specific aggravating movements and positions for each structure suspected to be a source of symptoms. Table 2.8 illustrates the possible responses of symptoms to aggravating factors.

Table 2.8 Possible aggravating factors for each of the symptoms

Symptoms	Lumbar spine		Sacroiliac joint		Nervous tissue		Hip
	Flexion	Walking	Sitting	Standing on one leg	Rolling over	Long sit in bed	Squat
Lumbar spine pain	+	−	+	−	−	−	−
Iliac crest pain	−	+	−	+	+	−	−
Buttock and posterior thigh pain	−	−	−	−	−	+	−

+, reproduction of symptoms; −, no production of symptoms.

The logical interpretation of the information on aggravating factors would be that the lumbar spine is producing the central lumbar spine pain, the left sacroiliac joint is producing the left iliac crest pain, and abnormal neurodynamics are producing the posterior buttock and left thigh pain.

Easing factors. The relationship between symptoms may be further confirmed by establishing the easing factors. The patient may find that the lumbar spine pain is eased by lying supine and that the iliac crest pain is eased by applying a tight belt around the pelvis. Provocation of the buttock and posterior thigh pain is reduced by avoiding any tensioning of the sciatic nerve, such as in long sitting or getting in or out of a car. This information would confirm the findings from the body chart and aggravating factors.

APPENDIX 2.3 COUNTERFEIT CLINICAL PRESENTATIONS (FROM GRIEVE 1994b)

Since clinicians are often 'first contact' clinicians, we have assumed greater responsibilities. While those interested in manipulation and allied treatments energetically improve their competence in the various techniques and applications, we might profitably spend a little time considering what we are doing all this to.

If we take patients off the street, we need more than ever to be awake for those conditions that may be other than benign neuromusculoskeletal. This is not 'diagnosis', only an enlightened awareness of when manual or other physical therapy may be more than merely foolish and perhaps dangerous.

There is also the factor of delaying more appropriate treatment. It is not in the patients' best interest to foster the notion that 'first contact clinician' also means 'diagnostician' (Grieve 1991). Pain distribution might confuse unwary or overconfident therapists, who may assume familiarity with a syndrome they recognise and then perhaps find themselves confronting the tip of a very different kind of iceberg.

Distribution of pain from visceral conditions, especially, can easily mislead, unless one maintains a lively awareness of how they can present. Some examples follow:

- Angina can affect face, neck and jaw only, and true anginal pain can on occasions be posterior thoracic as well as precordial. Simple thoracic joint problems often simulate angina, of course.
- Hiatus hernia may present with chest and bilateral shoulder pain, as may oesophageal spasm with, in this case, added radiation to the back.
- Virtually anything in the abdomen can present with back pain; examples are peptic ulcer, cancer of the colon or rectum, retroperitoneal disease (e.g. cancer of the pancreas) or abdominal arterial disease (Grieve 1994a). Some suggest that a peptic ulcer must be a gross lesion to refer pain to the back, yet individuals with an ulcer shallow enough to escape barium meal examination may have back pain from the ulcer. Even when the ulcer is healing, a glass of milk will ease the backache that follows gardening (Brewerton, personal communication, 1990). It is important to identify quickly non-neuromusculoskeletal conditions so these patients can receive appropriate treatment.

Provocation and relief

A common opinion is that benign neuromusculoskeletal conditions of the spine are recognisable because the clinical features are provoked by certain postures and activities (such as coughing and sneezing) and lessened by other (antalgic) postures and activities; this pattern of provocation and relief is the distinguishing factor. By contrast, the features of systemic, neoplastic or other (non-neuromusculoskeletal) conditions are said, in broad terms, to be identifiable in being less influenced by postures or activity.

This rule of thumb is too simplistic; many conditions, in either category, do not behave in this way.

The writer recalls two patients: one who, with a clear history of recent trauma to the left upper thorax, developed the classic features of a simple rib joint lesion, and another who presented with a watertight history of bouts of low-back pain, closely related to prolonged periods of sitting and stooping. In each case, the physical signs confirmed the opinion that these were simple benign lesions. Both were neoplasms. Both patients soon succumbed. Fortunately, treatment was not aggressive or enthusiastic and soon stopped.

References

Adams, C.B.T., Logue, V., 1971. Studies in cervical spondylotic myelopathy II. The movement and contour of the spine in relation to the neural complications of cervical spondylosis. Brain 94, 569–587.

Aroll, B., Khin, N., Kerse, N., 2003. Screening for depression in primary care with two verbally asked questions: cross sectional study. Br. Med. J. 327, 1144–1146.

Austen, R., 1991. The distribution and characteristics of lumbar-lower limb symptoms in subjects with and without a neurological deficit. In: Proceedings of the Manipulative Physiotherapists Association of Australia, 7th Biennial Conference, New South Wales, pp. 252–257.

Barrows, H.S., Feltovich, P., 1987. The clinical reasoning process. Med. Educ. 21, 86–91.

Bhatti, N., Law, M.R., Morris, J.K., et al., 1995. Increasing incidence of tuberculosis in England and Wales: a study of the likely causes. Br. Med. J. 310, 967–969.

Bogduk, N., 1994. Cervical causes of headache and dizziness. In: Boyling, J.D., Palastanga, N. (Eds.), Grieve's modern manual therapy, second ed. Churchill Livingstone, Edinburgh, p. 317.

Brem, H., Tomic-Canic, M., 2007. Cellular and molecular basis of wound healing in diabetes. J. Clin. Invest. 117, 1219–1222.

Butler, D., Moseley, L., 2003. Explain pain. Neuro Orthopaedic Institute, Adelaide, pp. 8–81, 100–101.

Cakir, M., Samanci, N., Balci, N., et al., 2003. Musculoskeletal manifestations in patients with thyroid disease. Clin. Endocrinol. 59, 162–167.

Clinical Standards Advisory Report, 1994. Report of a CSAG committee on back pain. HMSO, London.

Corrigan, B., Maitland, G.D., 1994. Musculoskeletal and sports injuries. Butterworth-Heinemann, Oxford.

Dalton, P.A., Jull, G.A., 1989. The distribution and characteristics of neck-arm pain in patients with and without a neurological deficit. Aust. J. Physiother. 35, 3–8.

Dickson, R.A., Wright, V., 1984. Musculoskeletal disease. Heinemann, London.

Doubell, T.P., Mannion, R.J., Woolf, C., 2002. The dorsal horn: state-dependent sensory processing, plasticity and the generation of pain. In: Melzack, R., Wall, P. (Eds.), Textbook of pain, fourth ed. Churchill Livingstone, Edinburgh, p. 165.

Edwards, I., Jones, M., Carr, J., et al., 2004. Clinical reasoning strategies in physical therapy. Phys. Ther. 84, 312–330.

Edwards, I., Jones, M., Hillier, S., 2006. The interpretation of experience and its relationship to body movement: a clinical reasoning perspective. Man. Ther. 11, 2–10.

Fields, H. (Ed.), 1995. Core curriculum for professional education in pain. second ed. Seattle, IASP.

Gifford, L., 1996. The clinical biology of ache and pains (course manual), fifth ed. Neuro-Orthopaedic Institute UK, Falmouth.

Gifford, L., Thacker, M., 2002. A clinical overview of the autonomic nervous system, the supply to the gut and the mind–body pathways. In: Gifford, L. (Ed.), Topical issues in pain 3. Physiotherapy Pain Association, Falmouth, p. 49.

Goodman, C.C., Boisonnault, W.G., 1998. Pathology: implications for the physical therapist. W B Saunders, Philadelphia.

Greenhalgh, S., Selfe, J., 2006. Red flags: a guide to identifying serious pathology of the spine. Elsevier, Edinburgh.

Grieve, G.P., 1981. Common vertebral joint problems. Churchill Livingstone, Edinburgh.

Grieve, G.P., 1991. Mobilisation of the spine, fifth ed. Churchill Livingstone, Edinburgh.

Grieve, G.P., 1994a. The masqueraders. In: Boyling, J.D., Palastanga, N. (Eds.), Grieve's modern manual therapy, second ed. Churchill Livingstone, Edinburgh, pp. 841.

Grieve, G.P., 1994b. Counterfeit clinical presentations. Manipulative Physiotherapist 26, 17–19.

Hakim, A., Grahame, R., 2003. A simple questionnaire to detect hypermobility; and adjunct to the assessment of patients with diffuse musculoskeletal pain. Int. J. Clin. Pract. 57, 163–166.

Harding, V., Williams, A.C., de C., 1995. Extending physiotherapy skills using a psychological approach: cognitive-behavioural management of chronic pain. Physiotherapy 81, 681–688.

Higgs, J., Jones, M. (Eds.), 2000. Clinical reasoning in the health professions, second ed. Butterworth Heinemann, Oxford.

Hinnant, D.W., 1994. Psychological evaluation and testing. In: Tollison, C.D. (Ed.), Handbook of pain management, second ed. Williams & Wilkins, Baltimore, pp. 18.

Huskisson, E.C., Dieppe, P.A., Tucker, A.K., et al., 1979. Another look at osteoarthritis. Ann. Rheum. Dis. 38, 423–428.

Jones, M.A., 1995. Clinical reasoning and pain. Man. Ther. 1, 17–24.

Jones, M.A., Rivett, D.A., 2004. Clinical reasoning for manual therapists. Butterworth-Heinemann, Edinburgh.

Jones, M., Jensen, G., Edwards, I., 2008. Clinical reasoning in physiotherapy. In: Higgs, J., Jones, M.A., Loftus, S. (Eds.), Clinical reasoning in the health professions, third ed. Butterworth Heinemann/Elsevier, Amsterdam, pp. 245–256.

Jull, G.A., 1986. Examination of the lumbar spine. In: Grieve, G.P. (Ed.), Modern manual therapy. Churchill Livingstone, Edinburgh, pp. 547.

Keefe, F.J., Block, A.R., 1982. Development of an observation method for assessing pain behaviour in chronic low back pain patients. Behav. Ther. 13, 363–375.

Kerry, R., Taylor, A., 2006. Cervical arterial dysfunction assessment and manual therapy. Man. Ther. 11, 243–253.

Kerry, R., Taylor, A., Mitchell, J., et al., 2008. Cervical arterial dysfunction and manual therapy: a critical literature review to inform professional practice. Man. Ther. 13, 278–288.

Lindsay, K.W., Bone, I., Callander, R., 1997. Neurology and neurosurgery illustrated, third ed. Churchill Livingstone, Edinburgh.

Magee, D.J., 2006. Orthopedic physical assessment, fourth ed. Saunders Elsevier, Philadelphia.

Main, C.J., Spanswick, C.C., 2000. Pain management, an interdisciplinary approach. Churchill Livingstone, Edinburgh.

Main, C.J., Wood, P.L., Hillis, S., 1992. The distress and risk assessment method. Spine 17, 42–52.

Maitland, G.D., Hengeveld, E., Banks, K., et al., 2005. Maitland's Peripheral Manipulation, fourth ed. Butterworth-Heinemann, Elsevier, London.

McGuire, D.B., 1995. The multiple dimensions of cancer pain: a framework for assessment and management. In: McGuire, D.B., Yarbro, C.H., Ferrell, B.R. (Eds.), Cancer pain management, second ed. Jones & Bartlett, Boston, pp. 1–17.

McKenzie, R.A., 1981. The lumbar spine: mechanical diagnosis and therapy. Spinal Publications, New Zealand.

Melzack, R., Wall, P., 1996. The challenge of pain, second ed. Penguin, London.

Mense, S., 1993. Nociception from skeletal muscle in relation to clinical muscle pain. Pain 54, 241–289.

Mooney, V., Robertson, J., 1976. The facet syndrome. Clin. Orthop. Relat. Res. 115, 149–156.

Nachemson, A., 1992. Lumbar mechanics as revealed by lumbar intradiscal pressure measurements. In: Jayson, M.I.V. (Ed.), The lumbar spine and back pain, fourth ed. Churchill Livingstone, Edinburgh, pp. 157.

Newham, D.J., Mills, K.R., 1999. Muscles, tendons and ligaments. In: Wall, P.D., Melzack, R. (Eds.), Textbook of pain, fourth ed. Churchill Livingstone, Edinburgh, p. 517.

O'Connor, M.I., Currier, B.L., 1992. Metastatic disease of the spine. Orthopaedics 15, 611–620.

Petty, N.J., Moore, A.P., 2001. Neuromusculoskeletal examination and assessment: a handbook for therapists, second ed. Churchill Livingstone, Edinburgh.

Price, D., 2000. Psychological mechanisms of pain and analgesia. International Association for the Study of Pain (IASP), Seattle.

Refshauge, K., Gass, E. (Eds.), 2004. Musculoskeletal physiotherapy: clinical science and evidence-based practice. Butterworth-Heinemann, Oxford.

Rivett, D.A., Higgs, J., 1997. Hypothesis generation in the clinical reasoning behavior of manual therapists. J. Phys. Ther. Educ. 11, 40–45.

Shorland, S., 1998. Management of chronic pain following whiplash injuries. In: Gifford, L. (Ed.), Topical issues in pain. Neuro-Orthopaedic Institute UK, Falmouth, pp. 115–134.

Simmonds, J., Keer, R., 2007. Hypermobility and the hypermobility syndrome. Man. Ther. 12, 298–309.

Siris, E., Miller, P., Barrett-Connor, E., 2001. Identification and fracture outcomes of undiagnosed low bone mineral density in postmenopausal women results from the national osteoporosis risk assessment. J. Am. Med. Assoc. 286, 2815–2822.

Solomon, L., Warwick, D., Nayagam, S., 2001. Apley's system of orthopaedics and fractures, eighth ed. Arnold, London.

Tagliati, M., Grinnell, J., Godbold, J., et al., 1999. Peripheral nerve function in HIV infection. Arch. Neurol. 56, 84–89.

van Cranenburgh, B., 1989. Inleiding in de toegepaste neurowetenschappen, deel 1, Neurofilosofie (Introduction to applied neuroscience, part 1, Neurophysiology), third ed. Uitgeversmaatschappij de Tijdstroom, Lochum.

van Griensven, H., 2005. Pain in practice theory and treatment strategies for manual therapists. Elsevier, Edinburgh.

Waddell, G., 2004. The back pain revolution, second ed. Churchill Livingstone, Edinburgh.

Woolf, C., 2004. Pain: moving from symptom control toward mechanism specific pharmacologic management. Ann. Intern. Med. 140, 441–451.

World Health Organization, 2001. International classification of functioning, disability and health. World Health Organization, Geneva.

Physical examination

3

Dionne Ryder

Introduction

The aim of the physical examination is to determine what structure(s) and/or factor(s) are responsible for producing the patient's symptoms. Physical testing procedures justified through clinical reasoning are carried out to collect evidence to confirm the clinician's hypotheses and negate other possible hypotheses. As has been clearly stated elsewhere, the physical examination 'is not simply the indiscriminate application of routine tests, but rather should be seen as an extension of the subjective examination . . . for specifically testing hypotheses considered from the subjective examination' (Jones & Jones 1994).

Two assumptions are made when carrying out the physical examination:

1. If symptoms are reproduced (or eased) then the test has somehow affected the structures at fault. The word 'structures' is used in its widest sense, and could include anatomical structures or physiological mechanisms. None of the tests stress individual structures in isolation – each test affects a number of tissues, both locally and at a distance. For example, knee flexion will affect the tibiofemoral and patellofemoral intra-articular and periarticular joint structures, surrounding muscles and nerves, as well as joints, muscles and nerves proximally at the hip and spine and distally at the ankle.

2. If an abnormality is detected in a structure, which theoretically could refer symptoms to the symptomatic area, then that structure is suspected to be a source of the symptoms and is fully examined in the physical examination. The abnormality is described as a 'comparable sign' (Maitland et al. 2005).

The term 'objective' is often applied to the physical examination but suggests that this part of the examination is not prejudiced and that the findings are valid and reliable. This is certainly misleading as most of the tests carried out rely on the skill of the clinician to observe, move and palpate the patient and, as stated earlier, these are not pure tests. The clinician needs to take account of this when making an assessment of a patient based on the findings of the physical examination. The clinician should use all the information obtained from the subjective and physical examination in order to make sense of the patient's overall presentation; that is, 'making features fit' (Maitland et al. 2001). The clinician must therefore keep an open mind, thinking logically throughout the physical examination, not quickly jumping to conclusions based on just one or two tests.

Table 3.1 Summary of the physical examination

Observation	Informal and formal observation of posture, muscle bulk and tone, soft tissues, gait, function and patient's attitude
Joint integrity tests	For example, knee abduction and adduction stress tests
Active physiological movements with overpressure	Active movements with overpressure
Passive physiological movements	
Muscle tests	Strength, control, length, isometric contraction, diagnostic
Nerve tests	Neurological integrity, neurodynamic, diagnostic
Special tests	Vascular, soft tissue, cardiorespiratory
Palpation	Superficial and deep soft tissues, bone, joint, ligament, muscle, tendon and nerve
Joint tests	Accessory movements, natural apophyseal glides, sustained natural apophyseal glides, mobilisations with movement

The physical examination is summarised in Table 3.1. Some of the tests that are common to a number of areas of the body, such as posture, muscle tests and neurological examination, are described in this chapter, rather than repeating them in each chapter. More specific tests, such as for cervical artery dysfunction, are described in the relevant chapters. Clinicians may have a personal preference for the order of testing, as demonstrated in subsequent regional chapters of this text, or may alter the order according to the patient and the condition.

Physical examination step by step

Observation

Informal and formal observation can give the clinician information about the following:

- the pathology, e.g. olecranon bursitis produces a localised swelling over the olecranon process
- whether the patient displays overt pain behaviour (see Box 2.2) and the possible factors contributing to the patient's problem, e.g. a difference in the height of the left and right anterior superior iliac spines in standing suggests a leg length discrepancy or pelvic dysfunction
- the physical testing procedures that need to be carried out, e.g. strength tests for any muscle that appears wasted on observation
- the possible treatment techniques, e.g. postural re-education for patients who suffer from headaches and who are observed to have a forward head posture.

It should be remembered, however, that the posture a patient adopts reflects a multitude of factors, including not only the state of bone, joint, muscle and neural tissue, but also the pain experienced and the patient's emotions and body awareness or lack thereof.

Informal observation

The clinician's observation of the patient begins from the moment they first meet. In the waiting area is the patient sitting or standing? How is the patient moving? A reluctance to move may demonstrate fear avoidance, an indication of possible illness behaviour. Does the patient appear in pain? During the subjective examination, is the patient comfortable or constantly shifting position? It may well be that this informal observation is as informative as the formal assessment, as a patient under such scrutiny may not adopt his/her usual posture. The clinician can also observe whether the patient is using aids (prescribed or non-prescribed) such as collars, sticks and corsets and whether they are being used in an appropriate way.

Formal observation

Observation of posture. The clinician observes posture by examining the anterior, lateral and posterior views of the patient. The ideal alignment is summarised in Figure 3.1. Typical postures that may be observed include:

- The kyphosis–lordosis posture (Kendall et al. 1993) where there is an anteriorly rotated pelvis, an increased lumbar lordosis and slight flexion of the hips. This is shown in Figure 3.2.
- Layer syndrome (Jull & Janda 1987; Janda 1994, 2002), shown in Figure 3.3, where there are alternate 'layers' of hypertrophic and hypotrophic

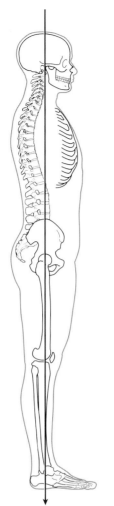

Figure 3.1 • Ideal alignment. (From Kendall et al. 1993 © Williams and Wilkins.)

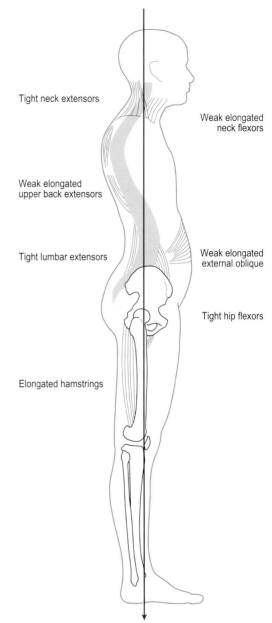

Tight neck extensors

Weak elongated neck flexors

Weak elongated upper back extensors

Tight lumbar extensors

Weak elongated external oblique

Tight hip flexors

Elongated hamstrings

Figure 3.2 • Kyphosis–lordosis posture. (After Kendall et al. 1993 © Williams & Wilkins.)

muscles when the patient is viewed from behind. There is weakness and then a possible hypotrophic presentation of the lower stabilisers of the scapula, lumbosacral erector spinae, gluteus maximus, rectus abdominis and transversus abdominis; there is hypertrophy of the cervical erector spinae, upper trapezius, levator scapulae, thoracolumbar erector spinae and hamstrings.

• The flat-back posture (Kendall et al. 1993), shown in Figure 3.4, which is characterised by a slightly extended cervical spine, flexion of the upper part of the thoracic spine (the lower part is straight), absent lumbar lordosis, a posterior pelvic tilt and extension of the hip joints and slight

plantarflexion of the ankle joints. This is thought to be due to elongated and weak hip flexors and short, strong hamstrings. Sahrmann (1993) additionally considers the lumbar paraspinal muscles to be long.

Muscle hypotrophy   Muscle hypertrophy

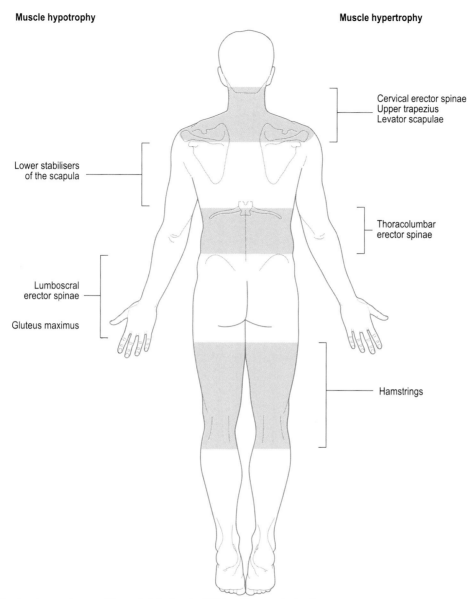

Figure 3.3 • Layer syndrome. (From Jull & Janda 1987, with permission.)

- The sway-back posture (Kendall et al. 1993), shown in Figure 3.5, which is characterised by a forward head posture, slightly extended cervical spine, increased flexion and posterior displacement of the upper trunk, flexion of the lumbar spine, posterior pelvic tilt, hyperextended hip joints with anterior displacement of the pelvis, hyperextended knee joints and neutral ankle joints. This posture is thought to be due to elongated and weak hip flexors, external obliques, upper-back extensors and neck flexors, short and strong hamstrings and upper fibres of the internal oblique abdominal muscles, and strong, but not short, lumbar paraspinal muscles. Individuals with joint hypermobility syndrome (JHS) tend to adopt end-of-range postures such as sway. If initial posture cues combined with subjective markers (see Chapter 2) indicate possible hypermobility,

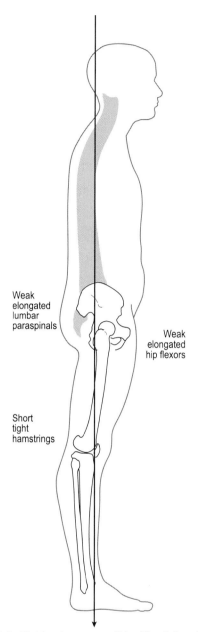

Figure 3.4 • Flat-back posture. (After Kendall et al. 1993 © Williams & Wilkins.)

Weak elongated lumbar paraspinals

Weak elongated hip flexors

Short tight hamstrings

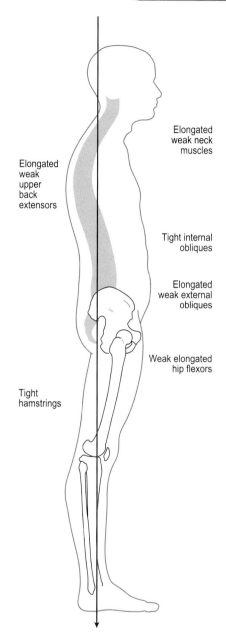

Figure 3.5 • Sway-back posture. (After Kendall et al. 1993 © Williams & Wilkins.)

Elongated weak neck muscles

Elongated weak upper back extensors

Tight internal obliques

Elongated weak external obliques

Weak elongated hip flexors

Tight hamstrings

then the nine-point Beighton score can be applied (Box 3.1). A score of 4 and above is indicative of JHS. Results can be incorporated into validated criteria, called the Brighton criteria; see Box 3.2 (Simmonds & Keer 2007). This genetically inherited disorder results in connective tissue differences and recognition is significant as the

patients may present with associated neural and muscle dysfunction and proprioceptive deficits.

- The handedness posture (Kendall et al. 1993), shown in Figure 3.6, which is characterised, for right-handed individuals, as a low right shoulder, adducted scapulae with the right scapula depressed, a thoracolumbar curve convex to the

Box 3.1

Beighton score (Beighton et al. 1973)

Passive dorsiflexion of little fingers beyond 90°
Passive apposition of the thumbs to the flexor aspects
of the forearm
Hyperextension of the elbows beyond 10°
Hyperextension of the knees beyond 10°
Forward flexion of the trunk with knees straight so that
palms rest easily of the floor.

The Beighton score is a 9-point scale with points awarded for
5 manoeuvres (1 point for each joint). Patients scoring 4 out of
9 or more are considered to have hypermobility syndrome.

Box 3.2

Brighton Criteria (Simmonds & Keer 2007)

Brighton criteria: diagnostic criteria for joint
hypermobility syndrome (JHS; Grahame et al. 2000)

Major criteria

1. A Beighton score of 4/9 or greater (either currently or
   historically)
2. Arthralgia for longer than 3 months in four or more joints

Minor criteria

1. A Beighton score of 1, 2 or 3/9 (0, 1, 2 or 3 if aged 50+)
2. Arthralgia (for 3 months or longer) in 1–3 joints or back
   pain (for 3 months or longer), spondylosis,
   sponylolysis/spondylolisthesis
3. Dislocation/subluxation in more than one joint, or in
   one joint on more than one occasion
4. Soft-tissue rheumatism: three or more lesions (e.g.
   epicondylitis, tenosynovitis, bursitis)
5. Marfanoid habitus (tall, slim, span/height ratio 41.03,
   upper:lower segment ratio less than 0.89,
   arachnodactyly (positive Steinberg/wrist signs)
6. Abnormal skin striae, hyperextensibility, thin skin,
   papyraceous scarring
7. Eye signs: drooping eyelids or myopia or
   antimongoloid slant
8. Varicose veins or hernia or uterine/rectal proplapse

JHS is diagnosed in the presence of *two major criteria* or
one major and *two minor criteria* or *four minor criteria*. Two
minor criteria will suffice where there is an unequivocally
affected first-degree relative. JHS is excluded by the
presence of Marfan or Ehlers–Danlos syndromes (EDS)
other than the EDS hypermobility type (formerly EDS III).

Note: criteria major 1 and minor 1 are mutually exclusive, as are
major 2 and minor 2.

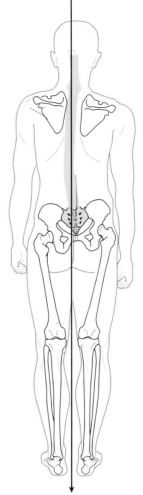

Figure 3.6 • Handedness posture. (After Kendall et al.
1993 © Williams & Wilkins.)

left, lateral pelvic tilt (high on the right), right hip
joint adducted with slight medial rotation, and
the left hip joint abducted with some pronation of
the right foot. It is thought to be due to the
following muscles being elongated and weak: left
lateral trunk muscles, hip abductors on the right,
left hip adductors, right peroneus longus and
brevis, left tibialis posterior, left flexor hallucis
longus and left flexor digitorum longus. The right
tensor fasciae latae may or may not be weak. There
are short and strong right lateral trunk muscles,
left hip abductors, right hip adductors, left
peroneus longus and brevis, right tibialis posterior,
right flexor hallucis longus and right flexor

digitorum longus. The left tensor fasciae latae is usually strong and there may be tightness in the iliotibial band. There is the appearance of a longer right leg.

Other postural presentations may include skin creases at various spinal levels. A common example would be a crease at the mid-cervical spine indicating a focus of movement at that level; this would be followed up later on in the examination with passive accessory intervertebral movement (PAIVM) and passive physiological intervertebral movement (PPIVM), which would uncover hypermobility at this level. Protracted and downward rotation of the scapula with internal rotation of the humerus is another common presentation, with associated reduced length of rhomboids, levator scapulae, pectoralis minor muscles as well as a lack of muscle control of mid-and lower fibres of trapezius and serratus anterior.

Any abnormal asymmetry in posture can be corrected to determine its relevance to the patient's problem. If the symptoms are changed by altering an asymmetrical posture, this suggests that the posture is related to the problem. If the symptoms are not affected then the asymmetrical posture is probably not relevant. Note the resting position of relevant joints as this may be indicative of abnormal length of the muscles (White & Sahrmann 1994).

For further details on examination of posture, readers are referred to Magee (2006), Kendall et al. (1993) and other similar textbooks.

The clinician can also observe the patient in sustained postures and during habitual/repetitive movement where these are relevant to the problem. Sustained postures and habitual movements are thought to have a major role in the development of dysfunction (Sahrmann 2001). A patient with neck pain when sitting, for example, may be observed to have an extended cervical spine and forward head posture as well as holding the pelvis in posterior pelvic tilt (Figure 3.7A). When the clinician

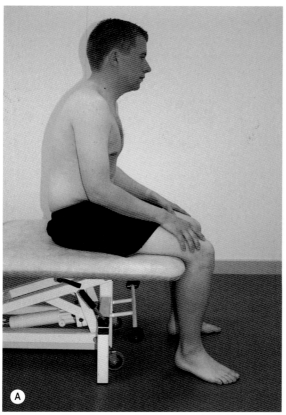 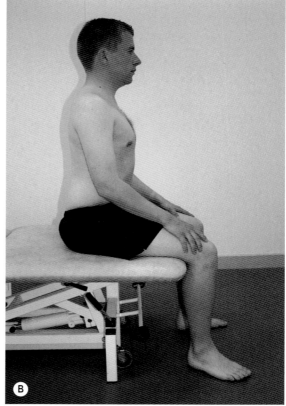

Figure 3.7 • The effect of pelvic tilt on cervical spine posture. A In posterior pelvic tilt the cervical spine is extended with a poking chin. B When the posterior pelvic tilt is reduced, the cervical spine is in a more neutral position.

corrects this posture to determine its relevance to the patient's problem, by guiding the pelvis into anterior pelvic tilt, the forward head posture may be lessened and the neck pain reduced (Figure 3.7B).

An example of habitual movement pattern may be a patient with lumbar spine pain who has pain on bending forwards. The patient may flex predominantly at the lumbar spine or predominantly at the hips (Figure 3.8). If movement mainly occurs at the lumbar spine then this region may be found to be hypermobile (tested by PAIVMs and PPIVMs later on in the examination) and the region where movement is least may be found to be hypomobile.

Observation of muscle form. The clinician observes the patient's muscle shape, bulk and tone, comparing the left and right sides. It must be remembered that handedness type and level and frequency of physical activity may produce differences in muscle bulk between sides.

Muscles produce and control movement, and normal movement is dependent on the strength and flexibility of the agonist and antagonist muscles acting over a joint. These muscles are listed in Table 3.2.

Observation of soft tissues. The local and general soft tissues can be observed, noting the colour and texture of the skin, the presence of scars, abnormal skin creases suggesting an underlying deformity, swelling of the soft tissues or effusion of the joints. Skin colour and texture can indicate the state of the circulation (a bluish tinge suggesting cyanosis or bruising and redness indicating inflammation), the state of the patient's general health, sympathetic changes such as increased sweating, bruising and the presence of other diseases. For example, complex regional pain syndrome (previously called reflex sympathetic dystrophy) may result in shiny skin that has lost its elasticity, excessive hair growth and nails which may become brittle and ridged. Scars may indicate injury or surgery and will be red if recent and white and avascular if old.

Observation of gait. This is often applicable for spinal and lower-limb problems. The clinician

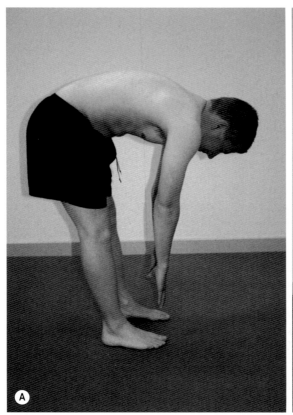 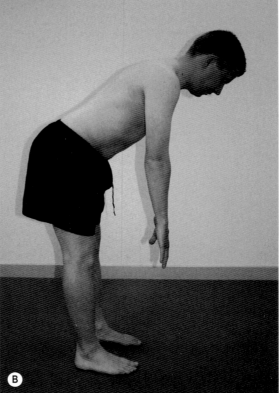

Figure 3.8 • On bending forwards the patient may bend predominantly at the lumbar spine (A) or at the hips (B).

Table 3.2 Reaction of muscles to stress (Jull & Janda 1987; Janda 1994; Comerford & Kinetic Control 2000)

Muscles prone to become tight	Muscles prone to become weak
Masseter, temporalis, digastric and suboccipital muscles, levator scapulae, rhomboid major and minor, upper trapezius, sternocleidomastoid, pectoralis major and minor scalenes, flexors of the upper limb, erector spinae (particularly thoracolumbar and cervical parts), quadratus lumborum, piriformis, tensor fasciae latae, rectus femoris, hamstrings, short hip adductors, tibialis posterior, gastrocnemius	Serratus anterior, middle and lower fibres of trapezius, deep neck flexors, mylohyoid, subscapularis, extensors of upper limb, gluteus maximus, medius and minimus, deep lumbar multifidus, iliopsoas, vastus medialis and lateralis, tibialis anterior and peronei

observes the gait from the front, behind and at the side, looking at the trunk pelvis, hips, knees, ankles and feet through all phases of the gait cycle. A detailed description of the observation can be found in Magee (2006). Common abnormalities of gait include the following:

- An antalgic gait due to pain at the hip, knee or foot is characterised by a shortened stance phase of the affected limb as compared with the non-affected limb.
- An arthrogenic gait, resulting from stiffness or deformity of the hip or knee, is characterised by exaggerated plantarflexion of the opposite ankle and circumduction of the stiff leg to clear the toes.
- A gluteus maximus gait, due to weakness of this muscle, produces a posterior thoracic movement during the stance phase to maintain hip extension.
- Trendelenburg's sign, which is due to weakness of gluteus medius, congenital dislocation of the hip or coxa vara, causes an excessive lateral movement of the thorax towards the affected limb during its stance phase of the gait cycle.
- A short-leg gait produces a lateral shift of the trunk towards the affected side during the stance phase.
- A drop-foot gait, due to weakness of the ankle and foot dorsiflexors, causes the patient to lift the knee higher than the unaffected limb.

Observation of the patient's attitude and feelings. The age, gender and ethnicity of patients and their cultural, occupational and social backgrounds may affect the attitudes and feelings they have towards themselves, their condition and the clinician. Patients may feel apprehensive, fearful, embarrassed, restless, resentful, angry or depressed in relation to their condition and/or the clinician. They may, for example, have had several, possibly conflicting, explanations of their problem. Unrealistic thoughts and beliefs affect patients' response to health problems and treatment (Shorland 1998; Zusman 1998). Clinicians should be aware of, and sensitive to, these attitudes and empathise and communicate appropriately throughout the physical examination. Agreeing treatment goals with the patient will enhance ownership and adherence by the patient.

Joint integrity tests

These are specific tests to determine the stability of the joint and will often be carried out early in the examination, as any instability found will affect, and may contraindicate, further testing. Specific tests are described in the relevant chapters.

Functional ability

Some functional ability may be tested in the observation section, but further testing may be carried out at this stage to examine gait analysis, stair climbing and lifting. There are a number of functional rating scales available for the different joints which will be briefly explored in relevant chapters. Assessment of general function using standardised tests is recommended, as it facilitates objectivity and can be used to evaluate treatment (Harding et al. 1994).

Active physiological movements

Active movements are general tests that affect joints, nerves and muscles. A detailed examination is made of the quality and range of active and passive (described later) physiological movement.

A physiological movement is defined as a movement that can be performed actively – examples include flexion, extension, abduction, adduction and medial and lateral rotation. These movements are examined actively; in other words, the patient produces the movement, which tests the function not only of the joint but also of the muscles that produce the movement and the relevant nerves. If the patient's symptoms allow, i.e. are non-severe, the clinician then applies an overpressure force to the movement to assess further the end of range of that movement. In this situation overpressure could be classified as a passive movement; however, normal convention would include overpressure within active movement testing.

The function of a joint is to allow full-range friction-free movement between the bones. A joint is considered to be normal if there is painless full active range of movement and if the resistance to movement felt by the clinician on applying overpressure is considered to be normal (Maitland et al. 2005). Joint dysfunction is manifested by a reduced (hypomobile) or increased (hypermobile) range of movement, abnormal resistance to movement (through the range or at the end of the range), pain and muscle spasm.

The aims of active physiological movements (Jull 1994) are to:

- reproduce all or part of the patient's symptoms – the movements that produce symptoms are then analysed to determine which structures are being stressed and these are then implicated as a source of the symptoms
- determine the pattern, quality, range, resistance and pain response for each movement
- identify factors that have predisposed to or arisen from the disorder
- obtain signs on which to assess effectiveness of treatment (reassessment 'asterisks' or 'markers').

This part of the examination offers confirmatory evidence (or not) as to the severity and irritability of the condition initially assessed in the subjective examination. The clinician must remain open-minded, as the assessment of severity and irritability needs to be refined at this stage.

The following information can be noted during the movements, and can be depicted on a movement diagram (described later in this chapter):

- the quality of movement
- the range of movement

- the presence of resistance through the range of movement and at the end of the range of movement
- pain behaviour (local and referred) through the range
- the occurrence of muscle spasm during the range of movement.

The procedure for testing active physiological movement is as follows:

- Resting symptoms prior to each movement should be established so that the effect of the movement on the symptoms can be clearly ascertained.
- The active physiological movement is carried out and the quality of this movement is observed, noting the smoothness and control of the movement, any deviation from a normal pattern of movement, the muscle activity involved and the tissue tension produced through range. Movement deviation can then be corrected to determine its relevance to the symptoms. A relevant movement deviation is one where symptoms are altered when it is corrected; if symptoms do not change on movement correction, this suggests that the deviation is not relevant to the patient's problem.
- Both the quality and quantity of movement can be tested further by altering part of the patient's posture during an active movement (White & Sahrmann 1994). For example, cervical movements can be retested with the clinician passively placing the scapula in various positions to determine the effect of length and stretch of the sternocleidomastoid, upper trapezius and levator scapulae.
- An alternative method of testing the quantity of movement in more detail is by palpating the proximal joint as the movement is carried out; for example, palpation of the cervical spinous processes during shoulder elevation may reveal excessive or abnormal spinal movement (White & Sahrmann 1994).
- Active physiological movements test not only the function of joints but also the function of muscles and nerves. This interrelationship is well explained by the movement system balance theory put forward by White & Sahrmann (1994). It suggests that there is an ideal mode of movement system function and that any deviation from this will be less efficient and more stressful to the components of the system.

Ideal movement system function is considered to be dependent on:

- The maintenance of precise movement of rotating parts; in other words, the instantaneous axis of rotation (IAR) follows a normal path. The pivot point about which the vertebrae move constantly changes during physiological movements and its location at any instant is referred to as the IAR. The shape of the joint surfaces and the mobility and length of soft-tissue structures (skin, ligament, tendon, muscle and nerves) are all thought to affect the position of the IAR (Comerford and Mottram 2001). There is some support for this theory, as several studies have found that some pathological conditions have been associated with an altered IAR (Frankel et al. 1971; Pennal et al. 1972; Amevo et al. 1992).

- Normal muscle length. As mentioned earlier, muscles can become shortened or lengthened and this will affect the quality and range of movement.
- Normal motor control, i.e. the precise and coordinated action of muscles.
- Normal relative stiffness of contractile and non-contractile tissue. It is suggested that the body takes the line of least resistance during movement – in other words, movement will occur where resistance is least. Thus, for instance, areas of hypomobility will often be compensated for by movement at other areas, which then become hypermobile. An example of this is seen in patients who have had a spinal fusion that is associated with hypermobility at adjacent segments. In the same way, hypomobility of hip extension may result in compensatory extension in the lumbar spine segments. With time, these movements become 'learned' and the soft tissues around the joint adapt to the new movement patterns such that muscles may become weak and lengthened or tight and shortened.
- Normal kinetics, i.e. the movement system function of joints proximal and distal to the site of the symptoms.

A movement abnormality may therefore be due to several factors (White & Sahrmann 1994):

- a shortened tissue, which may prevent a particular movement
- a muscle that is weak and unable to produce the movement
- a movement 'taken over' by a dominant muscle – this may occur with muscle paralysis, altered muscle length–tension relationship, pain inhibition, repetitive movements or postures leading to learned movement patterns
- pain on movement.

Joint range is measured clinically using a goniometer, tape measure or by visual estimation. Readers are directed to other texts on details of joint measurement (American Academy of Orthopaedic Surgeons 1990; Gerhardt 1992). It is worth mentioning here that range of movement is influenced by a number of factors – age, gender, occupation, date, time of day, temperature, emotional status, effort, medication, injury and disease – and there are wide variations in range of movement between individuals (Gerhardt 1992). The clinician has to determine what is normal for the patient, e.g. by comparing right and left sides.

Pain behaviour (both local and referred) throughout the joint range is recorded. The clinician asks the patient to indicate the point in the range where pain is first felt or is increased (if there is pain present before moving) and then how this pain is affected by further movement. The clinician can ask the patient to rate the intensity of pain as discussed in Chapter 2 and shown in Figure 2.8. The behaviour of the pain through the range can be clearly documented using a movement diagram, which is described later in this chapter.

The eliciting of any muscle spasm through the range of movement is noted. Muscle spasm is an involuntary contraction of muscle as a result of nerve irritation or secondary to injury of underlying structures, such as bone, joint or muscle, and occurs in order to prevent movement and further injury.

Overpressure is applied at the end of a physiological range to explore the extremes of range. Overpressure needs to be applied before declaring a joint range full, normal and ideal. Overpressure needs to be carried out carefully if it is to give accurate information; the following guidelines may help the clinician:

- The patient needs to be comfortable and suitably supported.
- The clinician needs to be in a comfortable position.
- The clinician uses body weight or the upper trunk to produce the force, rather than the intrinsic muscles of the hand, which can be uncomfortable for the patient.
- For accurate direction of the overpressure force, the clinician's forearm is positioned in line with the direction of the force.
- The force is applied slowly and smoothly to the end of the available range.
- At the end of the available range, the clinician can then apply small oscillatory movements to feel the resistance at this position.

There are a variety of ways of applying overpressure; the choice will depend on factors such as the size of the clinician, the size of the patient and the health and age of the patient. The overpressures demonstrated in each of the following chapters are given as examples only; it is the application of the principles that is more important.

While applying overpressure, the clinician will:

- feel the quality of the movement
- note the range of further movement
- feel the resistance through the latter part of the range and at the end of the range
- note the behaviour of pain (local and referred) through the overpressed range of movement
- feel the presence of any muscle spasm through the range.

Some clinicians do not add overpressure if the movement is limited by pain. However, it is argued here that the clinician cannot be certain that the movement is limited by pain unless the clinician applies the overpressure. The other reason why it can be informative to apply overpressure in the presence of pain is that one of three scenarios can occur: the overpressure can cause the pain to ease, to stay the same, or to get worse. This information can help the clinician to understand in more detail the movement and what is limiting it, and may also be helpful in selecting a treatment dose. For example, a rather more provocative movement may be chosen when on overpressure the pain eases or stays the same, compared with when the pain increases. What is vital when applying an overpressure to a movement that appears to be limited by pain is to apply the force extremely slowly and carefully, thereby only minimally increasing the patient's pain.

Normal movement should be painfree, smooth and resistance-free until the later stages of range when resistance will gradually increase until it limits further movement. Less than optimal quality of movement could be demonstrated by the patient's facial expression, e.g. excessive grimacing due to excessive effort or pain, by limb trembling due to muscle weakness or by substitution movements elsewhere due to joint restriction or muscle weakness – for instance, on active hip flexion the clinician may observe lumbar flexion and posterior rotation of the pelvis.

Movement is limited by one or more of a number of factors, such as articular surface contact, limit of ligamentous, muscle or tendon extensibility and apposition of soft tissue, and each of these factors will give a different quality of resistance. For example, wrist flexion and extension are limited by increasing tension in the surrounding ligaments and muscles; knee flexion is limited by soft-tissue apposition of the calf and thigh muscles; and elbow extension is limited by bony apposition. Thus different joints and different movements have different end-feels. The quality of this resistance felt at the end of range has been categorised by Cyriax (1982) and Kaltenborn (2002), as shown in Table 3.3. The resistance is considered abnormal if a joint does not have its characteristic normal end-feel, e.g. when knee flexion has a hard end-feel or if the resistance is felt too early or too late in what is considered normal range of movement. Additionally, Cyriax describes three abnormal end-feels: empty, springy and muscle spasm (Table 3.4).

The pain may increase, decrease or stay the same when overpressure is applied. This is valuable information as it can confirm the severity of the patient's pain and can help to determine the firmness with which manual treatment techniques can be applied.

Further information about the active range of movement can be gained in a number of ways (Box 3.3), as described below.

Combined movements. Combined movements are where movement in one plane is combined with movement in another plane; for example, shoulder abduction with lateral rotation. There are a number

Table 3.3 Normal end-feels (Cyriax 1982; Kaltenborn 2002)

Cyriax	Kaltenborn	Description
Soft-tissue approximation	Soft-tissue approximation or soft-tissue stretch	Soft end-feel, e.g. knee flexion or ankle dorsiflexion
Capsular feel	Firm soft-tissue stretch	Fairly hard halt to movement, e.g. shoulder, elbow or hip rotation due to capsular or ligamentous stretching
Bone to bone	Hard	Abrupt halt to the movement, e.g. elbow extension

Table 3.4 Abnormal end-feels (Cyriax 1982, Kaltenborn 2002). Abnormality is also recognised if a joint does not have its characteristic end-feel or if the resistance is felt too early or too late in what is considered the normal range

Cyriax	Kaltenborn	Description
Empty feel	Empty	No resistance offered due to severe pain secondary to serious pathology such as fractures, active inflammatory processes and neoplasm
Springy block		A rebound feel at end range, e.g. with a torn meniscus blocking knee extension
Spasm		Sudden hard end-feel due to muscle spasm

Box 3.3

Modifications to the examination of active physiological movements

- Repeated movements
- Speed of movement
- Combined movements
- Compression or distraction
- Sustained movements
- Injuring movements
- Differentiation tests
- Functional ability

of reasons why the clinician may choose to combine in this way and these include:

- to gain further information of a movement dysfunction
- to mimic a functional activity
- to increase the stress of the underlying tissues, particularly the joint.

A movement can be added prior to another movement; for example, the glenohumeral joint can be medially rotated prior to flexion. Alternatively, a movement can be added at the end of another movement; for example, the hip can be moved into flexion and then adduction can be added. The effect of altering the sequence of these movements might be expected to alter the symptom response.

Combining spinal movements has been thoroughly explored by Edwards (1999). Similar to the examples above, the lumbar spine can be moved into flexion and then lateral flexion, or it can be moved into lateral flexion and then flexion. Once again, the signs and symptoms will vary according to the order of these movements. A recording of the findings of combined movements for the lumbar spine is illustrated in Figure 3.9, which demonstrates that left rotation, extension and left lateral flexion in extension are limited to half normal range, both symptoms being produced in the left posterior part of the body. Following examination of the active movements and various combined movements, the patient can be categorised into one of three patterns (Edwards 1999):

1. Regular stretch pattern. This occurs when the symptoms are produced on the opposite side from that to which movement is directed. An example of this would be if left-sided cervical spine pain is reproduced on flexion, lateral flexion to the right and rotation to the right, and all other movements are full and painfree. In this case, the patient is said to have a regular stretch pattern. The term 'stretch' is used to describe the general stretch of spinal structures, in this example on the left-hand side of the cervical spine.

2. Regular compression pattern. This occurs when the symptoms are reproduced on the side to which the movement is directed. If left-sided cervical spine pain is reproduced on extension, left lateral flexion and left rotation and all other movements are full and painfree, the patient is said to have a regular compression pattern. The term 'compression' is used to describe the general compression of spinal structures, in this example on the left-hand side of the cervical spine.

3. Irregular pattern. Patients who do not clearly fit into a regular stretch or compression pattern are categorised as having an irregular pattern. In this case, symptoms are provoked by a mixture of stretching and compressing movements.

This information, along with the severity, irritability and nature (SIN) factors, can help to direct treatment. The clinician can position the patient in such a way as to increase or decrease the stretching or compression effect during palpation techniques. For example, accessory movements can be carried out with the spine at the limit of a physiological movement or in a position of maximum comfort.

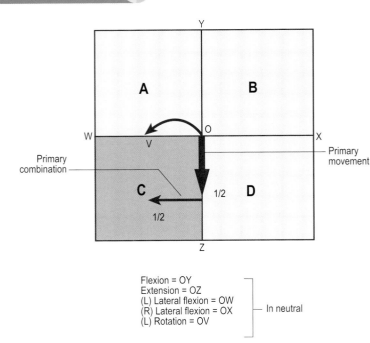

Figure 3.9 • Recording combined movements. Movements can be quickly and easily recorded using this box. It assumes that the clinician is standing behind the patient so that A and B refer to anterior, and C and D to posterior parts of the body; A and C are left side and B and D are right side. The box depicts the following information: left rotation is limited to half range; extension and left lateral flexion in extension range are half normal range. The symptoms are in the left posterior part of the body (represented by the shading). (From Edwards 1992, with permission.)

Flexion = OY
Extension = OZ
(L) Lateral flexion = OW
(R) Lateral flexion = OX
(L) Rotation = OV
— In neutral

To verify further whether the joint is a source of the patient's symptoms, accessory movements may be carried out (see later). The use of combined movements and accessory movements together forms what is sometimes referred to as 'joint clearing tests', referred to in this text as 'screening tests'. Normally, if strong end-of-range combined movements and accessory movements do not reproduce the patient's symptoms and reassessment asterisks remain the same, then the joint is not considered to be a source of the patient's symptoms; hence the joint has been screened. If symptoms are produced or there is reduced range of movement, the joint cannot be considered 'normal' and may need further examination. Suggested combined movements to 'clear' each joint are given in Table 3.5 and generally are the more stressful physiological movements.

Repeated movements. Repeating a movement several times may alter the quality and range of the movement. There may be a gradual increase in range with repeated movements because of the effects of hysteresis on the collagen-containing tissues such as joint capsules, ligaments, muscles and nerves (Gilmore 1986). If a patient with a Colles fracture who has recently come out of plaster was repeatedly to move his or her wrist into flexion, the range of movement would probably increase. Examining repeated movements may demonstrate

muscle fatigue and altered quality of movement. There may be an increase or decrease in symptoms as the movement is repeated.

The change in symptoms with repeated movements of the spine has been more fully described and redefined in McKenzie and May (2003, 2006). All joint problems of the spine are divided into six syndromes: reducible and irreducible derangement, dysfunction, adherent nerve root postural and other.

If movements cause symptoms at the end of range and repeated movements do not significantly alter the symptoms, the condition is classified as a dysfunction syndrome. This syndrome is thought to be caused by shortening of scar tissue such that, when movement puts the shortened tissue on stretch, pain is produced, but is relieved as soon as the stretch is taken off. It will occur whenever there is inadequate mobilisation following trauma or surgery where scar tissue has been laid down during the healing process. Of course, this scenario is commonly seen in the peripheral joints following a period of immobilisation, e.g. after a fracture.

If repeated movements produce phenomena known as peripheralisation and centralisation of symptoms, the condition is classified as a derangement syndrome. Peripheralisation occurs when symptoms arising from the spine and felt laterally from the midline or distally (into arms or legs) are

Table 3.5 Joint clearing tests

Joint	Physiological movement	Accessory movement
Temporomandibular joint	Open/close jaw, side-to-side movement, protraction/retraction	All movements
Cervical spine	Quadrants (flexion and extension)	All movements
Thoracic spine	Rotation and quadrants (flexion and extension)	All movements
Lumbar spine	Flexion and quadrants (flexion and extension)	All movements
Sacroiliac joint	Anterior and posterior gapping	
Shoulder girdle	Elevation, depression, protraction and retraction	
Shoulder joint	Flexion and hand behind back	
Acromioclavicular joint	All movements (particularly horizontal flexion)	
Sternoclavicular joint	All movements	
Elbow joint	All movements	
Wrist joint	Flexion/extension and radial/ulnar deviation	
Thumb	Extension carpometacarpal and thumb opposition	
Fingers	Flexion at interphalangeal joints and grip	
Hip joint	Squat and hip quadrant	
Knee joint	All movements	
Patellofemoral joint	Medial/lateral glide and cephalad/caudad glide	
Ankle joint	Plantarflexion/dorsiflexion and inversion/eversion	

increased or transferred to a more distal position when certain movements are performed. Centralisation occurs when symptoms arising from the spine and felt laterally from the midline or distally (into arms or legs) are reduced or transferred to a more central position when certain movements are performed. A patient with a reducible derangement will exhibit both phenomena – peripheralisation of symptoms on repeating a movement in one direction and centralisation on repeated movement in the opposite direction. For example, a patient may develop leg pain (peripheralisation) on repetitive lumbar spine flexion that eases on repetitive extension (centralisation); similarly, arm pain may be produced on repetitive cervical flexion that eases on repeated extension in irreducible derangement distal symptoms increase with no centralisation. (Figure 3.10).

The exact mechanisms underlying these phenomena are unclear. Repeated movements in the spine alter the position of the nucleus pulposus within the intervertebral disc (Shah et al. 1978) and it is thought that this increases or decreases pressure on pain-sensitive structures. McKenzie (1981, 1990) postulated that the nucleus pulposus may be displaced in any number of directions, and repeated movements have the effect of increasing this displacement. So, for example, it is suggested that if the nucleus pulposus lies anteriorly, then repeated extension would move the nucleus anteriorly and repeated flexion would move the nucleus posteriorly. The commonest nuclear displacement occurs in the posterior direction following, for example, prolonged periods of flexion; repetitive flexion is thought to move the nucleus pulposus even more posteriorly. This increases the pressure on the pain-sensitive structures around the posterior aspect of the intervertebral disc and is thought to cause referral of pain into the leg (peripheralisation). Repeated extension then causes the nucleus to move anteriorly and thus relieves the pressure on the pain-sensitive structures and eases

Peripheralisation

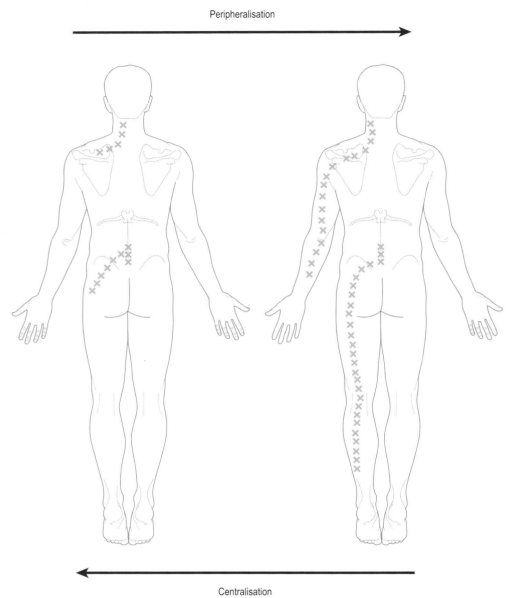

Centralisation

Figure 3.10 • Peripheralisation and centralisation phenomena.

the leg pain (centralisation). Research on the cervical intervertebral disc (Mercer & Jull 1996) details the mechanism by which repetitive movements alter the patient's pain remains unclear.

Speed of the movement. Movements can be carried out at different speeds, and symptoms are noted. Increasing the speed of movement may be necessary in order to replicate the patient's functional restriction and reproduce the patient's symptoms. For example, a footballer with knee pain may only feel symptoms when running fast and symptoms may only be reproduced with quick movements of the knee, and possibly only when weight-bearing. One of the reasons why the speed of the movement

can alter symptoms is because the rate of loading of viscoelastic tissues affects their extensibility and stiffness (Noyes et al. 1974).

Compression or distraction. Compression or distraction of the joint articular surfaces can be added during the movement. For example, compression or distraction of the shoulder joint can be applied with passive shoulder flexion. If the lesion is intra-articular then the symptoms are often made worse by compression and eased by distraction (Maitland 1985; Maitland et al. 2001).

Sustained movements. A movement is held at end of range or at a point in range and the effects on symptoms are noted. In this position, tissue creep will occur, whereby the soft-tissue structures that are being stretched lengthen (Kazarian 1972). Range of movement would therefore increase in normal tissue. This may be very valuable in assessing patients who have reported that their symptoms are aggravated by sustained postures.

Injuring movement. The movement carried out at the time of injury can be tested. This may be necessary when symptoms have not been reproduced by the previous movements described above or if the patient has momentary symptoms.

Differentiation tests. These tests are useful to distinguish between two structures suspected to be a source of the symptoms (Maitland et al. 2001, 2005). A position that provokes symptoms is held constant and then a movement that increases or decreases the stress on one of the structures is added and the effect on symptoms is noted. For example, in the straight-leg raise test, hip flexion with knee extension is held constant, which creates tension on the sciatic nerve and the hip extensor muscles (particularly hamstrings), and cervical flexion is then added. This increases the tension of the sciatic nerve without altering the length of the hip extensors.

This can help to differentiate symptoms originating from neural tissue from those of other structures around the lumbar spine.

Capsular pattern. In arthritic joint conditions affecting the capsule of the joint, the range of movement can become restricted in various directions and to different degrees. Each joint has a typical pattern of restricted movement (Table 3.6) and, because the joint capsule is involved, the phenomenon is known as a capsular pattern (Cyriax 1982). Where the capsular pattern involves a number of movements, these are listed in descending order of limitation; for instance, lateral rotation is the most limited range in the shoulder capsular pattern, followed by abduction and then medial rotation.

Passive physiological movements

A comparison of the response of symptoms to the active and passive movements can help to determine whether the structure at fault is non-contractile (articular) or contractile (extra-articular) (Cyriax 1982). If the lesion is of non-contractile tissue, such as ligamentous tissue, then active and passive movements will be painful and/or restricted in the same direction. For instance, if the anterior joint capsule of the proximal interphalangeal joint of the index finger is shortened, there will be pain and/or restriction of finger extension, whether this movement is carried out actively or passively. If the lesion is in a contractile tissue (i.e. muscle) then active and passive movements are painful and/or restricted in opposite directions. For example, a muscle lesion in the anterior fibres of deltoid will be painful on active flexion of the shoulder joint and on passive extension of the shoulder.

The range of active physiological movements of the spine is the accumulated movement at a number of vertebral segments and is thus a rather crude measure of range that does not in any way localise which segment is affected. For this reason, PPIVMs are carried out to determine the range of movement at each intervertebral level. To do this, the clinician feels the movement of adjacent spinous processes, articular pillars or transverse processes during physiological movements. A brief reminder of how to perform the technique is given in each relevant chapter and a full description can be found in Maitland et al. (2001). A quick and easy method of recording PPIVMs is shown in Figure 3.11. This method can also be used for a range of active movements.

Muscle tests

In the last 15 years or so there has been considerable interest in muscle examination, assessment and treatment (Janda 1986; Jull & Janda 1987; Jull & Richardson 1994; White & Sahrmann 1994; Hodges 1995; Hides et al. 1996; Hodges & Richardson 1996; Sahrmann 2001; Richardson et al. 2004).

Muscle function in relation to the lumbar spine was classified by Bergmark (1989) into local and global systems. This classification system was further refined by Comerford & Mottram (2001), who expanded the system under three broad headings: local stabiliser, global stabiliser and global mobiliser. Generally speaking, the local stabiliser muscles maintain a low, continuous activation in all joint positions

Table 3.6 Capsular patterns (Cyriax 1982). Movements are listed in descending order of limitation

Joint	Movement restriction
Temporomandibular joint	Opening mouth
Cervical spine	Side flexion and rotation are equally limited; flexion is full but painful, and extension is limited
Thoracic and lumbar spine	Difficult to detect capsular pattern
Sacroiliac, pubic symphysis and sacrococcygeal joints	Pain when the joint is stressed
Sternoclavicular and acromioclavicular joints	Pain at extremes of range
Shoulder joint	Lateral rotation then abduction then medial rotation
Elbow joint	More limitation of flexion than extension
Inferior radioulnar joint	Full range but pain at extremes of range
Wrist joint	Flexion and extension equally limited
Carpometacarpal joint of the thumb	Full flexion, limited abduction and extension
Thumb and finger joints	More limitation of flexion than extension
Hip joint	Medial rotation, extension, abduction, flexion, then lateral rotation
Knee joint	Gross limitation of flexion with slight limitation of extension Rotation full and painless in early stages
Tibiofibular joints	Pain when the joint is stressed
Ankle joint	More limitation of plantarflexion than dorsiflexion
Talocalcaneal joint	Limitation of inversion
Midtarsal joint	Limitation of dorsiflexion, plantarflexion, adduction and medial rotation; abduction and lateral rotation are full range
Metatarsophalangeal joint of the big toe	More limitation of extension than flexion
Metatarsophalangeal joint of the other four toes	Variable; tend to fix in extension with interphalangeal joints flexed

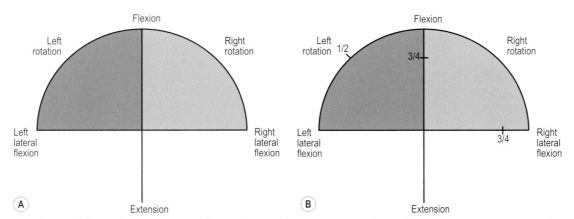

Figure 3.11 • A Recording passive physiological intervertebral movements (PPIVMs). B Example of a completed PPIVM recording for a segmental level. Interpretation: there is three-quarters range of flexion and right lateral flexion and one-half range of left rotation. There is no restriction of extension.

regardless of the direction of joint motion and tend to become inhibited when dysfunctional; examples include vastus medialis oblique, the deep neck flexors and transversus abdominis. The global stabilisers become activated on specific directions of joint movement, particularly eccentric control and rotation movement, and when dysfunctional tend to become long and weak; examples include gluteus medius, superficial multifidus and internal and external obliques. The global mobilisers are activated to produce specific directions of joint movement, particularly concentric movement, and when dysfunctional tend to become short and overactive; examples include rectus abdominis, hamstrings and levator scapulae. Further characteristics of each classification are given in Table 3.7. Normal muscle function requires normal muscle strength, length and coordination. A muscle does not function in isolation – it is also

Table 3.7 Classification of muscle function (Comerford & Kinetic Control 2000)

Local stabiliser	Global stabiliser	Global mobiliser
Examples		
Transversus abdominis	Internal and external obliques	Rectus abdominis
Deep lumbar multifidus	Superficial multifidus	Iliocostalis
Psoas major (posterior fasciculi)	Spinalis	Hamstrings
Vastus medialis oblique	Gluteus medius	Latissimus dorsi
Middle and lower trapezius	Serratus anterior	Levator scapulae
Deep cervical flexors	Longus colli (oblique fibres)	Scalenus anterior, medius and posterior
Function and characteristics		
Increases muscle stiffness to control segmental movement	Generates force to control range of movement	Generates torque to produce movement
Controls the neutral joint position. Contraction does not produce change in length and so does not produce movement. Proprioceptive function: information on joint position, range and rate of movement	Controls particularly the inner and outer ranges of movement. Tends to contract eccentrically for low-load deceleration of momentum and for rotational control	Produces joint movement, especially movements in the sagittal plane. Tends to contract concentrically. Absorbs shock
Activity is independent of direction of movement	Activity is direction-dependent	Activity is direction-dependent
Continuous activation throughout movement	Non-continuous activity	Non-continuous activity
Dysfunction		
Reduced muscle stiffness, loss of joint neutral position (segmental control). Delayed timing and recruitment	Poor control of inner and outer ranges of movement, poor eccentric control and rotation dissociation. Inner- and outer-range weakness of muscle	Muscle spasm. Loss of muscle length (shortened), limiting accessory and/or physiological range of movement
Becomes inhibited	Reduced low-threshold tonic recruitment	Overactive low-threshold, low-load recruitment
Local inhibition	**Global imbalance**	**Global imbalance**
Loss of segmental control	Increased length and inhibited stabilising muscles result in underpull at a motion segment	Shortened and overactive mobilising muscles result in overpull at a motion segment

dependent on the normality of its antagonist muscle as well as other local and distant muscle groups. The effect of muscle dysfunction can therefore be widespread throughout the neuromusculoskeletal system.

There is a close functional relationship between agonist and antagonist muscles. Muscle activation is associated with inhibition of its antagonist, so that overactivation of a muscle group, as occurs in muscle spasm, will be associated with inhibition of the antagonist group, which may then become weak. This situation produces what is known as muscle imbalance, i.e. a disruption of the coordinated interplay of muscles. Muscle imbalance can occur where a muscle becomes shortened and alters the position of the joint in such a way that the antagonist muscle is elongated and then becomes weak. Another example is where there is reflex inhibition of muscle and weakness in the presence of pain and/or injury, such as is seen with patellofemoral joint pain (Mariani & Caruso 1979; Voight & Wieder 1991) and low-back pain (Hodges 1995; Hides et al. 1996). Muscle testing therefore involves examination of the strength and length of both agonist and antagonist muscle groups.

The following tests are commonly used to assess muscle function: muscle strength, muscle control, muscle length, isometric muscle testing and some other muscle tests.

Muscle strength

This is usually tested manually with an isotonic contraction through the available range of movement and graded according to the Medical Research Council (MRC) scale (Medical Research Council 1976)

Table 3.8 Grades of muscle strength (Medical Research Council 1976)

Grade	Muscle activity
0	No contraction
1	Flicker or trace of contraction
2	Active movement, with gravity eliminated
3	Active movement against gravity
4	Active movement against gravity and resistance
5	Normal strength

Medical Research Council 1976 Aids to the investigation of peripheral nerve injuries. HMSO, London. Reproduced with kind permission of the Medical Research Council.

shown in Table 3.8. Groups of muscles are tested, as well as more specific testing of individual muscles. The strength of a muscle contraction will depend on the age, gender, build and usual level of physical activity of the patient. Details of these tests can be found in various texts, including Cole et al. (1988), Kendall et al. (1993) and Hislop & Montgomery (1995).

Some muscles are thought to be prone to inhibition and weakness and are shown in Table 3.2 (Jull & Janda 1987; Janda 1994, 2002; Comerford & Mottram 2001). They are characterised by hypotonia, decreased strength and delayed activation, with atrophy over a prolonged period of time (Janda 1993). While the mechanism behind this process is still unclear, it seems reasonable to suggest that the strength of these muscles in particular needs to be examined. White & Sahrmann (1994) suggest that the postural muscles tend to lengthen as a result of poor posture and that this occurs because the muscle rests in an elongated position. The muscles then appear weak when tested in a shortened position, although their peak tension in outer range is actually larger than the peak tension generated by a 'normal-length' muscle (Figure 3.12) (Gossman et al. 1982). Crawford (1973) found that the peak tension of the lengthened muscle in outer range may be 35% greater than normal muscle. In addition, muscles that lose their length will, over a period of time, become weak. Methods of testing the strength of individual muscles

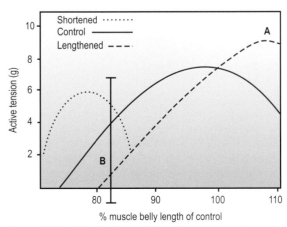

Figure 3.12 • Effects of muscle length on muscle strength. The normal length–tension curve (control) moves to the right for a lengthened muscle, giving it a peak tension some 35% greater than the control (point A). When tested in an inner-range position, however (point B), the muscle tests weaker than normal. (From Norris 1995, with permission.)

are outlined in Figure 3.13. The patient is asked to move against the resistance applied by the clinician.

Muscle control

Muscle control is tested by observing the recruitment and coordination of muscles during active movements. Some of these movements will have already been carried out (under joint tests) but there are other specific tests, which will be carried out here. The relative strength, endurance and control of muscles are considered to be more important than the overall strength of a muscle or muscle group (Jull & Janda 1987; Janda 1994, 2002; Jull & Richardson 1994; White & Sahrmann 1994; Sahrmann 2001). Relative strength is assessed by observing the pattern of muscle recruitment and the quality of movement and by palpating muscle activity in various positions. It should be noted that this relies on the observational skills of the clinician. A common term within the concept of muscle control is recruitment (or activation), which refers to timed onset of muscle activity. For a more indepth description of this concept the reader is directed to Sahrmann (2001).

Muscle length

Muscle length may be tested, in particular for those muscles that tend to become tight and thus lose their extensibility (Jull & Janda 1987; Janda 1994, 2002; Comerford & Mottram 2001) (Table 3.2). These muscles are characterised by hypertonia, increased strength and quickened activation time (Janda 1993). Methods of testing the length of individual muscles are outlined in Figure 3.14.

There are two important comments to make regarding muscle length tests. Firstly, while these tests are described according to individual muscles, it is clear that a number of muscles will be tested simultaneously. This awareness is important when interpreting a test: it cannot be assumed when testing upper trapezius muscle that it is this muscle and no other muscle that is reduced in length; for example, levator scapulae and scalene muscles may also be contributing to the reduced movement. Secondly, Figure 3.14 shows minimum muscle length test; further testing may often be appropriate for patients. For example, to test the length of the hamstring muscles fully, the clinician may investigate a number of different components such as hip flexion with some adduction/abduction and/or with some medial/lateral rotation. Similarly, for levator

scapulae, the clinician may examine varying degrees of cervical flexion, contralateral lateral flexion and contralateral rotation as well as varying the order of the movements. For further information on fully investigating muscle length tests, see Hunter (1998).

Muscle length is tested by the clinician stabilising one end of the muscle and slowly and smoothly moving the body part to stretch the muscle. The following information is noted:

- the quality of movement
- the range of movement
- the presence of resistance through the range of movement and at the end of the range of movement: the quality of the resistance may identify whether muscle, joint or neural tissues are limiting the movement
- pain behaviour (local and referred) through the range.

Reduced muscle length, i.e. muscle shortness or tightness, occurs when the muscle cannot be stretched to its normal length. This state may occur with overuse, which causes the muscle initially to become short and strong but later, over a period of time, to become weak (because of reduced nutrition). This state is known as stretch weakness (Janda 1993).

Isometric muscle testing

This may help to differentiate symptoms arising from inert rather than contractile tissues. The joint is put into a resting position (so that the inert structures are relaxed) and the patient is asked to hold this position against the resistance of the clinician. The clinician observes the quality of the muscle contraction to hold this position. If symptoms are reproduced on contraction, this suggests that symptoms may be coming from the muscle. However it must be appreciated that there will be some shearing and compression of the inert structures, so the test is not always conclusive. The patient may, for example, be unable to prevent the joint from moving or may hold with excessive muscle activity; either of these circumstances would suggest neuromuscular dysfunction. For a more thorough examination of muscle function the patient is asked to hold position in various parts of the physiological range.

Cyriax (1982) describes six possible responses to isometric muscle testing:

1. strong and painless – normal
2. strong and painful – suggests minor lesion of muscle or tendon, e.g. lateral epicondylalgia

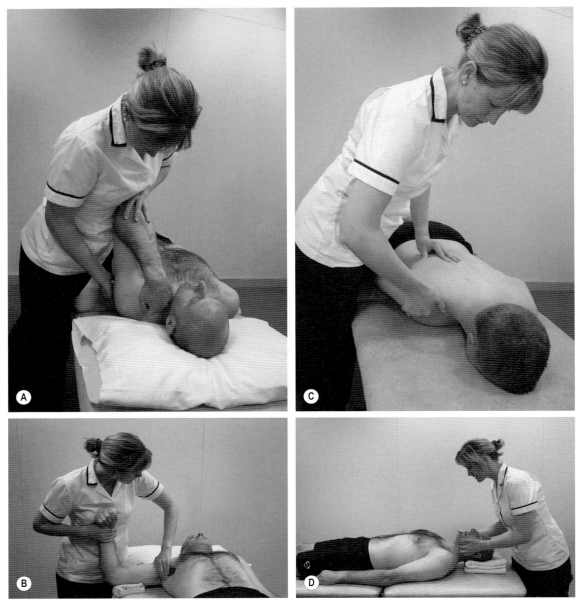

Figure 3.13 • Testing the strength of individual muscles prone to become weak (Cole et al. 1988; Janda 1994; Jull & Janda 1987). **A** Serratus anterior. The patient lies supine with the shoulder flexed to 90° and the elbow in full flexion. Resistance is applied to shoulder girdle protraction. **B** Subscapularis. In supine with the shoulder in 90° abduction and the elbow flexed to 90°. A towel is placed underneath the upper arm so that the humerus is in the scapular plane. The clinician gently resists medial rotation of the upper arm. The subscapularis tendon can be palpated in the axilla, just anterior to the posterior border. There should be no scapular movement or alteration in the abduction position. **C** Lower fibres of trapezius. In prone lying with the arm by the side and the glenohumeral joint placed in medial rotation, the clinician passively moves the coracoid process away from the plinth such that the head of the humerus and body of scapula lie horizontal. Poor recruitment of lower fibres of trapezius would be suspected from an inability to hold this position without substitution by other muscles such as levator scapulae, rhomboid major and minor or latissimus dorsi. **D** Deep cervical flexors. The patient lies supine with the cervical spine in a neutral position and is asked to tuck the chin in. If there is poor recruitment the sternocleidomastoid initiates the movement.

(Continued)

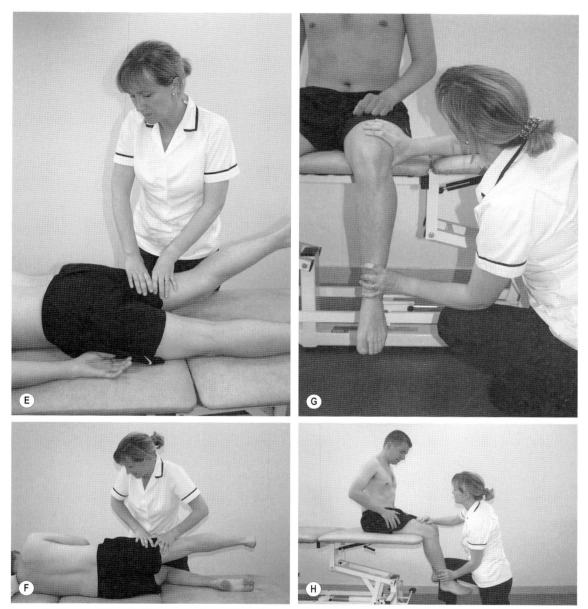

Figure 3.13—cont'd • E Gluteus maximus. The clinician resists hip extension. A normal pattern would be hamstring and gluteus maximus acting as prime movers and the erector spinae stabilising the lumbar spine and pelvis. Contraction of gluteus maximus is delayed when it is weak. Alternatively, the therapist can passively extend the hip into an inner-range position and ask the patient to hold this position isometrically (Jull & Richardson 1994). F Posterior gluteus medius. The patient is asked to abduct the uppermost leg actively. Resistance can be added by the clinician. Lateral rotation of the hip may indicate excessive activity of tensor fasciae latae, and using hip flexors to produce the movement may indicate a weakness in the lateral pelvic muscles. Other substitution movements include lateral flexion of the trunk or backward rotation of the pelvis. Inner-range weakness is tested by passively abducting the hip; if the range is greater than the active abduction movement, this indicates inner-range weakness. G Gluteus minimus. The clinician resists medial rotation of the hip. H Vastus lateralis, medialis and intermedius. The clinician resists knee extension.

(Continued)

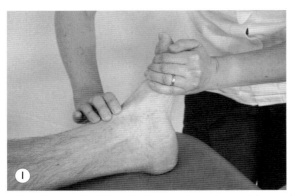
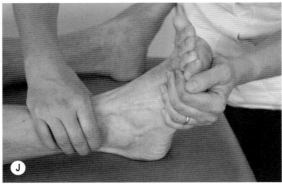

Figure 3.13—cont'd • I Tibialis anterior. The clinician resists ankle dorsiflexion and inversion. J Peroneus longus and brevis. The clinician resists ankle eversion.

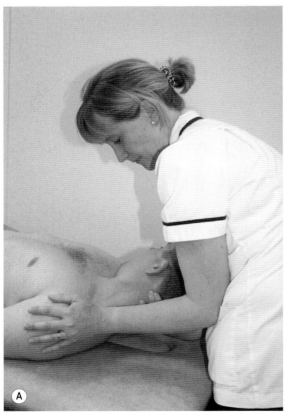
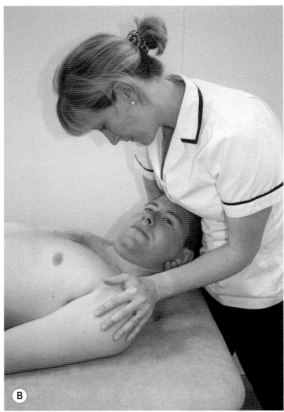

Figure 3.14 • Testing the length of individual muscles prone to becoming short (Jull & Janda 1987; Cole et al. 1988; Kendall et al. 1993; Janda 1994). **A** Levator scapulae. A passive stretch is applied by contralateral lateral flexion and rotation with flexion of the neck and shoulder girdle depression. Restricted range of movement and tenderness on palpation over the insertion of levator scapulae indicate tightness of the muscle. **B** Upper trapezius. A passive stretch is applied by passive contralateral lateral flexion, ipsilateral rotation and flexion of the neck with shoulder girdle depression. Restricted range of movement indicates tightness of the muscle.

(Continued)

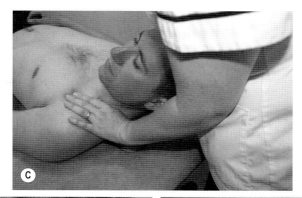

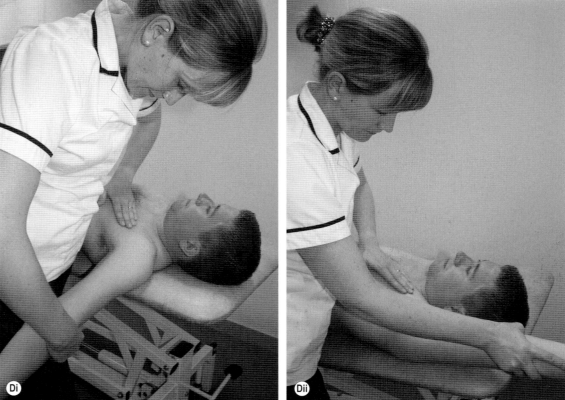

Figure 3.14—cont'd • C Sternocleidomastoid. The clinician tucks the chin in and then laterally flexes the head away and rotates towards the side of testing. The clavicle is stabilised with the other hand. **D** Pectoralis major. (i) Clavicular fibres – the clinician stabilises the trunk and abducts the shoulder to 90°. Passive overpressure of horizontal extension will be limited in range and the tendon becomes taut if there is tightness of this muscle. (ii) Sternocostal fibres – the clinician elevates the shoulder fully. Restricted range of movement and the tendon becoming taut indicate tightness of this muscle.

(Continued)

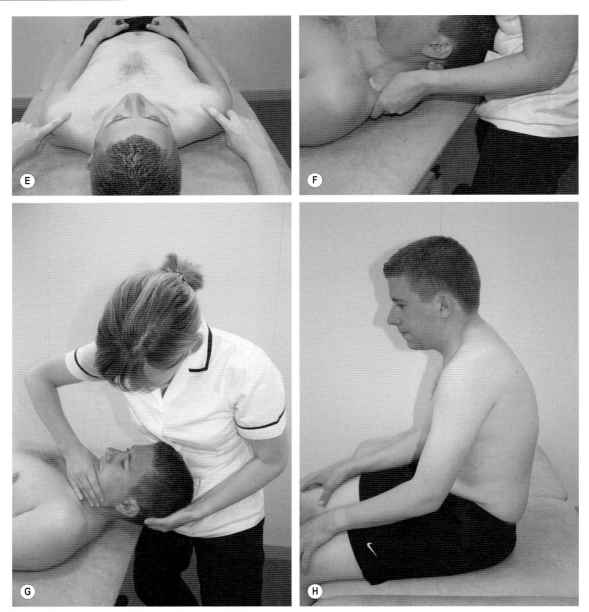

Figure 3.14—cont'd • E Pectoralis minor. With the patient in supine and arm by the side, the coracoid is found to be pulled anteriorly and inferiorly if there is a contracture of this muscle. In addition, the posterior edge of the acromion may rest further from the plinth on the affected side. F Scalenes. Fixing first and second ribs, the clinician laterally flexes the patient's head away and rotates towards the side of testing for anterior scalene; contralateral lateral flexion tests the middle fibres; contralateral rotation and lateral flexion test the posterior scalene muscle. G Deep occipital muscles. The right hand passively flexes the upper cervical spine while palpating the deep occipital muscles with the left hand. Tightness on palpation indicates tightness of these muscles. H Erector spinae. The patient slumps the shoulders towards the groin. Lack of flattening of the lumbar lordosis may indicate tightness (Lewit 1991).

(Continued)

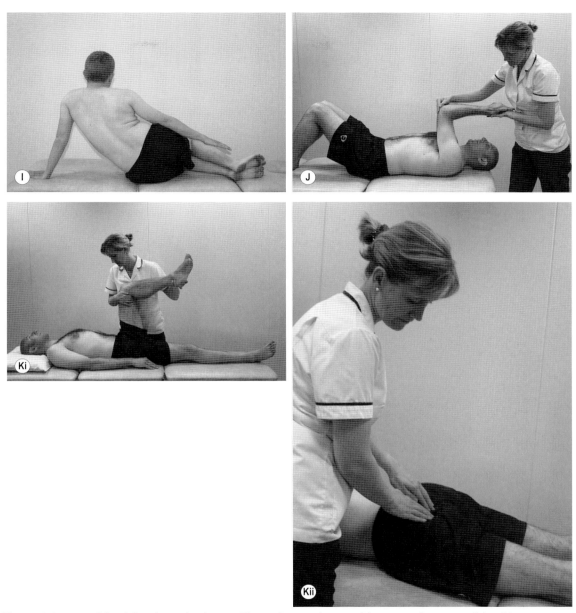

Figure 3.14—cont'd • I Quadratus lumborum. The patient pushes up sideways as far as possible without movement of the pelvis. Limited range of movement, lack of curvature in the lumbar spine and/or abnormal tension on palpation (just above the iliac crest and lateral to erector spinae) indicate tightness of the muscle. **J** Latissimus dorsi. With the patient in crook-lying with the lumbar spine flat against the plinth and the glenohumeral joints laterally rotated, the patient is asked to elevate the arms through flexion. Shortness of latissimus dorsi is evidenced by an inability to maintain the lumbar spine in against the plinth and/or inability to elevate the arms fully. **K** Piriformis. (i) The clinician passively flexes the hip to 90°, adducts it and then adds lateral rotation to the hip, feeling the resistance to the limit of the movement. There should be around 45° of lateral rotation. (ii) Piriformis can be palpated if it is tight by applying deep pressure at the point at which an imaginary line between the iliac crest and ischial tuberosity crosses a line between the posterior superior iliac spine and the greater trochanter.

(Continued)

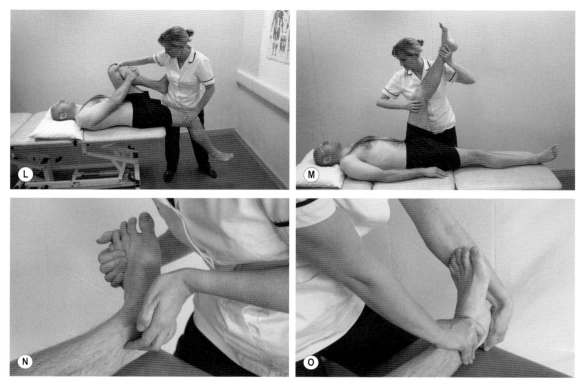

Figure 3.14—cont'd • L Iliopsoas, rectus femoris and tensor fasciae latae. The left leg is stabilised against the clinician's side. The free leg will be flexed at the hip if there is tightness of iliopsoas. An extended knee indicates tight rectus femoris. Abduction of the hip, lateral deviation of the patella and a well-defined groove on the lateral aspect of the thigh indicate tight tensor fasciae latae and iliotibial band. Overpressure to each of these movements, including hip abduction for the short adductors, will confirm any tightness of these muscles. M Hamstrings. With the patient lying supine, the clinician passively flexes the hip to 90° and then the knee is passively extended. N Tibialis posterior. The clinician dorsiflexes the ankle joint and everts the forefoot. Limited range of movement indicates tightness of the muscle. O Gastrocnemius and soleus. Gastrocnemius length can be tested by the range of ankle dorsiflexion with the knee extended and then flexed. If the range increases when the knee is flexed, this indicates tightness of gastrocnemius.

3. weak and painless – complete rupture of muscle or tendon or disorder of the nervous system
4. weak and painful – suggests gross lesion, e.g. fracture of patella
5. all movements painful – suggests emotional hypersensitivity
6. painful on repetition – suggests intermittent claudication.

Other muscle tests

For years clinicians have measured, with a tape measure, the circumference of the muscle bulk at a measured distance from a bony point and compared left and right sides. This test attempts to measure the size of a muscle in order to measure its strength.

There are a number of difficulties with this method. Firstly, it is not a pure measure of muscle size since it includes the subcutaneous fat (Stokes & Young 1986). Secondly, it assumes that the muscle fibres are running at right angles to the limb (so that the physiological cross-sectional area is being measured), but this is not the case for most muscles, which have a pennate structure (Newham 2001). Thirdly, there is no relationship between limb girth and muscle girth: a 22–33% reduction in the cross-sectional area of the quadriceps (measured by ultrasound scanning) may cause only a 5% reduction in the circumference of the limb using a tape measure (Young et al. 1982).

Specific regional muscle tests will be covered in relevant chapters.

Neurological tests

Neurological examination includes neurological integrity testing (the ability of the nervous system to conduct an action potential), neurodynamic tests (the ability of the nervous system to move) and the sensitivity of the nerves to palpation.

Integrity of the nervous system

The effects of compression of the peripheral nervous system are:

- reduced sensory input
- reduced motor impulses along the nerve
- reflex changes
- pain, usually in the myotome or dermatome distribution
- autonomic disturbance such as hyperaesthesia, paraesthesia or altered vasomotor tone.

Reduced sensory input

Sensory changes are due to compression or lesion of the sensory nerves anywhere from terminal branches in the receptor organ, e.g. joints, skin, to the spinal nerve root. Figure 3.15 serves to illustrate this. Knowledge of the cutaneous distribution of nerve roots (dermatomes) and peripheral nerves enables the clinician to distinguish the sensory loss due to a root lesion from that due to a peripheral nerve lesion. The cutaneous nerve distribution and dermatome areas are shown in Figures 3.16–3.19. It must be remembered, however, that there is a great deal of variability from person to person and an overlap between the cutaneous supply of peripheral nerves (Walton 1989) and dermatome areas (Hockaday & Whitty 1967). A sclerotome is the region of bone supplied by one nerve root; the areas are shown in Figure 3.20 (Inman & Saunders 1944; Grieve 1981).

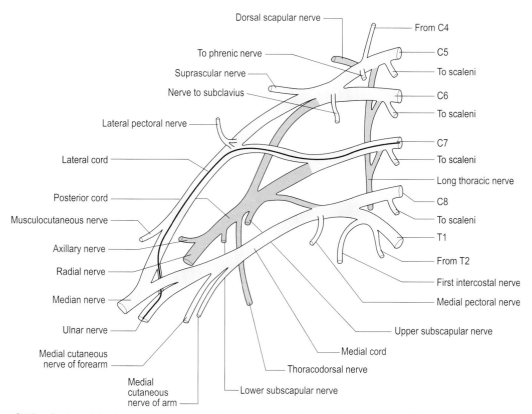

Figure 3.15 • A plan of the brachial plexus showing the nerve roots and the formation of the peripheral nerves. (From Williams et al. 1995, with permission.)

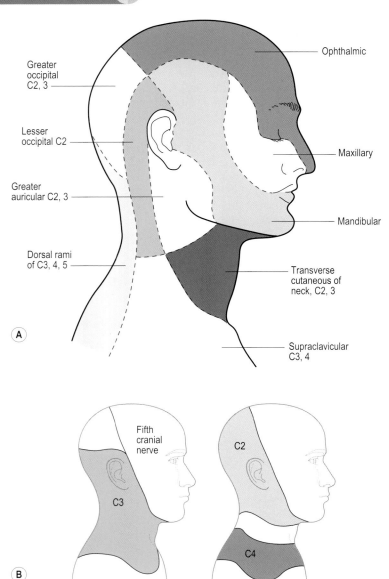

Figure 3.16 • A Cutaneous nerve supply to the face, head and neck. (From Williams et al. 1995, with permission.) **B** Dermatomes of the head and neck. (From Grieve 1981, with permission.)

Reduced motor impulses along the nerve

A loss of muscle strength is indicative of either a lesion of the motor nerve supply to the muscle(s) – located anywhere from the spinal cord to its terminal branches in the muscle – or a lesion of the muscle itself. If the lesion occurs at nerve root level then all the muscles supplied by the nerve root (the myotome) will be affected. If the lesion occurs in a peripheral nerve then the muscles that it supplies will be affected. A working knowledge of the muscular distribution of nerve roots

(myotomes) and peripheral nerves enables the clinician to distinguish the motor loss due to a root lesion from that due to a peripheral nerve lesion. The peripheral nerve distribution and myotomes are shown in Table 3.9 and Figures 3.21–3.23. It should be noted that most muscles in the limbs are innervated by more than one nerve root (myotome) and that the predominant segmental origin is given.

Over a period of time of motor nerve impairment there will be muscle atrophy and weakness, as is seen for example in the thenar eminence in carpal tunnel syndrome (median nerve entrapment).

Reflex changes

The deep tendon reflexes test the integrity of the spinal reflex arc consisting of an afferent or sensory neurone and an efferent or motor neurone. The reflexes test individual nerve roots, as shown in Table 3.9.

Procedure for examining the integrity of the nervous system. In order to examine the integrity of the peripheral nerves, three tests are carried out: skin sensation, muscle strength and deep tendon reflexes.

If a nerve root lesion is suspected, the tests carried out are referred to as dermatomal (area of skin supplied by one nerve root), myotomal (group of muscles supplied by one nerve root) and reflexal.

Testing sensation

There are five aspects of sensation that can be examined:

1. light touch
2. vibration: tests posterior-column large-diameter fibre patency
3. joint position sense
4. pinprick: tests spinothalamic small diameter
5. temperature fibre patency (Fuller 2004).

Loss of light touch is usually examined first. It is important that any diminished skin sensation is identified accurately and sensitively by the clinician. Cotton wool is often used to test the ability to feel light touch. The clinician strokes an unaffected area of the skin first so that the patient knows what to expect.

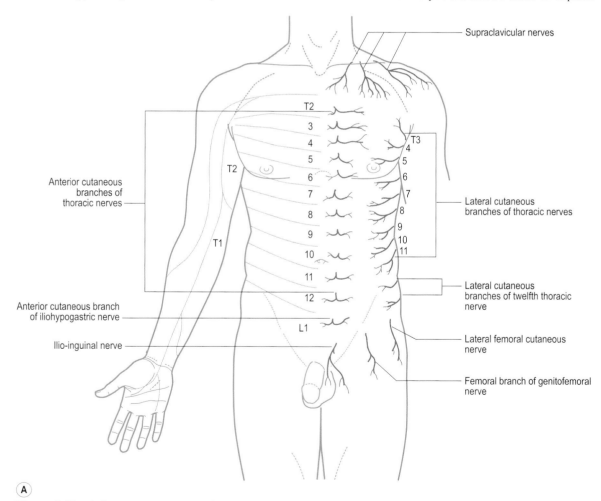

Figure 3.17 • A Cutaneous nerve supply to the trunk. (From Williams et al. 1995, with permission.)

(Continued)

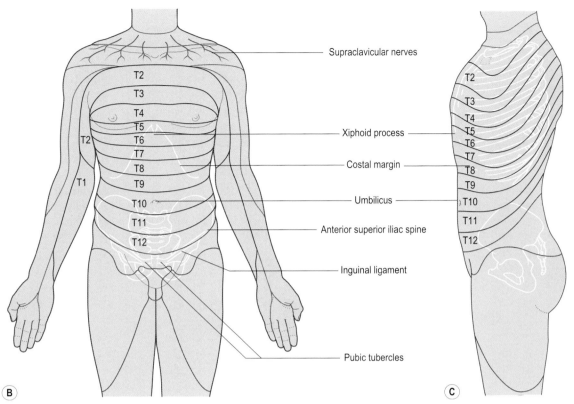

Figure 3.17—cont'd • B Anterior view of thoracic dermatomes associated with thoracic spinal nerves. C Lateral view of dermatomes associated with thoracic spinal nerves. (From Drake et al. 2005.)

The clinician then lightly strokes across the skin of the area being assessed and the patient is asked whether it feels the same as or different from the other side. An alternative and more standardised method of assessment of light touch to deep pressure is to use monofilaments (Semmes–Weinstein or West). Each monofilament relates to a degree of pressure, is repeatable and scales from loss of protective sensation through diminished light touch to normal sensation (Hunter 2002).

The clinician needs to identify and map out accurately the area of diminished sensation. The next step may be to explore further the area of diminished sensation, by testing pinprick (the ability to feel pain), vibration sensation, hot/cold sensation, joint position sense (proprioception) and stereognosis (in the hand). Vibration sense can be tested using a 128-Hz (some researchers advocate 256-Hz) tuning fork. With the patient's eyes closed the clinician strikes the fork before placing the flat end of the tuning fork on a bony prominence, e.g. medial malleolus. The patient is asked to confirm when s/he feels vibration (Leak 1998; Fuller 2004).

Areas of sensory abnormality should be documented on the body chart. Mapping out an area needs to be accurate, as a change, particularly an increase in the area, indicates a worsening neurological state and may require the patient to be referred to a medical practitioner; for example, progressive signs due to a prolapsed intervertebral disc pressing on the spinal cord or cauda equina may require immediate surgery. For this reason, sensation is often reassessed at each appointment, until it is established that the diminished sensation is stable.

Testing muscle strength

Muscle strength testing consists of carrying out an isometric contraction of a muscle group over a few seconds. The muscle is placed in mid-position and the patient is asked to hold the position against the resistance of the clinician. The resistance is applied slowly and smoothly to enable the patient to give the necessary resistance, and the amount of force applied must be appropriate to the specific muscle group and to the patient. Myotome testing is shown in Figures 3.24 and 3.25.

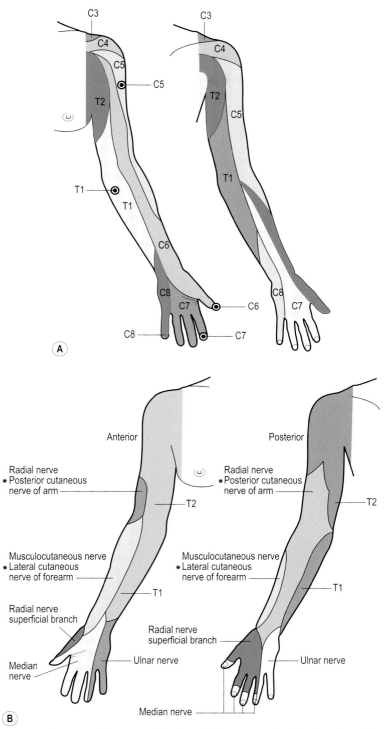

Figure 3.18 • Dermatomes and nerves of the upper limb. Dots indicate areas of minimal overlap. (From Drake et al. 2005.)

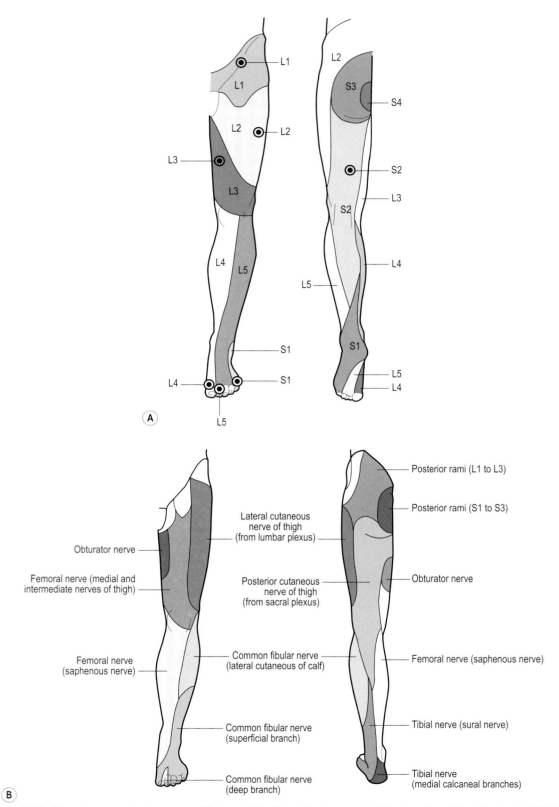

Figure 3.19 • Dermatomes and major nerves of the lower limb. Dots indicate areas of minimal overlap. (From Drake et al. 2005.)

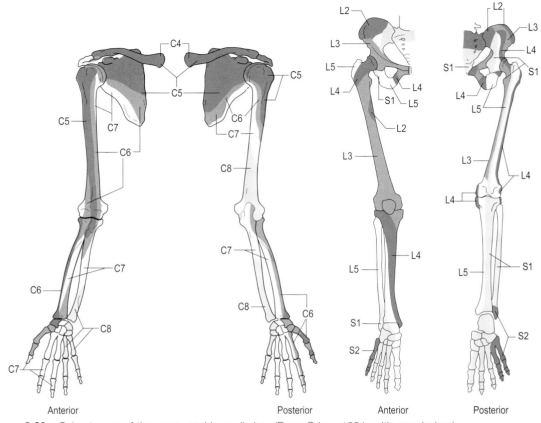

Anterior   Posterior   Anterior   Posterior

Figure 3.20 • Sclerotomes of the upper and lower limbs. (From Grieve 1991, with permission.)

If a peripheral nerve lesion is suspected, the clinician may test the strength of individual muscles supplied by the nerve using the MRC scale, as mentioned earlier. Further details of peripheral nerve injuries are beyond the scope of this text, but they can be found in standard orthopaedic and neurological textbooks.

Reflex testing

The deep tendon reflexes are elicited by tapping the tendon a number of times. The commonly used deep tendon reflexes are the biceps brachii, triceps, patellar and tendocalcaneus (Figure 3.26).

The reflex response may be graded as follows:

– or 0: absent
– or 1: diminished
+ or 2: average
++ or 3: exaggerated
+++ or 4: clonus.

A diminished reflex response can occur if there is a lesion of the sensory and/or motor pathways. An exaggerated reflex response suggests an upper motor lesion response, such as multiple sclerosis. Clonus is associated with exaggerated reflexes and is characterised by intermittent muscular contraction and relaxation produced by sustained stretching of a muscle. It is most commonly tested in the lower limb, where the clinician sharply dorsiflexes the patient's foot with the knee extended. If an upper motor neurone lesion is suspected the plantar response should be tested. This involves stroking the lateral plantar aspect of the foot and observing the movement of the toes. The normal response is for all the toes to plantarflex, while an abnormal response consists of dorsiflexion of the great toe and downward fanning out of the remaining toes (Walton 1989), which is known as the extensor or Babinski response.

Reflex changes alone, without sensory or motor changes, do not necessarily indicate nerve root involvement. Zygapophyseal joints injected with hypertonic saline can abolish ankle reflexes, which can then be restored by a steroid injection (Mooney

Table 3.9 Myotomes (Grieve 1991)

Root	Joint action	Reflex
V cranial (trigeminal N)	Clench teeth, note temporalis and masseter muscles	Jaw
VII cranial (facial N)	Wrinkle forehead, close eyes, purse lips, show teeth	
XI cranial (accessory N)	Shoulder girdle elevation and sternocleidomastoid	
C1	Upper cervical flexion	
C2	Upper cervical extension	
C3	Cervical lateral flexion	
C4	Shoulder girdle elevation	
C5	Shoulder abduction	Biceps jerk
C6	Elbow flexion	Biceps jerk
C7	Elbow extension	Triceps jerk and brachioradialis
C8	Thumb extension; finger flexion	
T1	Finger abduction and adduction	
T2–L1	No muscle test or reflex	
L2	Hip flexion	
L3	Knee extension	Knee jerk
L4	Foot dorsiflexion	Knee jerk
L5	Extension of the big toe	
S1	Eversion of the foot Contract buttock Knee flexion	Ankle jerk
S2	Knee flexion Toe standing	
S3–S4	Muscles of pelvic floor, bladder and genital function	

& Robertson 1976). For this reason, reflex changes alone may not be a relevant clinical finding. It should also be realised that all tendon reflexes can be exaggerated by tension and anxiety.

Neurodynamic tests

The mobility of the nervous system is examined by carrying out what are known as neurodynamic tests (Butler 2000). Some of these tests have been used by the medical profession for over 100 years (Dyck 1984), but they have been more fully developed by several therapists (Elvey 1985; Butler 2000; Maitland et al. 2001). A summary of the tests is given

here, but further details of the theoretical aspects of these tests and how the tests are performed can be found in Butler (2000) and Shacklock (2005). In addition to the mobility tests described overleaf, the clinician can also palpate the nerve with and without the nerve being under tension; details are given under palpation in relevant chapters. The testing procedures follow the same format as those of joint movement. Thus, resting symptoms are established prior to any testing movement and then the following information is noted:

- the quality of movement
- the range of movement

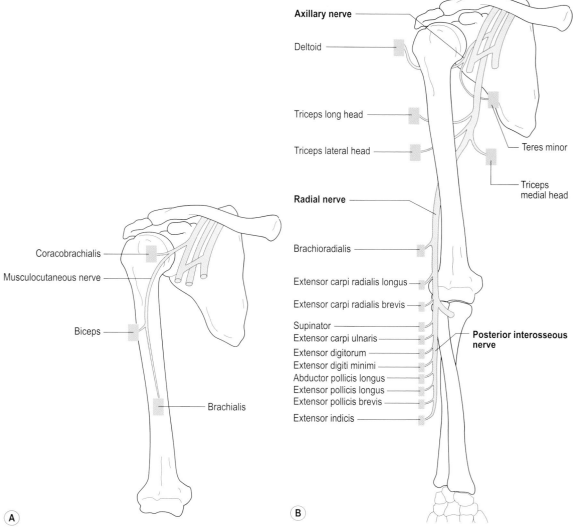

Axillary nerve

Deltoid

Triceps long head

Triceps lateral head

Teres minor

Triceps medial head

Radial nerve

Brachioradialis

Extensor carpi radialis longus

Extensor carpi radialis brevis

Supinator

Extensor carpi ulnaris

Extensor digitorum

Extensor digiti minimi

Abductor pollicis longus

Extensor pollicis longus

Extensor pollicis brevis

Extensor indicis

Posterior interosseous nerve

Coracobrachialis

Musculocutaneous nerve

Biceps

Brachialis

A

B

Figure 3.21 • The musculocutaneous (A), axillary and radial (B) nerves of the upper limb and the muscles that each supplies. (Medical Research Council 1976 Aids to the investigation of peripheral nerve injuries. HMSO, London. Reproduced with kind permission of the Medical Research Council.)

- the resistance through the range and at the end of the range
- pain behaviour (local and referred) through the range.

A test is considered positive if one or more of the following are found:

- All or part of the patient's symptoms have been reproduced.
- Symptoms different from the 'normal' response are produced.
- The range of movement in the symptomatic limb is different from that of the other limb.

As with all examination techniques the tests selected should be justified through sound clinical reasoning.

Patients are first informed what the purpose of the test is and to tell the clinician if they feel any symptoms during the movement. Single movements in one plane are then slowly added, gradually taking the upper or lower limb through a sequence of movements. The order of the test movements will influence tissue response (Coppieters et al. 2006). Taking up tension in the region of symptoms will test nerve tissue more specifically. For example, in a chronic ankle sprain with a possible peroneal nerve component, plantar flexion and inversion may be moved first, adding in straight-leg raise with additional sensitisers at the hip afterwards. If a patient's symptoms are very irritable, then adding local components first may prove to be too provocative. What matters is consistency in sequencing at each time of testing. Each movement is added on slowly and carefully and the clinician monitors the patient's symptoms continuously. If the patient's symptoms are reproduced then the clinician moves a part of the spine, or limb that is far away from where the symptoms are, either to increase the overall length of the nervous system (sensitising movement), also known as a tensioner technique, or to decrease the overall length of the nervous system (desensitising movement) or to examine the nerve's relationship with its interface and its ability to 'slide'. In order for

the test to be valid all other body parts are kept still. The clinician may assume a positive test if a desensitising movement eases the patient's symptoms. For example, for the patient in supine with hip flexion with knee extension when this produces posterior thigh pain, the clinician may then add cervical flexion if the thigh pain is increased with cervical flexion. This is a positive test and suggests a neurodynamic component to the thigh pain.

Neurodynamic tests include the following:

- passive neck flexion
- straight-leg raise
- prone knee bend
- femoral nerve slump test
- saphenous nerve test
- slump

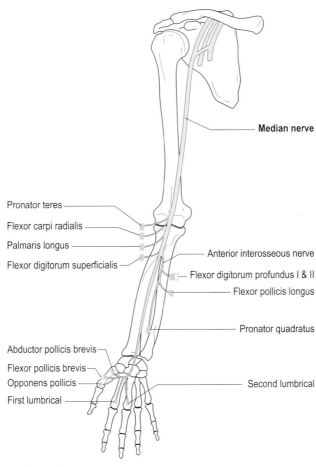

Pronator teres

Flexor carpi radialis

Palmaris longus

Flexor digitorum superficialis

Abductor pollicis brevis

Flexor pollicis brevis

Opponens pollicis

First lumbrical

Median nerve

Anterior interosseous nerve

Flexor digitorum profundus I & II

Flexor pollicis longus

Pronator quadratus

Second lumbrical

(A)

Figure 3.22 • Diagram of the median (A).

(Continued)

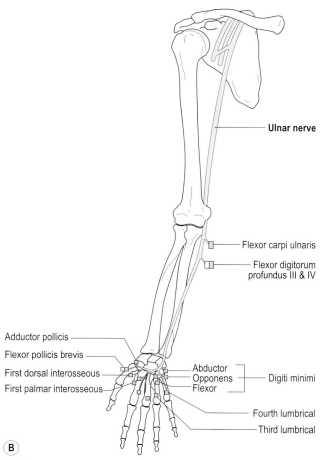

Ulnar nerve

Flexor carpi ulnaris

Flexor digitorum
profundus III & IV

Adductor pollicis

Flexor pollicis brevis

First dorsal interosseous

First palmar interosseous

Abductor
Opponens   Digiti minimi
Flexor

Fourth lumbrical

Third lumbrical

(B)

Figure 3.22—cont'd • ulnar (B) Ulnar nerves of the upper limb and the muscles that each supplies. (Medical Research Council 1976 Aids to the investigation of peripheral nerve injuries. HMSO, London. Reproduced with kind permission of the Medical Research Council.)

- obturator nerve test
- upper-limb neurodynamic tests (ULNT 1, 2a, 2b and 3).

Passive neck flexion

In the supine position, the head is flexed passively by the clinician (Figure 3.27). The normal response would be painfree full-range movement. Sensitising tests include the straight-leg raise or one of the upper-limb tension tests. Where symptoms are related to cervical extension, investigation of passive neck extension is necessary. Passively flexing the neck produces movement and tension of the spinal cord and meninges of the lumbar spine and of the sciatic nerve (Breig 1978; Tencer et al. 1985).

Straight-leg raise

The patient lies supine. The way in which the straight-leg raise is carried out depends on where the patient's symptoms are. The basic component movements of the straight-leg raise are hip adduction, hip medial rotation, hip flexion and knee extension (affecting sciatic nerve). The foot can be moved into any position, but ankle dorsiflexion/forefoot eversion would sensitise the tibial nerve and ankle plantarflexion/forefoot inversion, the common peroneal nerve. Additional movements of the forefoot may be used to bias the medial and lateral plantar nerves, which may be useful if symptoms are in the foot (Alshami et al. 2008). Neck flexion can be used to affect the spinal cord, meninges and sciatic nerve, and/or trunk lateral flexion to lengthen the spinal cord and sympathetic trunk on the contralateral side.

The straight-leg raise moves and tensions the nervous system (including the sympathetic trunk) from the foot to the brain (Breig 1978). The normal

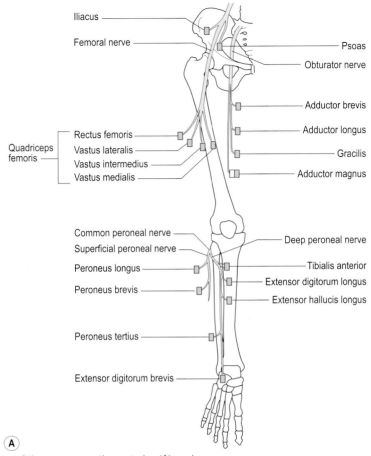

Iliacus

Femoral nerve

Psoas

Obturator nerve

Adductor brevis

Adductor longus

Rectus femoris

Quadriceps femoris

Vastus lateralis

Vastus intermedius

Vastus medialis

Gracilis

Adductor magnus

Common peroneal nerve

Superficial peroneal nerve

Deep peroneal nerve

Peroneus longus

Tibialis anterior

Extensor digitorum longus

Peroneus brevis

Extensor hallucis longus

Peroneus tertius

Extensor digitorum brevis

(A)

Figure 3.23 • Diagram of the nerves on the anterior (A) and

(Continued)

response to hip flexion/adduction/medial rotation with knee extension and foot dorsiflexion would be a strong stretching feeling or tingling in the posterior thigh, posterior knee and posterior calf and foot (Miller 1987; Slater 1994). Normal range of straight-leg raise can vary between 56° and 115° hip flexion (Sweetham et al. 1974); however the clinician identifies what is normal for a patient by comparing both limbs (Figure 3.28).

Prone knee bend

Traditionally, this test is carried out in the prone position, as the name suggests, with the test being considered positive if, on passive knee flexion, symptoms are reproduced. This does not, however, differentiate between nervous tissue (femoral nerve) and the hip flexor muscles, which are also being stretched. Normal range is between 110 and 150° with both limbs being compared.

Femoral nerve slump test

The femoral nerve can be more selectively tested with the patient in side-lying with the head and trunk flexed, allowing cervical extension to be used as a desensitising test (Figure 3.29). The test movements are as follows:

- The clinician determines any resting symptoms and asks the patient to say immediately if any of the symptoms are provoked during any of the movements.
- The patient is placed in side-lying with the symptomatic side uppermost with a pillow under the head (to avoid lateral flexion/rotation of the cervical spine). The patient is asked to hug both knees up on to the chest.
- The patient releases the uppermost knee to the clinician, who flexes the knee and then passively extends the hip, making sure the pelvis and trunk

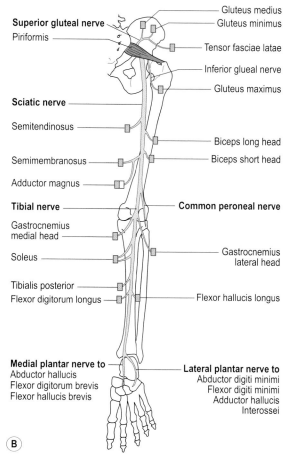

Superior gluteal nerve
Piriformis

Gluteus medius
Gluteus minimus
Tensor fasciae latae
Inferior glueal nerve
Gluteus maximus

Sciatic nerve

Semitendinosus

Biceps long head
Biceps short head

Semimembranosus

Adductor magnus

Tibial nerve

Common peroneal nerve

Gastrocnemius
medial head

Soleus

Gastrocnemius
lateral head

Tibialis posterior
Flexor digitorum longus

Flexor hallucis longus

Medial plantar nerve to
Abductor hallucis
Flexor digitorum brevis
Flexor hallucis brevis

Lateral plantar nerve to
Abductor digiti minimi
Flexor digiti minimi
Adductor hallucis
Interossei

(B)

Figure 3.23—cont'd • posterior (B) aspects of the lower limb and the muscles that they supply. (Medical Research Council 1976 Aids to the investigation of peripheral nerve injuries. HMSO, London. Reproduced with kind permission of the Medical Research Council.)

remain still. The clinician may need to add hip medial or lateral rotation and/or hip abduction/adduction movement to produce the patient's symptoms.

• At the point at which symptoms occur the patient is then asked to extend the head and neck while the clinician maintains the trunk and leg position. A typical positive test would be for the cervical extension to ease the patient's anterior thigh pain and for the clinician then to be able to extend the hip further into range. However, if cervical extension increases the patient's anterior thigh pain, this is also a positive test.

Saphenous nerve test

The patient lies prone and the hip is placed in extension and abduction with the knee extended.

The clinician then passively adds lateral rotation of the hip, dorsiflexion and inversion of the foot (Figure 3.30A). Shacklock (2005) suggests internal rotation of the hip because of the position of the sartorius muscle but advocates trying different positions. Butler (2000) suggests external rotation of the hip based on a study of saphenous nerve entrapments in adolescents (Nir-Paz et al. 1999). The clinician can sensitise the test by, for example, moving the foot into plantarflexion if symptoms are above the knee (Figure 3.30B) or by moving the hip into medial rotation if symptoms are below the knee, or by contralateral side flexion of the spine.

Slump

This test is fully described by Maitland et al. (2001) and Butler (2000) and is shown in Figure 3.31. The slump test can be carried out as follows:

• The clinician establishes the patient's resting symptoms and asks the patient to say immediately if any of the symptoms are provoked.
• The patient sits with thighs fully supported at the edge of the plinth with hands behind the back.
• The patient is asked to flex the trunk by 'slumping the shoulders towards the groin'.
• The clinician monitors trunk flexion.
• Active cervical flexion is carried out.
• The clinician monitors cervical flexion.
• Active knee extension is carried out on the asymptomatic side
• Active foot dorsiflexion is carried out on the asymptomatic side
• Return the foot and knee back to neutral.
• Active knee extension is carried out on the symptomatic side.
• Active foot dorsiflexion is carried out on the symptomatic side.
• Return the foot and knee back to neutral.
• Active bilateral foot dorsiflexion is carried out.
• Active bilateral knee extension is carried out.
• Return the foot and knee back to neutral.

Now that all the combinations of lower-limb movements have been explored, the clinician chooses the most appropriate movement to which to add a sensitising movement. This would commonly be as follows:

• Active knee extension on the symptomatic side is carried out.
• Active foot dorsiflexion on the symptomatic side is carried out.

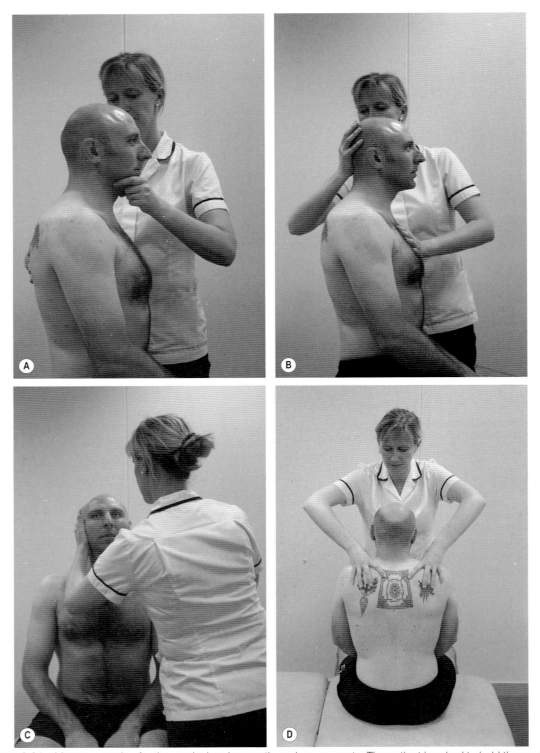

Figure 3.24 • Myotome testing for the cervical and upper thoracic nerve roots. The patient is asked to hold the position against the force applied by the clinician. A C1, upper cervical flexion. B C2, upper cervical extension. C C3, cervical lateral flexion. D C4, shoulder girdle elevation.

(Continued)

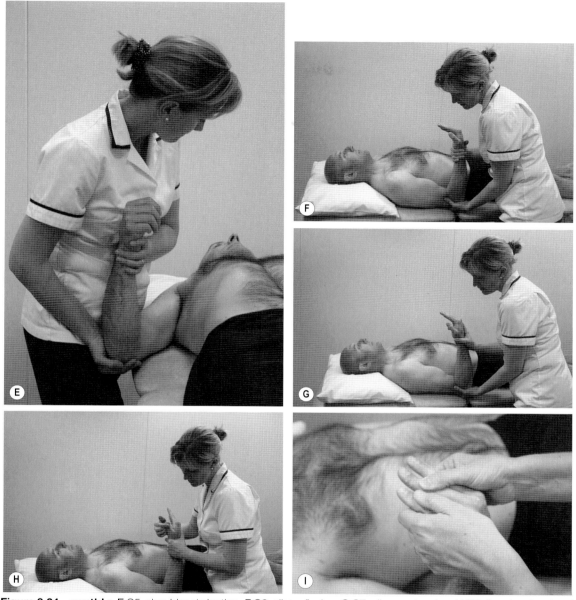

Figure 3.24—cont'd • E C5, shoulder abduction. F C6, elbow flexion. G C7, elbow extension. H C8, thumb extension. I T1, finger adduction.

• The patient is asked to extend the head to look upwards and report on any change in the symptoms. It is vital that there is no change in position of the trunk and lower limbs when the cervical spine is extended. A reduction in symptoms on cervical extension would be a typical positive test indicating a neurodynamic component to the patient's symptoms, but an increase in symptoms would also indicate a neurodynamic component.

The normal response might be:

• pain or discomfort in the mid-thoracic area on trunk and neck flexion

• pain or discomfort behind the knees or in the hamstrings in the trunk and neck flexion and knee

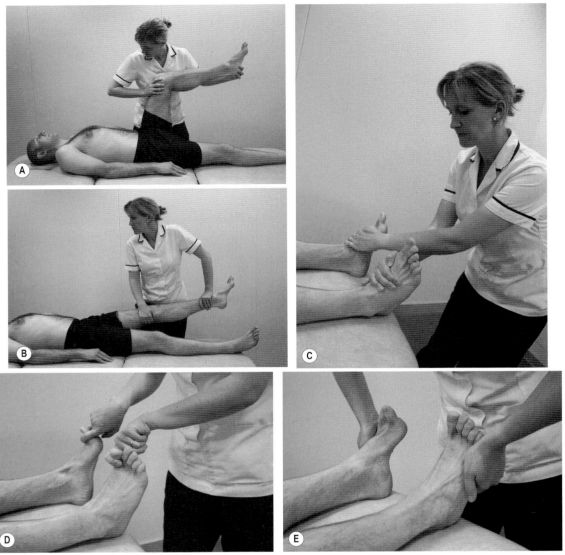

Figure 3.25 • Myotome testing for the lumbar and sacral nerve roots. A L2, hip flexion. B L3, knee extension. C L4, foot dorsiflexion. D L5, extension of the big toe. E S1, foot eversion.

(Continued)

extension position; symptoms are increased with ankle dorsiflexion

- some restriction of knee extension in the trunk and neck flexion position
- some restriction of ankle dorsiflexion in the trunk and neck flexion and knee extension position; this restriction should be symmetrical
- a decrease in pain in one or more areas with the release of the neck flexion

- an increase in the range of knee extension and/or ankle dorsiflexion with the release of the neck flexion.

The desensitising test is cervical extension. Sensitising tests can include cervical rotation, cervical lateral flexion, hip flexion, hip adduction, hip medial rotation, thoracic lateral flexion, altering foot and ankle movements as for the straight-leg raise test, or one of the upper-limb tension tests.

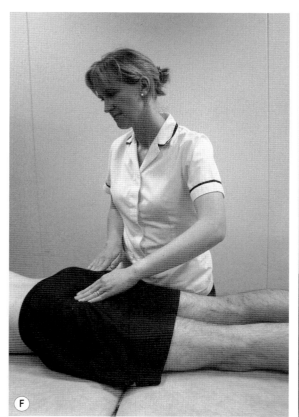

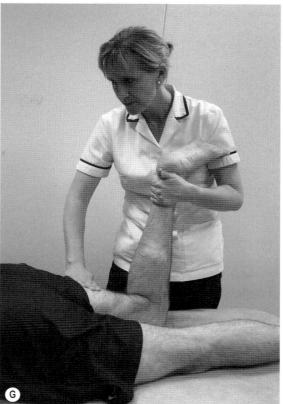

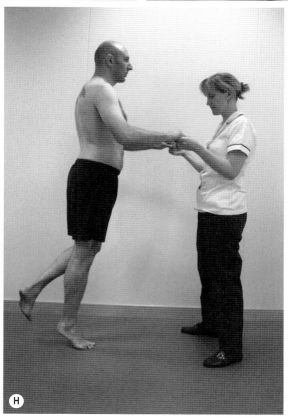

Figure 3.25—cont'd • F S1, contract buttock. G S1 and S2, knee flexion. H S2, toe standing.

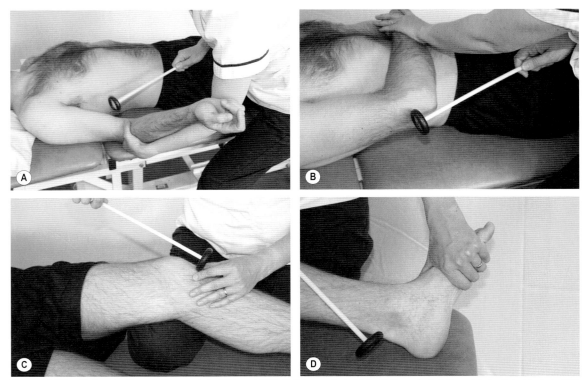

Figure 3.26 • Reflex testing. **A** Biceps jerk (C5 and C6). **B** Triceps jerk (C7). **C** Knee jerk (L3 and L4). **D** Ankle jerk (S1).

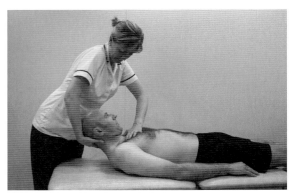

Figure 3.27 • Passive neck flexion.

Obturator nerve test

The slump position can be used further to differentiate muscle or nerve dysfunction as a cause of groin strain. By positioning the patient in sitting and abducting the hip to the onset of symptoms, slump and neck flexion are then added and if symptoms are increased this may suggest obturator nerve involvement; if there is no change in symptoms this may suggest a local groin strain.

Greater emphasis on the sympathetic chain can be tested by adding cervical extension and thoracic lateral flexion.

Upper-limb neurodynamic tests

There are four tests, each of which is biased towards a particular nerve:

1. ULNT 1 – median nerve
2. ULNT 2a – median nerve
3. ULNT 2b – radial nerve
4. ULNT 3 – ulnar nerve.

The test movements are outlined below. The following tests are described with the assumption that the symptoms are in the upper limb. The order of the movements has been chosen so that the last movement is the easiest for the clinician to measure by eye. The area of the patient's symptoms will help the clinician to decide which is the most appropriate ULNT. For example, where symptoms are mainly in the distribution of the radial nerve, ULNT 2b would be carried out.

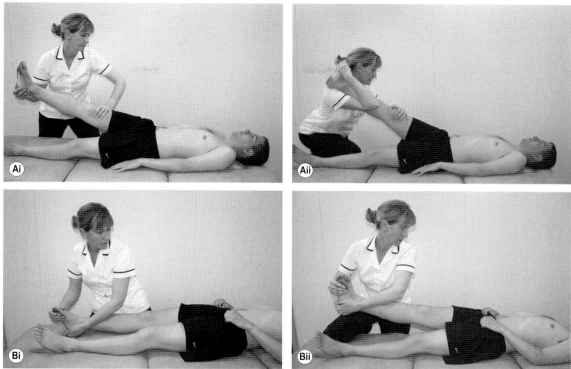

Figure 3.28 • A Straight-leg raise if, for example, symptoms are in the posterior thigh. (i) Hip adduction, medial rotation and then flexion to the onset of patient's posterior thigh symptoms. (ii) The clinician then adds ankle dorsiflexion and forefoot eversion. If the posterior thigh symptoms are increased (or decreased) with the dorsiflexion/eversion, this would be a positive test. B Straight-leg raise if, for example, symptoms are over lateral calf brought on with ankle plantarflexion and forefoot inversion. (i) Passive ankle plantarflexion and forefoot inversion to the onset of the patient's lateral calf symptoms. (ii) The clinician then adds hip adduction, medial rotation and flexion. If the lateral calf symptoms are increased (or decreased) with the addition of hip movements, this would be a positive test.

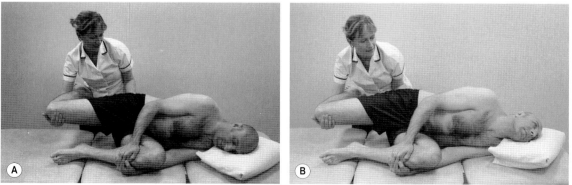

Figure 3.29 • Femoral nerve slump test (in side-lying). A With knee flexion, the clinician passively extends the hip to the point of onset of the patient's anterior thigh symptoms. B Patient extends the cervical spine. If the anterior thigh symptoms are reduced (or increased) with the neck movement, this would be a positive test.

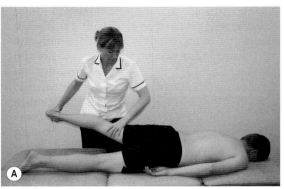
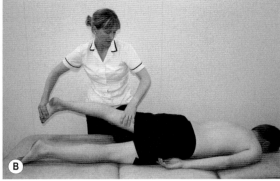

Figure 3.30 • Saphenous nerve length test. **A** With the hip in extension abduction and lateral rotation and the knee extended, the clinician moves the foot into dorsiflexion and eversion. **B** If symptoms are above the knee the clinician can then move the foot into plantarflexion and inversion. If the symptoms are reduced (or increased) with foot movement, this would be a positive test.

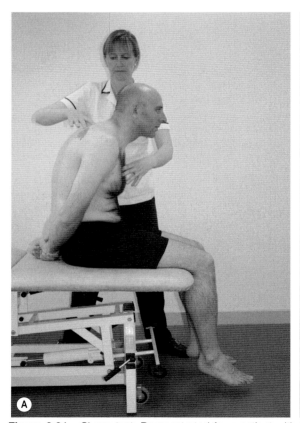
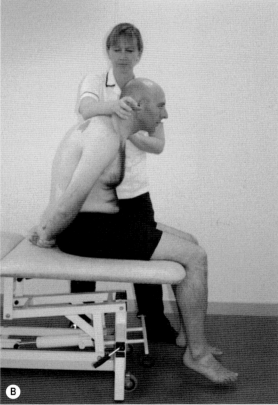

Figure 3.31 • Slump test. Demonstrated for a patient with left posterior thigh pain. **A** Active trunk flexion with arms behind back. **B** Monitoring trunk flexion.

(Continued)

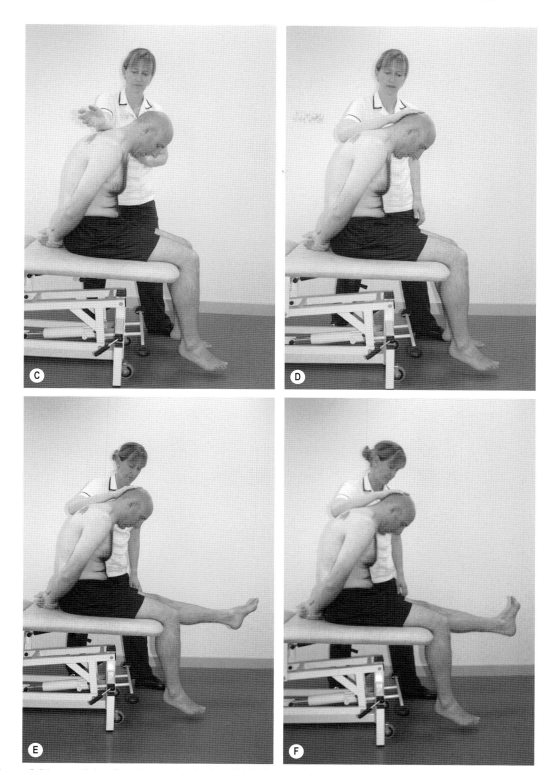

Figure 3.31—cont'd • C Active cervical flexion. D Monitoring of cervical flexion. E Left leg: knee extension. F Left leg: dorsiflexion.

(Continued)

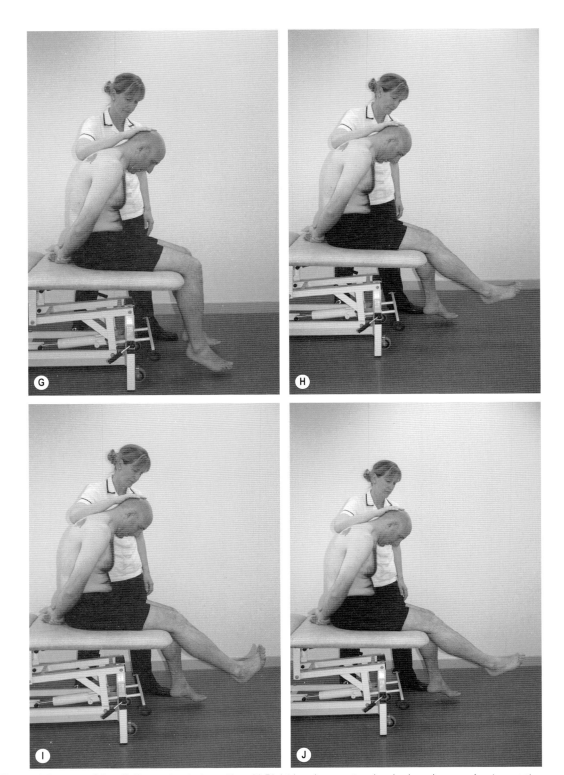

Figure 3.31—cont'd • G Return to start position. H Right leg: knee extension (reduced range due to onset of right thigh pain). I Right leg: knee extension (reduced range due to onset of left thigh pain); addition of dorsiflexion increases right thigh pain. J Right leg: release of dorsiflexion reduces right thigh pain.

(Continued)

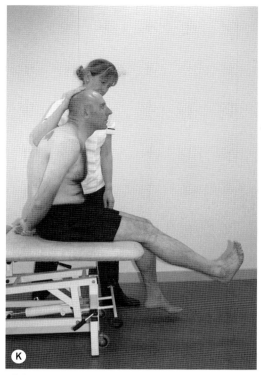
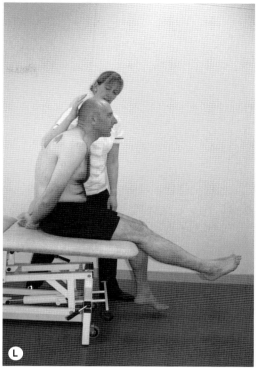

Figure 3.31—cont'd • K Active cervical extension. If cervical extension reduces (or increases) the patient's right posterior thigh pain, this would be a positive test. L Active cervical extension may produce an increase in range which would increase further on release of dorsiflexion.

ULNT 1: median nerve bias (Figure 3.32)

The following sequence of movements would be appropriate, if, for example, the patient has symptoms in the upper arm or below (in the forearm and hand):

1. neutral position of body on couch
2. contralateral lateral flexion of the cervical spine
3. shoulder girdle depression
4. shoulder abduction
5. wrist and finger extension
6. forearm supination
7. lateral rotation of the shoulder
8. elbow extension
9. ipsilateral lateral flexion of the cervical spine.

If symptoms are over the upper fibres of trapezius then:

10. wrist flexion would be used, instead of ipsilateral lateral flexion of the cervical spine.

The movement of ipsilateral lateral flexion of the cervical spine is used to test whether or not there is a neurodynamic component to the patient's symptoms. If there was a neurodynamic component, the patient's symptoms would be expected to be produced at some stage during the arm movements from 2 to 8, and that these symptoms would be reduced (or increased) by ipsilateral lateral flexion of the cervical spine. This principle will occur with each of the ULNT below.

ULNT 2a: median nerve bias (Figure 3.33)

This test is useful in cases where the patient has restricted glenohumeral range. The following sequence of movements would be appropriate if, for example, the patient has symptoms in the upper arm or below (in the forearm and hand):

1. neutral position of body on couch, but with shoulder girdle overhanging the edge
2. contralateral lateral flexion of the cervical spine
3. shoulder girdle depression
4. wrist, finger and thumb extension
5. forearm supination
6. elbow extension

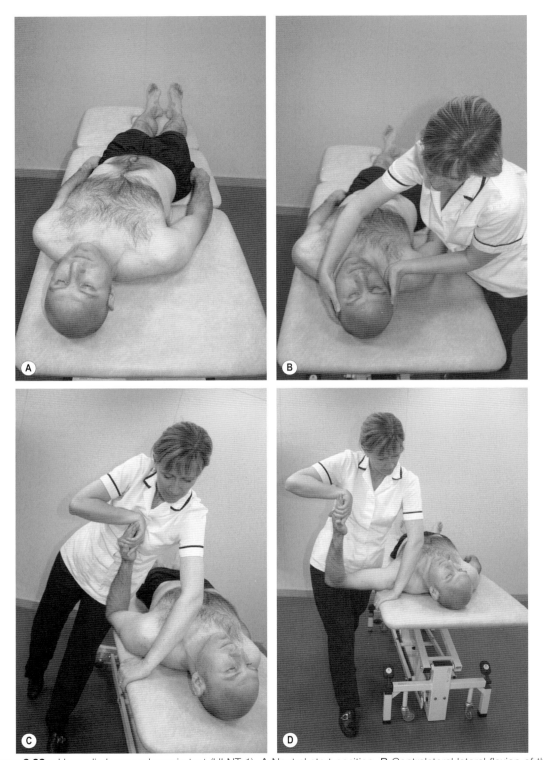

Figure 3.32 • Upper-limb neurodynamic test (ULNT 1). **A** Neutral start position. **B** Contralateral lateral flexion of the cervical spine. **C** Shoulder girdle depression. **D** Shoulder abduction.

(Continued)

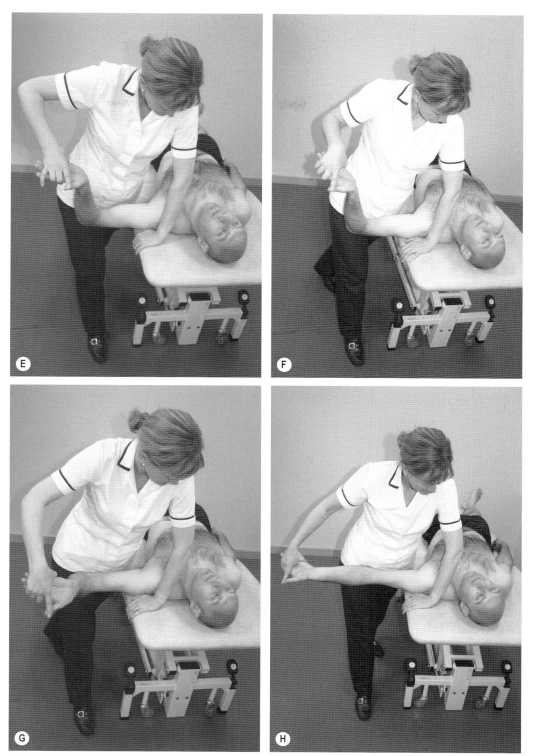

Figure 3.32—cont'd • E Wrist and finger extension. F Forearm supination. G Shoulder lateral rotation. H Elbow extension.

(Continued)

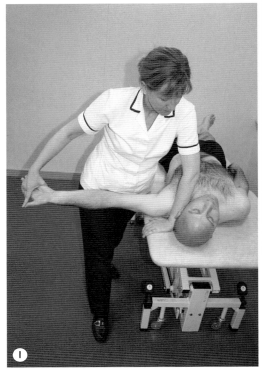 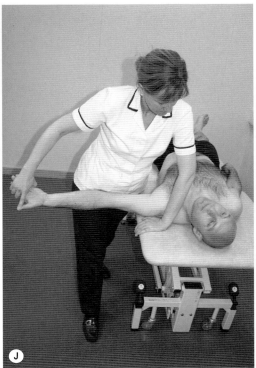

Figure 3.32—cont'd • I Ipsilateral lateral flexion of the cervical spine if symptoms are in the arm. If ipsilateral lateral flexion reduces (or increases) the patient's symptoms, this would be a positive test. J Wrist flexion may be used to desensitise the movement, if the patient's symptoms are close to the cervical spine such as over the upper fibres of trapezius. If wrist flexion reduces (or increases) the patient's neck symptoms this would be a positive test.

7. shoulder lateral rotation
8. shoulder abduction
9. desensitising movement of ipsilateral lateral flexion of the cervical spine.

If symptoms were near the cervical spine, for example over the upper fibres of trapezius, then the movement of wrist flexion, for example, could be used as the desensitising movement.

ULNT 2b: radial nerve bias (Figure 3.34)

The following sequence of movements would be appropriate if, for example, the patient has symptoms in the upper arm or below (in the forearm and hand):

1. neutral position of body on couch, but with shoulder girdle overhanging the edge
2. contralateral lateral flexion of the cervical spine
3. shoulder girdle depression
4. wrist, finger and thumb flexion
5. shoulder medial rotation
6. elbow extension

7. desensitising movement of ipsilateral lateral flexion of the cervical spine

or

8. wrist extension if symptoms are near the cervical spine, for example over the upper fibres of trapezius.

ULNT 3: ulnar nerve bias (Figure 3.35)

The following sequence of movements would be appropriate if, for example, the patient has symptoms in the upper arm or below (in the forearm and hand):

1. neutral position of body on couch
2. contralateral lateral flexion of the cervical spine
3. shoulder girdle stabilised
4. wrist and finger extension
5. forearm pronation
6. elbow flexion
7. shoulder abduction
8. shoulder lateral rotation
9. further shoulder abduction

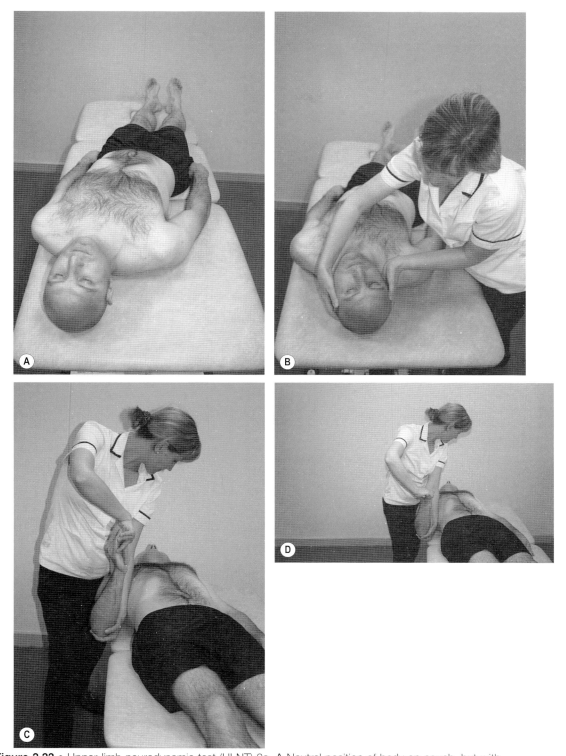

Figure 3.33 • Upper-limb neurodynamic test (ULNT) 2a. A Neutral position of body on couch, but with shoulder girdle overhanging the edge. B Contralateral lateral flexion of the cervical spine. C Shoulder girdle depression. D Wrist, finger and thumb extension.

(Continued)

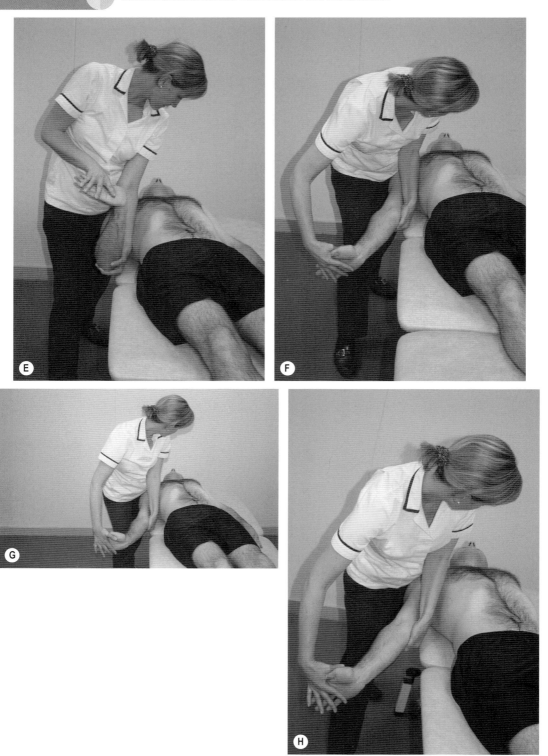

Figure 3.33—cont'd • E Forearm supination. F Elbow extension. G Shoulder lateral rotation. H Shoulder abduction.
(Continued)

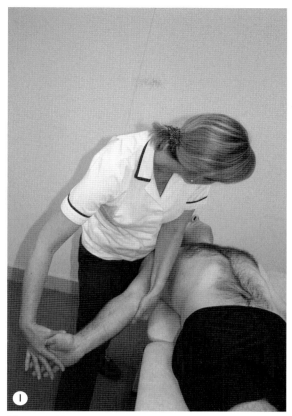

Figure 3.33—cont'd • I Desensitising movement of ipsilateral lateral flexion of the cervical spine.

10. desensitising movement of ipsilateral lateral flexion of the cervical spine

or

11. wrist flexion if symptoms are near the cervical spine, for example over the upper fibres of trapezius.

Normal responses to ULNT 1 (Kenneally et al. 1988) are a deep ache or stretch in the cubital fossa extending to the anterior and radial aspects of the forearm and hand, tingling in the thumb and first three fingers, and a stretching feeling over the anterior aspect of the shoulder. Contralateral cervical lateral flexion increased symptoms while ipsilateral cervical lateral flexion reduced the symptoms.

Normal responses to ULNT 2b (Yaxley & Jull 1993) on asymptomatic subjects are a feeling of stretching pain over the radial aspect of the proximal forearm; these symptoms are usually increased with the addition of contralateral cervical lateral flexion.

ULNT 3 normal responses are a stretching pain and pins and needles over the hypothenar eminence, ring and little finger (Flanagan 1993, cited in Butler 2000).

Additional tests for the upper-limb tension test include placing the other arm in a ULNT position and adding in either the straight-leg raise or the slump test. The tests can also be carried out with the subject in other starting positions; for instance, the ULNT can be performed with the patient prone, which allows accessory movements to be carried out at the same time. Other upper-limb movements can be carried out in addition to those suggested; for instance, pronation/supination or radial/ulnar deviation can be added to ULNT 1.

Nerve tissue palpation

Clinicians can further confirm neural tissue involvement through palpation of the nerves directly where they are superficial, and indirectly in and out of tension positions. Nerve tissue feels firmer and rounder than tendons and should be gently palpated. For further information on nerve palpation the reader is referred to Butler (2000).

Other neurological tests

These tests include various tests for spinal cord and peripheral nerve damage and are discussed in the relevant chapters.

Miscellaneous tests

These can include vascular tests, and tests of soft tissues (such as meniscal tears in the knee). These tests are all discussed in detail in the relevant chapters.

Palpation

It is useful to record palpation findings on a body chart (see Figure 2.3) and/or palpation chart for the vertebral column (Figure 3.36).

During the palpation of soft tissues and skeletal tissues, the following should be noted:

- the temperature of the area (increase is indicative of local inflammation)
- localised increased skin moisture (indicative of autonomic disturbance)
- the presence of oedema and effusion
- mobility and feel of superficial tissues, e.g. ganglions, nodules
- the presence or elicitation of muscle spasm

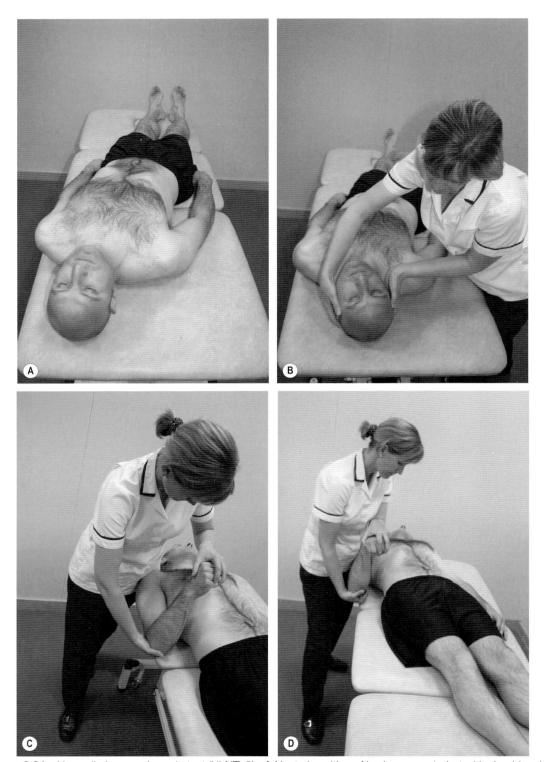

Figure 3.34 • Upper-limb neurodynamic test (ULNT) 2b. **A** Neutral position of body on couch, but with shoulder girdle overhanging the edge. **B** Contralateral lateral flexion of the cervical spine. **C** Shoulder girdle depression. **D** Wrist, finger and thumb flexion.

(Continued)

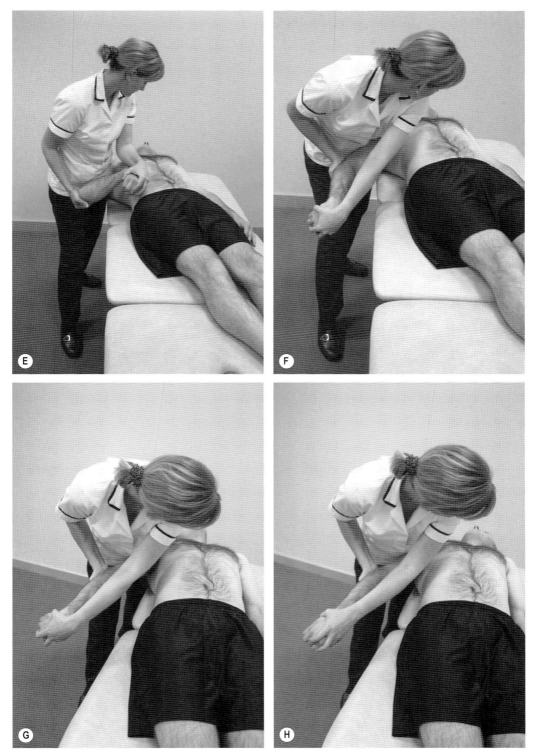

Figure 3.34—cont'd • E Shoulder medial rotation. F Elbow extension. G Desensitising movement of ipsilateral lateral flexion of the cervical spine, or H wrist extension would be used as a desensitising movement if symptoms are near the cervical spine, for example over the upper fibres of trapezius.

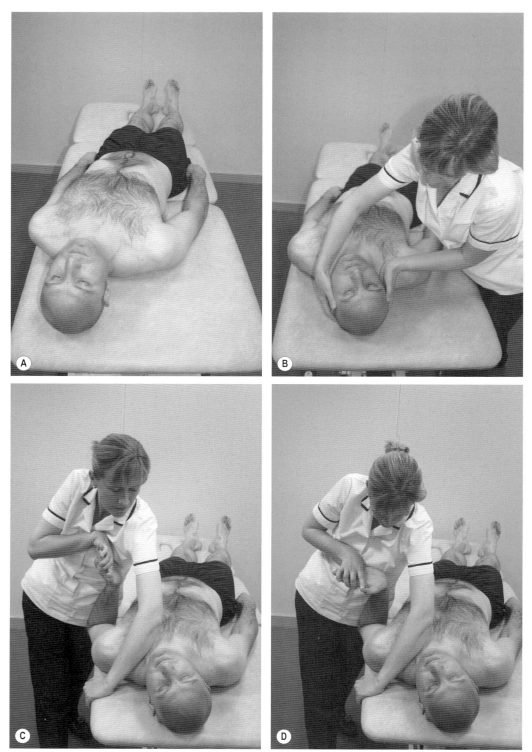

Figure 3.35 • Upper-limb neurodynamic test (ULNT) 3 (ulnar nerve bias). **A** Neutral position of body on couch. **B** Contralateral lateral flexion of the cervical spine. **C** Shoulder girdle stabilised. **D** Wrist and finger extension.

(Continued)

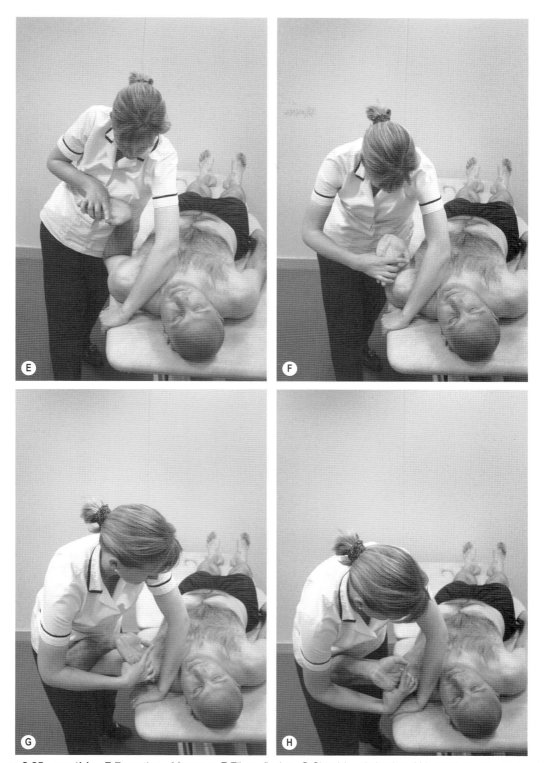

Figure 3.35—cont'd • E Pronation of forearm. F Elbow flexion. G Shoulder abduction. H Lateral rotation of shoulder.

(Continued)

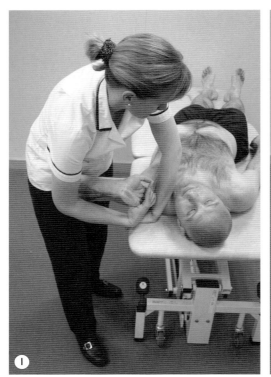

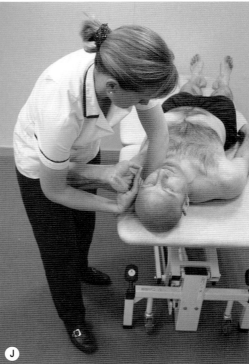

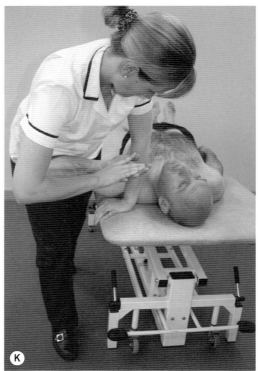

Figure 3.35—cont'd • I Further shoulder abduction. J Desensitising movement of ipsilateral lateral flexion of the cervical spine (if symptoms are in the forearm or hand), or K wrist flexion if symptoms are near the cervical spine or shoulder.

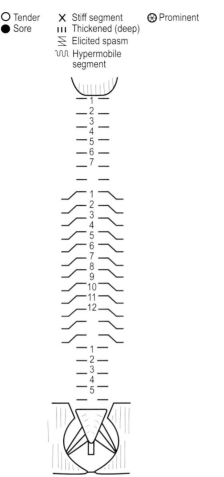

O Tender   X Stiff segment   ⊗ Prominent
● Sore   ııı Thickened (deep)
            ⩵ Elicited spasm
            ᚃᚃᚃ Hypermobile
                segment

Figure 3.36 • Palpation chart. (From Grieve 1991, with permission.)

- tenderness of bone, ligament, muscle, tendon, tendon sheath, trigger point and nerve
- increased or decreased prominence of bones
- joint effusion or swelling of a limb can be measured using a tape measure, and comparing left and right sides
- pain provoked or reduced on palpation.

Hints on the method of palpation are given in Box 3.4. Further guidance on palpation of the soft tissues can be found in Hunter (1998).

Trigger points

A trigger point is 'a focus of hyperirritability in a tissue that, when compressed, is locally tender and, if sufficiently hypersensitive, gives rise to referred pain and tenderness, and sometimes to referred autonomic phenomena and distortion of proprioception. Types include myofascial, cutaneous, fascial, ligamentous, and periosteal trigger points' (Travell & Simons 1983).

Trigger points can be divided into latent and active: a latent trigger point is where the tenderness is found on examination yet the person has no symptoms, while an active trigger point is one where symptoms are produced locally and/or in an area of referral. Active trigger points lead to shortening and weakening of the muscle and are thought to be caused by trauma to the muscle (Baldry 1993). Commonly found myofascial trigger points and their characteristic area of referral can be seen in Figure 3.37. In order to examine for a trigger point, the muscle is put on a slight stretch and the clinician searches for trigger points by firm pressure with the fingers over the muscle.

Accessory movements

Accessory movements are defined as those movements which a person cannot perform actively but which can be performed on that person by an external force (Maitland et al. 2001). They take the form of gliding (sometimes referred to as translation or sliding) of the joint surfaces (medially, laterally, anteriorly or posteriorly), distraction and compression of the joint surfaces and, in some joints, rotation movements where this movement cannot be performed actively, e.g. rotation at the metacarpal and interphalangeal joints of the fingers. These movements are possible because all joints have a certain amount of play or 'slack' in the capsule and surrounding ligaments (Kaltenborn 2002).

Limitation in physiological range of movement may be due to a limitation of the accessory range of movement at the joint. For example, during knee flexion in a non-weight-bearing position, the tibia rolls backwards and slides backwards on the femoral condyles; and during shoulder elevation through abduction, the head of the humerus rolls upwards and translates inferiorly on the glenoid cavity. The direction in which the bone glides during physiological movements depends upon the shape of the moving articular surface (Figure 3.38). When the joint surface of the moving bone is concave, the glide occurs in the same direction as the bone is moving, so that, with flexion of the knee joint (in non-weight-bearing), posterior glide of the tibia occurs on the femur; when the joint surface is convex, the glide is in the opposite direction to the bone movement, so that with

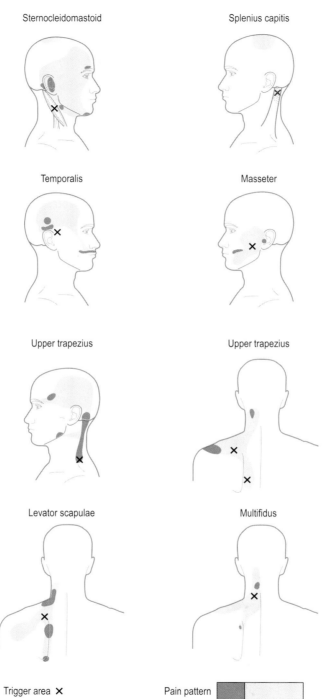

Figure 3.37 • Myofascial trigger points.

(Continued)

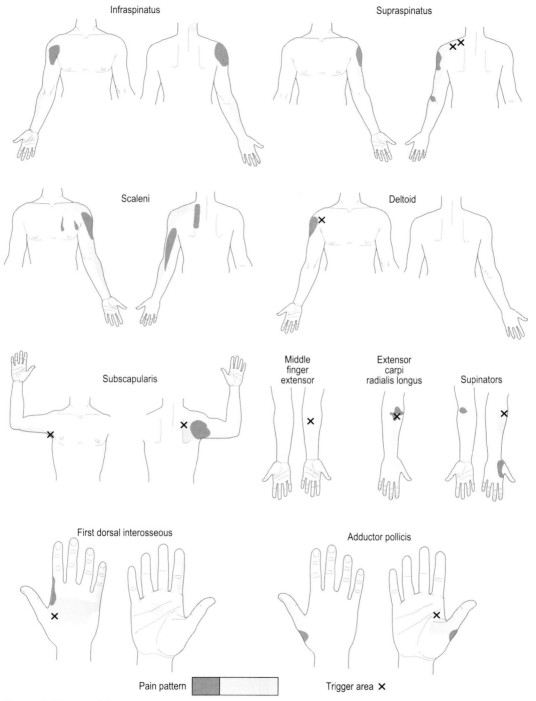

Figure 3.37—cont'd.

Pain pattern ▨▫   Trigger area ✗

Figure 3.37—cont'd.

(Continued)

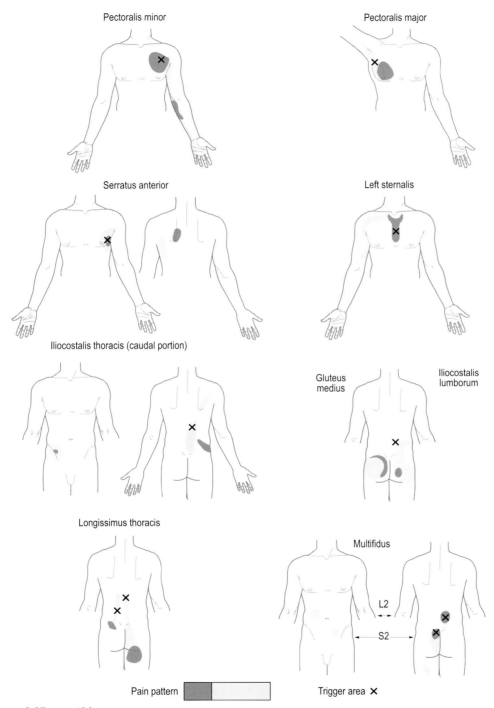

Pectoralis minor

Pectoralis major

Serratus anterior

Left sternalis

Iliocostalis thoracis (caudal portion)

Gluteus medius

Iliocostalis lumborum

Longissimus thoracis

Multifidus

L2

S2

Pain pattern

Trigger area ✕

Figure 3.37—cont'd.

(Continued)

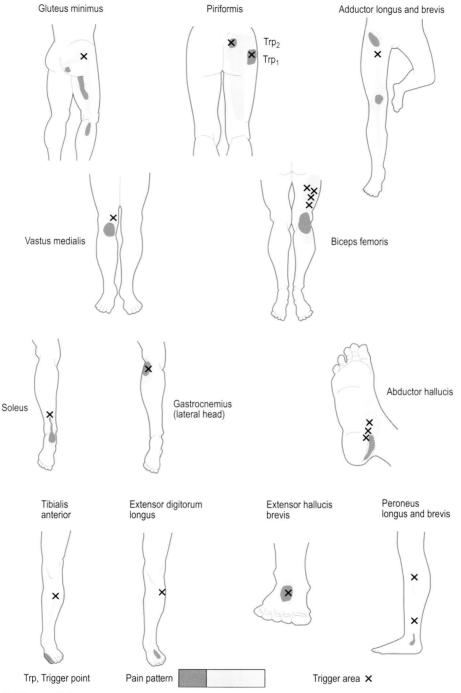

Gluteus minimus

Piriformis

Trp₂
Trp₁

Adductor longus and brevis

Vastus medialis

Biceps femoris

Soleus

Gastrocnemius
(lateral head)

Abductor hallucis

Tibialis
anterior

Extensor digitorum
longus

Extensor hallucis
brevis

Peroneus
longus and brevis

Trp, Trigger point   Pain pattern   Trigger area ✕

Figure 3.37—cont'd.

Box 3.4

Hints on palpation

- Palpate the unaffected side first and compare this with the affected side
- Palpate from superficial to deep
- Use just enough force to feel – excessive force can reduce feel
- Never assume that a relevant area does not need palpating

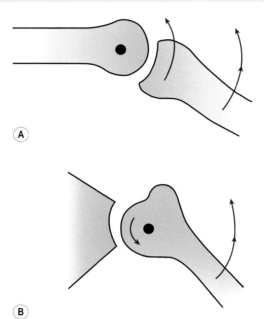

Figure 3.38 • Movement of articular surfaces during physiological movements. The single arrow depicts the direction of movement of the articular surface and the double arrow depicts the physiological movement. **A** With knee extension (non-weight-bearing), the concave articular surface of the tibia slides superiorly on the convex femoral condyles. **B** With shoulder elevation through abduction, the convex articular surface of the humerus slides inferiorly on the concave glenoid cavity. (From Kaltenborn 2002, with permission.)

shoulder abduction there is an inferior glide of the head of the humerus on the glenoid cavity.

Examination of the accessory movement is important as it can:

- identify and localise a symptomatic joint
- define the nature of a joint motion abnormality
- identify associated areas of joint motion abnormality

Box 3.5

Hints on performing an accessory movement

- Have the patient comfortably positioned
- Examine the joint movement on the unaffected side first and compare this with the affected side
- Initially examine the accessory movement without obtaining feedback from the patient about symptom reproduction. This helps to facilitate the process of learning to feel joint movement
- Have as large an area of skin contact as possible for maximum patient comfort
- The force is applied using the body weight of the clinician and not the intrinsic muscles of the hand, which can be uncomfortable for both the patient and the clinician
- Where possible, the clinician's forearm should lie in the direction of the applied force
- Apply the force smoothly and slowly through the range with or without oscillations
- At the end of the available movement, apply small oscillations to feel the resistance at the end of the range
- Use just enough force to feel the movement – the harder you press, the less you feel

- alter local muscle and nerve tissues and identify either source of the patient's symptoms or a contributing factor to the patient's condition
- provide a basis for the selection of treatment techniques (adapted from Jull 1994).

Pressure is applied to a bone close to the joint line and the clinician increases movement progressively through the range and notes the:

- quality of the movement
- range of the movement
- pain behaviour (local and referred) through the range, which may be provoked or reduced
- resistance through range and at the end of the range
- muscle spasm elicitation.

Hints on performing an accessory movement are given in Box 3.5. Findings can include the following:

- undue skeletal prominence
- undue tenderness
- thickening of soft tissues
- decreased mobility of soft tissues, such as periarticular tissues, muscles and nerves
- a point in the range of the accessory movement where symptoms are increased or reduced

- an indication as to the irritability of a problem (see Chapter 2)
- evidence of joint hypermobility
- evidence of joint hypomobility
- elicitation of muscle spasm
- joints that are not affected by the present problem
- the location(s) of the problem(s)
- the relationship of the problems to each other
- the possible nature of structures involved
- what is limiting the movement and the relationship of pain, resistance or muscle spasm within the available range of movement. A movement diagram (or joint picture) can be used to depict this information.

Movement diagrams

The movement diagram is useful for a student who is learning how to examine joint movement and is also a quick and easy way of recording information on joint movements. It was initially described by Maitland (1977) and then later refined by Margarey (1985) and Maitland et al. (2001).

A movement diagram is a graph that describes the behaviour of pain, resistance and muscle spasm, showing the intensity and position in range at which each is felt during a passive accessory or passive physiological movement of a joint (Figure 3.39).

The baseline AB is the range of movement of any joint. Point A is the beginning of range and point B is the end of the passive movement. The exact position of B will vary with the strength and boldness of the clinician. It is thus depicted on the diagram as a thick line.

The vertical axis AC depicts the intensity of pain, resistance or muscle spasm. Point A is the absence of any pain, resistance or spasm and point C is the maximum intensity that the clinician is prepared to provoke.

Procedure for drawing a movement diagram. *To draw resistance* (Figure 3.40). The clinician moves the joint and the first point at which resistance is felt is called R_1 and is marked on the baseline AB. A normal joint, when moved passively, has the feel of being well-oiled and friction-free until near the end of range, when some resistance is felt that increases to limit the range of movement. As mentioned previously, the resistance to further movement is due to bony apposition, increased tension in the surrounding ligaments and muscles or soft-tissue apposition.

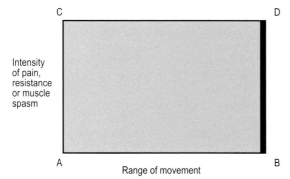

Figure 3.39 • A movement diagram. The baseline AB is the range of movement of any joint and the vertical axis AC depicts the intensity of pain, resistance or muscle spasm.

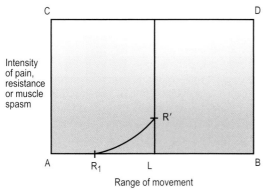 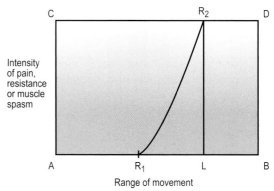

Figure 3.40 • Resistance depicted on a movement diagram for physiological movements. **A** The diagram describes a joint movement that is limited (L) to half range. Resistance is first felt at around one-quarter of full range (R_1) and increases a little at the end of the available range (R'). **B** The diagram describes a joint movement that is limited (L) to three-quarters range. Resistance is first felt at around half of full range (R_1) and gradually increases to the limit range of movement (R_2).

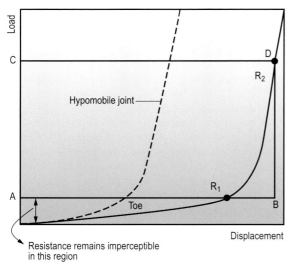

Figure 3.41 • Relationship of movement diagram (ABCD) to a load–displacement curve. (From Lee & Evans 1994, with permission.)

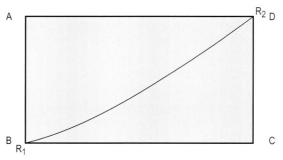

Figure 3.42 • A movement diagram of an accessory movement, where R_1 starts at the beginning of range (at A).

The joint is then taken to the limit of range and the point of limitation is marked by L on the baseline AB. If resistance limits the range, the point of limitation is marked by R_2 vertically above L on the CD line to indicate that it is resistance that limits the range. R_2 is the point beyond which the clinician is not prepared to push. The behaviour of the resistance between R_1 and R_2 is then drawn.

If, on the other hand, pain limits the range of movement, an estimate of the intensity of resistance is made at the end of the available range and is plotted vertically above L as R'. The behaviour of the resistance between R_1 and R' is then described by drawing a line between the two points.

The resistance curve of the movement diagram, during physiological movements, is essentially a part of the load–displacement curve of soft tissue (Panjabi 1992; Lee & Evans 1994) and is shown in Figure 3.41. In a normal joint, the initial range of movement has minimal resistance and this part is known as the toe region (Lee & Evans 1994) or neutral zone (Panjabi 1992). As the joint is moved further into range, resistance increases; this is known as the linear region (Lee & Evans 1994) or elastic zone (Panjabi 1992). R_1 is the point at which the therapist perceives an increase in the resistance and it will lie somewhere between the toe region/neutral zone and the linear region/elastic zone. The ease with which a therapist can feel this change in resistance might be expected to depend on the range of joint movement and the type of movement being examined. It seems reasonable to

suggest that it would be easier to feel R_1 when the range of movement is large and where there is a relatively long toe region, such as elbow flexion.

By contrast, accessory movements may only have a few millimetres of movement and no clear toe region (Petty et al. 2002); in this case R_1 may be perceived at the beginning of the range. For this reason, resistance occurs at the beginning of the range of movement for accessory movements, shown in Figure 3.42. A further complication in finding R_1 occurs with spinal accessory movements, because the movement is not localised to any one joint but produces a general movement of the spine (Lee & Svensson 1990).

To draw pain (Figure 3.43). In this case, the clinician must establish whether the patient has any resting pain before moving the joint.

The joint is then moved passively through range, asking the patient to report any discomfort immediately. Several small oscillatory movements are carried out, gradually moving further into range up to the point where the pain is first felt, so that the exact position in the range at which the pain occurs can be recorded on the diagram. The point at which pain first occurs is called P_1 and is marked on the baseline AB.

The joint is then moved passively beyond P_1 to determine the behaviour of the pain through the available range of movement. If pain limits range, the point of limitation is marked as L on the baseline AB. Vertically above L, P_2 is marked on the CD line to indicate that it is pain that limits the range. The behaviour of the pain between P_1 and P_2 is now drawn.

If, however, it is resistance that limits the range of movement, an estimate of the intensity of pain is made at the end of range and is plotted vertically above L as P'. The behaviour of the pain between P_1 and P' is then described by drawing a line between the two points.

To draw muscle spasm (Figure 3.44). The joint is taken through range and the point at which resistance

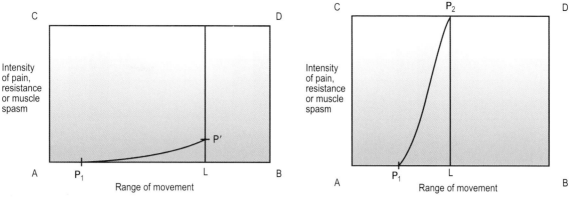

Figure 3.43 • Pain depicted on a movement diagram. **A** The diagram describes a joint movement that is limited to three-quarters range (L). Pain is first felt at around one-quarter of full range (P_1) and increases a little at the end of available range (P′). **B** The diagram describes a joint movement that is limited to half range (L). Pain is first felt at around one-quarter of full range (P_1) and gradually increases to limit range of movement (P_2).

due to muscle spasm is first felt is marked on the baseline AB as S_1.

The joint is then taken to the limit of range. If muscle spasm limits range, the point of limitation is marked as L on the baseline AB. Vertically above L, S_2 is marked on the CD line to indicate that it is muscle spasm that limits the range. The behaviour of spasm is then plotted between S_1 and S_2. When spasm limits range, it always reaches its maximum quickly and is more or less a straight line almost vertically upwards. The resistance from muscle spasm varies depending on the speed at which the joint is moved – as the speed increases, so the resistance increases.

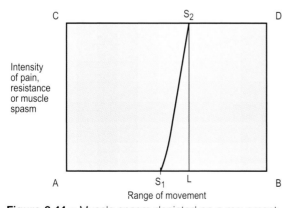

Figure 3.44 • Muscle spasm depicted on a movement diagram. The diagram describes a joint movement that is limited to three-quarters range (L). Muscle spasm is first felt just before three-quarters of full range (S_1) and quickly increases to limit the range of movement (S_2).

Examples of movement diagrams are given in Figure 3.45.

Joint pictures. Grieve (1981) uses 'joint pictures' to describe essentially the same information as movement diagrams, i.e. the behaviour of pain, resistance and muscle spasm throughout the available range of movement (Figure 3.46). A horizontal line depicts normal range, with the start of movement to the left. Pain is shown above the line, muscle spasm below, and resistance is shown as a number of vertical lines across the horizontal line. Limitation to movement is depicted by a vertical line from the dominant factor responsible for restricting the range of movement. A few examples of movement diagrams and joint pictures are shown for comparison in Figure 3.47.

Modifications to accessory movement examination

Accessory movements can be modified by altering the:

- speed of applied force; pressure can be applied slowly or quickly and it may or may not be oscillated through the range
- direction of the applied force
- point of application of the applied force
- resting position of the joint.

The joint can be placed in any number of resting positions; for example, accessory movements on the patella can be applied with the knee anywhere between full flexion and full extension, and accessory movements to any part of the spine can be performed

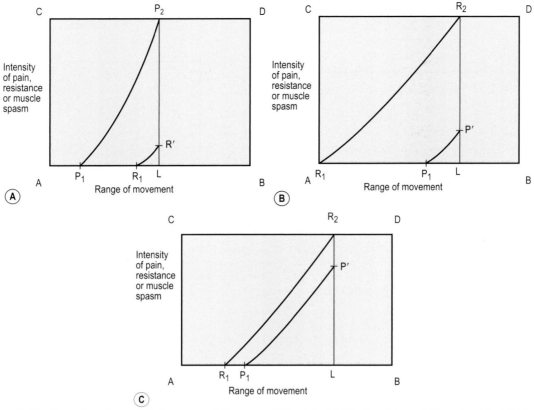

Figure 3.45 • Examples of completed movement diagrams. A Shoulder joint flexion. Interpretation: shoulder joint flexion is limited to just over half range (L). Pain first comes on at about one-quarter of full range (P_1) and increases to limit the range of movement (P_2). Resistance is first felt just before the end of the available range (R_1) and increases a little (R'). The movement is therefore predominantly limited by pain. B Central posteroanterior (PA) pressure on L3. Interpretation: the PA movement is limited to three-quarters range (L). Resistance is felt immediately, at the beginning of range (R_1), and increases to limit the range of movement (R_2). Pain is first felt just before the limit of the available range (P_1) and increases slightly (P'). The movement is therefore predominantly limited by resistance. C Left cervical rotation. Interpretation: left cervical rotation is limited to three-quarters range (L). Resistance is first felt at one-quarter of full range (R_1) and increases to limit range of movement (R_2). Pain is felt very soon after resistance (P_1) and increases (P') to an intensity of about 8/10 (where 0 represents no pain and 10 represents the maximum pain ever felt by the patient). Cervical rotation is therefore limited by resistance but pain is a significant factor.

(i) The horizontal line represents normal range and movement is from left to right

(ii) Pain is depicted above it

(iii) Spasm is depicted below it

(iv) Movement limitation is represented by a vertical line from the

dominant factor responsible

(v) Resistance (other than spasm) is represented by a number of vertical lines which always cross the range line

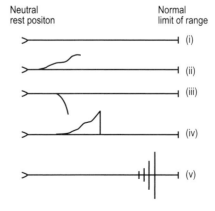

Figure 3.46 • Joint pictures. (From Grieve 1991, with permission.)

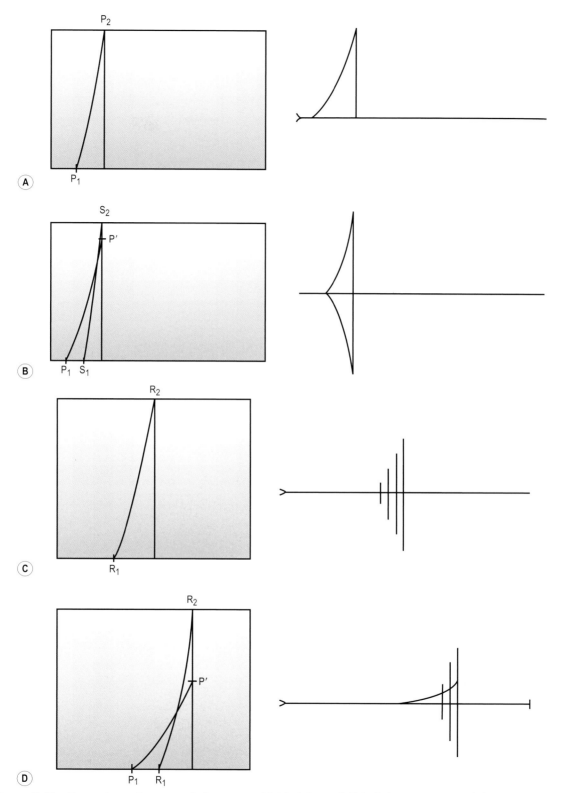

Figure 3.47 • Comparison of movement diagrams and joint pictures. **A** Pain limits movement early in the range. **B** Spasm and pain limit movement early in range. **C** Resistance limits movement halfway through range. **D** Limitation of movement to three-quarters range because of resistance, with some pain provoked from halfway through range.

with the spine in flexion, extension, lateral flexion or rotation, or indeed any combination of these positions. The effect of this positioning alters the effect of the accessory movement. For example, central postero-anterior pressure on C5 causes the superior articular facets of C5 to slide upwards on the inferior articular facets of C4, a movement similar to cervical extension; this upward movement can be enhanced with the cervical spine positioned in extension. Specific techniques have been described by Maitland et al. (2001), Maitland (1991) and Edwards (1999), and readers are referred to these authors for further information.

Accessory movements are carried out on each joint suspected to be a source of the symptoms. After each joint is examined in this way, all relevant asterisks are reassessed to determine the effect of the accessory movements on the signs and symptoms. For example, in a patient with cervical spine, shoulder and elbow pain, it may be found that, following accessory movements to the cervical spine, there is an increase in range and reduction in pain in both the cervical spine and the shoulder joint but that there is no change in elbow movement. Accessory movements to the elbow joint, however, may be found to improve the elbow range of movements. Such a scenario suggests that the cervical spine is giving rise to the pain in the cervical spine and the shoulder, and the local tissues around the elbow are responsible for producing the pain at the elbow. This process had been termed the 'analytical assessment' by Maitland et al. (2001) and is shown in Figure 3.48.

Accessory movements have been described by various authors (Cyriax 1982; Grieve 1991; Mulligan 1999; Maitland et al. 2001, 2005; Kaltenborn 2002, 2003). This text will deal mainly with those described by Maitland, Kaltenborn and Mulligan and they will be covered in the relevant chapters.

Developed from Kaltenborn's work (Kaltenborn 2002, 2003), the Mulligan concept is both an assessment and management approach to movement dysfunction (Mulligan 1999). As mentioned earlier, during normal physiological movements there is a combination of rolling and gliding of bony surfaces at the joint. The Mulligan approach proposes that movement dysfunction results from minor positional faults of a joint restricting movement and thus restoring the glide component of the movement facilitates full painfree movement at the joint. During examination, the clinician moves the bone parallel (translation) or at right angles (distraction/separation) to the treatment plane. The treatment plane passes through the joint and lies 'in' the concave articular

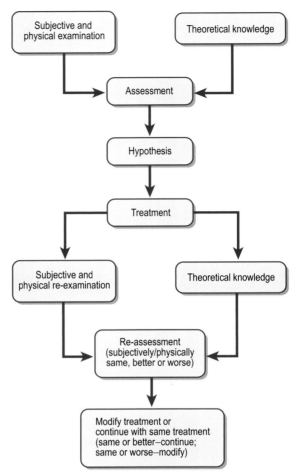

Figure 3.48 • Analytical assessment.

surface (Figure 3.49). During examination with these accessory movements, it is the relief of symptoms that implicates the joint as the source of symptoms, since the technique aims to facilitate movement (compare accessory movements used by Maitland et al. 2001 and Maitland 1991). The examination tests can be used as a treatment technique but details of these are outside the scope of this book.

Natural apophyseal glides (NAGs). These are mid-range passive oscillatory rhythmic mobilisations applied centrally or unilaterally in the cervical and upper thoracic spine (between C2 and T3). They are carried out in a weight-bearing position and the direction of the force is along the facet treatment plane (anterosuperiorly). They should eliminate the pain provoked during the movement.

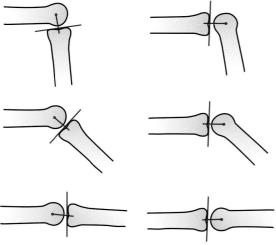

Figure 3.49 • The treatment plane is indicated by the line and passes through the joint and lies 'in' the concave articular surface. (From Kaltenborn & Evjenth 1989, with permission.)

Sustained natural apophyseal glides (SNAGs). These are end-range sustained mobilisations, which are combined with active movements and can be used for all areas of the spine. Like natural apophyseal glides, they are carried out in a weight-bearing position with the direction of the force along the facet treatment plane. They should eliminate the pain provoked during the movement.

Mobilisations with movement (MWM). These are sustained mobilisations carried out with active or passive movements or resisted muscle contraction and are used for the peripheral joints. They are generally applied close to the joint at right angles to the plane of the movement taking place. They should eliminate the pain provoked during the movement. It is proposed that the mobilisation affects and corrects a bony positional fault, which produces abnormal tracking of the articular surfaces during movement (Mulligan 1993, 1999; Exelby 1996).

Spinal mobilisation with limb movement (SMWLM). These can be useful differentiation tools where there is lower- or upper-limb movement restriction resulting from spinal or neurodynamic dysfunction. These complement other assessment approaches already described, i.e. symptom referral, active physiological lower-limb movements, PPIVMS and PAVIMS. These transverse glides can be applied to spine in weight-and non-weight-bearing positions with the addition of upper/lower limb movements.

Completion of the physical examination

Once all the above steps have been carried out, the physical examination is complete. It is vital at this stage to highlight with an asterisk (*) important findings from the examination. These findings must be reassessed at, and within, subsequent treatment sessions to evaluate the effects of treatment on the patient's condition. An outline examination chart that summarizes the physical examination is shown in Figure 3.50.

The physical testing procedures which specifically indicate joint, nerve or muscle tissues, as a source of the patient's symptoms, are summarised in Table 3.10. At one end of the scale the findings may provide strong evidence, and, at the other end, may provide weak evidence. A variety of presentations between these two extremes may, of course, be found.

The strongest evidence that a joint is the source of the patient's symptoms is that active and passive physiological movements, passive accessory movements and joint palpation all reproduce the patient's symptoms, and that, following a treatment dose, reassessment identifies an improvement in the patient's signs and symptoms. For example, let us assume a patient has lateral elbow pain caused by a radiohumeral joint dysfunction. In the physical examination, there is limited elbow flexion and extension movements due to reproduction of the patient's elbow pain, with some resistance. Active movement is very similar to passive movement in terms of range, resistance and pain reproduction. Accessory movement examination of the radiohumeral joint reveals limited posteroanterior and anteroposterior glide of the radius due to reproduction of the patient's elbow pain with some resistance. Following the examination of accessory movements, sufficient to be considered a treatment dose, reassessment of the elbow shows physiological movements are improved, in terms of range and pain. This scenario would indicate that there is a dysfunction at the radiohumeral joint, firstly because elbow movements, both active and passive physiological and accessory movements, reproduce the patient's symptoms, and, secondly, because following accessory movements the active elbow movements are improved. Even if the active movements are made worse, this would still suggest a joint dysfunction, since it is likely that the accessory movements would predominantly affect the joint, with much less effect on nerve and muscle tissues

Observation	Isometric muscle testing
Joint integrity tests	Other muscle tests
Active and passive physiological movements	Neurological integrity tests
	Neurodynamic tests
	Other nerve tests
Capsular pattern yes/no	Miscellaneous tests
Muscle strength	
	Palpation
Muscle control	
	Accessory movements and reassessment of each relevant region
Muscle length	

Figure 3.50 • Physical examination chart.

Table 3.10 Physical tests which, if positive, indicate joint, nerve and muscle as a source of the patient's symptoms

Test	Strong evidence	Weak evidence
Joint		
Active physiological movements	Reproduces patient's symptoms	Dysfunctional movement: reduced range, excessive range, altered quality of movement, increased resistance, decreased resistance
Passive physiological movements	Reproduces patient's symptoms; this test is the same as for active physiological movements	Dysfunctional movement: reduced range, excessive range, increased resistance, decreased resistance, altered quality of movement
Accessory movements	Reproduces patient's symptoms	Dysfunctional movement: reduced range, excessive range, increased resistance, decreased resistance, altered quality of movement
Palpation of joint	Reproduces patient's symptoms	Tenderness
Reassessment following therapeutic dose of accessory movement	Improvement in tests which reproduce patient's symptoms	No change in physical tests which reproduce patient's symptoms
Muscle		
Active movement	Reproduces patient's symptoms	Reduced strength Poor quality
Passive physiological movements	Do not reproduce patient's symptoms	
Isometric contraction	Reproduces patient's symptoms	Reduced strength Poor quality
Passive lengthening of muscle	Reproduces patient's symptoms	Reduced range Increased resistance Decreased resistance
Palpation of muscle	Reproduces patient's symptoms	Tenderness
Reassessment following therapeutic dose of muscle treatment	Improvement in tests which reproduce patient's symptoms	No change in physical tests which reproduce patient's symptoms
Nerve		
Passive lengthening and sensitising movement, i.e. altering length of nerve by a movement at a distance from patient's symptoms	Reproduces patient's symptoms and sensitising movement alters patient's symptoms	Reduced length Increased resistance
Palpation of nerve	Reproduces patient's symptoms	Tenderness

around the area. Collectively, this evidence would suggest there is a joint dysfunction, as long as this is accompanied by negative muscle and nerve tests.

Weaker evidence includes an alteration in range, resistance or quality of physiological and/or accessory movements and tenderness over the joint, with no alteration in signs and symptoms after treatment. One or more of these findings may indicate a dysfunction of a joint which may or may not be contributing to the patient's condition.

The strongest evidence that a muscle is the source of a patient's symptoms is if active movements, an isometric contraction, passive lengthening and palpation of a muscle all reproduce the patient's symptoms, and that, following a treatment dose, reassessment identifies an improvement in the patient's signs and symptoms. For example, let us assume that a patient has lateral elbow pain caused by lateral epicondylalgia, a primary muscle problem. In this case reproduction of the lateral elbow pain is found on active wrist and finger extension, isometric contraction of the wrist extensors and/or finger extensors, and passive lengthening of the extensor muscles to the wrist and hand. These signs and symptoms are found to improve following soft-tissue mobilisation examination, sufficient to be considered a treatment dose. Collectively, this evidence would suggest that there is a muscle dysfunction, as long as this is accompanied by negative joint and nerve tests.

Further evidence of muscle dysfunction may be suggested by reduced strength or poor quality during the active physiological movement and the isometric contraction, reduced range and/or increased/decreased resistance, during the passive lengthening of the muscle, and tenderness on palpation, with no alteration in signs and symptoms after treatment. One or more of these findings may indicate a dysfunction of a muscle which may or may not be contributing to the patient's condition.

The strongest evidence that a nerve is the source of the patient's symptoms is when active and/or passive physiological movements reproduce the symptoms, which are then increased or decreased with an additional sensitising movement, at a distance from the patient's symptoms. In addition, there is reproduction of the patient's symptoms on palpation of the nerve and neurodynamic testing, sufficient to be considered a treatment dose, results in an improvement in the above signs and symptoms. For example, let us assume this time that the lateral elbow pain is caused by a neurodynamic dysfunction of the radial nerve supplying this region. The patient's lateral elbow pain is reproduced during the component movements of ULNT 2b and is eased with ipsilateral cervical lateral flexion sensitising movement. There is tenderness over the radial groove in the upper arm and testing of ULNT 2b, sufficient to be considered a treatment dose, results in an improvement in the patient's signs and symptoms. Collectively, this evidence would suggest there is a neurodynamic dysfunction, as long as this is accompanied by negative joint and muscle tests. Further evidence of nerve dysfunction may be suggested by reduced range

(compared with the asymptomatic side) and/or increased resistance to the various arm movements, and tenderness on nerve palpation.

It can be seen that the common factor for identifying joint, nerve and muscle dysfunction as a source of the patient's symptoms is the reproduction of the patient's symptoms, the alteration in the patient's signs and symptoms following a treatment dose and the lack of evidence from other potential sources of symptoms. It is assumed that, if a test reproduces a patient's symptoms, then it is somehow stressing the structure at fault. As mentioned earlier, each test is not purely a test of one structure; every test, to a greater or lesser degree, involves all structures. For this reason, it is imperative that the treatment given proves its value by altering the patient's signs and symptoms. The other factor common in identifying joint, nerve or muscle dysfunction is the lack of positive findings in the other possible tissues; for example, a joint dysfunction is considered when joint tests are positive and muscle and nerve tests are negative. Thus the clinician collects evidence to implicate tissues and evidence to negate tissues: both are equally important.

Clinicians may find the treatment and management planning form shown in Figure 3.51 helpful in guiding them through what is often a complex clinical reasoning process. Figure 3.52 is a more advanced clinical reasoning form for more indepth analysis.

On completion of the physical examination the clinician:

- explains to the patient the findings of the physical examination and how these findings relate to the subjective assessment. Any misconceptions patients may have regarding their symptoms should be cleared up here.
- warns the patient of possible exacerbation up to 24–48 hours following the examination. With severe and/or irritable conditions, the patient may have increased symptoms following examination.
- requests the patient to report details on the behaviour of the symptoms following examination at the next attendance.
- evaluates the findings, formulates a clinical hypothesis and writes up a problem list, i.e. a concise numbered list of the patient's problems at the time of the examination. Signs and symptoms of patellofemoral dysfunction, for example, could include pain over the knee and difficulty ascending and descending stairs, inhibition of vastus medialis

What subjective and physical reassessment asterisks will you use?	
Subjective	Physical

What is your treatment plan for the:	
Source of symptoms	Contributing factors

What are your goals for discharge?

Figure 3.51 • Management planning form (to be completed after the physical examination). (After Maitland 1985.)

oblique, tightness of the iliotibial band and hamstring muscle group, and lateral tilt and external rotation of the patella. More general problems, such as lack of general fitness or coping behaviour, should also be included.

• determines the long- and short-term objectives for each problem in consultation with the patient. Short-term objectives for the above example might be relief of some of the knee pain,

increased contraction of vastus medialis oblique, increased extensibility of the iliotibial band and hamstrings, and correction of patellar malalignment by the end of the third treatment session. The long-term objective might be complete resolution of the patient's problem after six treatment sessions.

• through discussion with the patient devises an initial treatment plan in order to achieve the short- and long-term objectives. This includes the modalities and frequency of treatment and any patient education required. In the patellofemoral example, this might be treatment which may include passive stretches to the iliotibial band and hamstrings; passive accessory movements to the patella; taping to correct the patellar malalignment; and exercises with biofeedback to alter the timing and intensity of vastus medialis oblique contraction in squat standing, progressing to steps and specific functional exercises and activities.

By the end of the physical examination the clinician will have further developed the hypotheses categories initiated in the subjective examination (adapted from Jones & Rivett 2004).

In this way, the clinician will have developed the following hypotheses categories (adapted from Jones & Rivett 2004):

1.1 Source of symptoms

Symptomatic area	Structures under area	Structures which can refer to area	Supporting evidence

1.2 What is the mechanism of each symptom?
Explain from information from the subjective and physical examination findings

	Symptom	Symptom	Symptom	Symptom
Subjective				
Physical				

Figure 3.52 • Clinical reasoning form.

(Continued)

1.3 Following the physical examination, what is your clinical diagnosis?

2. Contributing factors

2.1 What factors need to be examined/explored in the physical examination?

2.2 How will you address each contributing factor?

3. Precautions and contraindications

3.1 Are any symptoms severe?   Yes   No
     Which symptoms, and explain why

3.2 Are any symptoms irritable?   Yes   No
     Which symptoms, and explain why

Figure 3.52—cont'd.

(Continued)

3.3 How much of each symptom are you prepared to provoke in the physical examination?

Symptom	Short of P$_1$	Point of onset or increase in resting symptoms	Partial reproduction	Total reproduction

3.4 Will a neurological examination be necessary in the physical?

           Yes   No   Explain why

3.5 Following the subjective examination, are there any precautions or contraindications?

           Yes   No   Explain why

4. Management

4.1 What tests will you do in the physical and what are the expected findings?

Physical tests	Expected findings

Figure 3.52—cont'd.

(Continued)

4.2   Were there any unexpected findings from the physical? Explain

4.3   What will be your subjective and physical reassessment asterisks?

4.4   What is your first choice of treatment (be exact) and explain why?

4.5   What do you expect the response to be over the next 24 hours following the 1st visit? Explain

4.6   How do you think you will treat and manage the patient at the 2nd visit, if the patient returns:

Same

Better

Worse

4.7   What advice and education will you give the patient?

Figure 3.52—cont'd.

(Continued)

4.8 What needs to be examined on the 2nd and 3rd visits?

2nd visit	3rd visit

5. Prognosis

5.1 List the positive and negative factors (from both the subjective and physical examination findings) in considering the patient's prognosis

	Positive	Negative
Subjective		
Physical		

5.2 Overall, is the patient's condition:

    Improving   Worsening   Static

5.3 What is your overall prognosis for this patient? Be specific

Figure 3.52—cont'd.

(Continued)

- activity capability/restriction/participant capability/restriction
- patients' perspectives on their experience
- pathobiological mechanisms, including the structure or tissue that is thought to be producing the patient's symptoms and the nature of the structure or tissues in relation to both the healing process and the pain mechanisms

- physical impairments and associated structures/tissue sources
- contributing factors to the development and maintenance of the problem; there may be environmental, psychosocial, behavioural, physical or heredity factors
- precautions/contraindications to treatment and management; this includes the severity and

6. After 3rd attendance

6.1 Has your understanding of the patient's problem changed from your interpretations made following the initial subjective and physical examination? If so, explain
6.2 On reflection, were there any clues that you initially missed, misinterpreted, under- or over-weighted? If so, explain

7. After discharge

7.1 Has your understanding of the patient's problem changed from your interpretations made following the 3rd attendance? If so, explain how
7.2 What have you learnt from the management of this patient which will be helpful to you in the future?

Figure 3.52—cont'd.

irritability of the patient's symptoms and the nature of the patient's condition
- management strategy and treatment plan
- prognosis – this can be affected by factors such as the stage and extent of the injury as well as the patient's expectation, personality and lifestyle.

For further information on treatment and management of patients with neuromusculoskeletal dysfunction, please see the companion to this text: *Principles of Neuromusculoskeletal Treatment and Management* (Petty 2011).

References

Alshami, A.M., Souvlis, T., Coppieters, M.W., 2008. A review of plantar heel pain of neural origin: differential diagnosis and management. Man. Ther. 13, 103–111.

American Academy of Orthopaedic Surgeons, 1990. Joint motion. Method of measuring and recording, third ed. Churchill Livingstone, New York.

Amevo, B., Aprill, C., Bogduk, N., 1992. Abnormal instantaneous axes of rotation in patients with neck pain. Spine 17, 748–756.

Baldry, P.E., 1993. Acupuncture, trigger points and musculoskeletal pain. Churchill Livingstone, Edinburgh.

Beighton, P.H., Solomon, l., Soskolne, C.L., 1973. Articular mobility in an African population. Ann. Rheum. Dis. 32, 413–418.

Bergmark, A., 1989. Stability of the lumbar spine. A study in mechanical engineering. Acta Orthop. Scand. 230 (Suppl.), 20–24.

Breig, A., 1978. Adverse mechanical tension in the central nervous system. Almqvist and Wiksell, Stockholm.

Butler, D.S., 2000. The sensitive nervous system. Neuro Orthopaedic Institute, Adelaide.

Cole, J.H., Furness, A.L., Twomey, L.T., 1988. Muscles in action: an approach to manual muscle testing. Churchill Livingstone, Edinburgh.

Comerford, M., Kinetic Control, 2000. Movement dysfunction focus on dynamic stability and muscle balance. Kinetic Control course notes.

Comerford, M., Mottram, S., 2001. Movement and stability dysfunction – contemporary developments. Man. Ther. 6, 15–26.

Coppieters, M.W., Alshami, A.M., Babri, A., et al., 2006. Strain and excursion of the sciatic, tibial and plantar nerves during a modified straight leg raising test. J. Orthop. Res. 24, 1883–1889.

Crawford, G.N.C., 1973. The growth of striated muscle immobilized in extension. J. Anat. 114, 165–183.

Cyriax, J., 1982. Textbook of orthopaedic medicine – diagnosis of soft tissue lesions, eighth ed. Baillière Tindall, London.

Drake, R.L., Vogl, W., Mitchell, A.W.M., 2005. Gray's anatomy for students. Churchill Livingstone, Philadelphia.

Dyck, P., 1984. Lumbar nerve root: the enigmatic eponyms. Spine 9, 3–6.

Edwards, B.C., 1992. Manual of combined movements: their use in the examination and treatment of mechanical vertebral column disorders. Churchill Livingstone, Edinburgh.

Edwards, B.C., 1999. Manual of combined movements: their use in the examination and treatment of mechanical vertebral column disorders, second ed. Butterworth-Heinemann, Oxford.

Elvey, R.L., 1985. Brachial plexus tension tests and the pathoanatomical origin of arm pain. In: Glasgow, E.F., Twomey, L.T., Scull, E.R. et al., (Eds.), Aspects of manipulative therapy, second ed. Churchill Livingstone, Melbourne, p. 116.

Exelby, L., 1996. Peripheral mobilisations with movement. Man. Ther. 1, 118–126.

Frankel, V.H., Burstein, A.H., Brooks, D.B., 1971. Biomechanics of internal derangement of the knee. Pathomechanics as determined by analysis of the instant centres of motion. J. Bone Joint Surg. 53A, 945–962.

Fuller, G., 2004. Neurological examination made easy. Churchill Livingstone, Edinburgh.

Gerhardt, J.J., 1992. Documentation of joint motion, third ed. Isomed, Oregon.

Gilmore, K.L., 1986. Biomechanics of the lumbar motion segment. In: Grieve, G.P. (Ed.), Modern manual therapy of the vertebral column. Churchill Livingstone, Edinburgh, p. 103.

Gossman, M.R., Sahrmann, S.A., Rose, S.J., 1982. Review of length-associated changes in muscle. Phys. Ther. 62, 1799–1808.

Grahame, R., Bird, H.A., Child, A., et al., 2000. The revised (Brighton 1998) criteria for the diagnosis of benign joint hypermobility syndrome (BJHS). J. Rheumatol. 27, 1777–1779.

Grieve, G.P., 1981. Common vertebral joint problems. Churchill Livingstone, Edinburgh.

Grieve, G.P., 1991. Mobilisation of the spine, fifth ed. Churchill Livingstone, Edinburgh.

Harding, V., Williams, A.C. de C., Richardson, P., et al., 1994. The development of a battery of measures for assessing physical functioning in chronic pain patients. Pain 58, 367–375.

Hides, J.A., Richardson, C.A., Jull, G.A., 1996. Multifidus muscle recovery is not automatic after resolution of acute, first-episode low back pain. Spine 21, 2763–2769.

Hislop, H., Montgomery, J., 1995. Daniels and Worthingham's muscle testing: techniques of manual examination, seventh ed. W B Saunders, Philadelphia.

Hockaday, J.M., Whitty, C.W.M., 1967. Patterns of referred pain in the normal subject. Brain 90, 481–496.

Hodges, P., 1995. Dysfunction of transversus abdominis associated with chronic low back pain. In: Proceedings of the Manipulative Physiotherapists Association of Australia, 9th biennial conference, Gold Coast, pp. 61–62.

Hodges, P.W., Richardson, C.A., 1996. Inefficient muscular stabilisation of the lumbar spine associated with low back pain, a motor control evaluation of transversus abdominis. Spine 21, 2640–2650.

Hunter, G., 1998. Specific soft tissue mobilization in the management of soft tissue dysfunction. Man. Ther. 3, 2–11.

Hunter, J.M. (Ed.), 2002. Rehabilitation of the hand and upper extremity, fifth ed. Mosby, St Louis.

Inman, V.T., Saunders, J.B. de C.M., 1944. Referred pain from skeletal structures. J. Nerv. Ment. Dis. 90, 660–667.

Janda, V., 1986. Muscle weakness and inhibition (pseudoparesis) in back pain syndromes. In: Grieve, G.P. (Ed.), Modern manual therapy of the vertebral column. Churchill Livingstone, Edinburgh, p. 197.

Janda, V., 1993. Muscle strength in relation to muscle length, pain and muscle imbalance. In: Harms-Ringdahl, K. (Ed.), Muscle strength. Churchill Livingstone, Edinburgh, p. 83.

Janda, V., 1994. Muscles and motor control in cervicogenic disorders: assessment and management. In: Grant, R. (Ed.), Physical therapy of the cervical and thoracic spine, second ed. Churchill Livingstone, Edinburgh, p. 195.

Janda, V., 2002. Muscles and motor control in cervicogenic disorders. In: Grant, R. (Ed.), Physical therapy of the cervical and thoracic spine, third ed. Churchill Livingstone, New York, p. 182.

Jones, M.A., Jones, H.M., 1994. Principles of the physical examination. In: Boyling, J.D., Palastanga, N. (Eds.), Grieve's modern manual therapy, second ed. Churchill Livingstone, Edinburgh, p. 491.

Jones, M.A., Rivett, D.A., 2004. Clinical reasoning for manual therapists. Butterworth-Heinemann, Edinburgh.

Jull, G.A., 1994. Examination of the articular system. In: Boyling, J.D., Palastanga, N. (Eds.), Grieve's modern manual therapy, second ed. Churchill Livingstone, Edinburgh, p. 511.

Jull, G.A., Janda, V., 1987. Muscles and motor control in low back pain: assessment and management. In: Twomey, L.T., Taylor, J.R. (Eds.), Physical therapy of the low back. Churchill Livingstone, Edinburgh, p. 253.

Jull, G.A., Richardson, C.A., 1994. Rehabilitation of active stabilization of the lumbar spine. In: Twomey, L.T., Taylor, J.R. (Eds.), Physical therapy of the low back. second ed. Churchill Livingstone, Edinburgh, p. 251.

Kaltenborn, F.M., 2002. Manual mobilization of the joints, vol I. The extremities, sixth ed. Olaf Norli, Oslo.

Kaltenborn, F.M., 2003. Manual mobilization of the joints, vol II. The spine, fourth ed. Olaf Norli, Oslo.

Kaltenborn, F.M., Evjenth, O., 1989. Manual mobilisation of the extremity joints: basis examination and treatment techniques, fourth ed. Olaf Norlis Bokhandel, Universitetsgaten, Sydney.

Kazarian, L., 1972. Dynamic response characteristics of the human vertebral column. Acta Orthop. Scand. 146, 54–117.

Kendall, F.P., McCreary, E.K., Provance, P.G., 1993. Muscles: testing and function, fourth ed. Lippincott, Williams & Wilkins, Baltimore.

Kenneally, M., Rubenach, H., Elvey, R., 1988. The upper limb tension test: the SLR test of the arm. In: Grant, R. (Ed.), Physical therapy of the cervical and thoracic spine. Churchill Livingstone, Edinburgh, p. 167.

Leak, S., 1998. Measurement of physiotherapists' ability to reliably generate vibration amplitudes and pressures using a tuning fork. Man. Ther. 3, 90–94.

Lee, R., Evans, J., 1994. Towards a better understanding of spinal posteroanterior mobilisation. Physiotherapy 80, 68–73.

Lee, M., Svensson, N.L., 1990. Measurement of stiffness during simulated spinal physiotherapy. Clin. Phys. Physiol. Meas. 11, 201–207.

Lewit, K., 1991. Manipulative therapy in rehabilitation of the locomotor system, second ed. Butterworth-Heinemann, Oxford.

Magee, D.J., 2006. Orthopedic physical assessment, fourth ed. Saunders Elsevier, Philadelphia.

Maitland, G.D., 1977. Vertebral manipulation, fourth ed. Butterworths, London.

Maitland, G.D., 1985. Passive movement techniques for intra-articular and periarticular disorders. Aust. J. Physiother. 31, 3–8.

Maitland, G.D., 1991. Peripheral manipulation, third ed. Butterworths, London.

Maitland, G.D., Hengeveld, E., Banks, K., et al., 2001. Maitland's vertebral manipulation, sixth ed. Butterworth-Heinemann, Oxford.

Maitland, G.D., Hengeveld, E., Banks, K., 2005. Maitland's peripheral manipulation, fourth ed. Elsevier, Edinburgh.

Margarey, M., 1985. Selection of passive treatment techniques. In: Proceedings of the Manipulative Therapists Association of Australia, 4th biennial conference, Brisbane, pp. 298–320.

Mariani, P.P., Caruso, I., 1979. An electromyographic investigation of subluxation of the patella. J. Bone Joint Surg. 61B, 169–171.

McKenzie, R.A., 1981. The lumbar spine: mechanical diagnosis and therapy. Spinal Publications, New Zealand.

McKenzie, R.A., 1990. The cervical and thoracic spine: mechanical diagnosis and therapy. Spinal Publications, New Zealand.

McKenzie R.A., May S., 2003. The Lumbar Spine: Mechanical Diagnosis and Therapy. (Vols. 1 and 2) Spinal Publications, Waikanae, New Zealand; 2nd Edition.

McKenzie R., and May S., 2006. The Cervical and Thoracic Spine: Mechanical Diagnosis and Therapy. volume 1. Spinal Publications, Waikanae, New Zealand.

Medical Research Council, 1976. Aids to the investigation of peripheral nerve injuries. HMSO, London.

Mercer, S.R., Jull, G.A., 1996. Morphology of the cervical intervertebral disc: implications for McKenzie's model of the disc derangement syndrome. Man. Ther. 1, 76–81.

Miller, A.M., 1987. Neuro-meningeal limitation of straight leg raising. In: Dalziel, B.A., Snowsill, J.C. (Eds.), Manipulative Therapists Association of Australia, 5th biennial conference proceedings, Melbourne, pp. 70–78.

Mooney, V., Robertson, J., 1976. The facet syndrome. Clin. Orthop. Relat. Res. 115, 149–156.

Mulligan, B.R., 1993. Mobilisations with movement (MWMs). J. Man. Manip. Ther. 1, 154–156.

Mulligan, B.R., 1999. Manual therapy 'NAGs', 'SNAGs', 'MWMs' etc., fourth ed. Plane View Services, New Zealand.

Newham, D.J., 2001. Strength, power and endurance. In: Trew, M., Everett, T. (Eds.), Human movement, fourth ed. Churchill Livingstone, Edinburgh, p. 105.

Nir-Paz, R., Luder, A.S., Cozacov, J.C., 1999. Saphenous nerve entrapment in adolescence. Paediatrics 103, 161–163.

Norris, C.M., 1995. Spinal stabilisation, muscle imbalance and the low back. Physiotherapy 81 (3), 127–138.

Noyes, F.R., Delucas, J.L., Torvik, P.J., 1974. Biomechanics of anterior cruciate ligament failure: an analysis of strain-rate sensitivity and mechanisms of failure in primates. J. Bone Joint Surg. 56A, 236–253.

Panjabi, M.M., 1992. The stabilising system of the spine: part II. Neutral zone and instability hypothesis. J. Spinal. Disord. 5, 390–396.

Pennal, G.F., Conn, G.S., McDonald, G., et al., 1972. Motion studies of the lumbar spine, a preliminary report. J. Bone Joint Surg. 54B, 442–452.

Petty, N.J., 2011. Principles of neuromusculoskeletal treatment and management: a guide for therapists, second ed. Churchill Livingstone, Edinburgh.

Petty, N.J., Maher, C., Latimer, J., et al., 2002. Manual examination of accessory movements – seeking R1. Man. Ther. 7, 39–43.

Richardson, C., Hodges, P.W., Hides, J., 2004. Therapeutic exercise for lumbopelvic stabilization. A motor control approach for the treatment and prevention of low back pain, second ed. Churchill Livingstone, Edinburgh.

Sahrmann, S.A., 1993. Diagnosis and treatment of movement system imbalances associated with musculoskeletal pain. Lecture notes. Washington University School of Medicine, Washington.

Sahrmann, S.A., 2001. Diagnosis and treatment of movement impairment syndromes. Mosby, St Louis.

Shacklock, M., 2005. Clinical neurodynamics. Churchill Livingstone, Edinburgh.

Shah, J.S., Hampson, W.G.J., Jayson, M.I.V., 1978. The distribution of surface strain in the cadaveric lumbar spine. J. Bone Joint Surg. 60B, 246–251.

Shorland, S., 1998. Management of chronic pain following whiplash injuries. In: Gifford, L. (Ed.), Topical issues in pain. NOI, Falmouth, pp. 115–134.

Simmonds, J.V., Keer, R.J., 2007. Hypermobility and the hypermobility syndrome. Man. Ther. 12, 298–309.

Slater, H., 1994. The dynamic nervous system. Examination and assessment using tension tests. In: Boyling, J.D., Palastanga, N. (Eds.), Grieve's modern manual therapy, second ed. Churchill Livingstone, Edinburgh.

Stokes, M., Young, A., 1986. Measurement of quadriceps cross-sectional area by ultrasonography: a description of the technique and its application in physiotherapy. Physiother. Theory Pract. 2, 31–36.

Sweetham, B.J., Anderson, J.A., Dalton, E.R., 1974. The relationships between little finger mobility, lumbar mobility straight leg raising and low back pain. Rheumatol. Rehabil. 13, 161–168.

Tencer, A.F., Allen, B.L., Ferguson, R.L., 1985. A biomechanical study of thoracolumbar spine fractures with bone in the canal: part III. Mechanical properties of the dura and its tethering ligaments. Spine 10, 741–747.

Travell, J.G., Simons, D.G., 1983. Myofascial pain and dysfunction: the trigger point manual. Williams & Wilkins, Baltimore.

Voight, M.L., Wieder, D.L., 1991. Comparative reflex response times of vastus medialis obliquus and vastus lateralis in normal subjects and subjects with extensor mechanism dysfunction. Am. J. Sports Med. 19, 131–137.

Walton, J.H., 1989. Essentials of neurology, sixth ed. Churchill Livingstone, Edinburgh.

White, S.G., Sahrmann, S.A., 1994. A movement system balance approach to musculoskeletal pain. In: Grant, R. (Ed.), Physical therapy of the cervical and thoracic spine, second ed. Churchill Livingstone, Edinburgh, p. 339.

Williams, P.L., Bannister, L.H., Berry, M.M., et al., (Eds.), 1995. Gray's anatomy, thirty-eighth ed. Edinburgh, Churchill Livingstone.

Yaxley, G.A., Jull, G.A., 1993. Adverse tension in the neural system. A preliminary study of tennis elbow. Aust. J. Physiother. 39, 15–22.

Young, A., Hughes, I., Round, J.M., et al., 1982. The effect of knee injury on the number of muscle fibres in the human quadriceps femoris. Clin. Sci. 62, 227–234.

Zusman, M., 1998. Structure orientated beliefs and disability due to back pain. Aust. J. Physiother. 44, 13–20.

Assessment

4

Laura Finucane

CHAPTER CONTENTS

The previous chapters described the clinical reasoning and assessment process within the step-by-step subjective and physical examination processes. Each aspect of the subjective and physical examination was explained in a bottom-up approach. This text uses a top-down approach, that is, the information is organised according to final decision-making prior to starting treatment. It is hoped that, taken together, the three chapters will provide an explicit account of the broad clinical reasoning process that leads to the treatment and management of patients with neuromusculoskeletal dysfunction.

The word 'assessment' is used to denote the analysis, or interpretation, of the examination findings by the clinician (Box 4.1). At the patient's first appointment, the subjective and physical examination is used, in part, to gather information about the patient. Assessment is the interpretation of this information and is used to guide the clinician in the treatment and management of the patient. Assessment is, in essence, the problem-solving and decision-making process involved in clinical practice and it can be referred to as clinical reasoning. Assessment and treatment are used together in every appointment the patient has with the clinician and can be depicted as shown in Figure 4.1. Only through assessment can the clinician decide on meaningful treatment, and the quality of treatment given will be directly related to the quality of assessment. To quote Maitland et al. (2005, p. 55): 'assessment is the keystone of effective, informative treatment, without which treatment successes and treatment failures lose all value as learning experiences. Like the keystone, assessment is at the summit of treatment, locking the whole together'. The subject of clinical reasoning as well as expertise is an expanding field and the reader is referred to two excellent texts: Higgs & Jones (2000) and Jensen et al. (1999).

With every piece of information gathered from the subjective and physical examination the clinician will make immediate judgements about the patient. Such judgements may or may not be correct. While a high level of expertise may enable a clinician to make correct judgements, and as a consequence provide effective and efficient care of the patient, there is also the possibility of error, leading to ineffective and inefficient care. An analogy may help to clarify this point. The process of examination and assessment is very similar to the work of a police detective. Let us assume that a man has been murdered. Statistically, the wife is the most likely murderer. On questioning the woman, the lack of an alibi and the fact that she had just had an argument with her husband may be sufficient evidence for an inexperienced detective to consider her guilty. Once this hypothesis has been made, the detective continues the

Box 4.1

Assessment is the analysis, or interpretation, of the examination findings by the clinician

Assessment ←——————————→ Treatment

Figure 4.1 • Relationship of assessment and treatment. (World Health Organisation 2001 International classification of functioning, disability and health. World Health Organisation, Geneva. http://www.who.int/classifications/icf/en/)

investigation, looking for information to support the hypothesis, and either not recognising or ignoring the evidence that would negate this hypothesis. In other words, the detective believes that the woman is guilty and is seeking evidence to support this belief. The consequence is that this woman may be wrongly convicted of murder. An experienced detective has a more open mind and acknowledges the lack of an alibi and the argument with the husband, and treats these aspects with suspicion by following this line of enquiry, but does not make the error of believing that these two pieces of information prove that the woman is guilty. This detective seeks out all the other possibilities, however unlikely. Every avenue must be fully explored, and substantial amounts of evidence must be collected to prove the guilt and, as importantly, to disprove the guilt, of every possible suspect. The assumption that the detective must make is that everyone is guilty until proven innocent. Compare this with a clinical situation: a patient presents with knee pain, the clinician collects information to identify a lateral ligament sprain of the knee and collects information to clarify that the pain in the knee is not coming from the spine or hip, and that it is not a muscle problem or a tibiofemoral or patellofemoral joint problem. In this way, during the examination the clinician explores all possible structures that could be a source of the patient's symptoms, and only once these structures have been seriously and fully explored can the clinician decide that they are not a source of the patient's symptoms (Box 4.2). Jones (1994) refers to this as the clinician developing 'multiple diagnostic hypotheses' and an 'evolving concept of the patient's problem'.

Clinical reasoning, clinical mileage and clinical expertise are essential in determining the amount and nature of evidence required to dismiss a structure as a possible source of the patient's symptoms. The clinical presentation of some patients will, of course, be very straightforward. For example, a patient may be referred following a Colles fracture and 6 weeks of immobilisation; in this instance the patient simply needs local rehabilitation of the forearm, wrist and hand; or a patient may be referred with a simple lateral ligament sprain of the ankle and, again, straightforward rehabilitation is all that is necessary. In these cases very little hunting for the source of the patient's symptoms is required. In cases of acute injury such as a sprained ankle, early treatment, not examination (on the first day of attendance), would be the priority. There are, however, a large number of patients who do not have a straightforward presentation. In these situations it is imperative that the clinician has a clear and logical strategy for examining and assessing the patient. This chapter attempts to make this strategy explicit.

The initial appointment will usually consist of a subjective examination and a physical examination and these have been more fully described in Chapters 2 and 3.

It cannot be emphasised enough that the subjective examination is a critical part of the overall examination (Box 4.3). The reason why this aspect of the subjective examination is reiterated here is that it is the subjective examination that decides the direction that the physical examination will follow and the procedures to be carried out and is therefore a vital decision in the overall examination process.

In order for the clinician to make the right decisions s/he needs to develop a rapport with the patient that will, among other things, enable the clinician to obtain an accurate and comprehensive understanding of the patient's problem. In order to do this the clinician needs a high level of skill in communication, which includes verbal, non-verbal and listening skills, as well as a thorough understanding of what needs to be asked and why.

The subjective examination clarifies the relative importance of various possible structures that could

Box 4.2

All possible structures that could be a source of the patient's symptoms need to be explored and excluded

Box 4.3

The subjective examination is a critical part of the overall examination be a source of the patient's symptoms. For example, a clinician may decide that the patient has a local problem around the knee and that this region is all that needs to be examined in the physical. In this case, clarifying that the patient has no symptoms in the lumbar spine, sacroiliac joint or hip region may provide sufficient evidence to satisfy the clinician that these regions do not need to be examined in the physical. If this evidence is going to be so influential as to negate physical examination of these regions, the clinician must be certain that they have been fully explored. For example, to enquire casually of the patient whether s/he has any pain in these regions is totally inadequate. If this is done, the patient may quietly dismiss a slight ache or stiffness and respond negatively, thus giving the clinician inaccurate information. The physical examination may then focus on inappropriate testing procedures. Rather than a casual enquiry about pain in these regions, it is suggested that the clinician asks the patient, in a deliberate way, 'do you have any pain or stiffness here (lumbar spine, or sacroiliac joint or hip)?', 'nothing at all?' Having obtained and double-checked the answer, and on some occasions triple-checked the answer, the clinician can now be satisfied that the patient has been given every opportunity to tell him or her about even the slightest symptom in that region which may be relevant to the patient's problem.

Inexperienced clinicians will be surprised how often the patient initially will negate any pain in an area, but when this is checked again, will say 'yes, actually it does sometimes ache a bit'. Establishing the relationship between structures will be required at this stage as the subjective examination will not readily separate out geographically close structures. For example, the clinician may suspect that a patient with pain over the lumbar spine, posterior superior iliac spine and groin has a lumbar spine, sacroiliac and/or hip problem. Information about the behaviour of the symptoms, functional limitations, 24-hour behaviour and recent history will probably not clarify for the clinician how much s/he needs to explore the lumbar spine, sacroiliac joint and hip region. The structures lie so close together that movement in one region will produce movement in the other region, and so distinctions are not easily made. The same is true of the cervical spine, scapular thoracic and shoulder regions. However, where a patient has back pain, and knee or foot pain, or neck pain, and elbow or hand pain, a clearer distinction may be able to be made between the regions. For

example, a patient may have had neck pain for 20 years, neck movements feel slightly sore with no pain in the wrist and the neck pain may have remained the same since the wrist was injured. The wrist pain may have come on recently, with simple active wrist movements producing the pain; this scenario would suggest two separate problems and the clinician could decide to look only at the wrist region on the first attendance. Any hint, however, in the subjective (or physical) examination that the wrist pain is being referred from the cervical spine will require examination of the spine.

By the end of the subjective examination the clinician should know:

- what physical examination procedures need to be carried out
- how the physical procedures should be carried out, in terms of symptom production
- of any precautions or contraindications to the physical examination or, later on, with treatment
- what other factors that might be contributing to the patient's symptoms need to be examined.

This information helps the clinician to plan the physical examination and this can be formalised using a physical examination planning form (Figure 4.2).

Once the testing procedures are decided, the physical examination simply requires the clinician to carry out those tests. Of course, the tests need to be evaluated, and modifications to the physical examination may need to be made. This point is made very well by Jones & Jones (1994), who state that 'the physical examination is not simply the indiscriminate application of routine tests'

Following the physical examination, the clinician is able to discuss with the patient the plan for treatment and management (Figure 4.3). The treatment and management must be patient-centred if it is to be successful and this requires the patient to take an active part in the planning through mutual decision-making (Higgs & Jones 2000).

Developing hypotheses

Following completion of the subjective and physical examinations of a patient, the clinician must decide on a number of hypotheses (Jones & Jones 1994). These include:

- source of the symptoms and/or dysfunction. This includes the structure(s) at fault and the mechanism of symptom production

	Symptom	Symptom	Symptom	Symptom
Is it severe?				
Is it irritable?				
Will you move: – short of production? – point of onset/increase in resting symptoms? – partial reproduction? – total reproduction?				
How will you reproduce symptom: – repeat? – alter speed? – combine? – sustain? – other? (state)				

Are there any precautions or contraindications? State   Yes   No
What other factors contributing to the patient's symptom(s) need to be examined?

Figure 4.2 • Physical examination planning form.

- factors contributing to the condition, be they environmental, behavioural, emotional, physical or biomechanical factors
- precautions or contraindications to physical examination and/or treatment
- prognosis of the condition
- plan of management of the patient's condition.

Clinicians may find it helpful to complete the more indepth clinical reasoning form of the overall management of the patient, shown in the Appendix, to help them identify these categories of hypotheses.

Developing each of these hypotheses requires the clinician to consider information from various aspects of the subjective and physical examination findings. There is never one piece of information from the subjective examination, or one test from the physical examination, that will fully develop any one of the above hypotheses. Rather, it is the weight of evidence, from a number of aspects from the subjective examination and physical examination, that enables the clinician to make a hypothesis. Ideally, all aspects of the subjective and physical examination findings should come together, logically, to formulate a hypothesis; that is, the clinician is 'making features fit' (Maitland et al. 2005, p. 57). Where this is not possible it may prompt the clinician for alternative

What subjective and physical reassessment asterisks will you use?

Subjective	Physical

What is your treatment plan for the:

Source of symptoms	Contributing factors

What are your goals for discharge?

Figure 4.3 • Treatment and management planning form.

explanations; for example, perhaps underlying the patient's problems there is a serious pathology which may require medical investigation. The information from the subjective and physical examinations, which may inform each category of hypothesis, is given below.

Source of the symptoms and/or dysfunction

The priority of day 1 examination is often to identify the source of the patient's symptoms. The word 'source' is used here in its widest sense, whether

Box 4.4

If the patient's symptoms are reproduced with a movement test, the structures being stressed are implicated as a potential source of symptoms

Box 4.5

If an abnormality is detected in a structure, which theoretically could refer symptoms to the symptomatic area, then that structure is suspected to be a source of the symptoms

there is an affective, physical, central or autonomic cause. The ability to identify the source of the patient's symptoms may, however, not always be possible. For example, a patient with an acute injury may not be able to be fully examined; in this situation the examination will occur over a period of time as the acute state settles.

There are two underlying assumptions used in the identification of the source of the symptoms. The first is that, if the patient's exact symptoms are reproduced when a structure is stressed, the symptoms are thought to arise from that structure (Box 4.4). The word 'exact' means that the quality or 'feel' to the patient is the symptom of which s/he is complaining, which is wholly or partially reproduced by a test. The difficulty with this, of course, is that there are no functional movements or physical testing procedures which stress individual structures. Active hip flexion, when climbing stairs for example, involves hip joint movement, isotonic activity of the muscles around the hip, alteration in length of the femoral and sciatic nerve, posterior pelvic tilt and knee flexion. It is therefore difficult to identify, with any movement, which structure is at fault and producing the patient's symptoms. Similarly, in the physical examination, hip flexion in supine alters the:

- lumbar spine (moved into flexion)
- sacroiliac joint (moved with posterior pelvic rotation and a shear force due to the weight of the thigh)
- hip joint (moved into end-range flexion)
- extensor muscles of hip and knee flexors (lengthened)
- sciatic nerve (lengthened).

If posterior thigh pain is produced on hip flexion overpressure, the clinician cannot be certain which of the above structures is producing this pain. Further testing, and in particular differentiation testing, is necessary to try to tease out which of the above structures is provoking the pain; for example, adding knee extension would increase the length of the sciatic nerve and hamstring muscle group and increase the longitudinal force through the femur

to the hip joint. Further differentiation could be achieved by the addition of ankle dorsiflexion, which would increase the length of the sciatic nerve without changing hamstring length or altering hip joint compression. If symptoms are increased with knee extension and dorsiflexion, this would suggest the sciatic nerve as the source of the symptoms; if symptoms are not altered with dorsiflexion this implicates the hamstring muscles or the hip joint. Isometric testing of the hamstring muscles and muscle palpation may then help to implicate the hamstring muscle group. In addition, negative physical testing procedures would be required to negate the other possible structures at fault, that is, the lumbar spine, sacroiliac joint, hip joint and other posterior hip muscles.

The second assumption, in identifying the source of the symptoms, is that if an abnormality is detected in a structure, which theoretically could refer symptoms to the symptomatic area, then that structure is suspected to be a source of the symptoms (Box 4.5). For example, if a patient has pain over the inner aspect of the forearm, wrist, and into the little and ring finger, the C8 and T1 nerve roots would be suspected as a source of the symptoms because this is the dermatomal area of these nerve roots. Clearly, further examination of the cervical spine would be needed to confirm or refute this.

Having identified the underlying assumptions, the information from the subjective and physical examinations, which informs the hypothesis category of source of symptoms, will now be discussed. Where relevant, reference will be made to the indepth clinical reasoning form (Appendix). Finding the source of the patient's symptoms may require information from the following.

Body chart

It is critical for the clinician to obtain accurate and comprehensive information for the body chart. This information includes the area, quality, depth, type and behaviour (in terms of intermittent or constant) of symptoms, as well as the all-important aspect of the relationship of symptoms. The body chart thus includes:

1. Area of symptoms. Structures underneath the area of symptoms, or structures which are known to refer to the area of symptoms, are automatically considered to be a possible source of the symptoms (section 1.1 of the clinical reasoning form, shown in the Appendix). A patient who complains of lateral elbow pain must be asked whether there is any pain or stiffness in the cervical spine, thoracic spine or shoulder, as these regions can refer pain to the lateral aspect of the elbow. Patients with neurological symptoms are more likely to report distal symptoms (Dalton & Jull 1989; Austen 1991).

2. Quality of the symptoms. The quality of symptoms for patients with and without neurological deficit is similar (Dalton & Jull 1989; Austen 1991).

3. Depth of symptoms, although – like quality – this can be misleading (Austen 1991).

4. Abnormal sensation – paraesthesia, for example – indicates a lesion of the sensory nerves. A knowledge of the cutaneous distribution of the nerve roots and peripheral nerves enables the clinician to distinguish the sensory loss due to a root lesion (dermatomal pattern) from that due to a peripheral nerve lesion.

5. Constant versus intermittent symptoms. For example, constant unremitting pain, along with unexplained weight loss, would suggest malignancy as a possible source of the symptoms. Where symptoms are constant the clinician will explore, in the physical examination, movements that ease the patient's symptoms. These may then be used to treat the patient.

6. Relationship of symptoms. This is an extremely useful piece of information to guide the clinician to a hypothesis of the source of the symptoms. Symptoms are related when they come on at the same time and ease at the same time. If right neck pain and right lateral elbow pain come on at the same time, and ease at the same time, this would suggest that the cervical spine may be a source of both symptoms. If the patient has only one symptom at any one time, neck pain without elbow pain, and elbow pain without neck pain, this would suggest that there may be two separate problems – perhaps at the cervical spine, producing the neck pain, and a structure around the elbow, producing

the elbow pain. However, it is possible to have elbow pain without neck pain and neck pain without elbow pain and still be related. The crucial information to ascertain whether they are related is from the onset of symptoms.

Sometimes, clinicians may ask the patient: 'do you think the symptoms are related?' This can be a useful initial question to ask patients as it may reflect their understanding of the symptoms and the condition. The question does not, however, provide accurate information as to the behavioural relationship of the patient's symptoms. Patients may think they are unrelated because:

- they do not know that forearm pain can come from the spine
- there is quite a different timescale in the history of the onset of each symptom
- they do not think their neck ache is relevant
- they really want you to understand that it is the forearm that bothers them, and that is why they have come for treatment.

Because of these alternative ways of understanding this question it is not helpful in determining the relationship of symptoms.

Simplicity is often the best strategy for obtaining accurate and meaningful information, by asking the patient 'when the neck pain comes on, what happens to the forearm pain?' and confirming a negative answer with: 'so you have the forearm pain without any neck pain?'. If the neck symptoms are constant, 'if your neck pain gets worse, what happens to your forearm pain?'

Behaviour of symptoms

Aggravating factors. The clinician asks the patient about his or her functional abilities and the effect of these activities on the symptoms. The clinician then analyses these movements to determine which structures are being stressed, and to what degree. Obviously, as has been mentioned earlier, each movement will stress a number of structures; the clinician therefore identifies the relative stress on each structure. The structure most stressed would be the most likely structure at fault, and the structure least stressed would be the least likely structure at fault. However, all structures stressed in any way, however minimal, could still be the source of the symptoms, and therefore the clinician cannot completely rule them out.

In addition to functional activities, the clinician asks the patient about theoretically known aggravating movements and postures, for structures which could be a source of the symptoms. For example, a patient may have one symptom, lateral elbow pain. This pain may be referred from the cervical or thoracic spine, from the shoulder region or from the elbow region; it could be joint, nerve or muscle. The clinician gathers evidence to support or refute each of these regions as a source of the lateral elbow pain. The following questions provide some examples of the types of question that could be asked:

- 'Are there any neck/thoracic/shoulder/elbow/ hand movements that you are now unable to do?' These areas would be asked individually.
- 'Do you have any pain or stiffness in your neck?'
- 'Does turning your head to look over your shoulder produce any of your elbow pain?'
- 'Does sitting reading or looking up at the ceiling produce any of your elbow pain?'
- 'Do you have any pain or stiffness twisting (such as when reversing the car)?'
- 'Do you have any pain when you cough or sneeze?'
- 'Do you have any pain or stiffness lifting your arms above your head?'
- 'Do you have any pain or stiffness when you put your hand behind your back (when you tuck your shirt in, or do up your bra)?'
- 'Do you have any pain or stiffness on bending or straightening your elbow?'
- 'Do you have any problem twisting your arm (pronation/supination)?'
- 'Do you have any problem gripping?'

If a patient finds that elbow pain comes on only with forearm pronation and gripping and responds negatively in relation to neck movements, this would suggest that there is a local problem and that the spine and shoulder are less likely to be implicated in the lateral elbow pain.

Easing factors. The clinician asks about movements or positions which ease the patient's symptoms. The clinician analyses the position and/or movement in terms of which structures are de-stressed. Again, a number of structures will be affected and the clinician needs to determine the relative de-stress of each structure in order to differentiate between possible structures. Positions and movements which ease the patient's symptoms are particularly useful for patients who have constant irritable symptoms (see section on precautions for physical examination and/or treatment, below).

Twenty-four-hour behaviour

If the patient's symptoms wake him or her at night, as a result of sustaining or changing a position, the clinician needs to analyse the position or movement in terms of the structures being stressed. This helps to determine the possible structures at fault which are giving rise to the patient's symptoms. For example, if the patient has left shoulder pain which wakes him or her when lying on the left shoulder, this could be due to compression of the shoulder region or it could be the position of the neck on the pillows. If, on further questioning, the clinician considers that the neck is well supported on pillows, and the patient wakes in the morning with no neck pain or stiffness, this might negate slightly the neck as the problem, and, by deduction, implicate the shoulder region.

History of present condition

The last part of the subjective examination, the history of present condition (HPC), can give very strong clues as to the source of the symptoms or dysfunction. In traumatic injuries in particular, the mechanism of the injury can help to clarify which structures are at fault. For example, if medial knee pain came after a kick on the lateral aspect of the knee, which forced the lower leg into abduction, the medial structures around the knee would be particularly suspect as a source of the patient's symptoms. In addition, the HPC can help to clarify the relationship of the symptoms; for example, the patient may complain of neck and lateral elbow pain which, up to this point in the examination, may have been considered to be related, with the cervical spine suspected of being a source of both symptoms. However, the history of onset of these two symptoms may suggest otherwise: the patient may have had the neck pain for 10 years, the elbow pain for 2 months and, when the elbow pain started, no change was felt in the neck pain. While this does not rule out the possibility of the neck as a source of the two symptoms, it would suggest that there may be two separate sources.

A hypothesis as to the source of symptoms and/or dysfunction is thus established from the various aspects of the subjective examination, the body chart, aggravating factors, easing factors, 24-hour behaviour of symptoms and HPC. This information will provide answers for section 1.1, in particular, of the clinical reasoning form (Appendix).

Production of symptoms

Patients often present with the symptom of pain. Pain is defined as 'an unpleasant sensory and emotional experience associated with actual or potential tissue damage, or described in terms of such damage' (Merskey et al. 1979). Pain has been classified into nociceptive (mechanical, inflammatory or ischaemic), peripheral neurogenic, central, autonomic and affective (Gifford 1998).

Briefly, these mechanisms of pain can be described as follows:

1. Nociceptive pain is due to mechanical, ischaemic, chemical or thermal effects on nociceptors; for example, lengthening or compressing tissue which contains nociceptors. The release of chemicals into the tissues sensitises the nociceptors and produces pain.
2. Peripheral neurogenic pain is pain arising from a peripheral nerve axon; this may be due to sustained stretch or pressure on an axon.
3. Autonomic pain is due to increased sensitivity of the nociceptors from the secretion of catecholamines (adrenaline (epinephrine) and noradrenaline (norepinephrine)) from the sympathetic nervous system.
4. Central sensitisation pain is a result of emotions and cognition (beliefs). Emotion (or affect) affects the way the brain processes information, sensations felt, and the body's physiology and can lead to a perception of pain.

The clinical features of each of these mechanisms are given in Table 4.1. More than one mechanism may co-exist; for example, a patient with severe low-back pain may have mechanical and inflammatory nociceptive pain with an affective component driven by the patient's emotional state. The clinician needs to be aware of the features of each mechanism to hypothesise which is responsible for producing the patient's pain. This information will provide answers for section 1.2 of the clinical reasoning form shown in the Appendix.

At the end of the subjective examination the clinician needs to develop a working hypothesis as to the likely source of the symptoms and/or dysfunction and the pain mechanism (section 1.3 of the clinical reasoning form in the Appendix). Positive and negating evidence, from throughout the subjective examination, needs to be considered. The clinician is then able to plan the physical examination, determining which physical tests need to be carried out in order to clarify the source of the patient's symptoms.

Physical testing includes observation, active movements, passive movements, muscle tests, nerve tests and palpation and accessory movements. It is worth mentioning here that each examination procedure is impure and does not test only what its name suggests. A joint test is not a pure joint test, a muscle test is not a pure muscle test and a nerve test is not a pure nerve test (Box 4.6). For example, isometric muscle testing predominantly tests the ability of a muscle to contract isometrically; however, to do this it requires normal neural input and any accompanying joint movement must be symptom-free. Thus, while isometric muscle testing is predominantly a test of muscle, it is also, to some degree, a test of nerve and joint function. Some further examples to highlight this are given in Table 4.2. The reason that this is emphasised is that it needs to underpin the analysis of physical examination findings. If the clinician assumes that the tests are pure, and that a muscle test only tests muscle, then a positive muscle test may be misinterpreted to be indicative of a muscle problem.

The aim of the physical examination is often to reproduce all, or part, of the patient's symptoms (if the symptoms are non-severe and non-irritable). If symptoms are severe and/or irritable then the aim of the physical examination is to find movements and positions that ease all, or some, of the symptoms. When a test reproduces or eases the patient's symptoms it implicates those structures being stressed or eased by that test. Analysis of the structures predominantly affected by the test will enable the clinician to narrow down the possible structure(s) at fault. By the end of the physical examination the clinician can use all the evidence from the subjective and physical examinations to develop a hypothesis as to the source of the symptoms and/or dysfunction. The clinician can arrive at a physical clinical diagnosis that will help to provide a basis for the treatment and management of the patient.

The diagnosis will identify where the symptoms are believed to be emanating from, and will vary with the tissue. For example, if a joint is felt to be the source of the patient's symptoms, the clinician may identify altered accessory or physiological movement. If a muscle is felt to be the source of the patient's symptoms, the clinician may hypothesise that there is a muscle or tendon tear, or a muscle contusion. If a nerve is felt to be the source of the patient's symptoms the clinician may hypothesise a reduction in nerve length or a nerve compression injury. Most of these descriptors provide some guidance for treatment and management, but are quite limited.

Table 4.1 Clinical features of pain mechanisms

Pain mechanism	Clinical features
Mechanical pain	Particular movements that aggravate and ease the pain, sometimes referred to as 'on/off pain'
Inflammatory pain	Redness, oedema and heat Acute pain and tissue damage Close relationship of stimulus response and pain Diurnal pattern with pain and stiffness worst at night and in the morning Signs of neurogenic inflammation (redness, swelling or symptoms in neural zone) Beneficial effect of anti-inflammatory medication
Ischaemic pain	Symptoms produced after prolonged or unusual activities Rapid ease of symptoms after a change in posture Symptoms towards the end of the day or after the accumulation of activity Poor response to anti-inflammatory medication Absence of trauma
Neuropathic pain	Persistent and intractable Stimulus-independent pain: shooting, lancinating or burning pain Paraesthesia Dysaesthesia
Autonomic pain	Cutaneous capillary vasodilation
Early-stage pain Associated with:	Increased temperature Increased sweating Oedema Trophic changes: glossy skin, cracking nails Feeling of heaviness or feeling of swelling
Chronic-stage pain Associated with:	Coldness Pallor Atrophy of skin – skin flaking Atrophy of soft tissue Joint stiffness Hair loss
Affective pain	Loneliness Hopelessness Sadness Fear Anger

Box 4.6

There is no pure joint, muscle or nerve test. Each test affects all tissues

Generally, the clinician examines the patient to identify a movement dysfunction. While there are a number of known pathological processes leading to specific signs and symptoms, for instance a tear of the medial meniscus of the knee or a lateral ligament sprain of the ankle, a large majority of patients with neuromusculoskeletal dysfunction have signs and symptoms which do not clearly identify a known pathology. Evidence includes the fact that normal

Table 4.2 Analysis of physical tests

Physical tests	Physical test	Involves/tests
Observation	Static and dynamic postures	Emotional state of patient Entire neuromusculoskeletal system
Active and passive movements	Active physiological movements	Patient's willingness to move Muscle strength and length Nerve input to muscle Motor control Joint function
	Passive physiological movements	Patient's willingness to move and be moved Muscle length Joint function
Muscle tests	Isometric muscle test	Patient's willingness and motivation to do this Muscle strength and endurance Nerve input to muscle Joint function
	Muscle strength	Patient's willingness and motivation to do this Muscle strength and endurance Nerve input to muscle Joint function
	Muscle control	Movement control of brain Muscle function
	Muscle length	Joint function to move Nerve function to movement
	Palpation of muscle	Includes palpation of skin and nerve tissue
Nerve tests	Nerve integrity tests	
	Neurodynamic tests	Muscle function to move Joint function to move
	Palpation of nerve	Includes palpation of skin and muscle
Joint test	Accessory movements	Affects any overlying soft tissues Affects muscles attaching to bone Affects local nerves
	Palpation of joint	Includes palpation of skin and overlying muscle

age-related changes seen on spinal radiograph are often not related to the patient's signs and symptoms (Clinical Standards Advisory Group 1994). It is also well known that approximately 30% of asymptomatic people will have a disc herniation on magnetic resonance imaging (Kaplan et al. 2001). This clearly emphasises the need for close clinical correlation with signs and symptoms (Gundry & Fritts 1997).

Knowledge of pathology and clinical syndromes is valuable to the clinician who is then able to recognise the signs and symptoms that suggest these conditions and, where necessary, refer to a medical practitioner.

The difficulty of linking signs and symptoms to pathology led to the concept of the permeable brick wall adapted from Maitland et al. (2005) and shown in Box 4.7. The left-hand column depicts the knowledge and skills that the clinician brings to the therapeutic relationship. The right-hand column depicts the knowledge and skills that the patient brings to the relationship. The internet has given patients easy access to information about their condition, and they may come with some knowledge of anatomy, biomechanics and physiology. The interrupted vertical line of 'bricks' between the clinician and the patient is the 'permeable brick wall' which identifies that sometimes the patient's clinical presentation will fit with a known textbook description of a disorder and the clinician is able to see the link between theory and practice. On other occasions the patient's presentation does not fit, the bricks are in the way

Box 4.7

Permeable brick wall (after Maitland et al. 2005, with permission)

The clinician		The patient
		Clinical presentation:
Beliefs		Beliefs
Values		Values
Experience		Experience
Skill		Skill
Anatomy		Anatomy
Biomechanics		Biomechanics
Physiology		Physiology
Pathology		Pathology
Diagnosis		Diagnosis
Theories		Theories
Research findings		Research findings

and the clinician cannot make features 'fit'. Where a patient presents with a known textbook description of, for example, a prolapsed intervertebral disc, then the wall is permeable, the clinician is able to link the textbook information to the patient's presentation. However, when a patient's presentation does not fit a known documented presentation, then the clinician is unable to make the link. Where this occurs, the concept states that the patient's presentation is true and sure, and is to be believed, regardless of the fact that the clinician is not able to link the presentation to any theoretical framework.

The clinical reasoning process advocated in this text assumes this model of thinking: the clinician is concerned with movement dysfunction, not pathology. Occasionally it may be possible to identify a known pathology, that is, where the brick wall is permeable, but more often than not the clinician identifies a movement dysfunction, with a hypothesis as to the structure causing the patient's symptoms and factors contributing to the onset and continuation of these symptoms. For this reason the reader is referred to the numerous pathology textbooks available for details of known pathologies and their clinical presentation.

The clinical diagnosis used by the expected reader of this text will be related to movement dysfunction, and treatment will aim to restore that movement. Clinical diagnosis can be defined as the history and signs and symptoms that are distinct to that individual and includes the identification of a mechanical cause (Refshauge & Gass 2004). The patient presents with pain, for example, and the clinician seeks to identify where that pain is emanating from. For this

reason other pieces of information are added to the clinical diagnosis to describe the movement dysfunction fully and this often involves simply identifying the positive physical tests. For example:

> A patellofemoral joint problem giving anterior knee pain which is a mechanical nociceptive pain, which is not severe and not irritable. There is a tight lateral retinaculum pulling the patella laterally during eccentric control of knee flexion, which is eased with a medial glide of the patella.

> A right C4/5 zygapophyseal joint dysfunction giving one area of pain in the right side of the neck and the lateral upper arm, which is an inflammatory and mechanical nociceptive pain and is not severe and not irritable. A component of the pain is thought to be a neural interface, as there is a positive upper-limb tension test 2a, biasing the median nerve (ULNT 2a [upper-limb neurodynamic test 2a]). Cervical movements exhibit a regular compression pattern.

It can be seen that the above descriptions provide a summary of the main findings of the examination. The descriptions revolve around the physical testing procedures, which are by nature tests of movement.

Having noted this, there are exceptions, such as identifying a possible torn meniscus, a spondylolisthesis, a prolapsed intervertebral disc, as well as identifying serious pathology that may require medical intervention; these are considered in the section on precautions for physical examination and/or treatment, below.

The patient generally understands diagnoses such as 'meniscal tear' but the above descriptions may not be meaningful or understandable. It is important therefore that these descriptions are translated into a language that patients understand if they are to be compliant with treatment.

Factors contributing to the condition

These factors include environmental, behavioural, emotional, physical or biomechanical factors (Jones 1994). One or more factors may be responsible for the development, or maintenance, of the patient's problem. Environmental factors, such as the patient's work station or tennis racket, will be identified in the social history of the subjective examination. Behavioural and emotional factors will be identified throughout the subjective and physical examination as the clinician becomes aware of the patient's attitude towards him- or herself, the clinician and the condition. Physical and biomechanical factors, such as a short leg, poor posture or reduced muscle length, will be identified from the physical testing procedures carried out in the physical examination. At the end of the subjective and physical examination, the clinician needs to develop a hypothesis as to which, if any, of these factors may be contributing to the patient's problem. This information would inform section 2 of the clinical reasoning form shown in the Appendix. The extent to which these factors are thought to be contributing to the patient's condition will determine when they are addressed in the management of the patient.

Precautions for physical examination and/or treatment

This hypothesis serves a number of purposes. It helps to identify patients who are appropriate for neuromusculoskeletal treatment, whether there are any precautions for examination and treatment, to avoid exacerbation of their condition and to avoid unnecessary discomfort for patients. These aspects will be discussed in turn.

Screening patients for neuromusculoskeletal treatment

The first overarching purpose is to identify patients who are appropriate for treatment and to screen out those who are not. The clinician determines whether the patient's symptoms are emanating from a mechanical neuromusculoskeletal disorder or whether the symptoms are due to some other disease process. If the symptoms are being produced from a neuromusculoskeletal disorder then treatment is appropriate; if not then neuromusculoskeletal therapy may not be appropriate, and referral to a medical practitioner may be needed. Visceral structures can masquerade as musculoskeletal disorders and an understanding of how to differentiate these structures from musculoskeletal conditions is important. For further information on the clinical presentation of pathological conditions the reader is referred to suitable pathology textbooks such as Goodman & Boissonnault (1998) and Grieve (1981).

Having identified that the patient is suitable for treatment, the clinician must then decide how the physical examination, and later treatment, needs to be tailored to the patient's presentation.

Precautions for examination and treatment

Information from the subjective examination provides vital information on any precautions to joint and nerve mobilisation, and this is summarised in Table 4.3. A brief explanation of the possible causes underlying the finding is given and, where appropriate, the implications for examination and/or

Table 4.3 Precautions to spinal and peripheral passive joint mobilisations and nerve mobilisations

Aspects of subjective examination	Subjective information	Possible cause/implication for examination and/or treatment
Body chart	Constant unremitting pain Symptoms in the upper limb below the acromion or symptoms in the lower limb below the gluteal crease	Malignancy, systemic, inflammatory cause Nerve root compression. Carry out appropriate neurological integrity tests in physical examination
	Widespread sensory changes and/or weakness in upper or lower limb	Compression on more than one nerve root, metabolic (e.g. diabetes, vitamin B_{12}), systemic (e. g. rheumatoid arthritis)
Aggravating factors	Symptoms severe and/or irritable	Care in treatment to avoid unnecessary provocation or exacerbation
Special questions	Feeling unwell	Systemic or metabolic disease

(Continued)

Aspects of subjective examination	Subjective information	Possible cause/implication for examination and/or treatment
	General health: – history of malignant disease, in remission	Not relevant
	– active malignant disease if associated with present symptoms	Contraindicates neuromusculoskeletal treatment, may do gentle maintenance exercises
	– active malignant disease not associated with present symptoms	Not relevant
	– hysterectomy	Increased risk of osteoporosis
	Recent unexplained weight loss	Malignancy, systemic
	Diagnosis of bone disease (e.g. osteoporosis, Paget's, brittle bone)	Bone may be abnormal and/or weakened Avoid strong direct force to bone, especially the ribs
	Diagnosis of rheumatoid arthritis or other inflammatory joint disease	Avoid accessory and physiological movements to upper cervical spine and care with other joints
	Diagnosis of infective arthritis	In active stage immobilisation is treatment of choice
	Diagnosis of spondylolysis or spondylolisthesis	Avoid strong direct pressure to the subluxed vertebral level
	Systemic steroids	Osteoporosis, poor skin condition requires careful handling, avoid tape
	Anticoagulant therapy	Increase time for blood to clot. Soft tissues may bruise easily
	Human immunodeficiency virus (HIV) Pregnancy	Check medication and possible side-effects Ligament laxity, may want to avoid strong forces
	Diabetes Bilateral hand/feet pins and needles and/or numbness	Delayed healing, peripheral neuropathies Spinal cord compression, peripheral neuropathy
	Difficulty walking	Spinal cord compression, peripheral neuropathy, upper motor neurone lesion
	Disturbance of bladder and/or bowel function	Cauda equina syndrome
	Perineum (saddle)	Cauda equina syndrome
	Anaesthesia/paraesthesia For patients with cervicothoracic symptoms: dizziness, altered vision, nausea, ataxia, drop attacks, altered facial sensation, difficulty speaking, difficulty swallowing, sympathoplegia, hemianaesthesia, hemiplegia	Vertebrobasilar insufficiency, upper cervical instability, disease of the inner ear
	Heart or respiratory disease	May preclude some treatment positions
	Oral contraception	Increased possibility of thrombosis – may avoid strong techniques to cervical spine
	History of smoking	Circulatory problems – increased possibility of thrombosis
Recent history	Trauma	Possible undetected fracture, e.g. scaphoid

treatment. This information would guide the response to section 3 of the clinical reasoning form shown in the Appendix.

As well as identifying any precautions for neuro-musculoskeletal examination and treatment, the clinician needs to identify, as early as possible, how best to examine the patient. The clinician needs to make every effort to avoid exacerbating the patient's condition, and this is done by identifying the severity and irritability of the symptoms. The clinician also needs to be able to explore fully the patient's neuromusculoskeletal system without provoking unnecessary discomfort for the patient; this is done by identifying the severity of the patient's symptoms.

Severity of the symptoms

The clinician determines the severity of every symptom. Whether the symptoms are constant or intermittent, the symptoms are deemed to be severe if the patient reports that a single movement, which increases this pain, is so severe that the movement has to be stopped. Severe symptoms will limit the extent of the physical examination. The clinician would, in this situation, aim to examine the patient as fully as possible, but within the constraints of the patient's symptoms. The effect of severe pain on active movements is given below as an example of how a physical test has to be adapted.

Active movements would involve the patient moving to a point just before the onset of (or increase in) the symptom, or just to the point of onset (or increase), and would then immediately return to the starting position. No overpressures would be applied. This requires the clinician to give clear instructions to the patient. For example, if active shoulder flexion is being examined the clinician may instruct the patient in the following way (emphasis is in italics):

Intermittent severe symptom: 'Lift your arm up in front of you, and *as soon as you think you are about to get your arm pain*, bring your arm down again' or 'Lift your arm up in front of you, and *as soon as you get your arm pain*, bring your arm down again'.

Constant severe symptom: 'Lift your arm up in front of you, and *as soon as you think your arm pain is going to increase*, bring your arm down again' or 'Lift your arm up in front of you, and *as soon as your arm pain increases*, bring your arm down again'.

For passive movements, patients may be asked to say as soon as they think they are about to feel their symptom (intermittent), or feel it is about to increase (constant). In both cases, pain is avoided. Alternatively, the patient may be able to tolerate movement just to the onset (or increase) of the symptom. The clinician would carry out the passive movement and, under the instruction of the patient, take the movement to only the first point of pain – and then immediately return to the starting point. In both situations the clinician must give clear instructions to the patient. For example, for passive shoulder flexion, the clinician may instruct the patient in the following way (emphasis is in italics):

Intermittent symptoms: 'I want to move your arm, but I want you to tell me *as soon as you think you are about to get your arm pain*, and I'll bring your arm down'.

'I want to move your arm, but I want you to tell me *as soon as you get your arm pain*, and I will bring your arm down'.

Constant symptoms: 'I want to move your arm, but I want you to tell me *as soon as you think you are about to get more of your arm pain*, and I'll bring your arm down'.

'I want to move your arm up, but I want you to tell me *as soon as you get more of your arm pain*, and I will bring your arm down'.

The clinician must be able to control the movement and carry it out very slowly. This is necessary in order to avoid overshooting and causing unnecessary symptoms and to obtain an accurate measure of range of movement for reassessment purposes. This process is depicted in Figure 4.4.

Irritability of the symptoms

The irritability of the symptoms is the degree to which the symptoms increase and reduce with provocation. When a movement is performed, and pain is provoked, for example, and this provoked pain continues to be present for a length of time, then the pain is said to be irritable. In the context of an examination, any period of time that is required for symptoms to return to their resting level is classified as irritable. If symptoms are provoked and require a time delay before the examination can recommence, this will increase the appointment time, which may not be possible in a busy department. As well as this, repeatedly provoking symptoms and then waiting for them to settle will add little to the clinician's understanding of the patient's

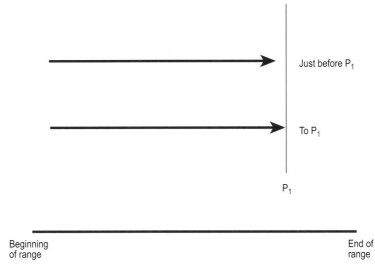

Figure 4.4 • A passive movement is carried out just prior to, or at, the first point of onset (or increase) of the symptom (P_1).

condition. For this reason, an alternative strategy is used whereby movements are carried out within the symptom-free range; irritable symptoms are not provoked at all.

For the examination of active movements for a patient with intermittent symptoms, the patient would move to a point just before the onset of the symptoms and then immediately return to the start position. In this way, symptoms are not provoked and therefore there will be no lingering symptoms. For example, if active shoulder flexion is being examined, the clinician may instruct the patient in the following way (emphasis is in italics):

Intermittent symptoms: 'Lift your arm up in front of you, and *as soon as you think you are about to get your arm pain*, bring your arm down again'.

Constant symptoms: 'Lift your arm up in front of you and *as soon as you think your arm pain is going to increase*, bring your arm down again'.

For passive movements, patients may be asked to say as soon as they think they are about to feel the symptom (intermittent), or feel that it is about to increase (constant). In both cases, pain is avoided. The clinician must give clear instructions to the patient. For example, for passive shoulder flexion, the clinician may instruct the patient in the following way (emphasis is in italics):

Intermittent symptoms: 'I want to move your arm, but I want you to tell me *as soon as you think you are about to get your arm pain*, and I'll bring your arm down'.

Constant symptoms: 'I want to move your arm, but I want you to tell me *as soon as you think you are about to get more of your arm pain*, and I'll bring your arm down'.

For irritable symptoms, whether intermittent or constant, it is particularly important that the clinician clarifies after each movement the patient's resting symptoms, to avoid exacerbating symptoms.

Special questions

This section of the subjective examination is concerned with identifying precautions to examination and treatment, and is summarised in Table 4.3. The special questions ask about known pathological conditions of the patient as well as those symptoms which may suggest a pathological condition. The implication of such pathologies and symptoms on the examination and treatment of the patient is suggested. Some of this information has been obtained from pathology textbooks, for example Goodman & Boissonnault (1998), and some is from clinical experience and simply suggested by the author. The reader should note this limitation.

Malignancies can present as neuromusculoskeletal disorders. Increasingly the therapists are the first clinicians to carry out a thorough examination, therefore it is important that they have the skills to differentiate these pathologies from neuromusculoskeletal disorders. There are a number of patients who have a past history of malignancy; this in itself does not contraindicate examination or treatment. However the clinician needs to clarify whether or not the presenting symptoms are being caused by a malignancy or whether there is a separate neuromusculoskeletal disorder. It has been suggested that the following factors may predispose a patient to sinister pathology: previous history of cancer, failed conservative treatment, unexplained weight loss and aged over 50 years (Deyo & Diehl 1988). However other factors may need to be considered, including night pain and severity of symptoms. Equally, clinical judgement in these cases has been shown to be important and cannot, and should not, be ignored (Henschke et al. 2007). If the symptoms are thought to be associated with the malignancy then this may contraindicate most neuromusculoskeletal treatment techniques, although gentle maintenance exercises may be given.

Red flags are often regarded as a sign of serious pathologies. For more detailed information regarding red flags the reader is referred to Greenhalgh & Selfe (2006).

Osteoporosis can be caused by a number of factors, including long-term use of steriods, early menopause or hysterectomy. Osteoporosis and Paget's disease produce abnormal and weakened bone which would increase the risk of fractures, particularly over the ribs. For this reason the presence of bone disease would contraindicate strong direct forces applied to bone.

A diagnosis of inflammatory joint disease such as rheumatoid arthritis would contraindicate accessory and physiological movements to the upper cervical spine and care is needed in applying forces to other joints. The reason for this is that inflammatory arthritis weakens ligaments, particularly in the upper cervical spine. This increases the risk of subluxation or dislocation of the C1/C2 joint, which may cause spinal cord compression.

A diagnosis of infective arthritis, in the active stage, requires immobilisation. For this reason, neuromusculoskeletal therapy is contraindicated.

The presence of spondylolysis or spondylolisthesis would contraindicate strong direct pressure to the implicated vertebral level as this might increase the slip and cause spinal cord or cauda equina compression.

Anticoagulant therapy causes an increase in the time for blood to clot. The clinician needs to be aware that this may cause soft tissues to bruise when force is applied. Similarly the use of long-term steroids may weaken the skin and careful handling may be required.

If a patient has been diagnosed with human immunodeficiency virus (HIV), his or her medication may have side-effects that will affect neuromusculoskeletal treatment.

If a patient is pregnant there will be ligament laxity. This may cause a reduction in joint stiffness and an increase in range of joint movement. Excessive forces may be inadvisable.

Diabetes can cause delayed healing and so affect the patient's prognosis. Diabetes is also associated with peripheral neuropathies and patients may complain of bilateral pins and needles or numbness in both hands and/or both feet. This may need to be distinguished from other causes for these symptoms, including spinal cord compression or vitamin B_{12} deficiency.

There are obviously many reasons why a patient may have difficulty walking; of concern here is the possibility of spinal cord compression, an upper motor neurone lesion or peripheral neuropathy. These may be further tested in the physical examination by carrying out neurological integrity tests, including the plantar response.

Disturbance of bladder or bowel function may be due to compression on the cauda equina. Loss of sensation or paraesthesia in the perineum is also suggestive of cauda equina compression.

Dizziness, altered vision, nausea, ataxia, drop attacks, altered facial sensation, difficulty speaking, difficulty swallowing, sympathoplegia, hemianaesthesia and hemiplegia indicate vertebrobasilar insufficiency (VBI), upper cervical instability or disease of the inner ear. A lack of blood supply to the vestibular nuclei in the brainstem causes dizziness, the most common symptom of VBI (Bogduk 1994).

Heart or respiratory disease may preclude some treatment positions; for example, the patient may not tolerate lying flat.

Oral contraception and smoking are each associated with an increased risk of thrombosis. For this reason strong techniques to the cervical spine are inadvisable for patients taking oral contraceptives.

A traumatic onset of symptoms may give helpful clues as to the source of the patient's symptoms as the mechanism of the injury is analysed in detail. There is the possibility of a fracture underlying a traumatic incident; for example, a fall on the outstretched hand may cause a scaphoid fracture which is sometimes difficult to identify on radiograph.

The reader is referred to pathology textbooks for further information on pathological conditions and their clinical presentation. The reader is then encouraged to read an excellent chapter that highlights the challenge of clinical practice to distinguish benign neuromusculoskeletal conditions from serious pathologies (Grieve 1994). Safe clinical practice requires a constant awareness by the clinician that what appears straightforward may not be.

Prognosis of the condition

The clinician needs to develop a hypothesis as to whether the patient's condition is suitable for neuromusculoskeletal treatment and management, and the likely prognosis. A large number of positive and negative factors from throughout the subjective examination will inform this hypothesis. These factors include patients' age, general health, lifestyle, attitude, personality, expectations and attitude towards their condition, towards themselves and towards the clinician, as well as the mechanical versus inflammatory nature of the symptoms, severity and irritability of the symptoms, degree of tissue damage and length of time and progression of the condition. By considering all of these factors, the clinician is then able to provide the patient with a hypothesis as to how long and to what extent the symptoms may be eased with treatment. The prognosis is as specific as possible for the patient. At discharge, it is useful for the clinician to compare the final outcome with the predicted outcome; this reflection will help clinicians to learn and enhance their ability to hypothesise in the future. A hypothesis could, for example, be: 'will restore full range of movement in the shoulder region, and completely alleviate the shoulder pain; neck pain and stiffness will be reduced by 50%'. This information would provide answers for section 5 of the clinical reasoning form shown in the Appendix.

Management

The use of an outcome tool may help the clinician to direct treatment and assess its effect, for example the Patient-specific Functional Scale. This questionnaire can be used to assess any limitation of activity and measure functional outcome (Stratford et al. 1995). It has been validated in a number of conditions, including back and neck pain (Pietrobon et al. 2002).

Management can be considered in two phases: the initial appointment on day 1 and the follow-up appointments.

Initial appointment

The clinician develops a plan as to how to treat and manage the patient and the condition. The first step in this process occurs between the subjective and physical examinations. At this point, the clinician must decide what structures are suspected to be a source of the symptoms and need to be examined in the physical examination. Along with any precautions or contraindications, a plan of the physical examination is developed. The aims of the physical examination are to:

- identify the source of the patient's symptoms
- confirm, if necessary, any precautions or contraindications; for example, identify the presence of spinal cord compression
- explore further, if relevant, any factors contributing to the patient's condition; for example, measure leg length.

In order to identify the source of the symptoms the clinician uses the information from the subjective examination to predict the findings of the physical examination. This includes:

- the structures thought to be at fault
- which tests are likely to reproduce/alter the patient's symptoms
- how the tests need to be performed to reproduce/alter the patient's symptoms; for example, combined movements may be required
- what other structures need to be examined in order to disprove them as a source of the symptoms.

The process then involves putting the possible structures at fault in priority order and planning the physical examination accordingly. The information would provide answers for question 4.1 in the clinical reasoning form shown in the Appendix.

At the end of the physical examination the clinician needs to reflect on all the information from both the subjective and physical examinations and develop a treatment and management plan. Almost all the information obtained will be used in this process. The information would provide answers for questions 4.2–4.8 of the clinical reasoning form shown in the Appendix.

The physical testing procedures which specifically indicate joint, nerve or muscle tissues as a source of the patient's symptoms are summarised

Table 4.4 Physical tests which, if positive, indicate joint, nerve and muscle as a source of the patient's symptoms

Test	Strong evidence	Weak evidence
Joint		
Active physiological movements	Reproduces patient's symptoms	Dysfunctional movement: reduced range, excessive range, altered quality of movement, increased resistance, decreased resistance
Passive physiological movements	Reproduces patient's symptoms; this test same as for active physiological movements	Dysfunctional movement: reduced range, excessive range, increased resistance, decreased resistance, altered quality of movement
Accessory movements	Reproduces patient's symptoms	Dysfunctional movement: reduced range, excessive range, increased resistance, decreased resistance, altered quality of movement
Palpation of joint	Reproduces patient's symptoms	Tenderness
Reassessment following therapeutic dose of accessory movement	Improvement in tests which reproduce patient's symptoms	No change in physical tests which reproduce patient's symptoms
Muscle		
Active movement	Reproduces patient's symptoms	Reduced strength Poor quality
Passive physiological movements	Do not reproduce patient's symptoms	
Isometric contraction	Reproduces patient's symptoms	Reduced strength Poor quality
Passive lengthening of muscle	Reproduces patient's symptoms	Reduced range Increased resistance Decreased resistance
Palpation of muscle	Reproduces patient's symptoms	Tenderness
Reassessment following therapeutic dose of muscle treatment	Improvement in tests which reproduce patient's symptoms	No change in physical tests which reproduce patient's symptoms
Nerve		
Passive lengthening and sensitising movement, i.e. altering length of nerve by a movement at a distance from patient's symptoms	Reproduces patient's symptoms and sensitising movement alters patient's symptoms	Reduced length Increased resistance
Palpation of nerve	Reproduces patient's symptoms	Tenderness

in Table 4.4. At one end of the scale the findings may provide strong evidence, and at the other end they may provide weak evidence. Of course, one may find a variety of presentations between these two extremes.

The strongest evidence that a joint is the source of the patient's symptoms is that active and passive physiological movements, passive accessory movements and joint palpation all reproduce the patient's symptoms, and that, following a treatment dose, reassessment identifies an improvement in the patient's signs and symptoms. For example, let us assume a patient has lateral elbow pain caused by a radiohumeral joint dysfunction. In the physical examination there are limited elbow flexion and extension movements due to reproduction of the patient's elbow pain, with some resistance. Active movement is very similar to passive movement in terms of range, resistance and pain reproduction. Accessory movement examination of the radiohumeral joint reveals limited posteroanterior and anteroposterior glide of the radius due to reproduction of the patient's elbow pain with some resistance. Following the examination of accessory movements, sufficient to be considered a treatment dose, reassessment of the elbow physiological movements are improved, in terms of range and pain. This scenario would indicate that there is a dysfunction at the radiohumeral joint – first, because elbow movements, both active and passive physiological, and accessory movements, reproduce the patient's symptoms, and, second, because, following accessory movements, the active elbow movements are improved. Even if the active movements are made worse, this would still suggest a joint dysfunction because it is likely that the accessory movements would predominantly affect the joint, with much less effect on nerve and muscle tissues around the area. Collectively, this evidence would suggest that there is a joint dysfunction, as long as this is accompanied by negative muscle and nerve tests.

Weaker evidence includes an alteration in range, resistance or quality of physiological and/or accessory movements and tenderness over the joint, with no alteration in signs and symptoms after treatment. One or more of these findings may indicate a dysfunction of a joint which may, or may not, be contributing to the patient's condition.

The strongest evidence that a muscle is the source of a patient's symptoms is if active movements, an isometric contraction, passive lengthening and palpation of a muscle all reproduce the patient's symptoms, and that, following a treatment dose, reassessment identifies an improvement in the patient's signs and symptoms. For example, let us assume that a patient has lateral elbow pain caused by lateral epicondylalgia, a primary muscle problem. In this case reproduction of the patient's lateral elbow pain is found on active wrist and finger extension, isometric contraction of the wrist extensors and/or finger extensors, and passive lengthening of the extensor muscles to

the wrist and hand. These signs and symptoms are found to improve following soft-tissue mobilisation examination, sufficient to be considered a treatment dose. Collectively, this evidence would suggest that there is a muscle dysfunction, as long as this is accompanied by negative joint and nerve tests.

Further evidence of muscle dysfunction may be suggested by reduced strength or poor quality during the active physiological movement and the isometric contraction, reduced range and/or increased/decreased resistance, during the passive lengthening of the muscle, and tenderness on palpation, with no alteration in signs and symptoms after treatment. One or more of these findings may indicate a dysfunction of a muscle which may, or may not, be contributing to the patient's condition.

The strongest evidence that a nerve is the source of the patient's symptoms is when active and/or passive physiological movements reproduce the patient's symptoms, which are then increased or decreased with an additional sensitising movement, at a distance from the patient's symptoms. In addition, there is reproduction of the patient's symptoms on palpation of the nerve, and following neurodynamic testing – sufficient to be considered a treatment dose – an improvement in the above signs and symptoms. For example, let us assume this time that the lateral elbow pain is caused by a neurodynamic dysfunction of the radial nerve supplying this region. The patient's lateral elbow pain is reproduced during the component movements of the ULNT 2b and is eased with ipsilateral cervical lateral flexion sensitising movement. There is tenderness over the radial groove in the upper arm and, following testing of the ULNT 2b, sufficient to be considered a treatment dose, an improvement in the patient's signs and symptoms. Collectively, this evidence would suggest that there is a neurodynamic dysfunction, as long as this is accompanied by negative joint and muscle tests.

Further evidence of nerve dysfunction may be suggested by reduced range (compared with the asymptomatic side) and/or increased resistance to the various arm movements, and tenderness on nerve palpation.

It can be seen that the common factor for identifying joint, nerve and muscle dysfunction as a source of the patient's symptoms is reproduction of the patient's symptoms, alteration in the patient's signs and symptoms following a treatment dose and lack of evidence from other potential sources of symptoms. It is assumed that if a test reproduces a patient's symptoms then it is somehow stressing the structure at fault. As mentioned earlier, each test is not purely a test of one structure – every test, to a greater or lesser degree, involves all structures. For this reason, it is imperative that, whatever treatment is given, it is proved to be of value by altering the patient's signs and symptoms. The other factor common in identifying joint, nerve or muscle dysfunction is the lack of positive findings in the other possible tissues; for example, a joint dysfunction is considered when joint tests are positive and muscle and nerve tests are negative. Thus the clinician collects evidence to implicate tissues and evidence to negate tissues – both are equally important. The reader is reminded of the earlier analogy of the detective who must collect evidence to prove the guilt or innocence of all possible suspects. The classification of joint, nerve and muscle used in this textbook is summarised in Table 4.5.

The first priority of treatment will often be to address the source of the patient's symptoms, and later any relevant contributing factors. However, it may be necessary to treat a contributing factor intially in order to affect the source of symptoms. For example, the source of symptoms may be a hypermobile segment of the lumbar spine and treatment of the neighbouring hypomobile segment may improve symptoms. The types of treatment for joint, nerve and muscle are summarised in Table 4.6.

Table 4.5 Joint, muscle and nerve dysfunctions

Joint dysfunction	Muscle dysfunction	Nerve dysfunction
Hypomobility	Reduced length	Reduced length
Altered quality of movement Symptom production	Symptom production Reduced strength, power and endurance Altered motor control	Symptom production Altered nerve conduction

Table 4.6 Types of joint, muscle and nerve treatment techniques

Joint	Muscle	Nerve
Accessory movement	Strength, power and endurance training	
Physiological (active or passive) movement	Passive or active lengthening of muscle	Passive or active lengthening of nerve
Accessory with physiological (active or passive) movement Soft-tissue mobilisations (includes frictions)	Soft-tissue mobilisations (includes frictions)	Soft-tissue mobilisations (includes frictions)
Exercises to enhance motor control and coordination	Exercises to enhance motor control and coordination	Exercises to enhance motor control and coordination
PNF	PNF	PNF
Taping	Taping	Taping
Electrotherapy	Electrotherapy	Electrotherapy

PNF, proprioceptive neuromuscular facilitation.

Box 4.8

The clinician assesses and reassesses the patient's subjective and physical asterisks within and between appointments to determine the effects of treatment

Good clinical practice requires that clinicians know the effects of their treatment. This involves continual assessment of the patient at each attendance, so that the effect of the previous treatment is known, and after the application of each treatment technique within a treatment session (Box 4.8). Any significant finding relevant to the patient's problem, in the subjective and physical examinations, is highlighted in the clinical notes by using asterisks (*) for ease of reference. These subjective and physical findings are referred to as 'asterisks' (Maitland et al. 2005) or 'markers'. Rather than fully re-examine the patient at each attendance, the clinician simply checks with the patient any change in these asterisks from the subjective examination, and retests the physical asterisks. In this way, the clinician obtains an overview of any change in the patient's condition by looking at the key features of the patient's presentation. Aspects of the subjective findings, which may be used as reassessment asterisks, include:

- information from the body chart
- aggravating factors
- easing factors
- functional ability
- drug therapy
- 24-hour behaviour.

Aspects of the physical examination will include any abnormal joint, nerve and muscle test.

Follow-up appointments

Following treatment, both within and between treatment sessions, the subjective and physical asterisks may alter. However, they may not change in the same way: some may improve, some may worsen and some may remain the same. The clinician has to make an overall judgement as to whether the patient has improved, worsened or stayed the same. It can be useful, when making this judgement, to consider the weighting of each test.

A change in subjective asterisks would seem to be fairly strong evidence that there has been a change. A patient who is able to increase the time ironing or walking, or is able to sleep better, for example, seems fairly clear, although the response will depend, in part, on the patient's attitude to the problem, to the clinician and towards treatment, which may positively or negatively affect the patient's response. Further questioning of any change is always needed to clarify that it is the condition that has improved and not something else. For example, if sleeping has improved, the clinician checks the details of the nature of that improvement, and whether there is any other explanation, such as a new mattress or a change in analgesia that would explain the improvement.

The change in the physical findings also needs careful and unbiased analysis by the clinician. A test must be carried out in a reliable way for the clinician to consider that a change in the test is a real change. That is, a test must, as far as possible, be replicated within and between treatment sessions so that any change in the test result can be considered a real change. Clearly, some of the tests carried out are easier to replicate than others. For example, a change in an active movement is rather more convincing than the clinician's 'feel' of a passive physiological intervertebral movement (PPIVM). Clinicians will do well to evaluate critically their reassessment asterisks and consider carefully how much weight they can place upon them when they interpret a change.

At each attendance, the clinician needs to obtain a detailed account of the effect of the last treatment on the patient's signs and symptoms. This will involve the immediate effects after the last treatment, the relevant activities of the patient since the last treatment, and enquiring how they are presenting on the day of treatment. Patients who say they are worse since the last treatment need to be questioned carefully as this may be due to some activity they have been involved with rather than any treatment that has been given. Patients who say they are better also need to be questioned carefully as the improvement may not be related to treatment. If the patient remains the same, following the subjective and physical reassessment, the clinician may consider altering the treatment dose

Figure 4.5 • Modification, progression and regression of treatment.

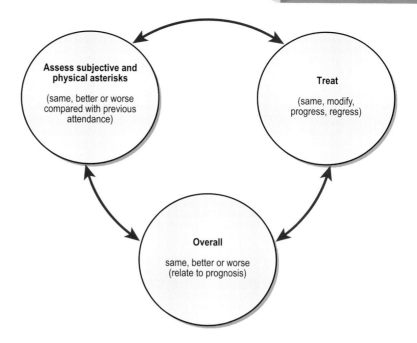

and then seeing whether this alteration has been effective. The process of assessment, treatment and assessment is depicted in Figure 4.5. After, perhaps, the third attendance it may be useful to reflect on the response of the patient to treatment. Suggested prompts are given in section 6 of the clinical reasoning form shown in the Appendix.

The more long-term effects of treatment are determined by comparing the subjective and physical asterisks at a follow-up appointment with the findings at the initial assessment. The clinician's hypotheses from the initial examination of the patient are often rather tenuous and are strengthened at each subsequent treatment session as the effects of treatment become known. Critical in this process is the reassessment of all joint, nerve and muscle asterisks following a treatment, as this allows the clinician to develop a hypothesis of the relationship between the structures. For example, a unilateral posteroanterior pressure to C4 that improves both cervical movements, and a positive neurodynamic test, would suggest a common source of symptoms and a possible neurodynamic interface

problem; where this treatment improves only cervical movements, with no change to the neurodynamic test, it may suggest two separate problems. For further information the reader is referred to the relevant chapter on assessment by Maitland et al. (2005).

After the patient has been discharged it may be useful for the clinician to reflect on the overall management of the patient by completing section 7 of the clinical reasoning form shown in the Appendix.

This completes the discussion on assessment. Two case studies now follow to help clarify the development and implementation of treatment and the management of two patients. The case studies are organised such that the left-hand column provides the clinical examination findings of the patient. The right-hand column provides the thoughts and thus the interpretation of the clinician; these are not firm conclusions – they simply provide the ongoing generation of hypotheses as the information is revealed. It is hoped that, in this way, the clinical reasoning process will be made very explicit.

Case study 1

Patient with arm and hand symptoms

32-year-old woman

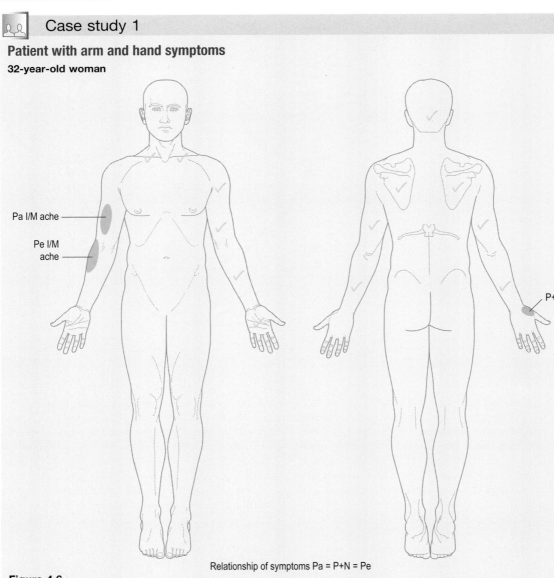

Pa I/M ache

Pe I/M ache

P+N

Relationship of symptoms Pa = P+N = Pe

Figure 4.6

Clinical reasoning

Area of symptoms suggests that the following structure may be implicated. For upper-arm pain: cervical spine (somatic or radicular); shoulder: upper-limb nerves or underlying muscles; for forearm pain: cervical spine (somatic or radicular), elbow or superior radioulnar joint, radial or median nerves or underlying muscles.

P + N: radial nerve, or radicular referral from cervical spine (?C5, C6)

All symptoms are intermittent; this suggests a mechanical nociceptive pain, but the presence of P+N may suggest a peripheral neurogenic component

Relationship of symptoms
Pe can occur independently of P+N and Pa. P+N occur only in the presence of Pe. Pa occurs with worsening Pe and P+N

The onset of each symptom is linked, which suggests a single source of symptoms, i.e. cervical spine nerve root (? C5 or C6) or neurodynamic component

Aggravating factors
Typing for 5 min Pe, increases after 20 min and onset of P+N. After 2 hours Pa

Identifies source of symptoms as follows: cervical spine (somatic or radicular), shoulder, elbow or superior radioulnar joint, radial or median nerves or underlying muscles

Cutting bread (gripping) Pe immediately, P+N occasionally, no Pa

Arm in coat Pe and P+N immediately, no Pa

Radial nerve, shoulder, elbow, superior radioulnar joint

Cervical spine movements ✓✓

Negates cervical spine

Cervical spine stiffness ✓✓

Negates cervical spine

Arm elevation ✓✓

Negates shoulder

Lying on shoulder ✓✓

Negates shoulder

Elbow movements ✓✓

Negates elbow

Supination/pronation ✓✓

Negates superior radioulnar

Because of the positive relationship of symptoms, the spine must continue to be suspected as a source of symptoms. However, because gripping does not involve movement of the cervical spine, peripheral structures must be fully examined

Severity
Typing – can continue after onset of symptoms
Cutting bread – can continue
Single movements do not reproduce symptoms

Not severe, as the patient can continue activities which reproduce her symptoms

In terms of the physical examination. Single movements do not reproduce symptoms. It will therefore be necessary to combine active movements in order to reproduce Pa, Pe and P+Ns

Irritability
Typing – eases immediately if ceased within 30 min
Cutting bread – eases immediately when stops
Arm in coat – eases immediately

Non-irritable, as the symptoms cease immediately unless they are reproduced for a prolonged period of time. Because the examination will not equate with more than 30 min of typing, this is considered to be non-irritable in terms of the physical examination

24-hour behaviour
Wakes 2× per night with P+N, ?? lying on arm, no Pe or Pa
No pain on waking
Pain activity dependent during day

Nerve pain can be worse at night, may be either cervical spine radicular or peripheral nerve

Special questions
None of note

No precautions or contraindications

History of present condition (HPC)
Onset of symptoms approximately 6 months ago. ?? cause. Patient noticed Pe first. Approx. 1 month later P+N onset at time of worsening Pe. Noticed Pa about 4 weeks ago during a period of increased typing at work and increase in Pe and P+N. Problem ISQ at present

Provides supporting evidence that all the symptoms are related

Past medical history
Nil of note, no history of musculoskeletal pain

First episode of pain, so good prognosis

(Continued)

Case study 1—cont'd

Social history

Touch typist, can be typing for up to 8 hours per day

Must assess and educate patient about keyboard positioning to try to prevent future recurrence if appropriate, as this may be a contributory factor

Plan of physical examination

Contradictory evidence was gained from the subjective examination. The relationship of symptoms and the HPC and aggravating factors suggested that there is a single source of symptoms. This, together with the body chart, would implicate the cervical spine. However, the aggravating factors for cervical spine were negative. Therefore, when examining the cervical spine it will be necessary to use combined movements

The aggravating factors, together with the body chart, implicate the elbow region and radial nerve as a source of symptoms

Although the aggravating factors could also have implicated the shoulder region, the area of symptoms, Pe and P+N and the relationship of symptoms negate this as a source

The plan for day 1 is therefore to examine fully the elbow and radial nerve and cervical spine. Clearing the shoulder region is not a priority. Because of P+N a neurological integrity test will be necessary

Physical examination

Observation in sitting

Increased thoracic kyphosis, protracted shoulder girdle and poking chin

Clinical reasoning

Very poor posture may increase the strain on the neuromusculoskeletal system. This may be a contributing factor

Cervical spine active movements

F/LLF/Lrot ✓✓
F/RLF/Rrot ✓✓
E/LLF/Lrot ✓✓
E/RLF/Rrot ✓✓

No symptom reproduction, suggesting that the cervical spine is not a source of symptoms. In order to exclude fully the cervical spine as a source of symptoms it will be necessary to perform accessory movements of the cervical spine, followed by reassessment of asterisks

Active movements

Elbow joint/radioulnar joint

F ✓✓
E ✓✓
Sup ✓✓
Pro ✓✓
F /FAbd/Add ✓✓
E abd ✓✓
E Add grinding of joint ++ and reproduction of Pe (20%)

This suggests that elbow structures are a source of symptoms for Pe. ?? May suggest more radiohumeral than superior radioulnar

Neurological integrity testing

Sensation ✓✓
Myotomes ✓✓
Reflexes ✓✓

Nothing abnormal
Negates cervical radiculopathy

ULTT 2b (radial nerve bias)

Left – Shoulder depression/medial rot/pronation/wrist flexion/elbow extension/abduction 40° – strong stretch in forearm – reduced with left cervical lateral flexion
Right – Shoulder depression/medial rot/pronation/wrist flexion/elbow extension – 45° Pe and P+N, decreased with right cervical lateral flexion

Suggests a neurodynamic component for production of Pe and P+Ns

Isometric muscle testing
Wrist extension – Pe (20%) – strength 50%
Middle finger extension – Pe (30%)
Wrist flexion ✓✓
Gripping – Pe (50%)

Suggests muscle as a source of symptoms
Suggests that extensor carpi radialis brevis may be a
source of symptoms

Cervical spine accessory movements
In neutral ✓✓
In combined positions ✓✓

Negates cervical spine

Reassessment
Active movements of elbow – ISQ
ULTT 2b – ISQ
Isometric muscle tests ISQ

Provides further evidence that the cervical spine is not
the source of symptoms or an interface for the
neurodynamic component

Palpation of elbow region
Tenderness around the right common extensor origin
Pe (10%). No tenderness left

With the result of isometric muscle tests, strongly
suggests extensor muscles as a source of symptoms

Accessory movements – elbow
Humeroulnar ✓✓

Suggests radiohumeral or superior radioulnar joint as a
source of Pe

Radial head ↕ reproduce Pe (20%) IV+

Suggests more radiohumeral than superior radioulnar as
amount of flexion changes response

Radial head ↕ in flexion – no Pe IV+
In ULTT 2b (radial nerve bias) ↕ radial head Pe (50%) and
P+N no Pa

Suggests mechanical interface to radial nerve for source of
Pe and P+N

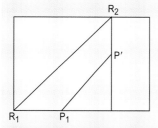

Figure 4.7

Reassess
E/Add elbow – Pe (10%)
ULTT 2b Right – Shoulder depression/medial rot/pronation/
wrist flexion/elbow extension – 30° Pe and P+N
Isometric muscle testing – ISQ

Suggests a local joint component
Provides further evidence that the radial head is a
mechanical interface affecting Pe and P+Ns
Suggests a separate muscular component

Impression
There is evidence to suggest wrist extensor muscles,
radiohumeral joint and radial nerve local to the elbow.
Evidence from the physical examination negates a cervical
component

Plan
Clear glenohumeral joint
Discuss work ergonomics and give advice on
alterations as necessary
In ULTT 2b (at P₁) ↕ radial head IV + 3× (30 s)

Because there is no strong evidence from the subjective
examination that the glenohumeral joint is not a source of
symptoms it will be necessary to clear this in the physical
examination D2

   This was the technique of choice because it was the
most provocative procedure and on reassessment asterisks
improved. Grade IV+ was chosen because it was a
resistance problem and in order to achieve the greatest effect
it is necessary to work as far into resistance as pain allows

(Continued)

Case study 1—cont'd

Day 2

Patient reports no change in subjective markers. No soreness after treatment

Discussed work position: patient will contact occupational health for an ergonomic assessment

E/Add elbow grinding of joint – Pe (20%)

ULTT 2b Right – Shoulder depression/medial rot/ pronation/wrist flexion/elbow extension – 45 degrees Pe and P+N

Isometric muscle testing – ISQ — No change

In ULTT 2b (radial nerve bias) ↕ radial head Pe (50%) and P+N no Pa

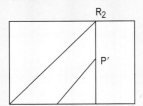

Figure 4.8

Glenohumeral joint

Combined movements in positions related to – aggravating factors ✓✓ — Negates glenohumeral joint
Accessory movements ✓✓
Reassessment of asterisks ISQ

Treatment

In ULTT 2b (at P_1) ↓ radial head IV+ 3× (30 s)

Reassessment

E/Add ✓✓

ULTT 2b Right – Shoulder depression/medial rot/pronation/ wrist flexion/elbow extension – 20° Pe and P+N

Isometric muscle testing – ISQ

— This suggests that the joint and nerve components are related (for example, the radial head and the radial nerve). With a separate muscle component

Day 3

Typing 10–15 min Pe, P+N after 30 min no Pa — Increased time before onset of Pe and P+Ns. No Pa. Indicates an improvement

Cutting bread ISQ

Arm in coat ✓✓

E/Add ✓✓

ULTT 2b Right – Shoulder depression/medial rot/pronation/wrist flexion/elbow extension – 30° Pe and P+N, decreased with right cervical lateral flexion

— Shows improvement in joint and nerve components, but muscle component remains ISQ. Will need to address muscle component separately

Isometric muscle testing – ISQ — Further assessment of muscle component

In ULTT 2b (radial nerve bias) ↓ Pe (30%) and P+N no Pa

Specific soft-tissue mobilisation assessment

Medial glide in elbow extension most provocative Pe (40%)

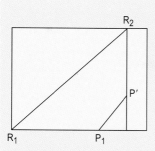

Figure 4.9

Treatment
In extension accessory (medial glide). SSTM to common
extensor origin IV+ 3× (30 s)

Reassessment

E/Add ✓✓	No change
ULTT 2b Right – Shoulder depression/medial rot/ pronation/wrist flexion/elbow extension – 30° Pe and P+N	No change
Isometric muscle testing	
Wrist extension Pe ✓✓	
Middle finger extension (20%)	
Gripping (30%)	Improved, and so supports a separate muscle component

Treatment 2

In ULTT 2b (at P_1) ↕ radial head IV+ 3× (60 s)	The duration of treatment has been increased in an attempt to gain quicker progress. It was felt that this treatment could be progressed despite adding a new treatment technique as the new technique aimed to address the muscle component and the initial technique had not affected the muscle component

Reassessment
ULTT 2b Right – Shoulder depression/medial rot/
pronation/wrist flexion/elbow extension Pe and P+N
Isometric muscle testing – ISQ

Plan

Progress both treatments (addressing all components) Assess effects of active neural/muscle mobilisation (ULTT 2b) and if appropriate teach for home exercise Ensure that ergonomic advice has been given	This would enable the patient to continue her own treatment and become less reliant on passive modalities

P+N, pins and needles; Pa, pain arm; Pe, pain elbow; ISQ, in status quo; F/LLF, flexion/left lateral flexion; F/RLF, flexion/right lateral flexion; E/LLF, extension/left lateral flexion; E/RLF, extension/right lateral flexion; ULTT, upper-limb tension test; SSTM, specific soft-tissue mobilisation.

Case study 2

Patient with back and lateral calf pain

43-year-old man

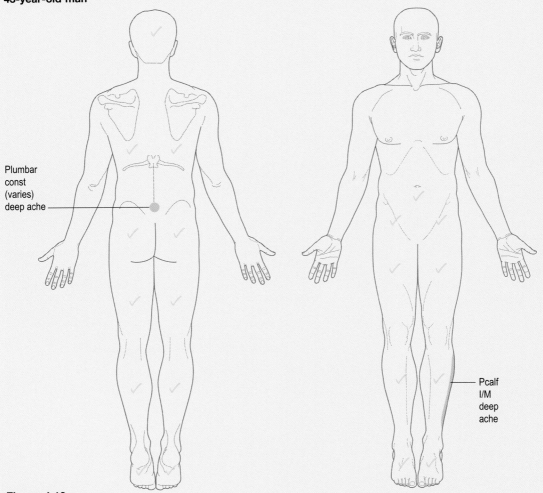

Plumbar
const
(varies)
deep ache

Pcalf
I/M
deep
ache

Figure 4.10

Relationship of symptoms
Plumbar and Pcalf come on together – they are related

Clinical reasoning
Area of symptoms suggests the following structures may be implicated. For lumbar pain: lumbar spine or SIJ; for calf pain: referral from lumbar spine or SIJ, low lumbar neurodynamic, L5 dermatome or sclerotome, or L5/S1 nerve root, superior tibiofibular joint, peroneal muscles, common peroneal nerve

Constant but varying lumbar spine pain suggests inflammatory and mechanical component

Lumbar spine and calf pain come on together, never separately: this suggests that symptoms are related and therefore implicates lumbar spine, SIJ, L5/S1 nerve root, or a neurodynamic component as source of both symptoms

Aggravating factors

Bending forward Plumbar, no Pcalf
Slump sitting: Plumbar immediately and, if knee extended, Pcalf
Sitting upright: no pains
Long sitting: both pains
Standing: no pains
Walking: no pains
Standing on one leg: no pains
Turning over in bed: no pains

Identifies the source of symptoms as follows:
Lumbar spine/SIJ

Lumbar spine/neurodynamic component
Extension eases lumbar pain
Lumbar spine/neurodynamic
Extension asymptomatic, negates L5/S1 nerve root
Extension asymptomatic, negates L5/S1 nerve root
Not SIJ

Because of the positive relationship of symptoms and aggravating factors linking lumbar spine/neurodynamic structures to all of the patient's symptoms, the superior tibiofibular joint and peroneal muscles are removed from the hypothesis of possible structures at fault

Severity

Bending forward – able to stay with pain

Not severe

Irritability

Returning to extension eases pain immediately
Easing factors:
lying prone eases both pains

Not irritable
Eased by extension ± not weight-bearing. Negates L5/S1 nerve root

24-hour behaviour

Not woken, first thing in morning stiff in lumbar spine for 15 min only

More mechanical than inflammatory

Special questions

Nil of note

No precautions or contraindications

History of present condition

Moving washing machine 10 days ago felt Plumbar as bending over and pushing with left foot in front of right. Next morning on rising felt Pcalf as well as Plumbar. Patient thinks just strained his back and wants some exercises to help reduce his pain

Recent onset with expected inflammatory component. Position of injury suggests neurodynamic component
Patient has positive attitude to his problem, appropriate expectations and is confident of improvement. Relationship again emphasises relationship of symptoms

Stage (or status) of condition

No change, still has both pains to same intensity

Need to try to produce a change with treatment

Past medical history

Nil of note. No history of LBP, calf pain

First episode of low-back pain, so good prognosis. Must educate patient about back pain to get a speedy recovery this time and educate to try to prevent a recurrence in the future

Social history

Services washing machines, full-time job, often having to move machines. Still working. Plays football 2× a week, not been playing since injury

Must educate patient on moving and handling. Need to make appointments convenient to his work. Need to encourage his return to football. Still at work – good prognostic indicator

Physical examination

Observation in standing: nil of note

(Continued)

Case study 2—cont'd

Active movements

lumbar:

*flex fingertips to base of patella, Plumbar overpressure increased Plumbar and produced Pcalf

with cervical flexion: increased calf pain

with pelvic compression: pain ISQ ext full range no pain on OP

lat flex L full range no pain on OP

lat flex R full range no pain on OP

rotation L full range no pain on OP

rotation R full range no pain on OP

*flex/R lat flex 1/4 range lat flex Pcalf OP increased Plumbar and Pcalf flex/L lat flex full range no pain on OP

Identifies source of symptoms as follows:
Lumbar spine/SIJ

With neurodynamic component
Not SIJ

As expected, negates L5/S1 nerve root
As expected, negates L5/S1 nerve root
As expected
As expected
As expected
Lumbar spine/neurodynamic component
Movements of flexion, contralateral lateral flexion suggest a regular stretch pattern

SIJ

Standing flex NAD

Sitting flex NAD

Hip flex ipsilateral NAD

contralateral NAD

Not SIJ
Not SIJ
Not SIJ
Not SIJ
Active movements confirm relationship of symptoms and a flexion-related problem

Neurological integrity

Sensation NAD

Strength NAD

Reflexes NAD

No neurological deficit, negates L5/S1 nerve root compromise

Neurodynamic tests

*SLR 60° Plumbar 70° Plumbar and Pcalf plantarflexion eased Pcalf

Neurodynamic component

Accessory movements

Central PA L4 and L5 stiff and tender

Unilateral PA left L4 tender

Unilateral PA left L5 stiff and Plumbar, with cephalad inclination increased Plumbar

Movement diagram of unilateral PA left L5

L5/S1 symptomatic level producing both pains
Resistance problem with a little pain. Treatment grade of movement could be IV or IV+

```
        R₂
 ┌────────┬──┐
 │       ╱│  │
 │      ╱ │  │
 │     ╱  ├─P'    Plumbar
 │    ╱  ╱│  │
 │   ╱  ╱ │  │
 │  ╱  ╱  │  │
 └────────┴──┘
 R₁     P₁
```

Figure 4.11

In lumbar flexion/R lat flex did unilateral PA L5 with ceph inclination: Plumbar, no Pcalf

Maximum pain provoked in combined position but calf pain not produced, suggests mechanism of pain production of Plumbar and Pcalf different; perhaps Plumbar mechanical nociceptive, Pcalf neurodynamic. In combined position more pain at L5 than L4: confirms L5/S1 level rather than L4/5

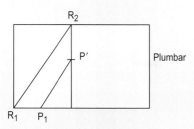

Figure 4.12
Lumbar flex fingertips 5 cm lower PISQ
Flex/R lat flex ISQ
SLR ISQ

On reassessment: some improvement, examination may
not have done sufficient to produce a strong therapeutic
effect

SIJ
AP/PA/Longitudinal caud/ceph NAD
Lumbar flex fingertips 5 cm below base patella PISQ
Flex/R lat flex ISQ
SLR ISQ

Not SIJ
On reassessment no improvement. Final confirmation not
SIJ

Source of symptoms
L5/S1 dysfunction with a neurodynamic component
giving rise to mechanical nociceptive pain in the
leg and inflammatory nociceptive ache in the lumbar spine

PPIVM reduced flexion/lat flex R and rotation L L5/S1,
otherwise NAD

Confirms flexion hypomobility L5/S1. May use rotation/
SLR as treatment technique
Explanation of above given to the patient. Discussed and
agreed treatment plan

Treatment day 1
Unilateral PA with ceph
Inclination left L5 Grade IV × 1 (1min)
Lumbar flex fingertips 7.5 cm below base patella increased
Plumbar OP increased Plumbar and produced Pcalf
Flex/R lat flex 1/4 range lat flex Pcalf OP increased
Plumbar and Pcalf
SLR ISQ
Unilateral PA with ceph inclination left L5 Grade IV × 1
(1 min)
Lumbar flex FT 7.5 cm below base of patella and Plumbar
'less', OP increased Plumbar and produced Pcalf
flex/R lat flex 1/3 range lat flex Pcalf OP increased Plumbar
and Pcalf but 'less'
SLR ISQ
Unilateral PA with ceph
Inclination left L5 Grade IV × 1 (1min)
Lumbar flex FT mid-calf increased Plumbar, OP increased
Plumbar and produced Pcalf
Flex/R lat flex 1/2 range lat flex no Pcalf OP increased
Plumbar and Pcalf but 'less than before'
SLR ISQ
Explained probable cause of back and leg pain and
explained natural history of back pain. Patient motivated to
look after his back

Try at the most symptomatic level. Grade IV to reduce
resistance and increase range
Slightly further lumbar flexion, pain the same
ISQ
ISQ

Try another repetition

Less pain now on lumbar flexion
Combined movement improved in range and pain
No change in SLR

Three repetitions of mobilisation treatment have improved
flexion and combined movement of flexion and lateral
flexion. No improvement on SLR, may need to treat
neurodynamic component next time

Must try to prevent a recurrence. Patient's motivation is
excellent; this may help to prevent this acute injury
becoming a chronic condition

Day 2
Patient felt less back and calf pain for 2 hours after last
treatment, then ISQ. Has not had to lift at work, on light
duties

Some lasting improvement for 2 hours; good sign that
further treatment will have longer symptomatic relief.
Patient must be looking after back, good

(Continued)

Case study 2—cont'd

Lumbar flex FT 7.5 cm above base patella increased
Plumbar, OP increased Plumbar and produced Pcalf
Flex/R lat flex 1/3 range lat flex no Pcalf OP increased
Plumbar and Pcalf
SLR ISQ
Movement diagram of unilat PA left L5

Maintained some improvement in flexion and combined
flex/lat flex range

SLR not changed by treatment yet
Movement diagram also maintained some improvement

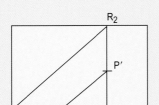

Figure 4.13
Unilateral PA with ceph inclination left L5 Grade IV+
× 3 (1 min)

Lumbar flex FT mid-calf increased Plumbar, OP increased
Plumbar and produced Pcalf
Flex/R lat flex 1/2 range lat flex no Pcalf OP increased
Plumbar and Pcalf
SLR ISQ
Unilateral PA with ceph inclination left L5 Grade IV+
× 3 (1 min) in flexion/R lat flex
Lumbar flex FT mid-calf increased Plumbar, OP increased
Plumbar and less Pcalf
Flex/R lat flex 1/2 range lat flex no Pcalf OP increased
Plumbar and Pcalf, but less intense
SLR ISQ
Mobilised SLR with hip flexion movement to
approx. 60°, producing lumbar spine and some calf
pain ×1 (1 min)

Lumbar flex ISQ as above flex/R lat flex ISQ as above SLR
70° increased
Plumbar, 80° increased Plumbar and produced Pcalf
Repeat SLR treatment as above × 1 (1 min)
Lumbar flex range ISQ but Plumbar and Pcalf 'less'
flex/R lat flex ISQ as above
SLR 75° increased Plumbar, 85° increased Plumbar and
produced Pcalf
Repeat SLR treatment as above ×1 (1 min)
Lumbar flex slight increase in range and Plumbar and Pcalf
'less'
flex/R lat flex ISQ as above
SLR 80° increased Plumbar, 85° increased Plumbar and
produced Pcalf
Patient agreed to do daily SLR stretches (every 2 hours)
Explanation given
Patient to attend 6-week back care classes in the
physiotherapy department

Need to progress treatment: increase grade to a
IV+ since pain eased and good response to last
treatment

Improved range
Improved range and no calf pain now at end of active
range. Still no change, need to treat neurodynamic
component

Fully progress joint treatment

Progression of joint treatment has improved lumbar
spine movements, but has had no effect on
neurodynamic component. Need to treat SLR directly

Start with a movement that provokes part of the calf pain,
don't want to exacerbate the calf pain. If no flare-up
progress to stronger movement

No effect on lumbar movements

SLR improved in range

SLR treatment eased calf pain on lumbar flexion; no
change to combined movement
SLR improved in range

SLR treatment increased range as well as reduced calf
pain; no change to combined movement

Further improvement in SLR range

Need to ask patient to continue treatment at home
Need to educate patient to prevent a recurrence

Day 3

Exercises feel they are 'loosening up the back and leg pains'. Back pain not constant anymore. Much less calf and back pain since last treatment. Able to bend forwards more easily and can slump sitting without just a little calf pain. In long sitting in the bath only has some calf pain, able to straighten left knee down now

Back feels less stiff in morning

No resting symptoms

Lumbar flex FT mid-calf Plumbar, OP increased Plumbar and produced Pcalf

flex/R lat flex 1/2 range lat flex OP increased Plumbar and Pcalf

SLR 80° Pcalf only

Movement diagram of unilat PA left L5

The patient is improving at a satisfactory rate. The inflammatory pain in the lumbar spine is settling, which is expected as it is 15 days postinjury

All original functional difficulties are improving

Maintained improvement

Maintained improvement

Improved with home exercises. Doing them correctly and frequently

Movement diagram also improved since last treatment

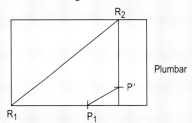

Figure 4.14

In flexion/right lateral flexion did unilateral PA with ceph inclination left L5 Grade IV+ × 3 (1 min)

Lumbar flex FT ankle joint, OP produced some Pcalf

flex/R lat flex full range lat flex OP some Pcalf

SLR 85° Pcalf

Grade V rotation R manipulation L5/S1

Lumbar flex FT ankle joint, OP no pain

flex/R lat flex full range lat flex OP some Pcalf, but less

SLR 85° Pcalf ISQ

mobilised SLR with hip flexion movement to approx. 60°, producing lumbar spine and some calf pain ×3 (1 min)

Lumbar flex FT ankle joint, OP no pain

flex/R lat flex full range lat flex OP slight Pcalf, 'much less than before'

SLR 85° Pcalf, 'less'

Home exercises checked, to continue to do exercises and see in 1 week

Continuing with back care classes

Progress treatment by applying PA in the symptomatic combined position

Range and pain improved

Range and pain improved

Improved range of SLR

Some improvement in lumbar spine movements

SLR treatment improved pain

SLR treatment improved pain

Less pain

Vast improvement, with home exercises the patient's condition should continue to improve

Day 4

No back or leg pain for last 4 days. Taking care of back and learnt how to move washing machines and generally how to look after back

Lumbar flex full range and no pain on OP

flex/R lat flex full range and no pain on OP

SLR full range and no pain on OP

Movement diagram of unilat PA left L5

This may help prevent recurrence

Asymptomatic

Asymptomatic

Asymptomatic

Asymptomatic

Emphasise must continue to look after back if to prevent a recurrence

(Continued)

Case study 2—cont'd

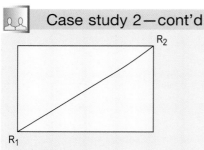

Figure 4.15
Discharged with advice

SIJ, sacroiliac joint; LBP, low-back pain; ISQ, in status quo; OP, overpressure; NAD, nothing abnormal detected; SLR, straight-leg raise; PISQ, pain in status quo; AP, anteroposterior; PA, posteroanterior; PPIVM, passive physiological intervertebral movements.

APPENDIX

CLINICAL REASONING FORM

1.1 Source of symptoms

Symptomatic area	Structures under area	Structures which can refer to area	Supporting evidence

1.2 What is the mechanism of each symptom? Explain from information from the subjective and physical examination findings

	Symptom	Symptom	Symptom	Symptom
Subjective				
Physical				

1.3 Following the physical examination what is your clinical diagnosis?

2. Contributing factors

2.1 What factors need to be examined/explored in the physical examination?

2.2 How will you address each contributing factor?

(Continued)

APPENDIX—cont'd

3. Precautions and contraindications

3.1 Are any symptoms severe?   Yes   No
Which symptoms, and explain why

3.2 Are any symptoms irritable?   Yes   No
Which symptoms, and explain why

3.3   How much of each symptom are you prepared to provoke in the physical examination?

Symptom	Short of P_1	Point of onset or increase in resting symptoms	Partial reproduction	Total reproduction

3.4 Will a neurological examination be necessary in the physical?
                        Yes   No   Explain why

3.5 Following the subjective examination are there any precautions or contraindications?
                        Yes   No   Explain why

4. Management

4.1 What tests will you do in the physical and what are the expected findings?

Physical tests	Expected findings

4.2 Were there any unexpected findings from the physical? Explain

4.3 What will be your subjective and physical reassessment asterisks?

4.4 What is your first choice of treatment (be exact) and explain why?

4.5 What do you expect the response to be over the next 24 hours following the 1st visit? Explain

(Continued)

APPENDIX—cont'd

4.6 How do you think you will treat and manage the patient at the 2nd visit, if the patient returns:

Same

Better

Worse

4.7 What advice and education will you give the patient?

4.8 What needs to be examined on the 2nd and 3rd visits?

2nd visit	3rd visit

5. Prognosis

5.1 **List the positive and negative factors (from both the subjective and physical examination findings) in considering the patient's prognosis?**

	Positive	Negative
Subjective		
Physical		

4.6 Overall, is the patient's condition:
                        Improving   Worsening   Static

5.3 What is your overall prognosis for this patient? Be specific

6. After 3rd attendance

6.1 Has your understanding of the patient's problem changed from your interpretations made following the initial subjective and physical examination? If so explain

6.2 On reflection, were there any clues that you initially missed, mis-interpreted, under- or over-weighted? If so explain

7. After discharge

7.1 Has your understanding of the patient's problem changed from your interpretations made following the 3rd attendance? If so explain how

7.2 What you have learnt from the management of this patient which will be helpful to you in the future?

References

Austen, R., 1991. The distribution and characteristics of lumbar-lower limb symptoms in subjects with and without a neurological deficit. In: Proceedings of the Manipulative Physiotherapists Association of Australia, 7th Biennial Conference, New South Wales, pp. 252–257.

Bogduk, N., 1994. Cervical causes of headache and dizziness. In: Boyling, J.D., Palastanga, N. (Eds.), Grieve's modern manual therapy, second ed. Churchill Livingstone, Edinburgh, pp. 317–331.

Clinical Standards Advisory Group, 1994. Report on back pain. HMSO, London.

Dalton, P.A., Jull, G.A., 1989. The distribution and characteristics of neck-arm pain in patients with and without a neurological deficit. Aust. J. Physiother. 35, 3–8.

Deyo, R.A., Diehl, A.K., 1988. Cancer as a cause of back pain: frequency, clinical presentation and diagnostic strategies. J. Gen. Intern. Med. 3, 230–238.

Gifford, L., 1998. Pain. In: Pitt-Brooke, J., Reid, H., Lockwood, J. (Eds.), Rehabilitation of movement, theoretical basis of clinical practice. W B Saunders, London, pp. 196–232.

Goodman, C.C., Boissonnault, W.G., 1998. Pathology: implications for the physical therapist. W. B. Saunders, Philadelphia.

Greenhalgh, S., Selfe, J., 2006. Red flags. A guide to identifying serious pathology of the spine. Churchill Livingstone, Edinburgh.

Grieve, G.P., 1981. Common vertebral joint problems. Churchill Livingstone, Edinburgh.

Grieve, G.P., 1994. The masqueraders. In: Boyling, J.D., Palastanga, N. (Eds.), Grieve's modern manual therapy, second ed. Churchill Livingstone, Edinburgh, pp. 841–856.

Gundry, C., Fritts, H., 1997. Magnetic resonance imaging of the musculoskeletal system. Part 8. The spine, section 2. Clin. Orthop. Relat. Res. 343, 260–271.

Henschke, N., Maher, C.G., Refshauge, K.M., 2007. Screening for malignancy in low back pain patients: a systematic review. Eur. Spine 16, 1673–1679.

Higgs, J., Jones, M., 2000. Clinical reasoning in the health professions, second ed. Butterworth-Heinemann, Oxford.

Jensen, G.M., Gwyer, J., Hack, L.M., et al., 1999. Expertise in physical therapy practice. Butterworth-Heinemann, Boston.

Jones, M.A., 1994. Clinical reasoning process in manipulative therapy. In: Boyling, J.D., Palastanga, N. (Eds.), Grieve's modern manual therapy, second ed. Churchill Livingstone, Edinburgh, pp. 471–489.

Jones, M.A., Jones, H.M., 1994. Principles of the physical examination. In: Boyling, J.D., Palastanga, N. (Eds.), Grieve's modern manual therapy, second ed. Churchill Livingstone, Edinburgh, pp. 491–501.

Kaplan, P., Helms, C., Dussalt, R., et al., 2001. Musculoskeletal MRI, second ed. W. B. Saunders, Philadelphia.

Maitland, G.D., Hengeveld, E., Banks, K., et al., 2005. Maitland's vertebral manipulation, seventh ed. Butterworth-Heinemann, Edinburgh.

Merskey, R., Albe-Fessard, D.G., Bonica, J.J., et al., 1979. Pain terms: a list with definitions and notes on usage. Pain 6, 249–252.

Pietrobon, R., Coeytaux, R.R., Carey, T.S., et al., 2002. Standard scales for measurement of functional outcome for cervical pain or dysfunction: a systematic review. Spine 27, 2299–2301.

Refshauge, K., Gass, E., 2004. Musculoskeletal physiotherapy clinical science and evidence-based practice, second ed. Butterworth Heinemann, Edinburgh.

Stratford, P., Gill, C., Westaway, M., et al., 1995. Assessing disability and change on individual patients; a report of a patient specific measure. Physiother. Can. 47, 258–263.

Examination of the temporomandibular region

5

Roger Kerry

Possible causes of pain and/or limitation of movement

- Muscle disorders:
  - masticatory muscle disorders
  - myofascial pain related to mouth-opening (pain/ache in jaw, temples, face, pre-auricular, intra-auricular)
- Disc displacements:
  - articular disc displacement with or without reduction (acute or chronic)
  - articular disc displacement with or without limited mandibular opening (acute or chronic)
  - retrodiscal tissue inflammation/dysfunction
  - subluxation
  - dislocation
- Diagnoses:
  - hypermobility
  - degenerative conditions: osteoarthrosis, arthralgia, or arthritis; polyarthritides
  - inflammatory conditions: synovitis or capsulitis
  - ankylosis: fibrous or bony ankylosis
  - neoplasm: malignant or benign
  - cranial neuralgia
- Other:
  - deviation in form (differentiate congenital from acquired)
  - referral of symptoms from the upper cervical spine, cervical spine, cranium, eyes, ears, nose, sinuses, teeth, mouth or other facial structures (Dworkin et al. 1992).

Disorders of the temporomandibular joint (TMJ) are common and offer an interesting diagnostic and therapeutic challenge for the clinician. Manual therapy for mechanical TMJ presentations has been shown to be effective in a number of studies (Cleland & Palmer 2004; McNeely et al. 2006; Medlicott & Harris 2006; Shin et al. 2007). Craniofacial pain is often a result of TMJ dysfunction; however, pain and TMJ disorders are also associated with symptoms from the upper cervical spine (C0–C3). The upper cervical spine can refer pain to the same areas as the TMJ, i.e. the frontal, retro-orbital, temporal and occipital areas of the head. The TMJ may also refer pain into the pre- or intra-auricular area, or along the mandible (Feinstein et al. 1954; Rocabado 1983). Symptoms in these areas can be mediated by both the upper cervical spine and the TMJ due to neural convergence in the trigeminocervical nucleus. This association is supported by assessing the effects of manual therapy of the cervical spine on the TMJ (Mansilla-Ferragut et al. 2009). For these reasons, it is suggested that examination of the temporomandibular region is always accompanied by examination of the upper cervical spine. Interested readers may like to read further and a textbook devoted to this region by von Piekartz & Bryden (2001) may prove useful.

Further details of the questions asked during the subjective examination and the tests carried out during the physical examination can be found in Chapters 2 and 3 respectively.

The order of the subjective questioning and the physical tests described below can be altered as appropriate for the patient being examined.

Subjective examination

Body chart

The following information concerning the area and type of current symptoms can be recorded on a body chart (see Figure 2.3).

Area of current symptoms

Be exact when mapping out the area of the symptoms. Symptoms can include crepitus, clicking (on opening and/or closing), grating, thudding sounds and joint locking, limitation or difficulty in jaw movement, as well as pain around the joint, head and neck. Ascertain the worst symptom and record the patient's interpretation of where s/he feels the symptoms are coming from.

Areas relevant to the region being examined

All other relevant areas are checked for symptoms; it is important to ask about pain or even stiffness, as this may be relevant to the patient's main symptom. Mark unaffected areas with ticks (✓) on the body chart. There are anatomical (Rocabado 1983; Ayub et al. 1984; Darling et al. 1987) links between the TMJ and the cervical spine, particularly the upper cervical spine, and so the clinician should

check carefully for any symptoms in the cervical spine. Symptoms in the thoracic spine, head, mouth and teeth should also be checked.

Ask whether the patient has ever experienced disequilibrium, dizziness or other symptoms associated with cervical arterial dysfunction (see Chapter 6). If these symptoms are a feature described by the patient, the clinician determines what factors aggravate and ease the symptoms, their duration and severity, and ultimately determines how likely these symptoms are related to serious neurovascular pathology. Suspicious presentations should be referred for medical investigation (Bogduk 1994; Kerry & Taylor 2006).

Quality of pain

Establish the quality of the pain. This is important information when attempting to determine the primary source of pain during differentiation between intra-/extra-articular, retrodiscal or muscular structures.

Intensity of pain

The intensity of pain can be measured using, for example, a visual analogue scale (VAS), as shown in Figure 2.8. A pain diary (see Chapter 2) may be useful for patients with chronic TMJ or cervical spine pain and/or headaches, to determine the pain patterns and triggering factors over a period of time.

Depth of pain

Establish the depth of the pain. Does the patient feel that it is on the surface or deep inside?

Abnormal sensation

Check for any altered sensation locally over the temporomandibular region and, if appropriate, over the face, cervical spine, upper thoracic spine or upper limbs.

Constant or intermittent symptoms

Ascertain the frequency of the symptoms, and whether they are constant or intermittent. If symptoms are constant, check whether there is variation in the intensity of the symptoms, as constant unremitting pain is indicative of neoplastic disease.

Relationship of symptoms

Determine the relationship between the symptomatic areas – do they come together or separately? For example, the patient may have pain over the jaw without neck pain, or the pains may always be present together.

Behaviour of symptoms

Aggravating factors

For each symptomatic area, establish what movements and/or positions aggravate the patient's symptoms, i.e. what brings them on (or makes them worse)? can this position or movement be maintained (severity)? what happens to other symptoms when this symptom is produced (or is made worse)? and how long does it take for symptoms to ease once the position or movement is stopped (irritability)? These questions help to confirm the relationship between the symptoms.

The clinician also asks the patient about theoretically known aggravating factors for structures that could be a source of the symptoms. Common aggravating factors for the temporomandibular region are opening the mouth, yawning, singing, shouting and chewing challenging foods such as nuts, meat, raw fruit, crusty bread and vegetables. Aggravating factors for other regions, which may need to be queried if they are suspected to be a source of the symptoms, are shown in Table 2.3.

The clinician ascertains how the symptoms affect function, such as: static and active postures, e.g. sitting, reading, writing (the patient may lean the hand on the jaw to support the head when reading or writing), using the telephone (it may be held between the head and shoulder), eating and drinking. The patient may have a habit of biting fingernails or chewing hair, pen or pencil tops, all of which may stress the temporomandibular region. Sports that might affect the TMJ could be shotputting and snooker. The clinician finds out if the patient is left- or right-handed as there may be increased stress on the dominant side.

Detailed information on each of the above activities is useful in order to help determine the structure(s) at fault and to identify functional restrictions. This information can be used to determine the aims of treatment and any advice that may be required. The most notable functional restrictions are highlighted with asterisks (*), explored in the physical examination, and reassessed at subsequent treatment sessions to evaluate treatment intervention.

Easing factors

For each symptomatic area, the clinician asks what movements and/or positions ease the patient's symptoms, how long it takes to ease them and what happens to other symptoms when this symptom is relieved. These questions help to confirm the relationship between the symptoms.

The clinician asks the patient about theoretically known easing factors for structures that could be a source of the symptoms. For example, symptoms from the TMJ may be eased by placing the joint in a particular position, whereas symptoms from the upper cervical spine may be eased by supporting the head or neck. The clinician can then analyse the position or movement that eases the symptoms, to help determine the structure at fault.

Twenty-four-hour behaviour

The clinician determines the 24-hour behaviour of symptoms by asking questions about night, morning and evening symptoms.

Night symptoms. The following questions may be asked:

- Do you have any difficulty getting to sleep?
- What position is most comfortable/ uncomfortable?
- What is your normal sleeping position?
- What is your present sleeping position?
- Do you grind your teeth at night?
- Do your symptoms wake you at night? If so,
  ○ Which symptom(s)?
  ○ How many times in the past week?
  ○ How many times in a night?
  ○ How long does it take to get back to sleep?
- How many and what type of pillows are used?

Morning and evening symptoms. The clinician determines the pattern of the symptoms first thing in the morning, through the day and at the end of the day. Patients who grind their teeth at night may wake up with a headache, and/or facial, jaw or tooth symptoms (Kraus 1994).

Stage of the condition

In order to determine the stage of the condition, the clinician asks whether the symptoms are getting better, getting worse or remaining unchanged.

Special questions

Special questions must always be asked, as they may identify certain precautions or contraindications to the physical examination and/or treatment (see

Table 2.4). As mentioned in Chapter 2, the clinician must differentiate between conditions that are suitable for conservative treatment and systemic, neoplastic and other non-neuromusculoskeletal conditions, which require referral to a medical practitioner. Readers are referred to Appendix 2.3 for details of various serious pathological processes that can mimic neuromusculoskeletal conditions (Grieve 1994).

The following information should be considered for TMJ patients.

Clicking

Establishing the nature of a click can assist diagnosis. The mandibular condyles normally translate anteriorly out of the mandibular fossa during opening. The condyle contacts with the articular disc which rotates relatively posteriorly into the fossa (in order to maintain condyle contact with its intermediate zone), thus allowing the condyles to translate fully. Clicking is associated with abnormal discocondylar mechanics.

- A single click on opening (no click on closing) is indicative of a bunched/adhered disc forcing the condyle to push past the posterior enlargement rapidly into the intermediate zone of the disc, whereby normal mechanics are restored. This click is heard early on in range of opening. A click further into range is indicative of probable anterior disc displacement (subluxation). When a click is heard in this case, normal mechanics have again been restored, i.e. the displacement has been reduced.
- A double (reciprocal) click, a click on opening and closing, is again indicative of anterior disc displacement with a retrusive (closing) component. The second click is usually a result of the disc being held too far anteriorly by the lateral pterygoid muscle.

Bruxism

The extent and nature of teeth grinding should be established, and its relationship to the present condition considered. The mechanical forces produced during grinding can contribute to TMJ dysfunction. Bruxism is often a manifestation of stress and as such it is important to consider associated psychological factors which may be causing, contributing to, and/or mediating the present condition.

Dental disorders

The association between upper and lower tooth contact (occlusion) and forces through the TMJ should be considered. A thorough history of all dental disorders, including surgery, tooth extraction, bracing, childhood developmental management and prolonged opening during dental examination/treatment, should be noted. Asymmetrical occlusion can affect the centric relationship between the mandible, maxilla and temporal bones. This can produce pathomechanical changes within and around the TMJ. The relevance of dental disorders with the presenting condition should be established.

Cranial nerve disorders

Signs and symptoms associated with TMJ dysfunction can be similar to those arising from frank cranial nerve disorders. It is therefore essential to establish whether or not there are cranial nerve disorders present which would require further medical investigation. Alternatively, known cranial nerve disorders may result in, or contribute to, TMJ dysfunction, and vice versa. The relevance of any disorder needs to be established. For example, pain and/or altered sensation in the forehead and face should be differentiated with trigeminal (cranial nerve (CN) V) neuralgia; consideration should be given to the trigeminal nerve innervation of masticating muscles for difficulties in opening and closing; facial asymmetries need to be differentiated from facial nerve (CN VII) palsies; aural symptoms should be differentiated from vestibulocochlear nerve (CN VIII) palsies – which may be related to serious neoplastic pathology; swallowing problems should be differentiated from glossopharyngeal (IX) and vagus (X) nerve palsies; tongue asymmetries should be differentiated from hypoglossal nerve (XII) disorder.

Cervical arterial dysfunction

The clinician should be able to identify symptoms suggestive of vasculopathy related to either the vertebral arteries (e.g. vertebrobasilar insufficiency (VBI)) or the internal carotid arteries. Pathology of these vessels can mimic craniofacial signs and symptoms associated with TMJ dysfunction (see Chapter 6). Symptoms include: disequilibrium, dizziness, altered vision (including diplopia), nausea, ataxia, drop attacks, altered facial sensation, difficulty speaking, difficulty swallowing, sympathoplegia, hemianaesthesia and hemiplegia (Bogduk 1994; Kerry & Taylor 2006).

Ptosis (drooping eyelid) is associated with internal carotid artery pathology and may be mistaken for facial asymmetry. Specifically, jaw claudication related to carotid pathologies can mimic mechanical TMJ dysfunction. If present, the clinician determines in the usual way the aggravating and easing factors. Similar symptoms can also be related to upper cervical instability and diseases of the inner ear. It is important to remember that, in their pre-ischaemic stage, cervical vasculopathies can present with just neck and head pain. Awareness of predisposing factors to vascular injury and information regarding the patient's blood pressure can assist in the diagnosis (Kerry & Taylor 2006, 2008, 2009). For presentations of temporofrontal headache, the clinician should also consider temporal arteritis as a differential diagnosis.

History of the present condition

For each symptomatic area, the clinician needs to discover how long the symptom has been present, whether there was a sudden or slow onset and whether there was a known cause that provoked the onset of the symptom, such as trauma, stress, surgery or occupation. If the onset was slow, the clinician should find out if there has been any change in the patient's lifestyle, e.g. a new diet, recent dental treatment or other factors contributing to increased stress felt by the patient. To confirm the relationship between symptoms, the clinician asks what happened to other symptoms when each symptom began.

Past medical history

The following information is obtained from the patient and/or dental/medical notes:

- The details of any relevant dental/medical history, particularly involving the teeth, jaw, cranium or cervical spine.
- The history of any previous attacks: how many episodes? when were they? what was the cause? what was the duration of each episode? and did the patient fully recover between episodes?
  If there have been no previous attacks, has the patient had any episodes of stiffness in the TMJ or cervical spine? Check for a history of trauma or recurrent minor trauma.
- Ascertain the results of any past treatment for the same or similar problem. Past treatment records may be obtained for further information.

Social and family history

Social and family history that is relevant to the onset and progression of the patient's problem is recorded. This includes the patient's perspectives, experience and expectations, age, employment, home situation and details of any leisure activities. Factors from this information may indicate direct and/or indirect mechanical influences on the TMJ. In order to treat the patient appropriately, it is important that the condition is managed within the context of the patient's social and work environment. TMJ disorders can have significant psychosocial associations and contributing factors. The clinician may ask the following types of question to elucidate psychosocial factors:

- Have you had time off work in the past with your pain?
- What do you understand to be the cause of your pain?
- What are you expecting will help you?
- How is your employer/co-workers/family responding to your pain?
- What are you doing to cope with your pain?
- Do you think you will return to work? When?

Although these questions are described in relation to psychosocial risk factors for poor outcomes for patients with low-back pain (Waddell 2004), they may be relevant to other patients.

Plan of the physical examination

When all this information has been collected, the subjective examination is complete. It is useful at this stage to highlight with asterisks (*), for ease of reference, important findings and particularly one or more functional restrictions. These can then be re-examined at subsequent treatment sessions to evaluate treatment intervention.

In order to plan the physical examination, the following hypotheses need to be developed from the subjective examination:

- The regions and structures that need to be examined as a possible cause of the symptoms, e.g. temporomandibular region, upper cervical spine, cervical spine, thoracic spine, muscles and nerves. Often, it is not possible to examine fully at the first attendance and so examination of the structures must be prioritised over subsequent treatment sessions.

- Other factors that need to be examined, e.g. working and everyday postures, vertebral artery, muscle weakness.
- In what way should the physical tests be carried out? Will it be easy or hard to reproduce each symptom? Will combined movements or repetitive movements need to be used to reproduce the patient's symptoms? Are symptoms severe and/or irritable? If symptoms are severe, physical tests may be carried out to just before the onset of symptom production or just to the onset of symptom production; no overpressures should be carried out, as the patient would be unable to tolerate this. If symptoms are irritable, physical tests may be examined to just before symptom production or just to the onset of provocation, with fewer physical tests being examined to allow for rest periods between tests.
- Are there any precautions and/or contraindications to elements of the physical examination that need to be explored further, such as VBI, neurological involvement, recent fracture, trauma, steroid therapy or rheumatoid arthritis? There may also be contraindications to further examination and treatment, e.g. symptoms of cord compression.

A planning form can be useful for clinicians to help guide them through the often complex clinical reasoning process (see Figure 2.10).

Physical examination

The information from the subjective examination helps the clinician to plan an appropriate physical examination. The severity, irritability and nature of the condition are the major factors that will influence the choice and priority of physical testing procedures. The first and overarching question the clinician might ask is: 'Is this patient's condition suitable for me to manage as a therapist?' For example, a patient presenting with obvious cranial nerve palsy may only need neurological integrity testing, prior to an urgent medical referral. The nature of the patient's condition will have a major impact on the physical examination. The second question the clinician might ask is: 'Does this patient have a neuromusculoskeletal dysfunction that I may be able to help?' To answer that, the clinician needs to carry out a full physical examination; however, this may not be possible if the symptoms are severe and/or irritable. If the patient's symptoms

are severe and/or irritable, the clinician aims to explore movements as much as possible, within a symptom-free range. If the patient has constant and severe and/or irritable symptoms, then the clinician aims to find physical tests that ease the symptoms. If the patient's symptoms are non-severe and non-irritable, then the clinician may want to find physical tests that reproduce each of the patient's symptoms.

Each significant physical test that either provokes or eases the patient's symptoms is highlighted in the patient's notes by an asterisk (*) for easy reference. The highlighted tests are often referred to as 'asterisks' or 'markers'.

The order and detail of the physical tests described below should be appropriate to the patient being examined; some tests will be irrelevant, some tests will be carried out briefly, while others will need to be investigated fully. It is important that readers understand that the techniques shown in this chapter are some of many; the choice depends mainly on the relative sizes of the clinician and patient, as well as the clinician's preference. For this reason, novice clinicians may initially want to copy what is shown, but then quickly adapt to what is best for them.

Observation

Informal observation

The clinician needs to observe the patient in dynamic and static situations; the quality of cervical and jaw movement is noted, as are the postural characteristics and facial expression. Informal observation will have begun from the moment the clinician begins the subjective examination and will continue to the end of the physical examination.

Formal observation

Observation of posture. The clinician observes both craniofacial and cervical posture. The myofascial relationships between the neck and the jaw mean that postural dysfunction in one may influence the other. For the cervical spine, the clinician observes the nature and extent of forward head posture, lateral tilting and rotation deformity, especially upper cervical rotation. For craniofacial observation, the clinician observes facial symmetry using anatomical landmarks shown in Figures 5.1 and 5.2.

Check whether optic, bipupital, otic and occlusive lines of the face are parallel (Figure 5.1). Note the patient's 'long side' and 'short side' using these

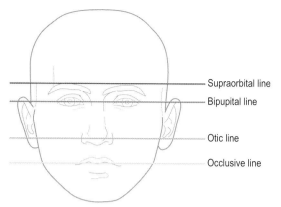

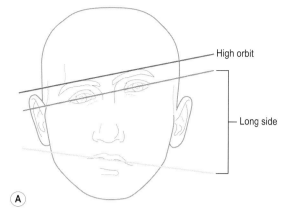

Figure 5.1 • Symmetry of the face can be tested comparing the supraorbital, bipupital, otic and occlusive lines, which should be parallel. (From Magee 2008, with permission)

marker lines. As a rule, a high orbit on the short side indicates mechanical craniovertebral dysfunction that may be amenable to manual therapy. A high orbit on a long side is indicative of a craniofacial dysfunction possibly requiring surgical/dental intervention (Figure 5.2). Additionally, the length (posterior–anterior) of the mandible can be measured from the TMJ joint line to the anterior notch of the chin, and any side-to-side differences noted.

Check vertical dimensions: note whether the distance between the outer corner of the eye and mouth, AB, is equal to the distance from nose to chin, CD (Figure 5.3); reduction of the latter distance by more than 1 mm indicates loss of teeth, overbite or temporomandibular dysfunction (Magee 2008). Check the wear of any false teeth and the state of the patient's gums.

The clinician checks the bony and soft-tissue contours of the face and TMJ. The clinician observes the resting position of the mandible (RPM), also known as the upper postural position of the mandible. In the RPM the back teeth are slightly apart, the mandible is in a relaxed position and the tip of the tongue lies against the palate just posterior to the inner surface of the upper central incisors. The clinician checks the intercuspal position, in which the back teeth are closed together, and observes the patient's teeth for malocclusion such as:

- underbite (mandibular teeth anterior to maxillary teeth, i.e. buccoversion)
- overbite (maxillary teeth anterior to mandibular teeth – 2 mm of overbite is normal). If overbite is apparent, the degree of overjet is noted (how far the maxillary incisors close down over the mandibular incisors (Magee 2008).

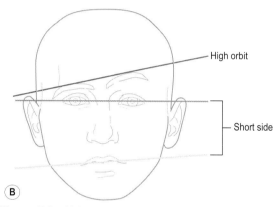

Figure 5.2 • Using the bipupital and occlusive lines to measure unilateral facial length and assessing the relative height of the orbit (supraorbital line), assessment can be made of the patient's suitability for manual therapy.
A Craniofacial dysfunction (surgical intervention more likely).
B Craniovertebral dysfunction (manual therapy likely to help).

- crossbite (deviation of the mandible to one side – use the interincisor gap between the two central incisors as reference points on both mandibular and maxillary sets).

Malocclusion and occlusal interference is noted, and is usually seen when teeth are very poorly formed, or when a dental brace is being worn.

It is useful to be aware that pure postural dysfunction rarely influences one region of the body in isolation and it will be necessary to examine the patient's posture when sitting and standing, noting the posture of head and neck, thoracic spine and upper limbs. The clinician passively corrects any asymmetry to determine its relevance to the patient's problem.

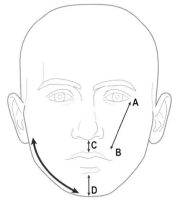

Figure 5.3 • Measurement of the vertical dimension of the face. Normally the distance AB is equal to CD. Left and right measurements of the mandible can be taken from the joint line to the anterior notch of the mandible (chin) (From Trott 1986, with permission.)

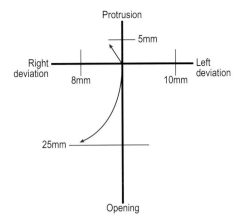

Figure 5.4 • Example of recording movement findings for the temporomandibular joint. Normally opening is around 35–45 mm. The joint mechanics normally function in a 4:1 ratio, i.e. 4 mm of opening to every 1 mm of lateral deviation/protrusion (Rocabado 2004).

Observation of muscle form. The muscles of mastication are the masseter, temporalis, medial pterygoid and lateral pterygoid. Only the masseter and temporalis are visible and may be enlarged or atrophied. If there is postural abnormality that is thought to be due to a muscle imbalance, then the muscles around the cervical spine and shoulder girdle may need to be inspected. Some of these muscles are thought to shorten under stress, while other muscles weaken, producing muscle imbalance (see Table 3.2).

Observation of soft tissues. The clinician observes the colour of the patient's skin, any swelling over the TMJ, face or gums, and takes cues for further examination.

Observation of the patient's attitudes and feelings. The age, gender and ethnicity of patients and their cultural, occupational and social backgrounds will all affect their attitudes and feelings towards themselves, their condition and the clinician. The clinician needs to be aware of and sensitive to these attitudes, and empathise and communicate appropriately so as to develop a rapport with the patient and thereby enhance the patient's compliance with the treatment.

Active physiological movements

For active passive physiological movements, the clinician notes the following:

- the quality of movement: deviation, minor subluxation, crepitus or a click on opening and/or closing the mouth

- the range of movement; excessive range, particularly opening, may indicate hypermobility of the TMJ
- the behaviour of pain through the range
- the resistance through the range of movement and at the end of the range of movement
- any provocation of muscle spasm.

TMJ movements can be recorded as shown in Figure 5.4. The active movements of opening/ closing, protraction/retraction and lateral deviation with overpressure listed in table 5 are shown in Figure 5.5 and can be tested with the patient sitting or lying supine. The clinician establishes the patient's symptoms at rest and prior to each movement, and corrects any movement deviation to determine its relevance to the patient's symptoms. Palpation of the movement of the condyles during active movements can be useful in feeling the quality of the movement. Excessive anterior movement of the lateral pole of the mandible may indicate TMJ hypermobility. During mouth opening, a small indent can normally be palpated posterior to the lateral pole. A large indentation may indicate hypermobility of the TMJ. If unilateral hypermobility is present, the mandible deviates towards the contralateral side of the hypermobile joint at the end of opening. Auscultation of the joint during jaw movements enables the clinician to listen to any joint sounds. The range of movement can be measured using a ruler.

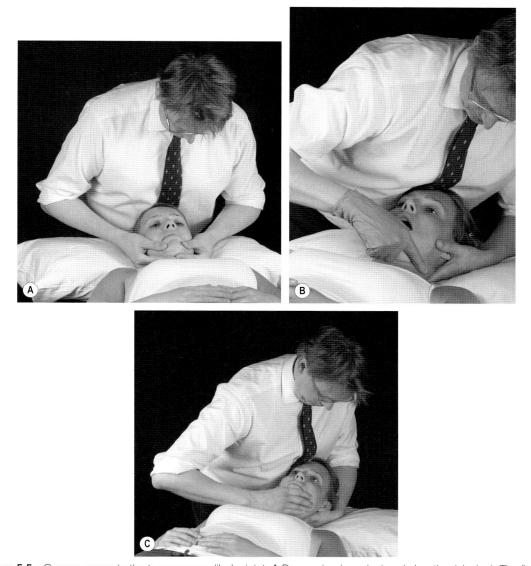

Figure 5.5 • Overpressures to the temporomandibular joint. **A** Depression (opening) and elevation (closing). The fingers and thumbs of both hands gently grasp the mandible to depress and elevate the mandible. **B** Protraction and retraction. A gloved thumb is placed just inside the mouth on the posterior aspect of the bottom front teeth. Thumb pressure can then protract and retract the mandible. **C** Lateral deviation. The left hand stabilises the head while the right hand cups around the mandible and moves the mandible to the left and right.

Movements of the TMJ and the possible modifications are given in Table 5.1. Various differentiation tests (Rocabado 2004; Maitland et al. 2005; Magee 2008) can be performed; the choice depends on the patient's signs and symptoms. For example, when cervical flexion reproduces the patient's TMJ pain in sitting, the addition of slump sitting (see Figure 3.31) or knee extension may help to differentiate the structures at fault. Slump sitting or knee extension, for example, may increase symptoms if there is a neurodynamic component to the patient's symptoms.

Other regions may need to be examined to determine their relevance to the patient's symptoms; they may be the source of the symptoms, or they may be contributing to the symptoms. The regions most

Table 5.1 Summary of active movements and their possible modification

Active movements	Modifications to active movements
Temporomandibular joint	Repeated
Depression (opening)	Speed altered
Elevation (closing)	Combined, e.g.
Protraction	– opening then lateral
Retraction	deviation
Depression in retracted	– lateral deviation then
Position	opening
Left lateral deviation	– protraction then opening
Right lateral deviation	– retraction then opening
?Upper cervical spine	Sustained
movements	Injuring movement
?Cervical spine movement	Differentiation tests
?Thoracic spine movements	Functional ability

likely are the upper cervical spine, cervical spine and thoracic spine. The joints within these regions can be tested fully (see relevant chapter) or partially with the use of screening tests (see Chapter 3 for further details).

Some functional ability has already been tested by the general observation of jaw movement as the patient has talked during the subjective examination. Any further testing can be carried out at this point in the examination and may include sitting and sleeping postures, using the telephone and brushing teeth. Clues for appropriate tests can be obtained from the subjective examination findings, particularly the aggravating factors.

Capsular pattern. The capsular pattern for the TMJ is restriction in opening the mouth (Cyriax 1982).

Passive physiological movements

The clinician can move the TMJ passively with the patient in the supine position. A comparison of the response of symptoms to the active and passive movements can help to determine whether the structure at fault is non-contractile (articular) or contractile (extra-articular) (Cyriax 1982). If the lesion is non-contractile, such as ligament, then active and passive movements will be painful and/or restricted in the same direction. If the lesion is in a contractile tissue (i.e. muscle) then active and passive movements are painful and/or restricted in opposite directions.

Other regions may need to be examined to determine their relevance to the patient's symptoms; they may be the source of the symptoms, or they may be contributing to the symptoms. The regions most likely are the upper cervical spine, cervical spine and thoracic spine.

Muscle tests

Muscle tests include examining muscle strength, control and isometric contraction.

Muscle strength

The clinician may test muscle groups that depress, elevate, protract, retract and laterally deviate the mandible and, if applicable, the cervical flexors, extensors, lateral flexors and rotators. For details of these general tests, readers are directed to Cole et al. (1988), Hislop & Montgomery (1995) or Kendall et al. (1993). Kraus (1994), however, considers mandibular muscle weakness to be rare in TMJ disorders and difficult to determine manually. Janda (1994) considers that suprahyoid and mylohyoid muscles have a tendency to weaken.

Muscle control

Excessive masticatory muscle activity is thought to be a factor in TMJ conditions. Muscle hyperactivity alters the normal sequence of swallowing because of an altered position of the tongue, which is thrust forward in the mouth (tongue thrust). The clinician can determine muscle hyperactivity indirectly by palpating the hyoid bone and suboccipital muscles (Figure 5.6) as the patient swallows some water (Kraus 1994). A slow and upward movement of the hyoid bone, as opposed to the normal quick up-and-down movement, and contraction of the suboccipital muscles suggest a tongue thrust and indicate hyperactivity of the masticatory muscles.

Testing the muscles of the cervical spine and shoulder girdle may be relevant for some patients.

Isometric muscle testing

Test the muscle groups that depress, elevate, protract, retract and laterally deviate the mandible in the resting position and, if indicated, in various parts of the physiological ranges. Also, if applicable, test the cervical flexors, extensors, lateral flexors and

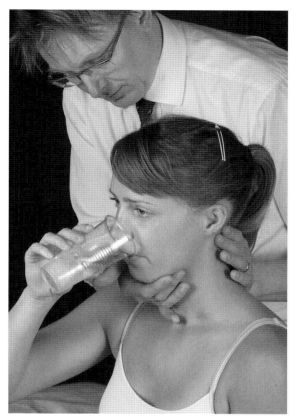

Figure 5.6 • The left hand palpates the suboccipital muscles and the right hand palpates the hyoid bone as the patient swallows some water.

rotators. In addition the clinician observes the quality of the muscle contraction necessary to hold this position (this can be done with the patient's eyes shut). The patient may, for example, be unable to prevent the joint from moving or may hold with excessive muscle activity; either of these circumstances would suggest a neuromuscular dysfunction.

Neurological tests

Neurological examination includes neurological integrity testing, neurodynamic tests and some other nerve tests.

Integrity of nervous system

Generally, if symptoms are localised to the upper cervical spine and head, neurological examination can be limited to cranial nerves and C1–C4 nerve roots.

Dermatomes/peripheral nerves. Light touch and pain sensation of the face, head and neck are tested using cotton wool and pinprick respectively, as described in Chapter 3. Knowledge of the cutaneous distribution of nerve roots (dermatomes) and peripheral nerves enables the clinician to distinguish the sensory loss due to a root lesion from that due to a peripheral nerve lesion. The cutaneous nerve distribution and dermatome areas are shown in Chapter 3.

Myotomes/peripheral nerves. The following myotomes are tested and are shown in Chapter 3:

- trigeminal (CN V): clench teeth, note temporalis and masseter muscles
- facial (CN VII): wrinkle forehead, close eyes, purse lips, show teeth
- accessory (CN XI): sternocleidomastoid and shoulder girdle elevation
- C1–C2: upper cervical flexion
- C2: upper cervical extension
- C3: cervical lateral flexion
- C4 and XI cranial nerve: shoulder girdle elevation.

A working knowledge of the muscular distribution of nerve roots (myotomes) and peripheral nerves enables the clinician to distinguish the motor loss due to a root lesion from that due to a peripheral nerve lesion.

Reflex testing. There are no deep tendon reflexes for C1–C4 nerve roots. The jaw jerk (CN V) is elicited by applying a sharp downward tap on the chin with the mouth slightly open. A slight jerk is normal; excessive jerk suggests bilateral upper motor neurone lesion.

Neurodynamic tests

The following neurodynamic tests may be carried out in order to ascertain the degree to which neural tissue is responsible for the production of the patient's symptom(s):

- passive neck flexion
- upper-limb neurodynamic tests
- straight-leg raise
- slump.

These tests are described in detail in Chapter 3.

Other nerve tests

Chvostek test for facial nerve palsy. To carry out this test, the clinician taps the parotid gland over the masseter muscle; twitching of the facial muscles indicates facial nerve palsy (Magee 2008).

Lingual mandibular reflex (CN V). The tongue is actively placed against the soft palate and a normal response is relaxation of masticatory muscles. Loss of this reflex is not necessarily serious, but rather an indication of sensorimotor dysfunction related to the TMJ/upper cervical dysfunction.

Plantar response to test for an upper motor neurone lesion (Walton 1989). Pressure applied from the heel along the lateral border of the plantar aspect of the foot produces flexion of the toes in the normal. Extension of the big toe with downward fanning of the other toes occurs with an upper motor neurone lesion.

Miscellaneous tests

To facilitate differential diagnosis, further testing may be undertaken as follows:

- Vertebral and carotid arterial examination (Kerry & Taylor 2006). This is described in detail in Chapter 6.
- Palpation of the temporal artery for suspected temporal arteries. A positive finding is a painful and exaggerated pulse.
- Further cranial nerve examination. Refer for medical investigation if frank nerve pathology is suspected.

Palpation

The TMJ and the upper cervical spine (see Chapter 6) are palpated. It is useful to record palpation findings on a body chart (see Figure 2.3) and/or palpation chart (see Figure 3.36).

The clinician should make a note of the following:

- the temperature of the area
- localised increased skin moisture
- the presence of oedema or effusion
- mobility and feel of superficial tissues, e.g. ganglions, nodules, thickening of deep suboccipital tissues
- position and prominence of the mandible and TMJ
- the presence or elicitation of any muscle spasm
- tenderness of bone, ligament, muscle (masseter, temporalis, medial and lateral pterygoids, splenius capitis, suboccipital muscles, trapezius, sternocleidomastoid, digastric), tendon, tendon sheath and nerve. Check for

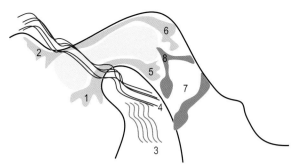

Figure 5.7 • Rocabado's joint pain map. Specific tissues can be palpated to assess for pain response: **1** anteroinferior synovial membrane; **2** anterosuperior synovial membrane; **3** lateral collateral ligament; **4** temporomandibular ligament; **5** posteroinferior synovial membrane; **6** posterosuperior synovial membrane; **7** posterior ligament; **8** retrodiscal tissue.

tenderness of the hyoid bone and thyroid cartilage. Test for the relevant trigger points shown in Figure 3.37
- symptoms (often pain) provoked or reduced on palpation.

Rocabado's joint pain map

Figure 5.7 shows a schematic pain map devised to facilitate structural diagnosis of joint dysfunction (Rocabado 2004). After locating the anterior pole of the mandibular condyle (protrusion during palpation of the lateral pole), the patient opens the mouth 10 mm. As the patient maintains this position, the clinician systematically palpates the points on the map. The patient raises a hand to signal pain. There is no evidence available to support or refute the utility of this procedure, but clinically it can provide valuable information.

Accessory movements

It is useful to use the palpation chart and movement diagrams (or joint pictures) to record findings. These are explained in detail in Chapter 3.

The clinician should make a note of the following:

- quality of movement
- range of movement
- resistance through the range and at the end of the range of movement
- behaviour of pain through the range
- provocation of any muscle spasm.

Temporomandibular joint

Dynamic loading and distraction. The clinician places a cotton roll between the upper and lower third molars on one side only and the patient is asked to bite on to the roll, noting any pain produced. Pain may be felt on the left or right TMJ as there will be distraction of the TMJ on the side of the cotton roll and compression of the TMJ on the contralateral side (Hylander 1979). Pain on the side of the cotton roll is indicative of capsulitis (Kraus 1993).

Passive loading (retrusive overpressure). The patient is asked to hold the back teeth slightly apart. The clinician holds on to the chin with the thumb and index finger with one hand, and with the other hand supports the head to provide a counterforce. The clinician then applies a posterosuperior force on the mandible centrally and then with some lateral inclination to the right and left. This test can be positive, reproducing the patient's pain, in both capsulitis and synovitis (Kraus 1993).

TMJ accessory movements are listed in Table 5.2 and shown in Figure 5.8, and are as follows:

- anteroposterior
- posteroanterior
- medial transverse
- lateral transverse
- longitudinal caudad
- longitudinal cephalad
- helicoidal craniomandibuar activator.

Following accessory movements to the TMJ, the clinician reassesses all the physical asterisks (movements or tests that have been found to reproduce the patient's symptoms) in order to establish the effect of the accessory movements on the patient's signs and symptoms. Accessory movements can then be tested for other regions suspected to be a source of the symptoms. Again, following accessory movements the clinician reassesses all the physical asterisks. Regions likely to be examined are the upper cervical spine, cervical spine and thoracic spine.

Completion of the examination

Having carried out the above tests, the examination of the temporomandibular region is now complete. The subjective and physical examinations produce a large amount of information, which needs to be recorded accurately and quickly. An outline examination chart may be useful for some clinicians and one is suggested in Figure 5.9. It is important, however, that the clinician does not examine in a rigid manner, simply following the suggested sequence outlined in the chart. Each patient presents differently and this needs to be reflected in the examination process. It is vital at this stage to highlight with an asterisk (*) important findings from the examination. These findings

---

Table 5.2 Accessory movements, choice of application and reassessment of the patient's asterisks

Accessory movements	Choice of application	Identify any effect of accessory movements on patient's signs and symptoms
Temporomandibular joint ↕ Anteroposterior ↕ Posteroanterior ↢↣ Med Medial transverse ↢↣ Lat Lateral transverse ↢↣↣ Caud Longitudinal caudad ↢↣↣ Ceph Longitudinal cephalad	Start position, e.g. with the mandible depressed, elevated, protracted, retracted, laterally deviated, or a combination of these positions Speed of force application Direction of the applied force Point of application of applied force	Reassess all asterisks
?Upper cervical spine	As above	Reassess all asterisks
?Cervical spine	As above	Reassess all asterisks
?Thoracic spine		Reassess all asterisks

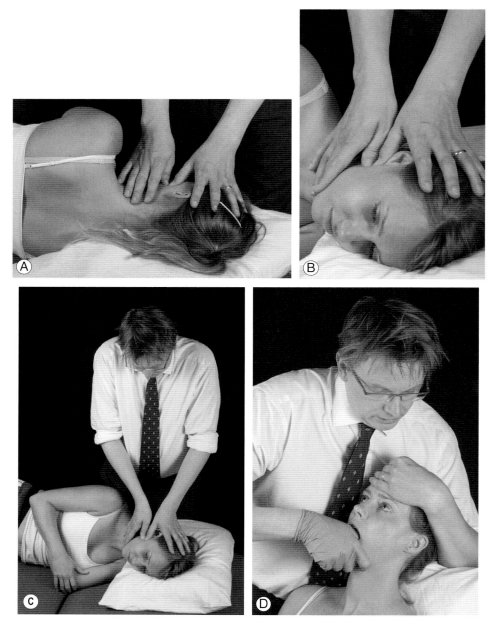

Figure 5.8 • Accessory movements to the temporomandibular joint. **A** Anteroposterior. With the patient in side-lying, thumbs apply an anteroposterior pressure to the anterior aspect of the head of the mandible. **B** Posteroanterior. With the patient in side-lying, thumbs apply a posteroanterior pressure to the posterior aspect of the head of the mandible. **C** Medial transverse. With the patient in side-lying, thumbs apply a medial pressure to the lateral aspect of the head of the mandible. **D** Lateral transverse. The patient is supported in sitting. The one hand supports the head while the gloved hand is placed inside the mouth so that the thumb rests along the medial surface of the mandible. Thumb pressure can then produce a lateral glide of the mandible.

(Continued)

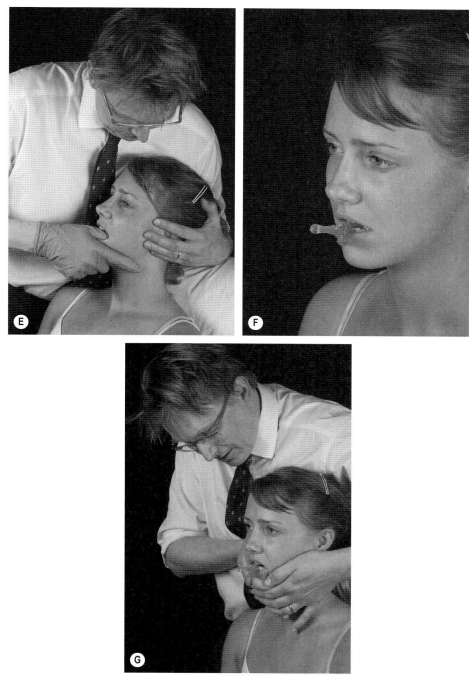

Figure 5.8—cont'd • E Longitudinal cephalad and caudad. With the patient sitting and the one hand supporting the head, the gloved hand is placed inside the mouth so that the thumb rests on the top of the lower back teeth.
The thumb and outer fingers then grip the mandible and apply a downward pressure (longitudinal caudad) and an upward pressure (longitudinal cephalad). **F** Rocabado helicoidal craniomandibular activator (RHCMA). The activator is placed between the central incisors to encourage normalisation of disc mechanics during active movement. **G** Example of RHCMA mobilisation with movement.

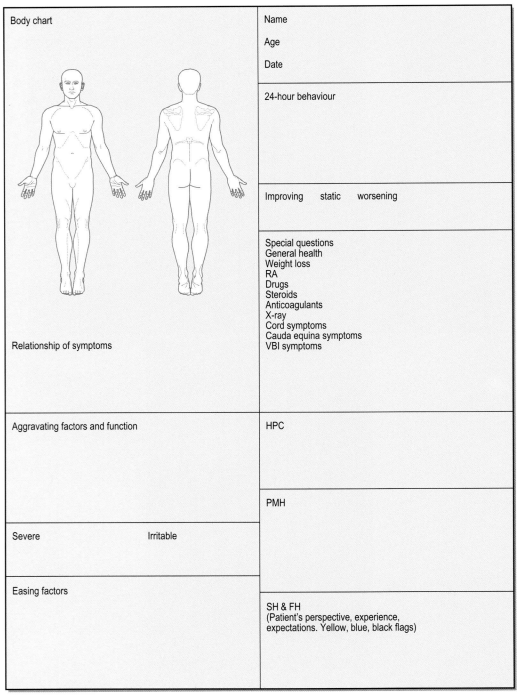

Body chart	Name
	Age
	Date
	24-hour behaviour
	Improving static worsening
	Special questions General health Weight loss RA Drugs Steroids Anticoagulants X-ray Cord symptoms Cauda equina symptoms VBI symptoms
Relationship of symptoms	
Aggravating factors and function	HPC
	PMH
Severe Irritable	
Easing factors	SH & FH (Patient's perspective, experience, expectations. Yellow, blue, black flags)

Figure 5.9 • Temporomandibular joint (TMJ) examination chart. RA, rheumatoid arthritis; HPC, history of presenting complaint; PMH, past medical history; SH, social history; FH, family history; VBI, vertebrobasilar insufficiency.

(Continued)

Observation	Isometric muscle testing
Joint integrity tests	Other muscle tests
Active and passive physiological movements	Neurological integrity tests
	Neurodynamic tests
	Other nerve tests
Capsular pattern yes/no	Miscellaneous tests
Muscle strength	
	Palpation
Muscle control	
	Accessory movements and reassessment of each relevant region
Muscle length	

Figure 5.9—cont'd.

must be reassessed at, and within, subsequent treatment sessions to evaluate the effects of treatment on the patient's condition.

The physical testing procedures which specifically indicate joint, nerve or muscle tissues, as a source of the patient's symptoms, are summarised in Table 3.10. The strongest evidence that a joint is the source of the patient's symptoms is that active and passive physiological movements, passive accessory movements and joint palpation all reproduce the patient's symptoms, and that, following a treatment dose, reassessment identifies an improvement in the patient's signs and symptoms. Weaker evidence includes an alteration in range, resistance or quality of physiological and/or accessory movements and tenderness over the joint, with no alteration in signs and symptoms after treatment. One or more of these findings may indicate a dysfunction of a joint which may or may not be contributing to the patient's condition.

The strongest evidence that a muscle is the source of a patient's symptoms is if active movements, an isometric contraction, passive lengthening and palpation of a muscle all reproduce the patient's symptoms, and that, following a treatment dose, reassessment identifies an improvement in the patient's signs and symptoms. Further evidence of muscle dysfunction may be suggested by reduced strength or poor quality during the active physiological movement and the isometric contraction, reduced range and/or increased/decreased resistance, during the passive lengthening of the muscle, and tenderness on palpation, with no alteration in signs and symptoms after treatment. One or more of these findings may indicate a dysfunction of a muscle which may, or may not, be contributing to the patient's condition.

The strongest evidence that a nerve is the source of the patient's symptoms is when active and/or passive physiological movements reproduce the patient's symptoms, which are then increased or decreased with an additional sensitising movement, at a distance from the patient's symptoms. In addition, there is reproduction of the patient's symptoms on palpation of the nerve and following neurodynamic testing, sufficient to be considered a treatment dose, results in an improvement in the above signs and symptoms. Further evidence of nerve dysfunction may be suggested by reduced range (compared with the asymptomatic side) and/or increased resistance to the various arm movements, and tenderness on nerve palpation.

On completion of the physical examination the clinician:

- explains the findings of the physical examination and how these findings relate to the subjective assessment. An attempt should be made to clear up any misconceptions patients may have regarding their illness or injury
- collaborates with the patient and via problem-solving together devise a treatment plan and discuss the prognosis
- warns the patient of possible exacerbation up to 24–48 hours following the examination
- requests the patient to report details on the behaviour of the symptoms following examination at the next attendance
- explains the findings of the physical examination and how these findings relate to the subjective assessment. It will be helpful to patients to clear up any misconceptions they may have regarding their illness or injury
- evaluates the findings, formulates a clinical diagnosis and writes up a problem list
- determines the objectives of treatment
- devises an initial treatment plan.

In this way, the clinician will have developed the following hypotheses categories (adapted from Jones & Rivett 2004):

- function: abilities and restrictions
- patient's perspective on his/her experience
- source of symptoms, including the structure or tissue that is thought to be producing the patient's symptoms, the nature of the structure or tissues in relation to the healing process and the pain mechanisms
- contributing factors to the development and maintenance of the problem. There may be environmental, psychosocial, behavioural, physical or heredity factors
- precautions/contraindications to treatment and management. This includes the severity and irritability of the patient's symptoms and the nature of the patient's condition
- management strategy and treatment plan
- prognosis – this can be affected by factors such as the stage and extent of the injury as well as the patient's expectation, personality and lifestyle
- for guidance on treatment and management principles, the reader is directed to the companion textbook (Petty 2011).

References

Ayub, E., Glasheen-Wray, M., Kraus, S., 1984. Head posture: a case study of the effects on the rest position of the mandible. J. Orthop. Sports Phys. Ther. 5 (4), 179–183.

Bogduk, N., 1994. Cervical causes of headache and dizziness. In: Boyling, J.D., Palastanga, N. (Eds.), Grieve's modern manual therapy, second ed. Churchill Livingstone, Edinburgh, p. 317.

Cleland, J., Palmer, J., 2004. Effectiveness of manual physical therapy, therapeutic exercise, and patient education on bilateral disc displacement without reduction of the temporomandibular joint: a single case design. J. Orthop. Sports Phys. Ther. 34 (9), 535–548.

Cole, J.H., Furness, A.L., Twomey, L.T., 1988. Muscles in action: an approach to manual muscle testing. Churchill Livingstone, Edinburgh.

Cyriax, J., 1982. Textbook of orthopaedic medicine – diagnosis of soft tissue lesions, eighth ed. Baillière Tindall, London.

Darling, D.W., Kraus, S., Glasheen-Wray, M.B., 1987. Relationship of head posture and the rest position of the mandible. In: Tenth International Congress of the World Confederation for Physical Therapy. pp. 203–206.

Dworkin, S.M., Friction, J.R., Hollender, L., et al., 1992. Research diagnostic criteria for temporomandibular disorders: review, criteria, examinations and specific critique. J. Craniomandib. Disord. 6, 301–355.

Feinstein, B., Langton, J.N.K., Jameson, R.M., et al., 1954. Experiments on pain referred from deep somatic tissues. J. Bone Joint Surg. 36A (5), 981–997.

Grieve, G.P., 1994. Counterfeit clinical presentations. Manipulative Physiotherapist 26, 17–19.

Hislop, H., Montgomery, J., 1995. Daniels and Worthingham's muscle testing, techniques of manual examination, seventh ed. W B Saunders, Philadelphia.

Hylander, W.L., 1979. An experimental analysis of temporomandibular joint reaction forces in macaques. Am. J. Phys. Anthropol. 51, 433.

Janda, V., 1994. Muscles and motor control in cervicogenic disorders: assessment and management. In: Grant, R. (Ed.), Physical therapy of the cervical and thoracic spine, second ed. Churchill Livingstone, Edinburgh, p. 195.

Jones, M.A., Rivett, D.A., 2004. Clinical reasoning for manual therapists. Butterworth-Heinemann, Edinburgh.

Kendall, F.P., McCreary, E.K., Provance, P.G., 1993. Muscles testing and function, fourth ed. Williams & Wilkins, Baltimore, MD.

Kerry, R., Taylor, A.J., 2006. Cervical arterial dysfunction assessment and manual therapy. Man. Ther. 11 (3), 243–253.

Kerry, R., Taylor, A.J., 2008. Arterial pathology and cervicocranial pain – differential diagnosis for manual therapists and medical practitioners. Int. Musculoskelet. Med. 30 (2), 70–77.

Kerry, R., Taylor, A.J., 2009. Cervical arterial dysfunction: knowledge and reasoning for manual physical therapists. J. Orthop. Sports Phys. Ther. 39 (5), 378–387.

Kraus, S., 1993. Evaluation and management of temporomandibular disorders. In: Saunders, H.D., Saunders, R. (Eds.), Evaluation, treatment and prevention of musculoskeletal disorders, vol 1. WB Saunders, Minneapolis, MN.

Kraus, S.L., 1994. Physical therapy management of TMD. In: Kraus, S.L. (Ed.), Temporomandibular disorders, second ed. Churchill Livingstone, Edinburgh.

Magee, D.J., 2008. Orthopedic physical assessment, fifth ed. W B Saunders, Philadelphia.

Maitland, G.D., Hengeveld, E., Banks, K., 2005. Maitland's peripheral manipulation, fourth ed. Elsevier, Edinburgh.

Mansilla-Ferragut, P., Fernández-de-Las Peñas, C., Alburquerque-Sendín, F., et al., 2009. Immediate effects of atlanto-occipital joint manipulation on active mouth opening and pressure pain sensitivity in women with mechanical neck pain. J. Manipulative Physiol. Ther. 32 (2), 101–106.

McNeely, M.L., Olivio, S.A., Magee, D.J., 2006. A systematic review of the effectiveness of physical therapy interventions for temporomandibular disorders. Phys. Ther. 86 (5), 710–725.

Medlicott, M.S., Harris, S.R., 2006. A systematic review of the effectiveness of exercise, manual therapy, electrotherapy, relaxation training, and biofeedback in the management of temporomandibular disorders. Phys. Ther. 86 (7), 955–973.

Petty, N.J., 2011. Principles of neuromusculoskeletal treatment and management: a guide for therapists, second ed. Churchill Livingstone, Edinburgh.

Rocabado, M., 1983. Biomechanical relationship of the cranial, cervical and hyoid regions. Cranio 1 (3), 62–66.

Rocabado, M., 2004. A university student with chronic facial pain. In: Jones, M.A., Rivett, D.A. (Eds.), Clinical reasoning in manual therapy. Butterworth Heinemann, Edinburgh, pp. 243–260.

Shin, B.C., Ha, C.H., Song, Y.S., et al., 2007. Effectiveness of combining manual therapy and acupuncture on temporomandibular dysfunction: a retrospective study. Am. J. Chin. Med. 35 (2), 203–208.

Trott, P.H., 1986. Examination of the temporomandibular joint. In: Grieve, G.P. (Ed.), Modern manual therapy of the vertebral column. Churchill Livingstone, Edinburgh, ch 48, p. 521.

von Piekartz, H., Bryden, L., 2001. Craniofacial dysfunction and pain: manual therapy, assessment and management. Butterworth-Heinemann, Oxford.

Waddell, G., 2004. The back pain revolution, second ed. Churchill Livingstone, Edinburgh.

Walton, J.H., 1989. Essentials of neurology, sixth ed. Churchill Livingstone, Edinburgh.

Examination of the upper cervical region

6

Roger Kerry

CHAPTER CONTENTS

Possible causes of pain and/or limitation of movement

- Trauma:
  - whiplash
  - sports/occupational injuries
  - fracture of vertebral body, spinous or transverse process
  - ligamentous sprain
  - muscular strain
  - degenerative conditions
  - spondylosis: degeneration of C2–C3 intervertebral disc
  - arthrosis: degeneration of zygapophyseal joints

- Inflammatory conditions:
  - rheumatoid arthritis
  - ankylosing spondylitis
- Neoplasm
- Infection
- Headache (Headache Classification Committee of the International Headache Society 1988, 2004; Sjaastad et al. 1998):
  - migraine
  - tension-type headache
  - cluster headache
  - miscellaneous headaches unassociated with structural lesion, e.g. cold stimulus headache, cough or exertional headache
  - headache associated with head trauma
  - headache associated with vascular disorders, e.g. transient ischaemic attack, intracranial haematoma, subarachnoid headache, arterial hypertension, carotid or vertebral artery pain
  - headache associated with non-vascular disorders, e.g. high or low cerebrospinal fluid pressure, intracranial infection or neoplasm
  - headache associated with substances or their withdrawal, e.g. monosodium glutamate, alcohol, analgesic abuse, caffeine, narcotics
  - headache associated with non-cephalic infection, e.g. bacterial or viral infection
  - headache associated with metabolic disorder, e.g. hypoxia, hypercapnia, sleep apnoea, hypoglycaemia
  - headache or facial pain associated with disorder of cranium, neck, eyes, ears, nose, sinuses, teeth, mouth or other facial or cranial

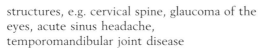
structures, e.g. cervical spine, glaucoma of the eyes, acute sinus headache, temporomandibular joint disease

- Cranial neuralgias, nerve trunk pain and deafferentation pain, e.g. diabetic neuritis, neck–tongue syndrome, herpes zoster, trigeminal neuralgia, occipital neuralgia
- Headache not classifiable
- Postural/repetitive activity syndromes
- Benign mechanical vertebral motion segment dysfunction.

For further information on the assessment and management of whiplash and headaches, readers are referred to Edeling (1994) and Jull et al. (2008a).

Further details of the questions asked during the subjective examination and the tests carried out in the physical examination can be found in Chapters 2 and 3 respectively.

The upper cervical spine is defined here as the articulations between the occiput and C1 (atlas), and also those between the upper three cervical vertebrae, C1 (atlas), C2 (axis) and C3, together with their surrounding soft tissues. For clarity, these segments are referred to as:

- C0–1 (also known as the atlanto-occipital joint – it is the craniovertebral junction between the occiput and C1)
- C1–2 (also known as the atlantoaxial joint)
- C2–3

It is important to remember that there is a nerve root exiting between the occiput and C1. This is referred to as the C1 nerve root. In contrast to the thoracolumbar spine, nerve roots are named in relation to the vertebra below. There is no disc between the occiput and C1, nor between C1 and C2. The first intervertebral disc is found between C2 and C3, and this is referred to as the C2 disc; like the thoracolumbar spine, discs are named in relation to the vertebra above. Accordingly, C1 is unique in that it does not possess a vertebral body. It is best thought of as a ring-like structure, or a washer, separating the head from the rest of the spinal column. C2 also exhibits a unique form with a vertebral body which develops superiorly into an elongated vertical pillar (dens articularis, or odontoid peg). This forms a trochoidal (pivot) joint with C1, and acts as an axis for C1–2 rotation.

The order of the subjective questioning and the physical tests described below can be altered as appropriate for the patient being examined.

Subjective examination

The upper cervical spine is commonly a source, cause of, or contributing factor to pain, restriction of movement and many other symptoms affecting the craniovertebral region. The myofascial and neurological associations between the cranium, brain and upper cervical spine result in a fascinating clinical challenge for the clinician. The remit of the clinician is to diagnose and manage complex dysfunction in this region. Manual therapy for upper cervical spine dysfunction has been the subject of growing research and there is some support of its efficacy (e.g. Walker et al. 2008).

The association between the upper cervical spine and headaches has long been considered, to the extent of the formation of a specific international study group into this phenomenon (Sjaastad et al. 1998). A neuroanatamical explanation for cervicogenic headaches has been established (Bogduk 1994), and this explanation provides a theoretical basis for the wide-ranging and often complex presentation seen in patients with upper cervical dysfunction. Dizziness is often associated with upper cervical spine dysfunction and can respond well to manual therapy interventions (Reid & Rivett 2005; Reid et al. 2008).

Reference to Figure 3.18, showing the cutaneous nerve supply to the face, head and neck, will aid understanding of the pain distribution around the upper cervical spine and head. The fact that many patients with upper cervical spine dysfunction present with frontal headaches and face pain (trigeminal nerve distribution) supports the trigeminocervical convergence theory (Bogduk 1994; Jull & Niere 2005).

Body chart

The following information concerning the area and type of current symptoms can be recorded on a body chart (see Figure 2.3).

Area of current symptoms

Be exact when mapping out the area of the symptoms. Typically, patients with upper cervical spine disorders have neck pain high up around the occiput and pain over the head and/or face. Ascertain the worst symptom and record where the patient feels the symptoms are coming from.

Areas relevant to the region being examined

All other relevant areas are checked for symptoms; it is important to ask about pain or even stiffness, as this may be relevant to the patient's main symptom. Mark unaffected areas with ticks (✓) on the body chart. Check for symptoms in the lower cervical spine, thoracic spine, head and temporomandibular joint and if the patient has ever experienced any disequilibrium or dizziness. This is relevant for symptoms emanating from the cervical spine, where cervical arterial dysfunction (CAD) such as vertebrobasilar insufficiency may be present, or provoked. If symptoms suggestive of CAD are described by the patient, the clinician proceeds with a thorough assessment for potential neurovascular pathology (Barker et al. 2000; Kerry & Taylor 2006; Kerry et al. 2008).

Quality of pain

Establish the quality of the pain. Headaches of cervical origin are often described as throbbing or as a pressure sensation. If the patient suffers from headaches, find out if there is any associated blurred vision, loss of balance, tinnitus, auditory disturbance, swelling and stiffness of the fingers, tendinitis and capsulitis, which could be due to irritation of the sympathetic plexus surrounding the vertebral artery or to irritation of the spinal nerve (Jackson 1966). Patients who have suffered a hyperextension injury to the cervical spine may complain of a sore throat, difficulty in swallowing and a feeling of something stuck in their throat resulting from an associated injury to the oesophagus (Dahlberg et al. 1997).

Intensity of pain

The intensity of pain can also be measured using, for example, a visual analogue scale, as shown in Chapter 2. A pain diary may be useful for patients with chronic neck pain or headaches, in order to determine the pain patterns and triggering factors, which may be unusual or complex.

Depth of pain

Establish the depth of the pain. Does the patient feel it is on the surface or deep inside?

Abnormal sensation

Check for any altered sensation locally over the cervical spine and head, as well as the face and upper limbs. Common abnormalities are paraesthesia and numbness.

Constant or intermittent symptoms

Ascertain the frequency of the symptoms, and whether they are constant or intermittent. If symptoms are constant, check whether there is variation in the intensity of the symptoms, as constant unremitting pain may be indicative of neoplastic disease. Headaches may change in frequency from once a month, to once a week, to daily (Edeling 1994).

Relationship of symptoms

Determine the relationship between the symptomatic areas – do they come together or separately? For example, the patient could have a headache without the cervical pain, or the pains may always be present together.

Behaviour of symptoms

Aggravating factors

For each symptomatic area, discover what movements and/or positions aggravate the patient's symptoms, i.e. what brings the symptoms on (or makes them worse)? is the patient able to maintain this position or movement (severity)? what happens to other symptom(s) when this symptom is produced (or is made worse)? and how long does it take for symptoms to ease once the position or movement is stopped (irritability)? These questions help to confirm the relationship between the symptoms.

The clinician also asks the patient about theoretically known aggravating factors for structures that could be a source of the symptoms. Common aggravating factors for the upper cervical spine are sustained cervical postures and movements. Headaches can be brought on with eye strain, noise, excessive eating, drinking, smoking, stress or inadequate ventilation. Aggravating factors for other regions, which may need to be queried if they are suspected to be a source of the symptoms, are shown in Table 2.3.

The clinician ascertains how the symptoms affect function, such as: static and active postures, e.g. sitting, standing, lying, washing, ironing, dusting, driving, reading, writing, work, sport and social activities. Note details of the training regimen for any sports activities. The clinician finds out if the patient is left- or right-handed as there may be increased stress on the dominant side.

Detailed information on each of the above activities is useful in order to help determine the structure(s) at fault and identify functional restrictions. This information can be used to determine the aims of treatment and any advice that may be required. The most notable functional restrictions are highlighted with asterisks (*), explored in the physical examination and reassessed at subsequent treatment sessions to evaluate treatment intervention.

Easing factors

For each symptomatic area, the clinician asks what movements and/or positions ease the patient's symptoms, how long it takes to ease them and what happens to other symptom(s) when this symptom is relieved. These questions help to confirm the relationship between the symptoms.

The clinician asks the patient about theoretically known easing factors for structures that could be a source of the symptoms. For example, symptoms from the upper cervical spine may be eased by supporting the head or neck. The clinician can analyse the position or movement that eases the symptoms, in order to help determine the structure at fault.

Twenty-four-hour behaviour of symptoms

The clinician determines the 24-hour behaviour of the symptoms by asking questions about night, morning and evening symptoms.

Night symptoms. The following questions may be asked:

- Do you have any difficulty getting to sleep?
- What position is most comfortable/ uncomfortable?
- What is your normal sleeping position?
- What is your present sleeping position?
- Do your symptoms wake you at night? If so,
  - ○ Which symptoms?
  - ○ How many times in the past week?
  - ○ How many times in a night?
  - ○ How long does it take to get back to sleep?
- How many and what type of pillows are used? Is the mattress firm or soft?

Morning and evening symptoms. The clinician determines the pattern of the symptoms first thing in the morning, through the day and at the end of the day. Stiffness in the morning for the first few minutes might suggest cervical spondylosis; stiffness

and pain for a few hours are suggestive of an inflammatory process such as rheumatoid arthritis.

Stage of the condition

In order to determine the stage of the condition, the clinician asks whether the symptoms are getting better, getting worse or remaining unchanged.

Special questions

Special questions must always be asked, as they may identify certain precautions or contraindications to the physical examination and/or treatment (see Table 2.4). As mentioned in Chapter 2, the clinician must differentiate between conditions that are suitable for conservative management and systemic, neoplastic and other non-neuromusculoskeletal conditions, which require referral to a medical practitioner. The reader is referred to Appendix 2.3 for details of various serious pathological processes that can mimic neuromusculoskeletal conditions (Grieve 1994).

The following information is routinely obtained from patients.

Cervical arterial dysfunction. The clinician needs to ask about symptoms that may be related to pathologies of the arterial vessels which lie in the neck, namely the vertebral arteries and the internal carotid arteries. Pathology of these vessels can result in neurovascular insult to the brain (stroke). These pathologies are known to produce signs and symptoms similar to neuromusculoskeletal dysfunction of the upper cervical spine (Bogduk 1994; Kerry & Taylor 2006). Care needs to be taken to differentiate vascular sources of pain from neuromusculoskeletal sources. Urgent medical investigation is indicated if frank vascular pathology is identified.

CAD can present initially with pain in the upper cervical spine and head. This is referred to as the pre-ischaemic stage. If the pathology develops, signs and symptoms of brain ischaemia may develop. Table 6.1 shows typical pre-ischaemic and ischaemic presentations for vertebral artery and internal carotid artery pathologies.

Risk factors associated with CAD are given in Box 6.1. The clinician uses further screening questions to help establish the nature and possible causes and sources of the patient's complaints.

Many patients present with treatable neuromusculoskeletal causes of symptoms, but also with many of the risk factors identified in Box 6.1. This does not

Table 6.1 Signs and symptoms during preischaemic and ischaemic stages for vertebral artery pathology and internal carotid artery pathology
Vertebral artery pathology

Preischaemic signs and symptoms	Ischaemic signs/symptoms
Ipsilateral posterior neck pain/occipital headache C2–C6 cervical root impairment (rare)	Hindbrain TIA/TIE (dizziness, diplopia, dysarthria, dysphagia, drop attacks, nausea, nystagmus, facial numbness, ataxia, vomiting, hoarseness, loss of short-term memory, vagueness, hypotonia/limb weakness (arm or leg), anhidrosis (lack of facial sweating), hearing disturbances, malaise, perioral dysthaesia, photophobia, papillary changes, clumsiness and agitation other cranial nerve dysfunctions) Hindbrain stroke (e.g. Wallenberg's syndrome, locked-in syndrome)

Internal carotid artery pathology

Preischaemic signs/symptoms	Ischaemic signs/symptoms
Horner's syndrome, pulsatile tinnitus Cranial nerve palsies (most commonly CN IX–XII)	TIA Ischaemic stroke (usually middle cerebral artery territory) Retinal infarction

TIA, transient ischaemic attack; TIE, transient ischaemic event; CN, cranial nerve.

Box 6.1

Risk factors for cervical arterial dysfunction (Barker et al. 2000; Kerry & Taylor 2006; Kerry et al. 2008)

- Past history of trauma to cervical spine/cervical vessels
- History of migraine-type headache
- Hypertension
- Hypercholesterolaemia/hyperlipidaemia
- Cardiac disease, vascular disease, previous cerebrovascular accident or transient ischaemic attacks
- Diabetes mellitus
- Blood-clotting disorders/alterations in blood properties (e.g. hyperhomocysteinaemia)
- Anticoagulant therapy
- Oral contraceptives
- Long-term use of steroids
- A history of smoking
- Infection
- Immediately postpartum

necessarily exclude them from manual therapy treatment, and careful clinical reasoning and monitoring of signs and symptoms are required in the management of these patients (Kerry & Taylor 2009).

Upper cervical instability (UCI). A loss of osteoligamentous integrity between the occiput and C2, and the C1–2 trochoidal joint (formed between the odontoid process of C2 and the posterior aspect of the anterior arch of C1), can result in impingement of the spinal cord, and ultimately paralysis. The clinician establishes whether or not the patient is presenting with features indicative of UCI, and urgent medical referral is made, if instability is suspected.

Although it is often considered that the patient will present with signs of cord compression, e.g. bilateral hand and foot dysthaesia, metallic taste in mouth, lump in throat, gait disturbance, such presentations are very rare (Cattrysse et al. 1997). Initially, UCI presents as head/neck pain and stiffness. The clinician should consider more subtle, early signs and risk factors of instability in attempting to diagnose differentially the cause of symptoms (Cook et al. 2005).

Risk factors for UCI:

- history of trauma (e.g. whiplash, rugby neck injury)
- congenital collagenous compromise (syndromes: Down's, Ehlers–Danlos, Grisel; Morquio)

- inflammatory arthritides, e.g. rheumatoid arthritis, ankylosing spondylitis
- recent neck/head/dental surgery.

Early presentations of UCI:

- extreme neck stiffness
- anxiety
- poor muscular control
- excessive need for external support for neck (e.g. hands/collar)
- worsening and unpredictability of symptoms
- reports of neck catching/giving way/feeling unstable
- reports of repeated/self-manipulation.

Joint integrity testing (described below) can be performed to assist in differential diagnosis. These tests have varied known diagnostic utility (Forrester & Barlos 1999; Kaale et al. 2008). They should not be performed in acute or traumatic cases, and use of these tests in whiplash-associated disorder should be considered with great care (Moore et al. 2005).

History of the present condition

For each symptomatic area the clinician needs to discover how long the symptom has been present, whether there was a sudden or slow onset and whether there was a known cause that provoked the onset of the symptom. If the patient complains of headaches, the clinician needs to find out whether there have been any factors that precipitated the onset, such as trauma, stress, surgery or occupation. If the onset was slow, the clinician finds out if there has been any change in the patient's lifestyle, e.g. a new job or hobby or a change in sporting activity. There may be an increased mechanical stress on the cervical spine or an increase in the patient's stress levels, which might explain the increase in the patient's symptoms. To confirm the relationship between the symptoms, the clinician asks what happened to other symptoms when each symptom began.

Past medical history

The following information is obtained from the patient and/or medical notes:

- The details of any relevant medical history involving the cervical spine and related areas.

- The history of any previous attacks: how many episodes? when were they? what was the cause? what was the duration of each episode? and did the patient fully recover between episodes? If there have been no previous attacks, has the patient had any episodes of stiffness in the cervical spine, thoracic spine or any other relevant region? Check for a history of trauma or recurrent minor trauma.
- Ascertain the results of any past treatment for the same or similar problem. Past treatment records may be obtained for further information.

Social and family history

Social and family history relevant to the onset and progression of the patient's problem should be recorded. This includes the patient's perspectives, experience and expectations, age, employment, home situation and details of any leisure activities. Factors from this information may indicate direct and/or indirect mechanical influences on the cervical spine. In order to treat the patient appropriately, it is important that the condition is managed within the context of the patient's social and work environment.

The clinician may ask the following types of question to elucidate psychosocial factors:

- Have you had time off work in the past with your pain?
- What do you understand to be the cause of your pain?
- What are you expecting will help you?
- How is your employer/co-workers/family responding to your pain?
- What are you doing to cope with your pain?
- Do you think you will return to work? When?

Although these questions are described in relation to psychosocial risk factors for poor outcomes for patients with low-back pain (Waddell 2004), they may be relevant to other patients.

Plan of the physical examination

When all this information has been collected, the subjective examination is complete. It is useful at this stage to highlight with asterisks (*), for ease of reference, important findings and particularly one or more functional restrictions. These can then be re-examined at subsequent treatment sessions to evaluate treatment intervention.

In order to plan the physical examination, the following hypotheses need to be developed from the subjective examination:

- The regions and structures that need to be examined as a possible cause of the symptoms, e.g. temporomandibular region, upper cervical spine, cervical spine, thoracic spine, muscles and nerves. Often it is not possible to examine fully at the first attendance and so examination of the structures must be prioritised over subsequent treatment sessions.

- Other factors that need to be examined, e.g. working and everyday postures, vertebral artery, muscle weakness.

- In what way should the physical tests be carried out? Will it be easy or hard to reproduce each symptom? Will combined movements and repetitive movements be necessary to reproduce the patient's symptoms? Are symptoms severe and/or irritable? If symptoms are severe, physical tests may be carried out to just before the onset of symptom production or just to the onset of symptom production; no overpressures will be carried out, as the patient would be unable to tolerate this. If symptoms are irritable, physical tests may be examined to just before symptom production or just to the onset of provocation with fewer physical tests being examined to allow for a rest period between tests.

Are there any precautions and/or contraindications to elements of the physical examination that need to be explored further, such as vertebrobasilar insufficiency, neurological involvement, recent fracture, trauma, steroid therapy or rheumatoid arthritis? There may also be certain contraindications to further examination and treatment, e.g. symptoms of cord compression.

A physical examination planning form can be useful for clinicians to help guide them through the clinical reasoning process (see Figure 2.10).

Physical examination

The information from the subjective examination helps the clinician to plan an appropriate physical examination. The severity, irritability and nature of the condition are the major factors that will influence the choice and priority of physical testing procedures. The first and overarching question the clinician might

ask is: 'Is this patient's condition suitable for me to manage as a therapist?' For example, a patient presenting with CAD may only need brief and focused neurovascular testing, prior to an urgent medical referral. The nature of the patient's condition has had a major impact on the physical examination. The second question the clinician might ask is: 'Does this patient have a neuromusculoskeletal dysfunction that I may be able to help?' To answer that, the clinician must carry out a full physical examination; however, this may not be possible if the symptoms are severe and/or irritable. If the patient's symptoms are severe and/or irritable, the clinician aims to explore movements as much as possible, within a symptom-free range. If the patient has constant and severe and/or irritable symptoms, then the clinician aims to find physical tests that ease the symptoms. If the patient's symptoms are non-severe and non-irritable, then the clinician aims to find physical tests that reproduce each of the patient's symptoms.

Each significant physical test that either provokes or eases the patient's symptoms is highlighted in the patient's notes by an asterisk (*) for easy reference. The highlighted tests are often referred to as 'asterisks' or 'markers'.

The order and detail of the physical tests described below need to be appropriate to the patient being examined; some tests will be irrelevant, some tests will be carried out briefly, while others will need to be fully investigated. It is important that readers understand that the techniques shown in this chapter are some of many; the choice depends mainly on the relative size of the clinician and patient, as well as the clinician's preference. For this reason, novice clinicians may initially want to copy what is shown, but then quickly adapt to what is best for them.

Observation

Informal observation

The clinician needs to observe the patient in dynamic and static situations; the quality of movement is noted, as are the postural characteristics and facial expression. Informal observation will have begun from the moment the clinician begins the subjective examination and will continue to the end of the physical examination.

Formal observation

Observation of posture. The clinician examines spinal posture in sitting and standing, noting the posture of head and neck, thoracic spine and upper limbs. The clinician passively corrects any asymmetry to determine its relevance to the patient's problem.

A specific abnormal posture relevant to the upper cervical spine is the shoulder crossed syndrome (Janda 1994, 2002), which is described in Chapter 3. Patients who experience headaches may have a forward head posture (Watson 1994).

It is worth noting that pure postural dysfunction rarely influences one region of the body in isolation and it may be necessary to observe the patient more fully for a full postural examination.

Observation of muscle form. The clinician observes the muscle bulk and muscle tone of the patient, comparing left and right sides. It must be remembered that handedness and level and frequency of physical activity may well produce differences in muscle bulk between sides. Some muscles are thought to shorten under stress, while other muscles weaken, producing muscle imbalance (see Table 3.2). Patterns of muscle imbalance are thought to be the cause of the shoulder crossed syndrome mentioned above, as well as other abnormal postures, outlined in Table 6.1.

Observation of soft tissues. The clinician observes the colour of the patient's skin and notes any swelling over the cervical spine or related areas, taking cues for further examination.

Observation of the patient's attitudes and feelings. The age, gender and ethnicity of patients and their cultural, occupational and social backgrounds will all affect their attitudes and feelings towards themselves, their condition and the clinician. The clinician needs to be aware of and sensitive to these attitudes, and to empathise and communicate appropriately so as to develop a rapport with the patient and thereby enhance the patient's compliance with the treatment.

Joint integrity tests (Pettman 1994)

These tests are applicable for patients suspected of mild UCI. It is recommended that specific training is undertaken prior to using these tests (Pettman 2004; Moore et al. 2005). Care must be taken during the tests, and the tests are not indicated in the presence of acute trauma, or where subjective indicators of instability are obvious. The tests described below are considered positive if the patient experiences one or more of the following symptoms: a loss of balance in relation to head movement, unilateral pain along the length of the tongue, facial lip paraesthesia, bilateral or quadrilateral limb paraesthesia or nystagmus.

However, the diagnostic utility of the tests has not been consistently demonstrated in research. The patient may require further diagnostic investigations of the upper cervical spine if the clinician finds instability during the tests below, or if subjective indicators are suggestive of instability.

Distraction tests. With the head and neck in neutral position, the clinician gently distracts the head. If this is symptom-free then the test is repeated with the head flexed on the neck. Reproduction of symptoms suggests upper cervical ligamentous instability, particularly implicating the tectorial membrane (Pettman 1994).

Sagittal stress tests. The forces applied to test the stability of the spine are directed in the sagittal plane and are therefore known as sagittal stress tests. They include anterior and posterior stability tests for the atlanto-occipital joint and two anterior stability tests for the atlantoaxial joint.

Posterior stability test of the atlanto-occipital joint. With the patient supine, the clinician applies an anterior force bilaterally to the atlas and axis on the occiput (Figure 6.1).

Anterior stability of the atlanto-occipital joint. With the patient supine, the clinician applies a posterior force bilaterally to the anterolateral aspect of the transverse processes of the atlas and axis on the occiput (Figure 6.2).

Sharp–Perser test. With the patient sitting and the head and neck flexed, the clinician fixes the spinous process of C2 and gently pushes the head posteriorly through the forehead to translate the occiput and atlas posteriorly. The test is considered positive, indicating anterior instability of the atlantoaxial joint, if the patient's symptoms are provoked on head and neck flexion and relieved by posterior pressure on the forehead (Figure 6.3).

Anterior translation stress of the atlas on the axis. With the patient supine, the clinician fixes C2 (using

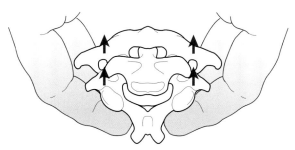

Figure 6.1 • Posterior stability test of the atlanto-occipital joint. (From Pettman 1994, with permission.)

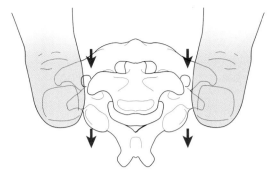

Figure 6.2 • Anterior stability of the atlanto-occipital joint. (From Pettman 1994, with permission.)

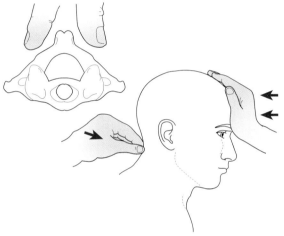

Figure 6.3 • Sharp–Perser test of the atlantoaxial joint. (From Pettman 1994, with permission.)

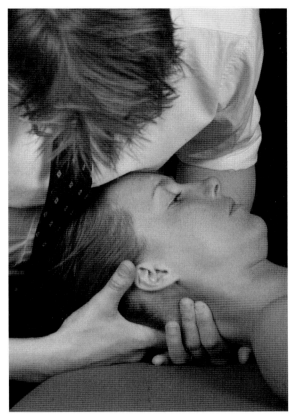

Figure 6.4 • Anterior stress test of the atlas on the axis. The left hand grips around the anterior edge of the transverse processes of the axis while the right hand lifts the occiput upwards.

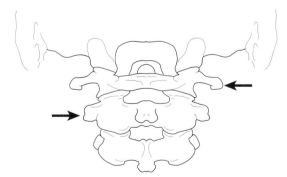

Figure 6.5 • Lateral stability stress test for the atlantoaxial joint. (From Pettman 1994, with permission.)

thumb pressure over the anterior aspect of the transverse processes) and then lifts the head and atlas vertically (Figure 6.4).

Coronal stress tests. The force applied to test the stability of the spine is directed in the coronal plane and is therefore known as a coronal stress test.

Lateral stability stress test for the atlantoaxial joint. With the patient supine, the clinician supports the occiput and the left side of the arch of the atlas, for example, with the other hand resting over the right side of the arch of the axis. A lateral shear of the atlas and occiput on the axis to the right is attempted. The test is then repeated to the other side. Excessive movement or reproduction of the patient's symptoms suggests lateral instability of this joint (Figure 6.5).

Alar ligament stress tests. Two stress tests apply a lateral flexion and a rotation stress on the alar ligament (which attaches to the odontoid peg and foramen magnum). The alar ligaments limit contralateral

lateral flexion and rotation movement of the occiput on the cervical spine.

Lateral flexion stress test for the alar ligaments. With the patient supine, the clinician fixes C2 along the neural arch and attempts to flex the craniovertebral joint laterally. No movement of the head is possible if the contralateral alar ligament is intact. The test is repeated with the upper cervical spine in flexion, neutral and extension. If motion is available in all three positions, the test is considered positive, suggesting an alar tear or arthrotic instability at the C0–C1 joint.

Rotational stress test for the alar ligament. This test is carried out if the previous lateral flexion stress test is positive, to determine whether the instability is due to laxity of the alar ligament or due to instability at the C0–C1 joint. In sitting, the clinician fixes C2 by gripping the lamina and then rotates the head. More than 20–30° of rotation indicates a damaged contralateral alar ligament (Figure 6.6). When the excessive rotational motion is in the same direction as the excessive lateral flexion (from the test above), this suggests damage to the alar ligament; when the excessive motions are in opposite directions, this suggests arthrotic instability (Pettman 1994).

Active physiological movements

For active physiological movements, the clinician notes the:

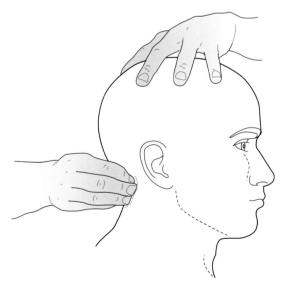

Figure 6.6 • Rotational stress test for the alar ligament (From Pettman 1994, with permission.)

- quality of movement (includes clicking or joint noises through the range)
- range of movement
- behaviour of pain through the range of movement
- resistance through the range of movement and at the end of the range of movement
- provocation of any muscle spasm.

A movement diagram can be used to depict this information. The active movements with overpressure listed below and shown in Figure 6.7 for the upper cervical spine (and in Chapter 7 for the cervicothoracic spine) are often tested with the patient sitting. The clinician establishes the patient's symptoms at rest and prior to each movement and corrects any movement deviation to determine its relevance to the patient's symptoms.

Movements of the upper cervical spine and possible modifications are shown in Table 6.2. Numerous differentiation tests (Maitland et al. 2001) can be performed; the choice depends on the patient's signs and symptoms. For example, when cervical flexion reproduces the patient's headache in sitting, the addition of slump sitting (see Chapter 3) or knee extension may help to differentiate the structures at fault. Slump sitting or knee extension may increase symptoms if there is a neurodynamic component to the patient's headache. The clinician is constantly aware of the body's attempts to protect hypersensitive neural tissue. For example, a reduction in upper cervical flexion could be due to neural hypersensitivity, not just articular restriction.

Observing the quality of movement can give important information regarding motor strategies and gross articular dysfunction. The clinician should be aware of the quality of sagittal movements whilst considering the eccentric control offered by the deep cervical flexors and extensors. During rotation, the clinician notes any obvious loss of C1/2 rotation evident by the patient 'carrying' the head on the upper cervical spine (dominant mid/lower cervical rotation), rather than a more natural 'spinning' of the head on the upper cervical spine (dominant early C1/2 rotation).

Other regions may need to be examined to determine their relevance to the patient's symptoms; they may be the source of the symptoms, or they may be contributing to the symptoms. The most likely regions are the temporomandibular, lower cervical spine and thoracic spine. The joints within these regions can be tested fully (see relevant chapter) or partially with the use of screening tests (see Chapter 3 for further details).

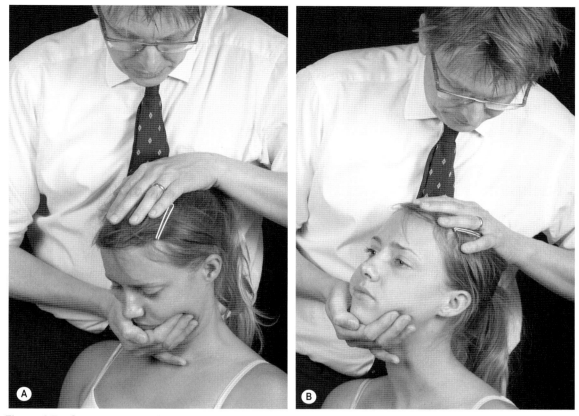

Figure 6.7 • Overpressures to the upper cervical spine. **A** Flexion. The left hand cups around the anterior aspect of the mandible while the right hand grips over the occiput. Both hands then apply a force to cause the head to rotate forwards on the upper cervical spine. **B** Extension. The right hand holds underneath the mandible while the left hand and forearm lie over the head. The head and neck are displaced forwards and then both hands apply a force to cause the head to rotate backwards on the upper cervical spine.

(Continued)

Some functional ability has already been tested by the general observation of the patient during the subjective and physical examinations, e.g. the postures adopted during the subjective examination and the ease or difficulty of undressing prior to the examination. Any further functional testing can be carried out at this point in the examination and may include sitting postures or certain movements of the upper limb. Clues for appropriate tests can be obtained from the subjective examination findings, particularly aggravating factors.

Palpation. The cervical spine is palpated, as well as the head, face, thoracic spine and upper limbs, as appropriate. It is useful to record palpation findings on a body chart (see Figure 2.3) and/or palpation chart (see Figure 3.36).

The clinician notes the:

- temperature of the area
- localised increased skin moisture
- presence of oedema or effusion
- mobility and feel of superficial tissues, e.g. ganglions, nodules, thickening of deep suboccipital tissues
- presence or elicitation of any muscle spasm
- tenderness of bone, ligaments, muscle, tendon, tendon sheath and nerve. Check for tenderness in the suboccipital region. Test for the relevant trigger points shown in Figure 3.37
- increased or decreased prominence of bones
- symptoms (often pain) provoked or reduced on palpation.

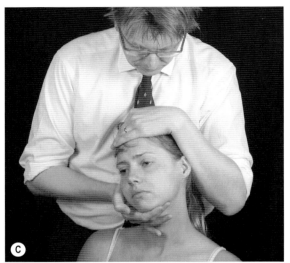

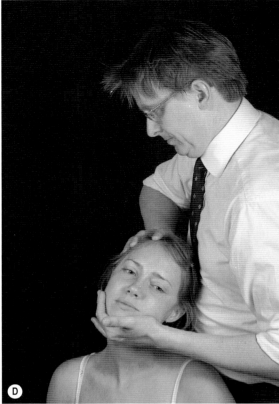

Figure 6.7—cont'd • C Lateral flexion. The hands grasp around the head and mandible and apply a force to tilt the head laterally on the upper cervical spine. D Left upper cervical quadrant. The hand position is the same as for upper cervical extension. The head is moved into upper cervical extension and then moved into left rotation and then left lateral flexion.

Passive intervertebral examination

Passive intervertebral examination of the cervical spine is intended to produce information regarding the quantity (range) and quality (through range and end-feel) of specific motion segments. The validity and reliability of this concept have been challenged in recent years, demonstrating varying results (Pool et al. 2004; Piva et al. 2006). Despite this variance, there is continuing use of these techniques, with a belief that findings from passive examination contribute towards clinical decision-making and management-planning (van Trijffel et al. 2005, 2009; Haxby Abbott et al. 2009). For the cervical spine, these manual examination techniques have been shown to be particularly important in decision-making when used with a cluster of tests (De Hertogh et al. 2007).

Passive physiological movements

This can take the form of passive physiological intervertebral movements (PPIVMs), which examine the movement at each segmental level of the spine. PPIVMs can be a useful adjunct to passive accessory intervertebral movements to identify segmental hypomobility and hypermobility. It can be performed with the patient supine or sitting. The clinician palpates between adjacent spinous processes or articular pillars to feel the range of intervertebral movement during the following physiological movements: upper cervical flexion and extension, lateral flexion and rotation. Assessment can be enhanced with the use of combined movements (Figure 6.8). Figure 6.9 demonstrates upper cervical flexion PPIVM in lying.

Table 6.2 Active physiological movements and possible modifications

Active movement	Modification to active movements
Cervical spine	Repeated
Cervical flexion	Speed altered
Upper cervical flexion	Combined (Edwards 1994, 1999) e.g.
Cervical extension Upper cervical extension Left lateral flexion Right lateral flexion Left rotation	– upper cervical flexion then rotation – upper cervical flexion, rotation and lateral flexion – upper cervical extension then rotation – rotation then flexion – rotation then extension
Right rotation	Compression or distraction
Compression	Sustained
Distraction	Injuring movement
?Temporomandibular	Differentiation tests
?Lower cervical spine	Function
?Thoracic spine	

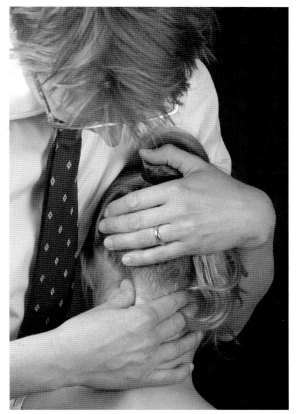

Figure 6.8 • Combined movements to the upper cervical spine. The head is supported by the clinician's left hand and forearm and the right hand palpates the upper cervical spine. The left hand then rotates the patient's head and adds flexion while the right hand feels the movement.

Specifically, a C1–2 flexion–rotation test (FRT) can determine segmental dysfunction even in the presence of normal active range of movement (Hall & Robinson 2004). The FRT has very high diagnostic utility in relation to differentiating cervicogenic (C1–2) headaches (Ogince et al. 2007). Average range of C1–2 rotation in asymptomatic subjects is between 39° and 42° (Amiri et al. 2003; Hall & Robinson 2004). The FRT has a cut-off point of 32° of C1–2 rotation for a positive test, although many subjects with cervicogenic headache have a unilateral (towards side of pain) range of around 20° (Hall & Robinson 2004). It has been shown that therapists can detect these differences reliably (Ogince et al. 2007). Figure 6.10 demonstrates the FRT in lying.

Other regions may need to be examined to determine their relevance to the patient's symptoms; they may be the source of the symptoms, or they may be contributing to the symptoms. The most likely regions are the temporomandibular region, lower cervical spine and thoracic spine.

Passive accessory intervertebral movements

It is useful to use the palpation chart and movement diagrams (or joint pictures) to record findings. These are explained in detail in Chapter 3.

The clinician notes the:

- quality of movement
- range of movement
- resistance through the range and at the end of the range of movement
- behaviour of pain through the range
- provocation of any muscle spasm.

Upper cervical spine (C1–C4) accessory movements are listed in Table 6.3 and for the C1 level are shown in Figure 6.11 (other levels are shown in Chapter 7).

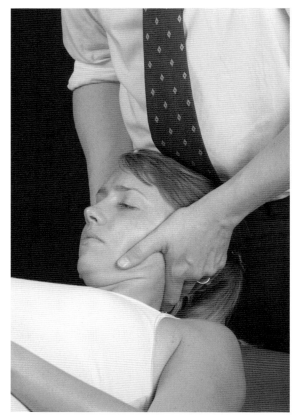

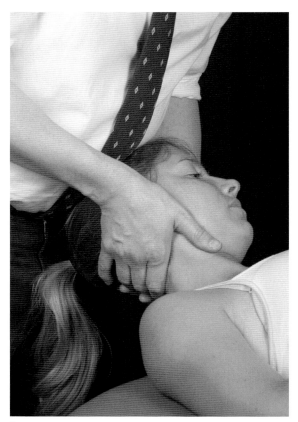

Figure 6.9 • Upper cervical flexion passive physiological intervertebral movement. The patient lies supine with the head over the end of the couch and supported on the clinician's stomach. The hands are placed so that the index and middle finger lie directly underneath the occiput and between the transverse process of C1 and the mastoid process. The head is then moved into upper cervical flexion and the palpating fingers feel the range of movement.

Figure 6.10 • The flexion–rotation test in lying. Gross cervical flexion is maintained whilst stabilising C2 and performing passive C1–C2 rotation with the head. This test can aid differentiation of cervicogenic headache, as well as being an accurate examination of upper cervical rotation.

A number of ways of combining movements have been documented (Edwards 1994, 1999) and are described below.

Atlanto-occipital joint. Apply anteroposterior (AP) and/or posteroanterior (PA) unilateral pressures on C1 with the spine positioned in flexion and rotation or extension and rotation, so as to increase and/or decrease the compressive or stretch effect at the atlanto-occipital joint:

• A PA on the right of C1 with the spine in flexion and right rotation will increase the stretch at the right C0–C1 joint (Figure 6.12); an AP on the right of C1 will decrease the stretch.

• An AP on the left of C1 with the spine in extension and right rotation will increase the stretch on the left C0–C1 joint; a PA on the left of C1 will decrease the stretch.

Atlantoaxial joint. Apply AP and/or PA unilateral vertebral pressures on C1 and/or C2 with the spine positioned in rotation and flexion or rotation and extension so as to increase and/or decrease the compressive or stretch effect at the atlantoaxial joint:

• A PA on the left of C1 with the head in right rotation and flexion will increase the stretch at the left C1–C2 joint; a PA on C2 will decrease this stretch.

• A PA on the left of C2 with the head in left rotation and extension will increase the rotation at the C1–C2 joint; a PA on C1 will decrease the rotation.

Table 6.3 Accessory movements, choice of application and reassessment of the patient's asterisks

Accessory movements	Choice of application	Identify any effect of accessory movements on patient's signs and symptoms
Upper cervical spine ↕ Central posteroanterior ⌐°°⌐ Unilateral posteroanterior →•→ Med transverse for C1 →•→ Med/lat transverse for C2–C4 �lↄ Unilateral anteroposterior	Start position, e.g. in flexion, extension, etc. — speed of force application — direction of the applied force — point of application of applied force	Reassess all asterisks
?Temporomandibular joint	As above	Reassess all asterisks
?Lower cervical spine	As above	Reassess all asterisks
?Thoracic spine	As above	Reassess all asterisks

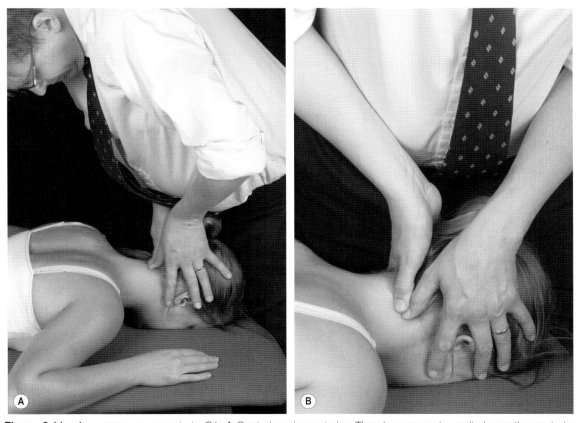

Figure 6.11 • Accessory movements to C1. A Central posteroanterior. Thumb pressure is applied over the posterior arch of C1 and directed upwards and forwards towards the patient's eyes. B Unilateral posteroanterior. Thumb pressure is applied laterally over the posterior arch of C1.

(Continued)

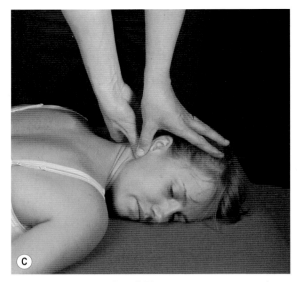

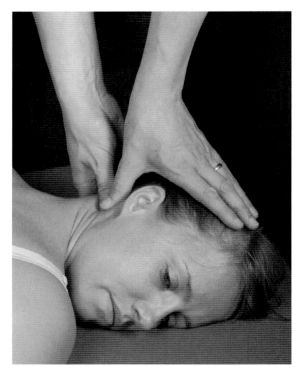

Figure 6.11—cont'd • C Transverse pressure on the right. The head is rotated to the right and thumb pressure is applied to the transverse process of C1.

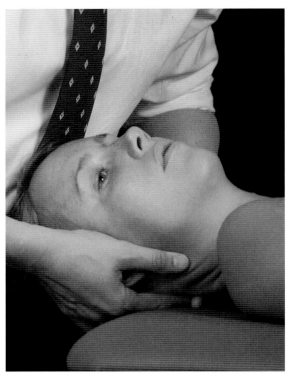

Figure 6.13 • Palpation for the C0–C1 joint using combined movements. Thumb pressure over the anterior aspect of the atlas on the right is applied with the head in right rotation and extension.

- An AP on the left of C2 with the head in right rotation and flexion will increase the rotation at the C1–C2 joint; an AP on C1 will decrease the rotation.
- An AP on the right of C1 with the head in right rotation and extension will increase the rotation at the C1–C2 joint (Figure 6.13); an AP on C2 will decrease the rotation.

Following accessory movements to the upper cervical spine the clinician reassesses all the physical asterisks (movements or tests that have been found to reproduce the patient's symptoms) in order to establish the effect of the accessory movements on the patient's signs and symptoms. Accessory movements can then be tested for other regions suspected to be a source of, or contributing to, the symptoms. Again, following accessory movements the clinician reassesses all the physical asterisks. Regions likely to be examined are the temporomandibular joint, lower cervical spine and upper thoracic spine (Table 6.2).

Figure 6.12 • Palpation for the C0–C1 joint using combined movements. Thumb pressure over the right of the posterior arch of the atlas is applied with the patient's head in flexion and right rotation.

Sustained natural apophyseal glides (SNAGs)

The painful cervical spine movements are examined in sitting. Pressure is applied by the clinician to each spinous process and/or transverse process of the cervical vertebrae as the patient moves slowly towards the pain (Mulligan 1999). Figure 6.14 demonstrates a SNAG to the spinous process of C4 as the subject moves into cervical flexion. The symptomatic level will be one in which the pressure reduces the pain. For further information, see Chapter 3.

For patients complaining of headaches, Mulligan (1999) describes four examination techniques.

Headache SNAGs. The clinician applies a PA pressure to C2 on a stabilised occiput with the patient in sitting (Figure 6.15). The pressure is sustained for at least 10 seconds while the patient remains still; there is no active movement. The test is considered positive if the headache is relieved, which would indicate a mechanical joint problem.

Reverse headache SNAGs. The clinician moves the occiput anteriorly on the stabilised C2 with

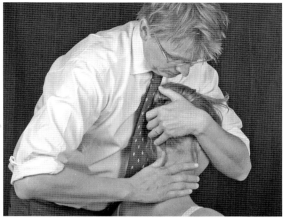

Figure 6.15 • Headache sustained natural apophyseal glide. A posteroanterior pressure is applied to C2 using the heel of the right hand. The left hand supports the head.

the patient in sitting (Figure 6.16). The movement is sustained for at least 10 seconds while the patient remains still; there is no active movement. Again the test is considered positive if the headache is relieved, which would indicate a mechanical joint problem.

Upper cervical traction. The clinician maintains the patient's cervical lordosis by placing a forearm under the cervical spine with the patient supine

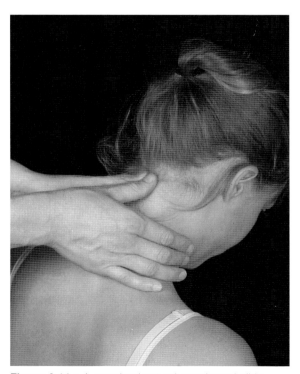

Figure 6.14 • A sustained natural apophyseal glide. A posteroanterior pressure is applied to C2 as the subject moves into cervical flexion.

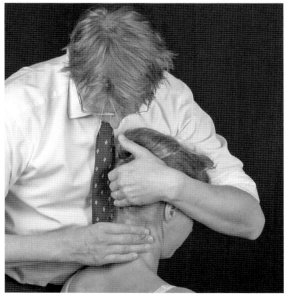

Figure 6.16 • Reverse headache sustained natural apophyseal glide. The right hand palpates the transverse processes of C2. The left hand supports and moves the head anteriorly on the stabilised C2.

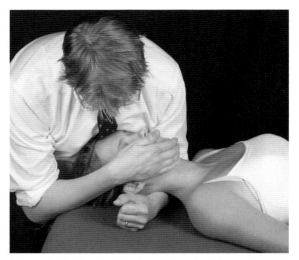

Figure 6.17 • Cervical traction. The patient lies supine and the clinician's forearm is placed under the patient's cervical spine. The right hand grips the mandible and applies a gentle traction force.

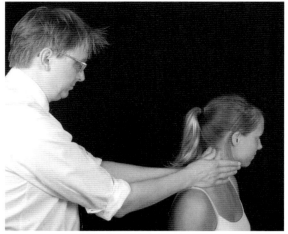

Figure 6.18 • Sustained natural apophyseal glides for restricted cervical rotation at C1–C2. A posteroanterior pressure is applied to the right articular pillar of C1 as the patient moves slowly into left rotation.

(Figure 6.17). Pronation of the forearm and a gentle pull on the chin produce cervical traction. The position is held for at least 10 seconds; relief of symptoms indicates a positive test, which would indicate a mechanical joint problem.

SNAGs for restricted cervical rotation at C1–C2. The painful cervical spine movements are examined in sitting. Pressure to the left or right side of the posterior arch of C1 is applied by the clinician as the patient slowly rotates to the right or left side towards the pain (Figure 6.18). Painfree movement indicates a positive test and would indicate a mechanical joint problem.

Muscle tests

Muscle tests include examining muscle strength, control, length and isometric muscle testing.

Muscle strength

The clinician may test the cervical flexors, extensors, lateral flexors and rotators. For details of these general tests, readers are directed to Cole et al. (1988), Hislop & Montgomery (1995) or Kendall et al. (1993).

Greater detail may be required to test the strength of muscles, in particular those thought prone to become weak (Janda 1994, 2002; Sahrmann 2002), which include serratus anterior, middle and lower fibres of trapezius and the deep neck flexors. Testing the strength of these muscles is described in Chapter 3.

Muscle control

The relative strength of muscles is considered to be more important than the overall strength of a muscle group (Janda 1994, 2002; Sahrmann 2002). Relative strength is assessed indirectly by observing posture, as already mentioned, by the quality of active movement, noting any changes in muscle recruitment patterns, and by palpating muscle activity in various positions. Additionally, specific muscle testing can be undertaken in the upper cervical spine.

Deep cervical muscle testing. Deep muscles in the cervical spine are important in the support and control of the head and neck (Jull et al. 2005). Weak deep neck flexors have been found to be associated with cervicogenic headaches (Watson 1994). These muscles are tested by the clinician observing the pattern of movement that occurs when the patient flexes his/her head from a supine position. When the deep neck flexors are weak, the sternocleidomastoid muscle initiates the movement, causing the jaw to lead the movement, and the upper cervical spine hyperextends. Owing to their high muscle spindle density, these muscles have a significant role in proprioception of head-on-neck movement, and also mediation of pain via their neurological associations with the brain (Treleaven 2008; O'Leary et al. 2009).

Poor motor strategies between groups of muscles, and between deep and superficial muscles in the cervical region, have been shown to be associated with upper cervical spine symptoms (Jull 2000; Falla et al. 2004).

Deep cervical flexors. Assessment of the deep cervical flexors (longus colli, longus capitis, rectus capitis anterior and lateralis) is made using the low-load cervicocranial flexion test (CCFT) (Jull et al. 2008b). A pressure biofeedback unit (PBU; Chattanooga, Australia) is used to measure the function of the deep neck flexors; the patient lies supine-crook with the clinician using towels to ensure the head and neck are in a neutral position. The PBU is placed under the cervical spine, abutted against the occiput and inflated to 20 mmHg (Figure 6.19). The patient is then taught the correct nodding action of upper cervical flexion, as if indicating 'yes'. It is important that the head is not lifted or retracted. Testing is then undertaken in two stages. As pain inhibits deep cervical flexor activity, testing should never induce symptoms (Falla & Farina 2008; Arendt-Nielsen & Falla 2009).

Stage 1 – analysis of movement patterning. This is a five-level test whereby the patient attempts progressively to increase the pressure on the PBU in a correct motor strategy. Using visual feedback from the PBU, the patient attempts to hold a nod at 22, 24, 26, 28 and 30 mmHg with a few seconds' rest between each stage. Ideally, subjects are able to progress through all five levels (Falla et al. 2003). Observation and palpation for overuse of superficial muscles (sternocleidomastoid, plus the scalene and hyoid groups) are made. These muscles may be active, but not dominant (Falla et al. 2004). A positive test is recorded when a patient is unable to achieve a level without either initiating a retraction

movement and/or recruiting superficial flexors as the dominant group. A recording is made of both the level achieved and the quality of movement.

Stage 2 – holding capacity of deep neck flexors. This stage is only undertaken when training in stage 1 has resulted in normal patterning at all five levels (Jull et al. 2008b). Beginning at 22 mmHg (2 mmHg above a baseline of 20 mmHg), the patient attempts to hold the test position (nod) for 10 seconds. Ten by 10-second repetitions are aimed for at each level. The number of 10-second repetitions is recorded and used as the patient's baseline score. A performance index (PI) may be used to quantify the performance (Jull et al. 1999). This is calculated by multiplying the pressure (mmHg) increase in performance from baseline (20 mmHg) by the number of correct 10-second holds at that level, e.g. if at 26 mmHg (i.e. 6 mmHg above baseline) five repetitions were achieved, the PI would be 6 × 5 = 30. Rehabilitation is aimed towards achieving 10 holds at 10 mmHg above baseline (level 5 – 30 mmHg), i.e. a PI of 100. As in stage 1, a positive finding is when there is superficial muscle dominance or retraction of the neck. The clinician also observes the quality of movement, looking for jerky, poor control of the head.

Deep cervical extensors. Although most clinical and research attention has been towards the deep cervical flexors, the deep extensors also contribute towards mechanical and neural (proprioception) control of the head on neck. The deepest of the extensors (semispinalis cervicis) cannot be palpated, but activity can be encouraged within these muscles by maintaining upper cervical neutral during full cervical extension (sagittal rotation around a C7 axis). Maintenance of upper cervical neutral will bias muscle activity towards semispinalis capitis, and discourage activity in the superficial semispinalis capitis and splenius capitis (Jull et al. 2008b).

The rectus capitis posterior and obliquus capitis groups are palpable and thus clinician and patient tactile feedback can be gained when re-educating motor strategies for these muscles. Simultaneous palpation and observation of these muscles with splenius capitis during through-range upper cervical nodding (into extension if pain allows) will allow assessment of extensor motor strategies. Although the validity or reliability is not known at present, a craniocervical extension test can allow quantification of extensor strategies. This can be undertaken as per the CCFT, but with the pressure cuff placed under the head rather than the neck. Alternatively, in prone lying, with the face in a breathing hole, the patient's forehead is rested on the PBU sensor (Figure 6.20). The

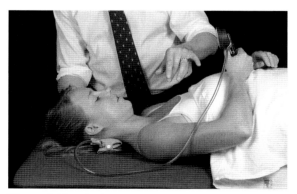

Figure 6.19 • Testing the strength of the deep neck flexors.

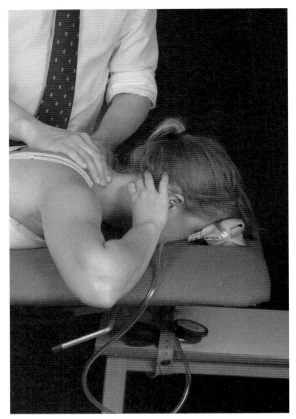

Figure 6.20 • The craniocervical extension test is used to assess motor strategies of the deep and superficial cervical extensors and rotators.

unit is inflated to 20 mmHg, by which time the sensor is taking the whole of the weight of the head. Visual feedback from the PBU is accessed through the breathing hole as the patient is instructed to perform upper cervical extension (nod) whilst both the clinician and the patient receive tactile feedback from deep muscle palpation. The patient repeatedly attempts fluidly to decrease pressure to 10 mmHg whilst maintaining a correct motor strategy. The test can be repeated in varying degrees of C1–2 rotation to bias the obliquus groups.

Axioscapular muscles. Owing to their attachments at the upper cervical spine and the occiput, activity of the upper fibres of the trapezius, levator scapulae, scalenae group and sternocleidomastoid will influence movement patterns in the upper cervical spine. Assessment of control and patterning of these muscles should be considered. Additionally, scapular control is considered to be associated with cervical dysfunction, specifically following whiplash

trauma (Jull et al. 2008a). Therefore assessment of scapular control via the middle and lower fibres of trapezius, together with the serratus muscles, may also be undertaken.

Sensorimotor assessment (Jull et al. 2008a; Treleaven 2008)

Afferents from neuromusculoskeletal structures of the upper cervical spine (nerve roots, deep muscles, joint structures) influence and mediate central and reflex activity. Functionally, these neurological connections manifest in the optimum coordinated stability of the head, eyes and posture. Pain and dysfunction in the upper cervical spine can result in altered reflex activity, which in turn can perpetuate a sensorimotor dysfunction. Clinically, alteration in sensorimotor function is associated with lasting pain, loss of movement, altered oculomotor function, dizziness, nausea, visual disturbance, hearing disturbances and loss of postural stability. Sensorimotor disturbances can be assessed using simple tests, summarised in Table 6.4.

Muscle length

The clinician tests the length of muscles, in particular those thought prone to shorten (Janda 1994); that is, levator scapulae, upper trapezius, sternocleidomastoid, pectoralis major and minor, scalenes and the deep occipital muscles. Testing the length of these muscles is described in Chapter 3.

Isometric muscle testing

Test the cervical spine flexors, extensors, lateral flexors and rotators in resting position and, if indicated, in different parts of the physiological range. This is usually carried out with the patient sitting but may be done supine. In addition the clinician observes the quality of the muscle contraction to hold this position (this can be done with the patient's eyes shut). The patient may, for example, be unable to prevent the joint from moving or may hold with excessive muscle activity; either of these circumstances would suggest a neuromuscular dysfunction.

Neurological tests

Neurological examination includes neurological integrity testing, neurodynamic tests and some other nerve tests.

Table 6.4 Summary of sensorimotor testing. All tests are positive if there is reproduction of symptoms, especially dizziness. The clinician aims to avoid inducing pain or other symptoms during testing

Assessment	Proposed primary reflex/central activity	Method	Positive finding
Head-righting (eyes open)	Cervicocollic reflex Vestibulocollic reflex Tonic neck reflex Cervicoocular reflex	Maintain stable head position whilst moving body	Excessive movement of head Overactivity of Cx Mm Poor-quality movement Difficulty initiating movement
Head-righting (eyes closed)	Labyrinthine; +a/a	a/a with eyes closed	a/a
Cervical joint position sense (JPS)	Cervicocollic reflex Vestibulocollic reflex	Sit 90 cm from wall Find head neutral and position marker centrally Move head and return to neutral	>4 cm error more than 3/10 Poor-quality movement
Oculomotor 1: smooth pursuit (SP)	Cervicocollic reflex Vestibulo-ocular reflex Optokinetic reflex	Head stable (neutral) Eyes follow target	Inability to keep up with target (eyes play 'catch up') Loss of smoothness
Oculomotor 2: smooth-pursuit neck torsion (SPNT)	a/a + Cervicocollic reflex	a/a but sat with 45° trunk rotation	a/a – especiallly when target crosses midline Difference between SP and SPNT = probable neck afferent dysfunction
Oculomotor 3: gaze stability	a/a	Maintain gaze whilst moving head	Inability to focus Loss of movement quality
Oculomotor 4: saccadic eye movement	a/a Bias to optokinetic reflex	Fix and follow fast-moving target/separate targets	Inability to change gaze/focus quickly Nystagmus
Oculomotor 5: Eye–head coordination	a/a Bias to cervicocollic reflex and cervico-ocular reflex	Move eyes and head together to maintain focus on moving target	a/a
Oculomotor 6: peripheral vision	a/a	Focus on target (e.g. number); read target on periphery	Inability to read peripheral target number
Postural stability	Cervicocollic reflex Tonic neck reflex Cervico-ocular reflex	Stand (prog to compromise) ± eyes closed	Significant difference between eyes open and eyes closed

Cx Mm, cervical muscle (superficial); a/a, as above; a/a+, as above, plus the following information.

Integrity of the nervous system

Generally, if symptoms are localised to the upper cervical spine and head, neurological examination can be limited to cranial nerves (CNs) and C1–C4 nerve roots.

Dermatomes/peripheral nerves. Light touch and pain sensation of the face, head and neck are tested using cotton wool and pinprick respectively, as described in Chapter 3. Knowledge of the cutaneous distribution of nerve roots (dermatomes) and peripheral nerves enables the clinician to distinguish the sensory loss due to a root lesion from that due to a peripheral nerve lesion. The cutaneous nerve distribution and dermatome areas are shown in Chapter 3.

Myotomes/peripheral nerves. The following myotomes are tested and shown in Chapter 3.

- CN V (trigeminal): clench teeth, note temporalis and masseter muscles
- CN VII (facial): wrinkle forehead, close eyes, purse lips, show teeth
- CN XI (accessory): sternocleidomastoid and shoulder girdle elevation
- C1–C2: upper cervical flexion
- C2: upper cervical extension
- C3: cervical lateral flexion
- C4 and CN XI: shoulder girdle elevation.

A working knowledge of the muscular distribution of nerve roots (myotomes) and peripheral nerves enables the clinician to distinguish the motor loss due to a root lesion from that due to a peripheral nerve lesion.

Reflex testing. There are no deep tendon reflexes for C1–C4 nerve roots. The jaw jerk (CN V) is elicited by applying a sharp downward tap on the chin with the mouth slightly open. A slight jerk is normal; excessive jerk suggests bilateral upper motor neurone lesion.

Neurodynamic tests

The following neurodynamic tests may be carried out in order to ascertain the degree to which neural tissue is responsible for the production of the patient's symptom(s):

- passive neck flexion
- upper-limb neurodynamic tests
- straight-leg raise
- slump.

These tests are described in detail in Chapter 3.

Other nerve tests

Plantar response to test for an upper motor neurone lesion (Walton 1989). Pressure applied from the heel along the lateral border of the plantar aspect of the foot produces flexion of the toes in the normal. Extension of the big toe with downward fanning of the other toes occurs with an upper motor neurone lesion.

Cervical arterial dysfunction testing. If vascular dysfunction is suspected following the subjective examination (see above), further information regarding the integrity of the cervical arterial system can be gained from the following examination procedures. Further reading (Kerry & Taylor 2006) is recommended to support understanding of the following procedures.

Blood pressure. In the event of acute arterial dysfunction, it is likely that there will be a systematic cardiovascular response manifesting in dramatic change in blood pressure (usually increasing). Blood pressure is taken using appropriate, validated procedures and equipment, in either sitting or lying.

Functional positional testing. Passive repositioning of the head has been classically considered a test for vertebrobasilar insufficiency (VBI). A minimum requirement of a passive 10-second hold into cervical rotation has been proposed (Magarey et al. 2004). A positive test is considered if reproduction of symptoms suggestive of hindbrain ischaemia is found. The diagnostic utility of this procedure is, however, not certain (Thiel & Rix 2004; Kerry 2006), and, like any of the individual parts of CAD testing, reliance on one result alone is not indicative of pathology.

Pulse palpation. The verterbral artery pulses are difficult to palpate due to their size and depth. The internal carotid artery is easily accessible at the mid-cervical level, medial to the sternocleido-mastoid muscle. Gross pathologies, such as aneurysm formation, are characteristic in the nature of their pulse, that is, a pulsatile, expandable mass. Pain and exaggerated pulse on palpation of the temporal artery may support a hypothesis of temporal arteritis.

Cranial nerve examination. Cranial nerve dysfunction can be a component part of arterial compromise in the neck and head, and this is an indication of possible vascular dysfunction. Careful screening for gross asymmetries and variations from the norm in cranial nerve function is indicated if CAD is suspected (Kerry & Taylor 2008).

Proprioception tests. Hindbrain ischaemia associated with VBI can result in gross loss of proprioceptive function. Simple proprioception testing such as tandem gait, heel-to-knee, Rhomberg's test and Hautant's test is undertaken to assess proprioception dysfunction.

Differentiation between dizziness produced from the vestibular apparatus of the inner ear and that from the neck movement (due to cervical vertigo or compromised vertebral artery) may be required. In standing, the clinician maintains head position while the patient moves the trunk to produce cervical rotation. Rotation to left and right is each held for at least 10 seconds, with at least a 10-second rest period between directions. The test is completed with repetitive trunk rotation movements to left and right (Magarey et al. 2000). The test is considered positive and stopped immediately if dizziness, nausea or any other symptom associated with vertebrobasilar insufficiency is provoked, which suggests that the patient's symptoms are not caused by a disturbance of the vestibular system. A positive vertebral artery test contraindicates certain treatment techniques to the cervical spine (see Table 2.4).

Completion of the examination

Having carried out the above tests, the examination of the upper cervical spine is now complete. The subjective and physical examinations produce a large amount of information, which needs to be recorded accurately and quickly. An outline examination chart may be useful for some clinicians and one is suggested in Figure 6.21. It is important, however, that the clinician does not examine in a rigid manner, simply following the suggested sequence outlined in the chart. Each patient presents differently and this should be reflected in the examination process. It is vital at this stage to highlight with an asterisk (*) important findings from the examination. These findings must be reassessed at, and within, subsequent treatment sessions to evaluate the effects of treatment on the patient's condition.

The physical testing procedures which specifically indicate joint, nerve or muscle tissues, as a source of the patient's symptoms, are summarised in Table 3.10. The strongest evidence that a joint is the source of the patient's symptoms is that active and passive physiological movements, passive accessory movements and joint palpation all reproduce the patient's symptoms, and that, following a treatment dose, reassessment identifies an improvement in the patient's signs and symptoms. Weaker evidence includes an alteration in range, resistance or quality of physiological and/or accessory movements and tenderness over the joint, with no alteration in signs and symptoms after treatment. One or more of these findings may indicate a dysfunction of a joint which may or may not be contributing to the patient's condition.

The strongest evidence that a muscle is the source of a patient's symptoms is if active movements, an isometric contraction, passive lengthening and palpation of a muscle all reproduce the symptoms, and that, following a treatment dose, reassessment identifies an improvement in the patient's signs and symptoms. Further evidence of muscle dysfunction may be suggested by reduced strength or poor quality during the active physiological movement and the isometric contraction, reduced range and/or increased/decreased resistance, during the passive lengthening of the muscle, and tenderness on palpation, with no alteration in signs and symptoms after treatment. One or more of these findings may indicate a dysfunction of a muscle which may, or may not, be contributing to the patient's condition.

The strongest evidence that a nerve is the source of the patient's symptoms is when active and/or passive physiological movements reproduce the patient's symptoms, which are then increased or decreased with an additional sensitising movement, at a distance from the patient's symptoms. In addition, there is reproduction of the patient's symptoms on palpation of the nerve and following neurodynamic testing, sufficient to be considered a treatment dose, results in an improvement in the above signs and symptoms. Further evidence of nerve dysfunction may be suggested by reduced range (compared with the asymptomatic side) and/or increased resistance to the various arm movements, and tenderness on nerve palpation.

On completion of the physical examination, the clinician will:

- explain the findings of the physical examination and how these findings relate to the subjective assessment. An attempt should be made to clear up any misconceptions patients may have regarding their illness or injury
- collaborate with the patient and via problem-solving together devise a treatment plan and discuss the prognosis
- warn the patient of possible exacerbation up to 24–48 hours following the examination
- request the patient to report details on the behaviour of the symptoms following examination at the next attendance
- explain the findings of the physical examination and how these findings relate to the subjective assessment. An attempt should be made to clear up any misconceptions patients may have regarding their illness or injury
- evaluate the findings, formulate a clinical diagnosis and write up a problem list
- determine the objectives of treatment
- devise an initial treatment plan.

In this way, the clinician develops the following hypotheses categories (adapted from Jones & Rivett 2004):

- function: abilities and restrictions
- patient's perspective on his/her experience

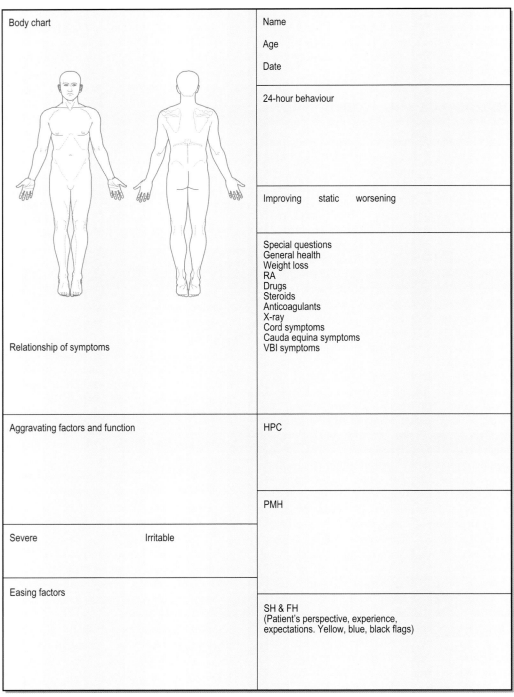

Body chart	Name
	Age
	Date
	24-hour behaviour
	Improving static worsening
	Special questions
	General health
	Weight loss
	RA
	Drugs
	Steroids
	Anticoagulants
	X-ray
	Cord symptoms
	Cauda equina symptoms
Relationship of symptoms	VBI symptoms
Aggravating factors and function	HPC
	PMH
Severe Irritable	
Easing factors	
	SH & FH
	(Patient's perspective, experience,
	expectations. Yellow, blue, black flags)

Figure 6.21 • Upper cervical spine examination chart. RA, rheumatoid arthritis; VBI, vertebrobasilar insufficiency; HPC, history of the present condition; PMH, past medical history; SH, social history; FH, family history.

(Continued)

Observation	Isometric muscle testing
Joint integrity tests	Other muscle tests
Active and passive physiological movements	Neurological integrity tests
	Neurodynamic tests
	Other nerve tests
Capsular pattern yes/no	Miscellaneous tests
Muscle strength	
	Palpation
Muscle control	
	Accessory movements and reassessment of each relevant region
Muscle length	

Figure 6.21—cont'd.

- source of symptoms, including the structure or tissue that is thought to be producing the patient's symptoms, the nature of the structure or tissues in relation to the healing process and the pain mechanisms
- contributing factors to the development and maintenance of the problem. There may be environmental, psychosocial, behavioural, physical or heredity factors
- precautions/contraindications to treatment and management. This includes the severity and irritability of the patient's symptoms and the nature of the patient's condition
- management strategy and treatment plan
- prognosis – this can be affected by factors such as the stage and extent of the injury as well as the patient's expectation, personality and lifestyle.

For guidance on treatment and management principles, the reader is directed to the companion textbook (Petty 2011).

References

Amiri, M., Jull, G., Bullock-Saxton, J., 2003. Measuring range of active cervical rotation in a position of full head flexion using the 3D Fastrack measurement system: an intra-tester reliability study. Man. Ther. 8 (3), 176–179.

Arendt-Nielsen, L., Falla, D., 2009. Motor control adjustments in musculoskeletal pain and the implications for pain recurrence. Pain 142 (3), 171–172.

Barker, S., Kesson, M., Ashmore, J., et al., 2000. Guidance for pre-manipulative testing of the cervical spine. Man. Ther. 5 (1), 37–40.

Bogduk, N., 1994. Cervical causes of headache and dizziness. In: Boyling, J.D., Palastanga, N. (Eds.), Grieve's modern manual therapy, second ed. Churchill Livingstone, Edinburgh, p. 317.

Cattrysse, E., Swinkels, R., Oostendorp, R., et al., 1997. Upper cervical instability: are clinical tests reliable? Man. Ther. 2 (2), 91–97.

Cole, J.H., Furness, A.L., Twomey, L.T., 1988. Muscles in action, an approach to manual muscle testing. Churchill Livingstone, Edinburgh.

Cook, C., Brismee, J.M., Fleming, R., et al., 2005. Identifiers suggestive of clinical cervical spine instability: a Delphi study of physical therapists. Phys. Ther. 85 (9), 895–906.

Dahlberg, C., Lanig, I.S., Kenna, M., et al., 1997. Diagnosis and treatment of esophageal perforations in cervical spinal cord injury. Top. Spinal Cord Inj. Rehabil. 2 (3), 41–48.

De Hertogh, W., Vaes, P., Duquet, W., 2007. The validity of the manual examination in the assessment of patients with neck pain. Spine 7 (5), 628–629.

Edeling, J., 1994. Manual therapy for chronic headache, second ed. Butterworth-Heinemann, Oxford.

Edwards, B.C., 1994. Examination of the high cervical spine (occiput–C2) using combined movements. In: Boyling, J.D., Palastanga, N. (Eds.), Grieve's modern manual therapy, second ed. Churchill Livingstone, Edinburgh, p. 555.

Edwards, B.C., 1999. Manual of combined movements: their use in the examination and treatment of mechanical vertebral column disorders, second ed. Butterworth-Heinemann, Oxford.

Falla, D., Farina, D., 2008. Neuromuscular adaptation in experimental and clinical neck pain. J. Electromyogr. Kinesiol. 18 (2), 255–261.

Falla, D., Campbell, C.D., Fagan, A.E., et al., 2003. Relationship between cranio-cervical flexion range of motion and pressure change during the cranio-cervical flexion test. Man. Ther. 8 (2), 92–96.

Falla, D., Jull, G.A., Hodges, P.W., 2004. Patients with neck pain demonstrate reduced electromyographic activity of the deep cervical flexor muscles during performances of the craniocervical flexion test. Spine 29 (19), 2108–2114.

Forrester, G.A., Barlas, P., 1999. Reliability and validity of the Sharp–Purser test in the assessment of atlantoaxial instability in patients with rheumatoid arthritis. Physiotherapy 85 (7), 376.

Grieve, G.P., 1994. Counterfeit clinical presentations. Manipulative Physiotherapist 26, 17–19.

Hall, T., Robinson, K., 2004. The flexion–rotation test and active cervical mobility – a comparative measurement in cervicogenic headache. Man. Ther. 9 (4), 197–202.

Haxby Abbott, J., Flynn, T.W., Fritz, J.M., et al., 2009. Manual physical assessment of spinal segmental motion: intent and validity. Man. Ther. 14 (1), 36–44.

Headache Classification Committee of the International Headache Society, 1988. Classification and diagnostic criteria for headache disorders, cranial neuralgias and facial pain. Cephalalgia 8 (7), 9–96.

Headache Classification Committee of the International Headache Society, 2004. The international classification of headache disorders, second ed. Cephalalgia 24 (Suppl.), 1–151.

Hislop, H., Montgomery, J., 1995. Daniels and Worthingham's muscle testing, techniques of manual examination, seventh ed. W B Saunders, Philadelphia.

Jackson, R., 1966. The cervical syndrome, third ed. Charles C Thomas, Springfield, IL.

Janda, V., 1994. Muscles and motor control in cervicogenic disorders: assessment and management. In: Grant, R. (Ed.), Physical therapy of the cervical and thoracic spine, second ed. Churchill Livingstone, New York, p. 195.

Janda, V., 2002. Muscles and motor control in cervicogenic disorders. In: Grant, R. (Ed.), Physical therapy of the cervical and thoracic spine, third ed. Churchill Livingstone, New York, p. 182.

Jones, M.A., Rivett, D.A., 2004. Clinical reasoning for manual therapists. Butterworth-Heinemann, Edinburgh.

Jull, G.A., 2000. Deep cervical flexor dysfunction in whiplash. J. Musculoskelet. Pain 8, 1–2, 143–154.

Jull, G.A., Niere, R.K., 2005. The cervical spine and headache. In: Boyling, J., Jull, G.A. (Eds.), Grieve's modern manual therapy, third ed. Elsevier, London.

Jull, G.A., Barrett, C., Magee, R., et al., 1999. Further clinical clarification of the muscle dysfunction in cervical headache. Cephalalgia 19, 179–185.

Jull, G.A., Falla, D., Treleaven, J., et al., 2005. A therapeutic exercise approach for cervical disorders. In: Boyling, J., Jull, G.A. (Eds.), Grieve's modern manual therapy, third ed. Elsevier, London, pp. 451–470.

Jull, G.A., Sterling, M., Falla, D., et al., 2008a. Whiplash, headache and neck pain. Elsevier, London.

Jull, G.A., O'Leary, S.P., Falla, D.L., 2008b. Clinical assessment of the deep cervical flexor muscles: the craniocervical flexion test. J. Manipulative Physiol. Ther. 31 (7), 525–533.

Kaale, B.R., Krakenes, J., Albrektsen, G., et al., 2008. Clinical assessment techniques for detecting ligament and membrane injuries in the upper cervical spine region – a comparison with MRI results. Man. Ther. 13 (5), 397–403.

Kendall, F.P., McCreary, E.K., Provance, P.G., 1993. Muscles testing and function, fourth ed. Williams & Wilkins, Baltimore, MD.

Kerry, R., 2006. Vertebral artery testing: how certain are you that your pre-cervical manipulation and mobilisation tests are safe and specific? In: HES 2nd International Evidence Based Practice Conference, London.

Kerry, R., Taylor, A.J., 2006. Masterclass: Cervical arterial dysfunction assessment and manual therapy. Man. Ther. 11 (3), 243–253.

Kerry, R., Taylor, A.J., 2008. Arterial pathology and cervicocranial pain – differential diagnosis for manual therapists and medical practitioners.

Int. Musculoskelet. Med. 30 (2), 70–77.

Kerry, R., Taylor, A.J., 2009. Cervical arterial dysfunction: knowledge and reasoning for manual physical therapists. J. Orthop. Sports Phys. Ther. 39 (5), 378–387.

Kerry, R., Taylor, A.J., Mitchell, J.M., et al., 2008. Cervical arterial dysfunction and manual therapy: a critical literature review to inform professional practice. Man. Ther. 13 (4), 278–288.

Magarey, M., Coughlan, B., Rebbeck, T., 2000. APA pre-manipulative testing protocol for the cervical spine: researched and renewed, part 2 – revised clinical guidelines. International Federation of Orthopaedic Manipulative Therapists, Perth.

Magarey, M.E., Rebbeck, T., Coughlan, B., et al., 2004. Pre-manipulative testing of the cervical spine review, revision and new clinical guidelines. Man. Ther. 9 (2), 95–108.

Maitland, G.D., Hengeveld, E., Banks, K., et al., 2001. Maitland's vertebral manipulation, sixth ed. Butterworth-Heinemann, Oxford.

Moore, A., Jackson, A., Jordan, J., et al., 2005. Clinical guidelines for the physiotherapy management of whiplash associated disorder. Chartered Society of Physiotherapy, London.

Mulligan, B.R., 1999. Manual therapy 'NAGs', 'SNAGs', 'MWMs' etc., fourth ed. Plane View Services, New Zealand.

Ogince, M., Hall, T., Robinson, K., et al., 2007. The diagnostic validity of the cervical flexion-rotation test in C1/2-related cervicogenic headache. Man. Ther. 12 (3), 256–262.

O'Leary, S., Fall, D., Elliot, M.E., et al., 2009. Muscle dysfunction in cervical spine pain: implications for assessment and management. J. Orthop. Sports Ther. 39 (5), 324–333.

Pettman, E., 1994. Stress tests of the craniovertebral joints. In: Boyling, J.D., Palastanga, N. (Eds.), Grieve's modern manual therapy, second ed. Churchill Livingstone, Edinburgh, p. 529.

Pettman, E., 2004. Craniovertebral dysfunction following a motor vehicle accident. Clinical reasoning for

manual therapy. In: Jones, M.A., Rivett, D.A. (Eds.), Butterworth Heinemann, London, Ch 15, pp. 215–228.

Petty, N.J., 2011. Principles of neuromusculoskeletal treatment and management: a guide for therapists, second ed. Churchill Livingstone, Edinburgh.

Piva, S.R., Erhard, R.E., Childs, J.D., et al., 2006. Inter-tester reliability of passive intervertebral and active movements of the cervical spine. Man. Ther. 11 (4), 321–330.

Pool, J.J., Hoving, J.L., de Vet, H.C., et al., 2004. The interexaminer reproducibility of physical examination of the cervical spine. J. Manipulative Physiol. Ther. 27 (2), 84–90.

Reid, S.A., Rivett, D.A., 2005. Manual therapy treatment of cervicogenic dizziness: a systematic review. Man. Ther. 10 (1), 4–13.

Reid, S.A., Rivett, D.A., Katekar, M.G., et al., 2008. Sustained natural apophyseal glides (SNAGs) are an effective treatment for cervicogenic dizziness. Man. Ther. 13 (4), 357–366.

Sahrmann, S.A., 2002. Diagnosis and treatment of movement impairment syndromes. Mosby, St Louis.

Sjaastad, O., Fredriksen, A., Pfaffenrath, V., 1998. Cervicogenic headache: diagnostic criteria. The CGHA International Study Group. Headache 38 (6), 442–445.

Thiel, H., Rix, G., 2004. Is it time to stop functional pre-manipulative testing of the cervical spine? Man. Ther. 10 (2), 154–1148.

Treleaven, J., 2008. Sensorimotor disturbances in neck disorders affecting postural stability, head and eye movement control. Man. Ther. 13 (1), 2–11.

van Trijffel, E., Anderegg, Q., Bossuyt, P.M.M., et al., 2005. Inter-examiner reliability of passive assessment of intervertebral motion in the cervical and lumbar spine: a systematic review. Man. Ther. 10 (4), 256–269.

van Trijffel, E., Oostendorp, R.A.B., Lindeboom, R., et al., 2009. Perceptions and use of passive intervertebral motion assessment of the spine: a survey among physiotherapists specializing in manual therapy. Man. Ther. 14 (3), 243–251.

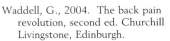

Waddell, G., 2004. The back pain revolution, second ed. Churchill Livingstone, Edinburgh.

Walker, M.J., Boyles, R.E., Young, B.A., et al., 2008. The effectiveness of manual physical therapy and exercise for mechanical neck pain: a randomized clinical trial. Spine 33 (22), 2371–2378.

Walton, J.H., 1989. Essentials of neurology, sixth ed. Churchill Livingstone, Edinburgh.

Watson, D.H., 1994. Cervical headache: an investigation of natural head posture and upper cervical flexor muscle performance. In: Boyling, J.D., Palastanga, N. (Eds.), Grieve's modern manual therapy, second ed. Churchill Livingstone, Edinburgh, p. 349.

Examination of the cervicothoracic region

7

Roger Kerry

CHAPTER CONTENTS

Possible causes of pain and/or limitation of movement

The cervicothoracic region is defined here as the region between C3 and T4, and includes the joints and their surrounding soft tissues.

- Trauma:
  - whiplash
  - fracture of vertebral body, spinous or transverse process
  - ligamentous sprain
  - muscular strain
- Degenerative conditions:
  - spondylosis: degeneration of intervertebral disc
  - arthrosis: degeneration of zygapophyseal joints
  - osteochondrosis (Scheuermann's disease)
  - costochondrosis (Tietze's disease)
- Inflammatory conditions:
  - rheumatoid arthritis
  - ankylosing spondylitis
- Neoplasm, e.g. Pancoast tumour
- Infection, e.g. tuberculosis
- Cervical rib
- Torticollis
- Hypermobility syndrome
- Referral from the upper cervical spine
- Thoracic outlet syndrome
- First/second rib dysfunction
- Cardiovascular disease/trauma: angina, aortic dissection.

Further details of the questions asked during the subjective examination and the tests carried out in the physical examination can be found in Chapters 2 and 3 respectively.

The order of the subjective questioning and the physical tests described below can be altered as appropriate for the patient being examined.

Subjective examination

Body chart

The following information concerning the area and type of current symptoms can be recorded on a body chart (see Chapter 2).

Area of current symptoms

Be exact when mapping out the area of the symptoms. Patients may have symptoms over a large area. As well as symptoms over the cervical spine, they may have symptoms over the head and face, thoracic spine and upper limbs. Ascertain which is the worst symptom and record where the patient feels the symptoms are coming from.

Areas relevant to the region being examined

All other relevant areas are checked for symptoms; it is important to ask about pain or even stiffness, as this may be relevant to the patient's main symptom. Mark unaffected areas with ticks (✓) on the body chart. Check for symptoms in the head, temporomandibular joint, thoracic spine, shoulder, elbow, wrist and hand and ascertain if the patient has ever experienced any disequilibrium or dizziness. This is relevant for symptoms emanating from the cervical spine where cervical arterial dysfunction (CAD), such as vertebrobasilar insufficiency (VBI), may be present, or provoked. If symptoms suggestive of CAD are described by the patient, the clinician proceeds with a thorough assessment for potential neurovascular pathology (Barker et al. 2000; Kerry & Taylor 2006; Kerry et al. 2008).

Quality of pain

Establish the quality of the pain. If the patient suffers from associated headaches, consider carrying out a full upper cervical spine examination (see Chapter 6). Patients who have suffered a hyperextension injury to the cervical spine may complain of a sore throat, difficulty in swallowing and a feeling of something stuck in their throat resulting from an associated injury to the oesophagus (Dahlberg et al. 1997).

Intensity of pain

The intensity of pain can be measured using, for example, a visual analogue scale, as shown in Chapter 2. A pain diary may be useful for patients with chronic neck pain with or without headaches to determine the pain patterns and triggering factors.

Depth of pain

Establish the depth of the pain. Does the patient feel it is on the surface or deep inside?

Abnormal sensation

Check for any altered sensation locally in the cervical spine and in other relevant areas such as the upper limbs or face.

Constant or intermittent symptoms

Ascertain the frequency of the symptoms, whether they are constant or intermittent. If symptoms are constant, check whether there is variation in the intensity of the symptoms, as constant unremitting pain may be indicative of neoplastic disease.

Relationship of symptoms

Determine the relationship between the symptomatic areas – do they come together or separately? For example, the patient could have shoulder pain without cervical pain, or the pains may always be present together.

Behaviour of symptoms

Aggravating factors

For each symptomatic area, discover what movements and/or positions aggravate the patient's symptoms, i.e. what brings them on (or makes them worse)? is the patient able to maintain this position or movement (severity)? what happens to other symptoms when this symptom is produced (or is made worse)? and how long does it take for symptoms to ease once the position or movement is stopped (irritability)? These questions help to confirm the relationship between the symptoms.

The clinician also asks the patient about theoretically known aggravating factors for structures that could be a source of the symptoms. Common aggravating factors for the cervical spine are cervical extension, cervical rotation and sustained flexion. Aggravating factors for other regions, which may need to be queried if they are suspected to be a source of the symptoms, are shown in Table 2.3.

The clinician ascertains how the symptoms affect function, such as: static and active postures, e.g. sitting, standing, lying, washing, ironing, dusting, driving, reading, writing, work, sport and social activities. Note details of the training regimen for any sports activities. The clinician finds out if the patient is left- or right-handed as there may be increased stress on the dominant side.

Detailed information on each of the above activities is useful in order to help determine the structure(s) at fault and identify functional restrictions. This information can be used to determine the aims of treatment and any advice that may be required. The most notable functional restrictions are highlighted with asterisks (*), explored in the physical examination and reassessed at subsequent treatment sessions to evaluate treatment intervention.

Easing factors

For each symptomatic area, the clinician asks what movements and/or positions ease the patient's symptoms, how long it takes to ease them and what happens to other symptom(s) when this symptom is relieved. These questions help to confirm the relationship between the symptoms.

The clinician asks the patient about theoretically known easing factors for structures that could be a source of the symptoms. For example, symptoms from the cervical spine may be eased by supporting the head or neck, whereas symptoms arising from a cervical rib may be eased by shoulder girdle elevation and/or depression. The clinician can then analyse the position or movement that eases the symptoms, to help determine the structure at fault.

Twenty-four-hour behaviour of symptoms

The clinician determines the 24-hour behaviour of symptoms by asking questions about night, morning and evening symptoms.

Night symptoms. The following questions may be asked:

- Do you have any difficulty getting to sleep?
- What position is most comfortable/uncomfortable?
- What is your normal sleeping position?
- What is your present sleeping position?
- Do your symptom(s) wake you at night? If so,
  ○ Which symptom(s)?
  ○ How many times in the past week?
  ○ How many times in a night?
  ○ How long does it take to get back to sleep?
- How many and what type of pillows are used?
- Is your mattress firm or soft?
- Has the mattress been changed recently?

Morning and evening symptoms. The clinician determines the pattern of the symptoms first thing in the morning, through the day and at the end of the day. Stiffness in the morning for the first few minutes might suggest cervical spondylosis; stiffness and pain for a few hours are suggestive of an inflammatory process such as rheumatoid arthritis.

Stage of the condition

In order to determine the stage of the condition, the clinician asks whether the symptoms are getting better, getting worse or remaining unchanged.

Special questions

Additional to the routine special questions identified in Chapter 3, are the following areas.

Cervical arterial dysfunction. The clinician needs to ask about symptoms that may be related to pathologies of the arterial vessels which course through the neck, namely the vertebral arteries and the internal carotid arteries. Pathologies of these vessels can result in neurovascular insult to the brain (stroke). These pathologies are known to produce signs and symptoms similar to neuromusculoskeletal dysfunction of the upper cervical spine (Bogduk 1994; Kerry & Taylor 2006). Care is taken to differentiate vascular sources of pain from neuromusculoskeletal sources. Urgent medical investigation is indicated if frank vascular pathology is identified.

CAD can present initially with pain in the upper cervical spine and head. This is referred to as the pre-ischaemic stage. If the pathology develops, signs and symptoms of brain ischaemia may develop. Table 6.1 shows typical preischaemic and ischaemic presentations for vertebral arteries and internal carotid artery pathologies.

Risk factors associated with CAD are given in Box 7.1. The clinician uses further screening questions to help establish the nature and possible causes and sources of the patient's complaints.

Many patients present with treatable neuromusculoskeletal causes of symptoms, but also with many of the risk factors identified in Box 7.1. This does not necessarily exclude them from manual therapy treatment, and careful clinical reasoning and monitoring of signs and symptoms are required in the management of these patients (Kerry & Taylor 2009).

History of the present condition

For each symptomatic area, the clinician needs to know how long the symptom has been present, whether there was a sudden or slow onset and whether there was a known cause that provoked

Box 7.1

Risk factors for cervical arterial dysfunction (Barker et al. 2000; Kerry & Taylor 2006; Kerry et al. 2008)

- Past history of trauma to cervical spine/cervical vessels
- History of migraine-type headache
- Hypertension
- Hypercholesterolaemia/hyperlipidaemia
- Cardiac disease, vascular disease, previous cerebrovascular accident or transient ischaemic attacks
- Diabetes mellitus
- Blood-clotting disorders/alterations in blood properties (e.g. hyperhomocysteinaemia)
- Anticoagulant therapy
- Oral contraceptives
- Long-term use of steroids
- A history of smoking
- Infection
- Immediately postpartum

the onset of the symptom. If the onset was slow, the clinician should find out if there has been any change in the patient's lifestyle, e.g. a new job or hobby or a change in sporting activity, which may have affected the stresses on the cervical spine and related areas. To confirm the relationship between the symptoms, the clinician asks what happened to other symptoms when each symptom began.

Past medical history

The following information is obtained from the patient and/or the medical notes:

- The details of any relevant medical history, particularly related to the cervical spine, cranium and face.
- The history of any previous attacks: how many episodes? when were they? what was the cause? what was the duration of each episode? and did the patient fully recover between episodes? If there have been no previous attacks, has the patient had any episodes of stiffness in the cervical or thoracic spine? Check for a history of trauma or recurrent minor trauma.
- Ascertain the results of any past treatment for the same or similar problem. Past treatment records may be obtained for further information.

Social and family history

Social and family history relevant to the onset and progression of the patient's problem is recorded. This includes the patient's perspectives, experience and expectations, age, employment, home situation and details of any leisure activities. Factors from this information may indicate direct and/or indirect mechanical influences on the cervical spine. In order to treat the patient appropriately, it is important that the condition is managed within the context of the patient's social and work environment.

The clinician may ask the following types of questions to elucidate psychosocial factors:

- Have you had time off work in the past with your pain?
- What do you understand to be the cause of your pain?
- What are you expecting will help you?
- How is your employer/co-workers/family responding to your pain?
- What are you doing to cope with your pain?
- Do you think you will return to work? When?

Although these questions are described in relation to psychosocial risk factors for poor outcomes for patients with low-back pain (Waddell 2004), they may be relevant to other patients.

Plan of the physical examination

When all this information has been collected, the subjective examination is complete. It is useful at this stage to highlight with asterisks (*), for ease of reference, important findings and particularly one or more functional restrictions. These can then be re-examined at subsequent treatment sessions to evaluate treatment intervention.

In order to plan the physical examination, the following hypotheses need to be developed from the subjective examination:

- The regions and structures that need to be examined as a possible cause of the symptoms, e.g. temporomandibular region, upper cervical spine, cervical spine, thoracic spine, acromioclavicular joint, sternoclavicular joint, glenohumeral joint, elbow, wrist and hand, muscles and nerves. Often, it is not possible to examine fully at the first attendance and so examination of the structures must be prioritised over the subsequent treatment sessions.

- Other factors that need to be examined, e.g. working and everyday postures, vertebral artery, muscle weakness.
- In what way should the physical tests be carried out? Will it be easy or hard to reproduce each symptom? Will it be necessary to use combined movements or repetitive movements to reproduce the patient's symptoms? Are symptoms severe and/or irritable? If symptoms are severe, physical tests may be carried out to just before the onset of symptom production or just to the onset of symptom production; no overpressures should be carried out, as the patient would be unable to tolerate this. If symptoms are irritable, physical tests may be examined to just before symptom production or just to the onset of provocation with fewer physical tests being examined to allow for a rest period between tests.

Are there any precautions and/or contraindications to elements of the physical examination that need to be explored further, such as CAD (e.g. VBI), neurological involvement, recent fracture, trauma, steroid therapy or rheumatoid arthritis? There may also be certain contraindications to further examination and treatment, e.g. symptoms of spinal cord compression.

A physical planning form can be useful for clinicians to help guide them through the clinical reasoning process (see Figure 2.10).

Physical examination

The information from the subjective examination helps the clinician to plan an appropriate physical examination. The severity, irritability and nature of the condition are the major factors that will influence the choice and priority of physical testing procedures. The first and overarching question the clinician might ask is: 'Is this patient's condition suitable for me to manage as a therapist?' For example, a patient presenting with symptoms suggestive of frank cervical radiculopathy may only need neurological integrity testing, prior to an urgent medical referral. The nature of the patient's condition has had a major impact on the physical examination. The second question the clinician might ask is: 'Does this patient have a neuromusculoskeletal dysfunction that I may be able to help?' To answer that, the clinician needs to carry out a full physical examination;

however, this may not be possible if the symptoms are severe and/or irritable. If the patient's symptoms are severe and/or irritable, the clinician aims to explore movements as much as possible, within a symptom-free range. If the patient has constant and severe and/or irritable symptoms, then the clinician aims to find physical tests that ease the symptoms. If the patient's symptoms are non-severe and non-irritable, then the clinician aims to find physical tests that reproduce each of the patient's symptoms.

Each significant physical test that either provokes or eases the patient's symptoms is highlighted in the patient's notes by an asterisk (*) for easy reference. The highlighted tests are often referred to as 'asterisks' or 'markers'.

The order and detail of the physical tests described below need to be appropriate to the patient being examined; some tests will be irrelevant, some tests will be carried out briefly, while it will be necessary to investigate others fully. It is important that readers understand that the techniques shown in this chapter are some of many; the choice depends mainly on the relative size of the clinician and patient, as well as the clinician's preference. For this reason, novice clinicians may initially want to copy what is shown, but then quickly adapt to what is best for them.

Observation

Informal observation

The clinician needs to observe the patient in dynamic and static situations; the quality of movement is noted, as are the postural characteristics and facial expression. Informal observation will have begun from the moment the clinician begins the subjective examination and will continue to the end of the physical examination.

Formal observation

Observation of posture. The clinician examines the patient's spinal posture in sitting and standing, noting the posture of the head and neck, thoracic spine and upper limbs. The clinician passively corrects any asymmetry to determine its relevance to the patient's problem. A specific posture relevant to the cervicothoracic spine is the shoulder crossed syndrome (Janda 1994, 2002), which has been described in Chapter 3.

It should be noted that pure postural dysfunction rarely influences one region of the body in isolation and it may be necessary to observe the patient more fully for a full postural examination.

Observation of muscle form. The clinician observes the muscle bulk and muscle tone of the patient, comparing left and right sides. It must be remembered that handedness and level and frequency of physical activity may well produce differences in muscle bulk between sides. Some muscles are thought to shorten under stress, while other muscles weaken, producing muscle imbalance (see Table 3.2). Patterns of muscle imbalance are thought to be the cause of the shoulder crossed syndrome mentioned above, as well as other abnormal postures outlined in Table 7.1.

Observation of soft tissues. The clinician observes the quality and colour of the patient's skin and any area of swelling or presence of scarring, and takes cues for further examination.

Observation of the patient's attitudes and feelings. The age, gender and ethnicity of patients and their cultural, occupational and social backgrounds will all affect their attitudes and feelings towards themselves, their condition and the clinician. The clinician needs to be aware of and sensitive to these attitudes, and to empathise and communicate

appropriately so as to develop a rapport with the patient and thereby enhance the patient's compliance with the treatment.

Active physiological movements

For active physiological movements, the clinician notes the:

- quality of movement
- range of movement
- behaviour of pain through the range of movement
- resistance through the range of movement and at the end of the range of movement
- provocation of any muscle spasm.

A movement diagram can be used to depict this information. The active movements with overpressure listed below and shown in Figure 7.1 are tested with the patient in sitting. Assessment can be enhanced with the use of combined movements (Figure 7.2). The clinician establishes the patient's symptoms at rest and prior to each movement, and corrects any movement deviation to determine its relevance to the patient's symptoms.

For the cervical spine the active movements and possible modifications are shown in Table 7.2. It is worth mentioning here the work of Robin McKenzie. If all movements are full and symptom-free on overpressure and symptoms are aggravated by certain postures, the condition is categorised as a postural syndrome. McKenzie and May (2006) suggest that maintaining certain postures that place some structures under prolonged stress will eventually produce symptoms. If on repeated movements there is no change in area of symptoms then the condition is categorised as a dysfunction syndrome (McKenzie & May 2006). If, on repeated movements, peripheralisation and centralisation syndrome are manifested then this is characterised as a derangement syndrome; there are seven types of derangement syndromes described (Table 7.3).

Numerous differentiation tests (Maitland et al. 2001) can be performed; the choice depends on the patient's signs and symptoms. For example, when turning the head around to the left reproduces the patient's left-sided infrascapular pain, differentiation between the cervical and thoracic spine may be required. The clinician can increase and decrease the rotation at the cervical and thoracic regions to find out what effect this has on the infrascapular pain. The patient turns the head and trunk around to the left; the clinician maintains the position of

Table 7.1 Possible muscle imbalance causing altered posture (Janda 1994)

Posture	Muscle tightness
Straight neck–shoulder line (gothic-shaped shoulders) and elevation of the shoulder girdle	Levator scapula and upper trapezius
Prominence of pectoralis major, protraction of the shoulder girdles and slight medial rotation of the arms	Pectoral muscles
Prominence of the insertion of sternocleidomastoid and forward head posture	Sternocleidomastoid

Posture	Muscle weakness
Winging of the scapula	Serratus anterior
Flat or hollowed interscapular space	Rhomboids and middle trapezius
Forward head position	Deep neck flexors

the cervical spine and derotates the thoracic spine, noting the pain response. If symptoms remain the same or increase, this might suggest the cervical spine is the source of the symptoms. The position of cervical and thoracic rotation is then resumed and this time the clinician maintains the position of the thoracic spine and derotates the cervical spine, noting the pain response. If the symptoms remain the same or increase, this implicates the thoracic spine, and this may be further tested by increasing the overpressure to the thoracic spine, which would be expected to increase the symptoms.

It may be necessary to examine other regions to determine their relevance to the patient's symptoms; they may be the source of the symptoms, or they may be contributing to the symptoms. The most likely

regions are the temporomandibular, shoulder, elbow, wrist and hand. The joints within these regions can be tested fully (see relevant chapter) or partially with the use of screening tests (see Chapter 3 for further details).

Some functional ability has already been tested by the general observation of the patient during the subjective and physical examinations, e.g. the postures adopted during the subjective examination and the ease or difficulty of undressing prior to the examination. Any further functional testing can be carried out at this point in the examination and may include sitting postures and aggravating movements of the upper limb. Clues for appropriate tests can be obtained from the subjective examination findings, particularly aggravating factors.

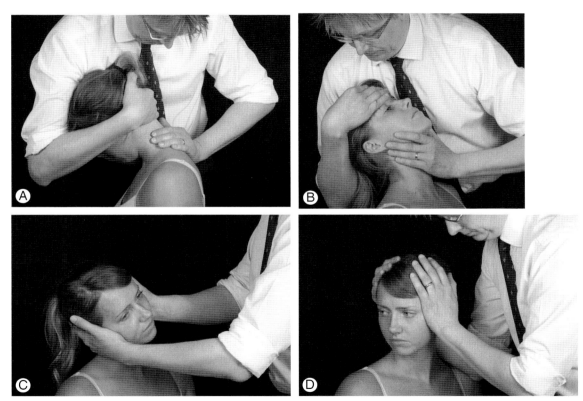

Figure 7.1 • Overpressures to the cervical spine. **A** Flexion. The left hand stabilises the trunk while the right hand moves the head down so that the chin moves towards the chest. **B** Extension. The right hand rests over the head to the forehead while the left hand holds over the mandible. Both hands then apply a force to cause the head and neck to extend backwards. **C** Lateral flexion. Both hands rest over the patient's head around the ears and apply a force to cause the head and neck to tilt laterally. **D** Rotation. The left hand lies over the zygomatic arch while the right hand rests over the occiput. Both hands then apply pressure to cause the head and neck to rotate.

(Continued)

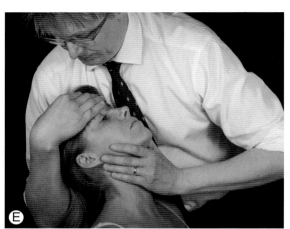

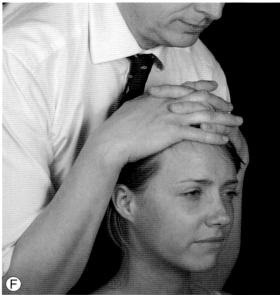

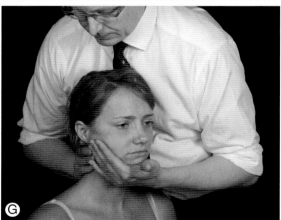

Figure 7.1—cont'd • E Left extension quadrant. This is a combination of extension, left rotation and left lateral flexion. The patient actively extends and, as soon as the movement is complete, the clinician passively moves the head into left rotation and then lateral flexion by applying gentle pressure over the forehead with the right hand and forearm. F Compression. The hands rest over the top of the patient's head and apply a downward force. G Distraction. The left hand holds underneath the mandible while the right hand grasps underneath the occiput. Both hands then apply a force to lift the head upwards.

Capsular pattern. The capsular pattern (Cyriax 1982) for the cervical spine is as follows: lateral flexion and rotation are equally limited, flexion is full but painful and extension is limited.

Palpation

The clinician palpates the cervicothoracic spine and, if appropriate, the patient's upper cervical spine, lower thoracic spine and any other relevant areas. It is useful to record palpation findings on a body chart (see Figure 2.3) and/or palpation chart (see Figure 3.36).

The clinician should note the following:

- the temperature of the area
- increased skin moisture
- the presence of oedema or effusion
- mobility and feel of superficial tissues, e.g. ganglions, nodules

Table 7.2 Active physiological movements with possible modifications

Active movements	Modifications
Cervical spine	Repeated movements
Flexion	Speed altered
Extension	Movements combined (Edwards 1980, 1985, 1999), e.g.
Left lateral flexion	— extension quadrant: extension, ipsilateral rotation and lateral flexion
Right lateral flexion	— flexion then rotation
Left rotation	— extension then rotation
Right rotation	— flexion then lateral flexion then rotation (Figure 7.2)
Compression	— extension then lateral flexion
Distraction	Compression or distraction sustained
Upper cervical extension/protraction (pro)	Injuring movement
Repetitive protraction (rep pro)	Differentiation tests
Repetitive flexion (rep flex)	Function
Upper cervical flexion/retraction (ret)	
Repetitive retraction (rep ret)	
Repetitive retraction and extension (rep ext)	
Left repetitive lateral flexion (rep lat flex)	
Right repetitive lateral flexion (rep lat flex)	
Left repetitive rotation (rep rot)	
Right repetitive rotation (rep rot)	
Retraction and extension lying supine	
Repetitive retraction and extension lying supine	
Static (maximum of 3 min) retraction and extension lying supine or prone	
?Temporomandibular	
?Shoulder	
?Elbow	
?Wrist and hand	

- the presence or elicitation of any muscle spasm
- tenderness of bone, ligaments, muscle, tendon, tendon sheath, trigger points (shown in Figure 3.37) and nerve; nerves in the upper limb can be palpated at the following points:
  ○ the suprascapular nerve along the superior border of the scapula in the suprascapular notch
  ○ the brachial plexus in the posterior triangle of the neck, at the lower third of sternocleidomastoid
  ○ the suprascapular nerve along the superior border of the scapula in the suprascapular notch
  ○ the dorsal scapular nerve medial to the medial border of the scapula
  ○ the median nerve over the anterior elbow joint crease, medial to the biceps tendon; also at the wrist between palmaris longus and flexor carpi radialis
  ○ the radial nerve around the spiral groove of the humerus, between brachioradialis and flexor carpi radialis; also in the forearm and at the wrist in the snuffbox
- increased or decreased prominence of bones
- symptoms (often pain) provoked or reduced on palpation.

Passive intervertebral examination

Passive intervertebral examination of the cervical spine is intended to produce information regarding the quantity (range) and quality (through range and end-feel) of specific motion segments. The validity and reliability of this concept have been challenged in recent years, demonstrating varying results (Pool et al. 2004; Piva et al. 2006). Despite this variance,

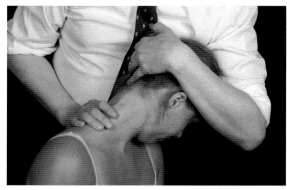

Figure 7.2 • Combined movement to the cervical spine. The right hand supports the trunk while the left hand moves the head into flexion, then lateral flexion then rotation.

there is continuing use of these techniques, with a belief that findings from passive examination contribute towards clinical decision-making and management-planning (van Trijffel et al. 2005, 2009; Haxby Abbott et al. 2009). For the cervical spine, these manual examination techniques have been shown to be particularly important in decision-making when used with a cluster of tests (De Hertogh et al. 2007).

Passive physiological movements

This can take the form of passive physiological intervertebral movements (PPIVMs), which examine the movement at each segmental level. PPIVMs can be a useful adjunct to passive accessory intervertebral movements to identify segmental hypomobility and hypermobility. With the patient supine, the clinician palpates the gap between adjacent spinous processes and articular pillars to feel the range of intervertebral movement during flexion, extension, lateral flexion and rotation. Figure 7.3 demonstrates a rotation PPIVM at the C4/5 segmental level. It may be necessary to examine other regions to determine their relevance to the patient's symptoms; they may be the source of the symptoms, or they may be contributing to the symptoms. The most likely regions are the temporomandibular region, shoulder, elbow, wrist and hand.

Passive accessory intervertebral movements

It is useful to use the palpation chart and movement diagrams (or joint pictures) to record findings. These are explained in detail in Chapter 3.

Table 7.3 Derangement syndromes of the cervical spine (McKenzie & May 2006)

Derangement	Clinical presentation
1	Central or symmetrical pain around C5–C7 Rarely scapula or shoulder pain No deformity Extension limited Rapidly reversible
2	Central or symmetrical pain around C5–C7 With or without scapula, shoulder or upper-arm pain Kyphotic deformity Extension limited Rarely rapidly reversible
3	Unilateral or asymmetrical pain around C3–C7 With or without scapula, shoulder or upper-arm pain No deformity Extension, rotation and lateral flexion may be individually or collectively limited Rapidly reversible
4	Unilateral or asymmetrical pain around C5–C7 With or without scapula, shoulder or upper-arm pain With deformity of torticollis Extension, rotation and lateral flexion limited Rapidly reversible
5	Unilateral or asymmetrical pain around C5–C7 With or without scapula or shoulder pain and with arm symptoms distal to the elbow No deformity Extension and ipsilateral lateral flexion limited Rapidly reversible
6	Unilateral or asymmetrical pain around C5–C7 With arm symptoms distal to the elbow with deformity – cervical kyphosis or torticollis Extension and ipsilateral lateral flexion limited With neurological motor deficit Not rapidly reversible
7	Symmetrical or asymmetrical pain around C4–C6 With or without anterior/anterolateral neck pain Dysphagia common No deformity Flexion limited Rapidly reversible

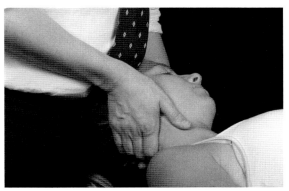

Figure 7.3 • Rotation passive physiological intervertebral movement at the C4–C5 segmental level. The clinician places the index finger, over the right C4–C5 zygapophyseal joint and feels the opening up at this level as the head is passively rotated to the left.

The clinician should note the following:
- quality of movement
- range of movement
- resistance through the range and at the end of the range of movement
- behaviour of pain through the range
- provocation of any muscle spasm.

The cervical and upper thoracic spine (C2–T4) accessory movements are shown in Figure 7.4 and listed in Table 7.4.

Following accessory movements to the cervicothoracic region, the clinician reassesses all the physical asterisks (movements or tests that have been found to reproduce the patient's symptoms) in order to establish the effect of the accessory movements on the patient's signs and symptoms. Accessory movements can then be tested for other regions suspected to be a source of, or contributing to, the patient's symptoms (Figure 7.5). Again, following accessory movements to any one region, the clinician reassesses all the asterisks. Regions likely to be examined are the upper cervical spine, lower thoracic spine, shoulder, elbow, wrist and hand (Table 7.4).

Natural apophyseal glides (NAGs)

These can be applied to the apophyseal joints between C2 and T3. The patient sits and the clinician supports the patient's head and neck and applies a static or oscillatory force to the spinous process or articular pillar in the direction of the facet joint plane of each vertebra (Mulligan 1999). Figure 7.6 demonstrates a unilateral NAG on C6. This is repeated 6–10 times. The patient should feel no pain, but may feel slight discomfort. The technique aims to facilitate the glide of the inferior facet of the vertebra upwards and forwards on the vertebra below. In the example given, if the C6 NAG on the right reduces pain on left lateral flexion, it suggests the symptomatic joint is the right C6–C7 apophyseal joint.

Reversed natural apophyseal glides

The patient sits and the clinician supports the head and neck and applies a force to the articular pillars of a vertebra using the index and thumb of the hand (Figure 7.7). A force is then applied to the pillars in the direction of the facet plane in order to facilitate the glide of the superior facet upwards and forwards on the inferior facet of the vertebra above. If a reversed NAG to C4 reduces the patient's pain on extension, for example, this would suggest that the symptomatic level is C3–C4.

Sustained natural apophyseal glides (SNAGs)

The painful cervical spine movements are examined in sitting. The clinician applies a force to the spinous process and/or transverse process in the direction of the facet joint plane of each cervical vertebra as the patient moves slowly towards the pain. All cervical movements can be tested in this way. Figure 7.8 demonstrates a C5 extension SNAG. The technique aims to facilitate the glide of the inferior facet of the vertebra upwards and forwards on the vertebra below. In the above example, if the C5 SNAG reduces the pain, it suggests that the symptomatic level is C5–C6. For further details on these techniques, see Chapter 3 and Mulligan (1999).

Muscle tests

Muscle tests include those examining muscle strength, control, length and isometric muscle contraction.

Muscle strength

The clinician tests the cervical flexors, extensors, lateral flexors and rotators and any other relevant muscle groups. For details of these general tests readers are directed to Cole et al. (1988), Hislop & Montgomery (1995) or Kendall et al. (1993).

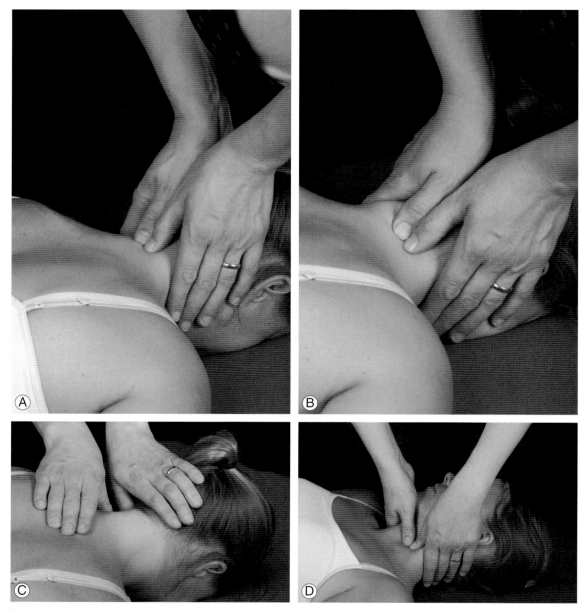

Figure 7.4 • Cervical accessory movements. **A** Central posteroanterior. Thumb pressure is applied to the spinous process. **B** Unilateral posteroanterior. Thumb pressure is applied to the articular pillar. **C** Transverse. Thumb pressure is applied to the lateral aspect of spinous process. **D** Unilateral anteroposterior. In the supine position, thumb pressure is applied to the anterior aspect of the transverse process. Care is needed to avoid pressure over the carotid artery (common or internal, depending on level).

Greater detail may be required to test the strength of muscles, in particular those thought prone to become weak (Janda 1994; Sahrmann 2002); these include serratus anterior, subscapularis, middle and lower fibres of trapezius and the deep neck flexors. Testing the strength of these muscles is described in Chapter 3.

Muscle control

The relative strength of muscles is considered to be more important than the overall strength of a muscle group (Janda 1994, 2002; Sahrmann 2002). Relative strength is assessed indirectly by observing posture, as already mentioned, by the quality of active

Table 7.4 Accessory movements, choice of application and reassessment of the patient's asterisks

Accessory movements		Choice of application	Identify any effect of accessory movements on patient's signs and symptoms
C2–T4		Alter speed of force application	Reassess all asterisks
	Central posteroanterior	Start position, e.g.	
	Unilateral posteroanterior	— in flexion	
	Transverse	— in extension	
	Unilateral anteroposterior (C2–T1 only)	— in lateral flexion	
Ribs 1–4			— in flexion and rotation
Caud	Longitudinal caudad 1st rib	— in flexion and lateral flexion	
	Anteroposterior	— in extension and rotation	
	Posteroanterior	— in extension and lateral flexion	
Med	Medial glide	Direction of the applied force	
		Point of application of applied force	
Upper cervical spine		As above	Reassess all asterisks
Lower thoracic spine		As above	Reassess all asterisks
Shoulder region		As above	Reassess all asterisks
Elbow region		As above	Reassess all asterisks
Wrist and hand		As above	Reassess all asterisks

movement, noting any changes in muscle recruitment patterns and by palpating muscle activity in various positions. Additionally, specific muscle testing can be undertaken in the upper cervical spine.

Deep cervical muscle testing. Deep muscles in the cervical spine are important in the support and control of the head and neck. See Chapter 6 for testing of the deep cervical flexors and extensors.

Scapular control. Muscle imbalance around the scapula has been described by a number of workers (Jull & Janda 1987; Janda 1994, 2002) and can be assessed by observation of upper-limb movements. For example, the clinician can observe the patient performing a slow push-up from the prone position. Any excessive or abnormal movement of the scapula is noted; muscle weakness may cause the scapula to rotate and glide laterally and/or move superiorly. Serratus anterior weakness, for example, will cause the scapula to wing (the medial border moves away from the thorax). Another movement that can be useful to analyse is shoulder abduction performed slowly, with the patient in sitting and the elbow flexed. Once again, the clinician observes the quality of movement of the shoulder joint and scapula and notes any abnormal or excessive movement.

Muscle length

The clinician tests the length of muscles, in particular those thought prone to shorten (Janda 1994); that is, levator scapulae, upper trapezius, sternocleidomastoid, pectoralis major and minor, scalenes and the deep occipital muscles. Testing the length of these muscles is described in Chapter 3.

Isometric muscle testing

Test neck flexors, extensors, lateral flexors and rotators in resting position and, if indicated, in different parts of the physiological range. In addition the clinician observes the quality of the muscle contraction to hold this position (this can be done with the patient's eyes shut). The patient may, for example, be unable to prevent the joint from moving or may hold with excessive muscle activity; either of these circumstances would suggest a neuromuscular dysfunction.

Neurological tests

Neurological examination includes neurological integrity testing, neurodynamic tests and some other nerve tests.

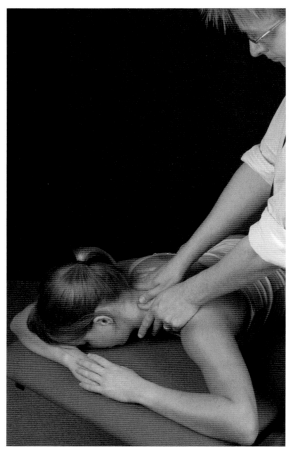

Figure 7.5 • Palpation of accessory movements using a combined movement. Thumb pressure over the left articular pillar of C5 is carried out with the cervical spine positioned in right lateral flexion.

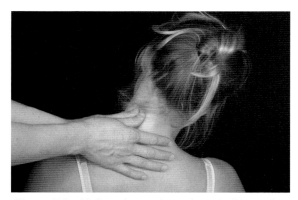

Figure 7.6 • Unilateral natural apophyseal glide on C6. Thumb pressure is applied to the left articular pillar of C6 (in the line of the facet joint plane) as the patient laterally flexes to the right.

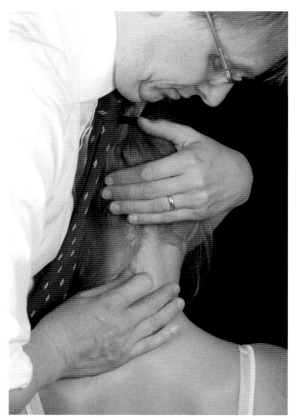

Figure 7.7 • Reversed flexion natural apophyseal glide to C4. The left hand supports the head and neck. The index and thumb of the right hand apply an anterior force to the articular pillars of C4 in the direction of the facet plane.

Integrity of nervous system

As a general guide, a neurological examination is indicated if symptoms are felt below the acromion.

Dermatomes/peripheral nerves. Light touch and pain sensation of the upper limb are tested using cotton wool and pinprick respectively, as described in Chapter 3. Knowledge of the cutaneous distribution of nerve roots (dermatomes) and peripheral nerves enables the clinician to distinguish the sensory loss due to a root lesion from that due to a peripheral nerve lesion. The cutaneous nerve distribution and dermatome areas are shown in Chapter 3.

Myotomes/peripheral nerves. The following myotomes are tested and are shown in Chapter 3:

- C4: shoulder girdle elevation
- C5: shoulder abduction
- C6: elbow flexion
- C7: elbow extension

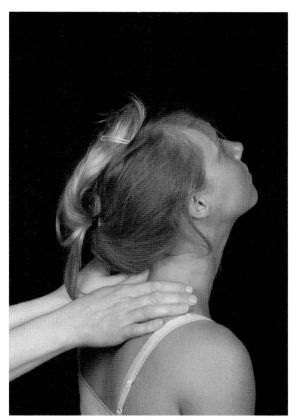

Figure 7.8 • Extension sustained natural apophyseal glide to C5. Thumb pressure is applied to the spinous process of C5, in the direction of the facet plane, as the patient slowly extends.

- C8: thumb extension
- T1: finger adduction.

A working knowledge of the muscular distribution of nerve roots (myotomes) and peripheral nerves enables the clinician to distinguish the motor loss due to a root lesion from that due to a peripheral nerve lesion. The peripheral nerve distributions are shown in Chapter 3.

Reflex testing. The following deep tendon reflexes are tested (see also Chapter 3):

- C5–C6: biceps
- C7: triceps and brachioradialis.

Neurodynamic tests

The following neurodynamic tests may be carried out in order to ascertain the degree to which neural tissue is responsible for the production of the patient's symptom(s):

- passive neck flexion
- upper-limb neurodynamic tests
- straight-leg raise
- slump.

These tests are described in detail in Chapter 3.

Other nerve tests

Plantar response to test for an upper motor neurone lesion (Walton 1989). Pressure applied from the heel along the lateral border of the plantar aspect of the foot produces flexion of the toes in the normal. Extension of the big toe with downward fanning of the other toes occurs with an upper motor neurone lesion.

Tinel's sign. The clinician taps the skin overlying the brachial plexus. Reproduction of distal pain/paraesthesia denotes a positive test indicating regeneration of an injured sensory nerve (Walton 1989).

Miscellaneous tests

Cervical arterial dysfunction testing. If vascular dysfunction is suspected following the subjective examination (see above), further information regarding the integrity of the cervical arterial system can be gained from the following examination procedures. Further reading (Kerry & Taylor 2006) is recommended to support understanding of these procedures.

Blood pressure. In the event of acute arterial dysfunction, it is likely that there will be a systematic cardiovascular response manifesting in dramatic change in blood pressure (usually increasing). Blood pressure is taken using appropriate, validated procedures and equipment, in either sitting or lying.

Functional positional testing. Passive repositioning of the head has been classically considered a test for VBI. A minimum requirement of a passive 10-second hold into cervical rotation has been proposed (Magarey et al. 2004). A positive test is considered if reproduction of symptoms suggestive of hindbrain ischaemia is found. The diagnostic utility of this procedure is, however, not certain (Thiel & Rix 2004; Kerry 2006) and, like any of the individual parts of CAD testing, reliance on one result alone is not indicative of pathology.

Pulse palpation. The verterbral artery pulses are difficult to palpate owing to their size and depth. The internal carotid artery is easily accessible at the mid-cervical level, medial to the sternocleido-mastoid muscle. Gross pathology, such as aneurysm formation, is characteristic in the nature of their pulse, that is, a pulsatile, expandable mass. Pain and exaggerated pulse on palpation of the temporal artery may support a hypothesis of temporal arteritis.

Cranial nerve examination. Cranial nerve dysfunction can be a component part of arterial compromise in the neck and head, and this may be an indication of vascular dysfunction. Careful screening for gross asymmetries and variations from the norm in cranial nerve function is indicated if CAD is suspected (Kerry & Taylor 2008).

Proprioception tests. Hindbrain ischaemia associated with VBI can result in gross loss of proprioceptive function. Simple proprioception testing such as tandem gait, heel-to-knee, Rhomberg's test and Hautant's test is undertaken to assess proprioception dysfunction.

Test for thoracic outlet syndrome. There are several tests for this syndrome, which are described in Chapter 9.

Completion of the examination

Having carried out the above tests, the examination of the cervical spine is now complete. The subjective and physical examinations produce a large amount of information, which needs to be recorded accurately and quickly. It is important, however, that the clinician does not examine in a rigid manner, simply following the suggested sequence outlined in the chart. Each patient presents differently and this needs to be reflected in the examination process. It is vital at this stage to highlight with an asterisk (*) important findings from the examination. These findings must be reassessed at, and within, subsequent treatment sessions to evaluate the effects of treatment on the patient's condition.

The physical testing procedures which specifically indicate joint, nerve or muscle tissues, as a source of the patient's symptoms, are summarised in Table 3.10. The strongest evidence that a joint is the source of the patient's symptoms is that active and passive physiological movements, passive accessory movements and joint palpation all reproduce the patient's symptoms, and that, following a treatment dose, reassessment identifies an improvement in the patient's signs and symptoms. Weaker evidence includes an alteration in range, resistance or quality of physiological and/or accessory movements and tenderness over the joint, with no alteration in signs and symptoms after treatment. One or more of these findings may indicate a dysfunction of a joint which may or may not be contributing to the patient's condition.

The strongest evidence that a muscle is the source of a patient's symptoms is if active movements, an isometric contraction, passive lengthening and palpation of a muscle all reproduce the patient's symptoms, and that, following a treatment dose, reassessment identifies an improvement in the patient's signs and symptoms. Further evidence of muscle dysfunction may be suggested by reduced strength or poor quality during the active physiological movement and the isometric contraction, reduced range and/or increased/decreased resistance, during the passive lengthening of the muscle, and tenderness on palpation, with no alteration in signs and symptoms after treatment. One or more of these findings may indicate a dysfunction of a muscle which may or may not be contributing to the patient's condition.

The strongest evidence that a nerve is the source of the patient's symptoms is when active and/or passive physiological movements reproduce the patient's symptoms, which are then increased or decreased with an additional sensitising movement, at a distance from the patient's symptoms. In addition, there is reproduction of the patient's symptoms on palpation of the nerve and neurodynamic testing, sufficient to be considered a treatment dose, results in an improvement in the above signs and symptoms. Further evidence of nerve dysfunction may be suggested by reduced range (compared with the asymptomatic side) and/or increased resistance to the various arm movements, and tenderness on nerve palpation.

On completion of the physical examination the clinician will:

- explain the findings of the physical examination and how these findings relate to the subjective assessment. An attempt should be made to clear up any misconceptions patients may have regarding their illness or injury
- collaborate with the patient and via problem-solving together devise a treatment plan and discuss the prognosis
- warn the patient of possible exacerbation up to 24–48 hours following the examination
- request the patient to report details on the behaviour of the symptoms following examination at the next attendance

- explain the findings of the physical examination and how these findings relate to the subjective assessment. An attempt should be made to clear up any misconceptions patients may have regarding their illness or injury
- evaluate the findings, formulate a clinical diagnosis and write up a problem list
- determine the objectives of treatment
- devise an initial treatment plan.

In this way, the clinician develops the following hypotheses categories (adapted from Jones & Rivett 2004):

- function: abilities and restrictions
- patient's perspective on his/her experience
- source of symptoms. This includes the structure or tissue that is thought to be producing the patient's symptoms, the nature of the structure or

tissues in relation to the healing process and the pain mechanisms involved

- contributing factors to the development and maintenance of the problem. There may be environmental, psychosocial, behavioural, physical or heredity factors
- precautions/contraindications to treatment and management. This includes the severity and irritability of the patient's symptoms and the nature of the patient's condition
- management strategy and treatment plan
- prognosis – this can be affected by factors such as the stage and extent of the injury as well as the patient's expectation, personality and lifestyle.

For guidance on treatment and management principles, the reader is directed to the companion textbook (Petty 2011).

References

Barker, S., Kesson, M., Ashmore, J., et al., 2000. Guidance for pre-manipulative testing of the cervical spine. Man. Ther. 5 (1), 37–40.

Bogduk, N., 1994. Cervical causes of headache and dizziness. In: Boyling, J.D., Palastanga, N. (Eds.), Grieve's modern manual therapy, second ed. Churchill Livingstone, Edinburgh, p. 317.

Cole, J.H., Furness, A.L., Twomey, L.T., 1988. Muscles in action, an approach to manual muscle testing. Churchill Livingstone, Edinburgh.

Cyriax, J., 1982. Textbook of orthopaedic medicine – diagnosis of soft tissue lesions, eighth ed. Baillière Tindall, London.

Dahlberg, C., Lanig, I.S., Kenna, M., et al., 1997. Diagnosis and treatment of esophageal perforations in cervical spinal cord injury. Top. Spinal Cord Inj. Rehabil. 2 (3), 41–48.

De Hertogh, W., Vaes, P., Duquet, W., 2007. The validity of the manual examination in the assessment of patients with neck pain. Spine 7 (5), 628–629.

Edwards, B.C., 1980. Combined movements in the cervical spine (C2–7): their value in examination and technique choice. Aust. J. Physiother. 26 (5), 165–169.

Edwards, B.C., 1985. Combined movements in the cervical spine (their use in establishing movement patterns). In: Glasgow, E.F., Twomey, L.T., Scull, E.R. et al., (Eds.) Aspects of manipulative therapy. Churchill Livingstone, Melbourne, ch 19, p. 128.

Edwards, B.C., 1999. Manual of combined movements: their use in the examination and treatment of mechanical vertebral column disorders, second ed. Butterworth-Heinemann, Oxford.

Haxby Abbott, J., Flynn, T.W., Fritz, J.M., et al., 2009. Manual physical assessment of spinal segmental motion: intent and validity. Man. Ther. 14 (1), 36–44.

Hislop, H., Montgomery, J., 1995. Daniels and Worthingham's muscle testing, techniques of manual examination, seventh ed. W B Saunders, Philadelphia.

Janda, V., 1994. Muscles and motor control in cervicogenic disorders: assessment and management. In: Grant, R. (Ed.), Physical therapy of the cervical and thoracic spine, second ed. Churchill Livingstone, New York, p. 195.

Janda, V., 2002. Muscles and motor control in cervicogenic disorders. In: Grant, R. (Ed.), Physical therapy of the cervical and thoracic spine,

third ed. Churchill Livingstone, New York, p. 182.

Jones, M.A., Rivett, D.A., 2004. Clinical reasoning for manual therapists. Butterworth-Heinemann, Edinburgh.

Jull, G.A., Janda, V., 1987. Muscles and motor control in low back pain: assessment and management. In: Twomey, L.T., Taylor, J.R. (Eds.), Physical therapy of the low back. Churchill Livingstone, New York, p. 253.

Kendall, F.P., McCreary, E.K., Provance, P.G., 1993. Muscles testing and function, fourth ed. Williams & Wilkins, Baltimore, MD.

Kerry, R., 2006. Vertebral artery testing: how certain are you that your pre-cervical manipulation and mobilisation tests are safe and specific? HES 2nd International Evidence Based Practice Conference, London.

Kerry, R., Taylor, A.J., 2006. Masterclass: Cervical arterial dysfunction assessment and manual therapy. Man. Ther. 11 (3), 243–253.

Kerry, R., Taylor, A.J., 2008. Arterial pathology and cervicocranial pain – differential diagnosis for manual therapists and medical practitioners. Int. Musculoskelet. Med. 30 (2), 70–77.

Kerry, R., Taylor, A.J., 2009. Cervical arterial dysfunction: knowledge and reasoning for manual physical therapists. J. Orthop. Sports Phys. Ther. 39 (5), 378–387.

Kerry, R., Taylor, A.J., Mitchell, J.M., et al., 2008. Cervical arterial dysfunction and manual therapy: a critical literature review to inform professional practice. Man. Ther. 13 (4), 278–288.

Magarey, M.E., Rebbeck, T., Coughlan, B., et al., 2004. Pre-manipulative testing of the cervical spine review, revision and new clinical guidelines. Man. Ther. 9 (2), 95–108.

McKenzie, R.A., May, S.J., 2006. The Cervical and Thoracic Spine: Mechanical Diagnosis and Therapy. Spinal Publications New Zealand Ltd. Waikanae, New Zealand.

Maitland, G.D., Hengeveld, E., Banks, K., et al., 2001. Maitland's vertebral manipulation, sixth ed. Butterworth-Heinemann, Oxford.

Mulligan, B.R., 1999. Manual therapy 'NAGs', 'SNAGs', 'MWMs' etc.,

fourth ed. Plane View Services, New Zealand.

Petty, N.J., 2011. Principles of neuromusculoskeletal treatment and management: a guide for therapists, second ed. Churchill Livingstone, Edinburgh.

Piva, S.R., Erhard, R.E., Childs, J.D., et al., 2006. Inter-tester reliability of passive intervertebral and active movements of the cervical spine. Man. Ther. 11 (4), 321–330.

Pool, J.J., Hoving, J.L., de Vet, H.C., et al., 2004. The interexaminer reproducibility of physical examination of the cervical spine. J. Manipulative Physiol. Ther. 27 (2), 84–90.

Sahrmann, S.A., 2002. Diagnosis and treatment of movement impairment syndromes. Mosby, St Louis.

Thiel, H., Rix, G., 2005. Is it time to stop functional pre-manipulative testing of the cervical spine? Man. Ther. 10 (2), 154–158.

van Trijffel, E., Anderegg, Q., Bossuyt, P.M.M., Lucas, C., 2005. Inter-examiner reliability of passive assessment of intervertebral motion in the cervical and lumbar spine: a systematic review. Man. Ther. 10 (4), 256–269.

van Trijffel, E., Oostendorp, R.A.B., Lindeboom, R., et al., 2009. Perceptions and use of passive intervertebral motion assessment of the spine: a survey among physiotherapists specializing in manual therapy. Man. Ther. 14 (3), 243–251.

Waddell, G., 2004. The back pain revolution, second ed. Churchill Livingstone, Edinburgh.

Walton, J.H., 1989. Essentials of neurology, sixth ed. Churchill Livingstone, Edinburgh.

Examination of the thoracic region

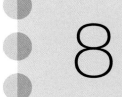

Linda Exelby

CHAPTER CONTENTS

Possible causes of pain and/or limitation of movement

- Trauma:
  - ○ fracture of spinous process, transverse process, vertebral arch, vertebral body or ribs; fracture dislocation
  - ○ ligamentous sprain
  - ○ muscular strain

- Degenerative conditions:
  - ○ spondylosis: degeneration of the intervertebral disc
  - ○ arthrosis: degeneration of the zygapophyseal, costovertebral or costotransverse joints
  - ○ Scheuermann's disease
- Inflammatory:
  - ○ ankylosing spondylitis
  - ○ costochondritis
  - ○ Tietze's syndrome
- Metabolic:
  - ○ osteoporosis
  - ○ Paget's disease
  - ○ osteomalacia
- Infections:
  - ○ tuberculosis of the spine
- Tumours, benign and malignant
- Syndromes:
  - ○ T4 syndrome
  - ○ thoracic outlet syndrome
- Neural:
  - ○ spinal cord compression
  - ○ intercostal neuralgia
- Postural thoracic pain
- Referral of symptoms from the cervical or lumbar spine or from the viscera (such as the gallbladder, heart, spleen, liver, kidneys, lung and pleura).

The thoracic spine and ribcage are an important source of local and referred pain. The curvature and mobility of the thoracic spine plays an important role in determining overall posture in the rest of the spine and shoulder girdle (Edmondston & Singer 1997).

An intact ribcage with its complex ligamentous attachments to the thoracic spine has been shown to play a significant role in thoracic spine stability (Oda et al. 2002). The ribcage also serves as a site for the attachment of a large number of cervical, lumbar and shoulder girdle muscles.

The thoracic spine examination is appropriate for patients with symptoms in the spine or thorax between T3 and T10. This region includes the intervertebral joints between T3 and T10 as well as the costovertebral, costotransverse, sternocostal, costochondral and interchondral joints with their surrounding soft tissues.

To test the upper thoracic spine above T4, it is more appropriate to carry out an adapted cervical spine examination. Similarly, to test the lower thoracic spine below T9, it is more appropriate to carry out an adapted lumbar spine examination.

Further details of the questions asked during the subjective examination and the tests carried out in the physical examination can be found in Chapters 2 and 3 respectively.

The order of the subjective questioning and the physical tests described below can be altered as appropriate for the patient being examined.

Subjective examination

Body chart

Perception of the patient's attitudes and feelings

The age, gender and ethnicity of patients and their cultural, occupational and social backgrounds will all affect their attitudes and feelings towards themselves, their condition and the clinician. The clinician needs to be aware of, and sensitive to, these attitudes to empathise and communicate appropriately so as to develop a rapport with the patient and thereby enhance the patient's compliance with the treatment. The structure of the session should be explained to the patient and consent gained.

The following information concerning the type and area of current symptoms can be recorded on a body chart (see Figure 2.4).

Area of current symptoms

Be exact when mapping out the area of the symptoms. The area of symptoms may follow the course of a rib or it may run horizontally across the chest; symptoms may be felt posteriorly over the thoracic spine and anteriorly over the sternum. The clinician needs to be aware that cervical spine structures (between C3 and C7) can refer pain to the scapula and upper arm (Cloward 1959; Bogduk & Marsland 1988). The upper thoracic spine can refer symptoms to the upper limbs, and the lower thoracic spine to the lower limbs. Ascertain which is the worst symptom and record where the patient feels the symptoms are coming from.

Areas relevant to the region being examined

All other relevant areas are checked for symptoms; it is important to ask about pain or even stiffness, as this may be relevant to the patient's main symptom. Mark unaffected areas with ticks (✓) on the body chart. Check for symptoms in the cervical spine and upper limbs if it is an upper thoracic problem, or in the lumbar spine and lower limbs if it is a lower thoracic problem. If the patient has symptoms that may emanate from these areas it may be appropriate to assess them more fully. See relevant chapters in this book.

Quality of pain

Establish the quality of the pain.

Intensity of pain

The intensity of pain can be measured using, for example, a visual analogue scale, as shown in Chapter 2. A pain diary may be useful for patients with chronic thoracic pain to determine the pain patterns and triggering factors over a period of time.

Depth of pain

Establish the depth of the pain. Does the patient feel it is on the surface or deep inside?

Abnormal sensation

Check for any altered sensation over the thoracic spine, ribcage and other relevant areas.

Constant or intermittent symptoms

Ascertain the frequency of the symptoms, whether they are constant or intermittent. If symptoms are constant, check whether there is variation in the intensity of the symptoms, as constant unremitting pain may be indicative of serious pathology.

Relationship of symptoms

Determine the relationship between the symptomatic areas – do they come together or separately? For example, the patient could have shoulder pain without thoracic spine pain, or the pains may always be present together. If one symptomatic area becomes more severe, what happens to the other symptomatic areas?

Behaviour of symptoms

Aggravating factors

For each symptomatic area, discover what movements and/or positions aggravate the patient's symptoms, i.e. what brings them on (or makes them worse)? is the patient able to maintain this position or movement (severity)? what happens to other symptoms when this symptom is produced (or is made worse)? and how long does it take for symptoms to ease once the position or movement is stopped (irritability)? These questions help to confirm the relationship between the symptoms.

The clinician also asks the patient about theoretically known aggravating factors for structures that could be a source of the symptoms. Common aggravating factors for the thoracic spine are rotation of the thorax and deep breathing. Aggravating factors for other regions, which may need to be queried if they are suspected to be a source of the symptoms, are shown in Table 2.3.

The clinician ascertains how the symptoms affect function, such as: static and active postures, e.g. sitting, standing, lying, performing domestic chores, driving (and reversing the car, which requires trunk rotation), work, sport and social activities. Note details of ergonomics at work and the training regimen for any sports activities. The clinician finds out if the patient is left- or right-handed as there may be increased stress on the dominant side. Check whether the patient is avoiding activities that exacerbate the symptoms as this may influence the severity and irritability rating.

Detailed information on each of the above activities is useful in order to help determine the structure(s) at fault and identify functional restrictions. This information can be used to determine the aims of treatment and any advice that may be required. The most notable functional restrictions are highlighted with asterisks (*), explored in the physical examination, and reassessed at subsequent treatment sessions to evaluate treatment intervention.

Easing factors

For each symptomatic area, the clinician asks what movements and/or positions ease the patient's symptoms, how long it takes to ease them and what happens to other symptom(s) when this symptom is relieved. These questions help to confirm the relationship between the symptoms.

The clinician asks the patient about theoretically known easing factors for structures that could be a source of the symptoms. The clinician can then analyse the position or movement that eases the symptoms to help determine the structure at fault.

Twenty-four-hour behaviour of symptoms

The clinician determines the 24-hour behaviour of each symptomatic area by asking questions about night, morning and evening symptoms.

Night symptoms. The following questions may be asked:

- Do you have any difficulty getting to sleep?
- What position is most comfortable/uncomfortable?
- What is your normal sleeping position?
- What is your present sleeping position?
- Do your symptoms wake you at night? If so,
  - ○ Which symptom(s)?
  - ○ How many times in the past week?
  - ○ How many times in a night?
  - ○ How long does it take to get back to sleep?
- How many and what type of pillows are used?
- Is your mattress firm or soft and has it been changed recently?

Morning and evening symptoms. The clinician determines the pattern of the symptoms in the morning (on waking and on rising), through the day and at the end of the day. The status of symptoms on first waking establishes whether the patient is better with rest. Pain/stiffness on waking would suggest an inflammatory component whereas no pain on waking but pain on rising would suggest a more mechanical origin. Stiffness in the morning for the first few minutes might suggest spondylosis; stiffness and pain for a few hours are suggestive of an inflammatory process such as ankylosing spondylitis.

Stage of the condition

In order to determine the stage of the condition, the clinician asks whether the symptoms are getting better, getting worse or remaining unchanged.

Special questions

A detailed medical history is important as certain precautions or contraindications to the physical examination and/or treatment can be identified (Table 2.4). As mentioned in Chapter 2, the clinician must differentiate between conditions that are suitable for conservative management and systemic, neoplastic, tuberculosis, osteomyelitis, human immunodeficiency virus (HIV) and other non-neuromusculoskeletal conditions, which require referral to a medical practitioner. The reader is referred to Appendix 2.3 for details of serious pathological processes that can mimic neuromusculoskeletal conditions (Grieve 1994).

The following information is routinely obtained from patients.

General health. The clinician ascertains the state of the patient's general health to find out if the patient suffers from any osteoporosis, respiratory disorders, cardiovascular disease, breathlessness, chest pain, malaise, fatigue, fever, abdominal cramps, nausea or vomiting, stress, anxiety or depression. Questions relating to change in visceral function may be appropriate owing to the referral pain patterns of these structures.

Weight loss. Has the patient noticed any recent unexplained weight loss?

Rheumatoid arthritis. Has the patient (or a member of his/her family) been diagnosed as having rheumatoid arthritis?

Drug therapy. Identify drugs being taken for any medical conditions patients may have. Do they control this condition? For example, if they have high blood pressure, is it controlled with the medication? If medication is taken specifically for the thoracic spine condition, is the patient taking the medication regularly? What effect does it have? How long before this appointment was the medication taken? Has the patient been prescribed long-term (6 months or more) medication/steroids? Has the patient been taking anticoagulants recently?

Radiograph and medical imaging. Has the patient been radiographed or had any other medical tests recently? Routine spinal radiographs are no longer considered necessary prior to conservative treatment as they only identify the normal age-related degenerative changes, which do not necessarily correlate with the patient's symptoms (Clinical Standards Advisory Report 1994). The medical tests may include blood tests, magnetic resonance imaging, myelography, discography or a bone scan.

Neurological symptoms. Has the patient experienced symptoms of spinal cord compression, which are bilateral tingling in hands or feet and/or disturbance of gait? Sympathetic function is difficult to measure but questions about changes in swelling, sweating, skin changes (pitting oedema, shiny and inelastic skin) and circulation should be included.

Vertebrobasilar insufficiency. For symptoms emanating from the cervical spine, the clinician should ask about symptoms that may be caused by vertebrobasilar insufficiency.

History of the present condition

For each symptomatic area, the clinician needs to know how long the symptom has been present, whether there was a sudden or slow onset and whether there was a known cause that provoked the onset of the symptom. The mechanism of injury gives some important clues as to the injured structure. If the onset was slow, the clinician finds out if there has been any change in the patient's lifestyle, e.g. a new job or hobby or a change in sporting activity, which may have affected the stresses on the thoracic spine and related areas. To confirm the relationship between symptoms, the clinician asks what happened to other symptoms when each symptom began. Clarify the progression and impact the symptoms have had on the patient's normal function from the initial onset of this episode to the present time. Find out full details about any treatment interventions and their effect.

Past medical history

The following information is obtained from the patient and/or the medical notes:

- The history of any previous attacks: symptom distribution, behaviour and cause of initial symptoms; since then how many episodes? when were they? what was the cause? what was the duration of each episode? and did the patient fully recover between episodes? If there have been no previous attacks, has the patient had any episodes of stiffness in the cervical, thoracic or lumbar spine or any other relevant region? Check for a history of trauma or recurrent minor trauma.
- Ascertain the results of any past treatment for the same or similar problem. Past treatment records may be obtained for further information.

Social and family history

Social and family history relevant to the onset and progression of the patient's problem is recorded. This includes patients' perspectives, experience and expectations, their age, employment, home situation and details of any leisure activities. Factors from this information may indicate direct and/or indirect mechanical influences on the thoracic spine. In order to treat the patient appropriately, it is important that the condition is managed within the context of the patient's social and work environment.

The clinician may ask the following types of question to elucidate psychosocial factors:

- Have you had time off work in the past with your pain?
- What do you understand to be the cause of your pain?
- What are you expecting will help you?
- How is your employer/co-workers/family responding to your pain?
- What are you doing to cope with your pain?
- Do you think you will return to work? When?

Although these questions are described in relation to psychosocial risk factors for poor outcomes for patients with low-back pain (Waddell 2004), they may be relevant to other patients. Validated, reliable questionnaires may be used to identify various psychosocial risk factors and may be useful in patients with more persistent pain. These help to guide assessment, management and prognosis.

Plan of the physical examination

When all this information has been collected, the subjective examination is complete. It is useful at this stage to highlight with asterisks (*), for ease of reference, important findings and particularly one or more functional restrictions. These can then be re-examined at subsequent treatment sessions to evaluate treatment intervention.

In order to plan the physical examination, the following hypotheses should be developed from the subjective examination:

- The regions and structures that need to be examined as a possible cause of the symptoms, e.g. thoracic spine, cervical spine, lumbar spine, upper-limb joints, lower-limb joints, muscles and nerves. Often, it is not possible to examine fully at the first attendance and so examination of the structures must be prioritised over subsequent treatment sessions.
- Other factors that need to be examined, e.g. working and everyday postures, breathing patterns and muscle weakness.
- In what way should the physical tests be carried out? Will it be easy or hard to reproduce each symptom? Will it be necessary to use combined movements or repetitive movements to reproduce the patient's symptoms? Are symptoms severe and/or irritable? If symptoms are severe, physical tests may be carried out to just before the onset of symptom production or just to the onset of symptom production; no overpressures will be carried out, as the patient would be unable to tolerate this. If symptoms are irritable, physical tests may be examined to just before symptom production or just to the onset of provocation with fewer physical tests being examined.

Are there any precautions and/or contraindications to elements of the physical examination that need to be explored further, such as vertebrobasilar insufficiency, neurological involvement, recent fracture, trauma, osteoporosis, steroid therapy and rheumatoid arthritis? There may also be certain contraindications to further examination and treatment, e.g. symptoms of cord compression.

A physical planning form can be useful for clinicians to help guide them through the clinical reasoning process (see Figure 2.10).

Physical examination

The information from the subjective examination helps the clinician to plan an appropriate physical examination. The severity, irritability, nature and pain mechanisms of the condition are the major factors that will influence the choice and priority of physical testing procedures. The first and overarching question the clinician might ask is: 'Is this patient's condition suitable for me to manage as a therapist?' For example, a patient presenting with cauda equina compression symptoms may only need neurological integrity testing, prior to an urgent medical referral. The nature of the patient's condition has a major impact on the physical examination. The second question the clinician might ask is: 'Does this patient have a neuromusculoskeletal dysfunction that I may be able to help?' To answer that, the clinician needs to carry out a full physical examination;

however, this may not be possible if the symptoms are severe and/or irritable. If the patient's symptoms are severe and/or irritable, the clinician aims to explore movements as much as possible, within a symptom-free range. If the patient has constant and severe and/or irritable symptoms, then the clinician aims to find physical tests that ease the symptoms. If the patient's symptoms are non-severe and non-irritable, then the clinician aims to find physical tests that reproduce each of the patient's symptoms.

Each significant physical test that either provokes or eases the patient's symptoms is highlighted in the patient's notes by an asterisk (*) for easy reference.

The order and detail of the physical tests described below should be appropriate to the patient being examined; some tests will be irrelevant, some tests will be carried out briefly, while it will be necessary to investigate others fully. It is important that readers understand that the techniques shown in this chapter are only some of many.

Observation

Informal observation

The clinician should observe the patient in dynamic and static situations; the quality of movement is noted, as are the postural characteristics and facial expression. Informal observation will have begun from the moment the clinician begins the subjective examination and will continue to the end of the physical examination.

Formal observation

Observation of posture. The clinician examines the spinal posture of the patient in sitting and standing, noting the level of the pelvis, scoliosis, kyphosis or lordosis and the posture of the upper and lower limbs. Common postural types are described in more detail in Chapter 3.

The clinician passively corrects any asymmetry to determine its relevance to the patient's problem. In addition, the clinician observes for any chest deformity, such as pigeon chest, where the sternum lies forward and downwards; funnel chest, where the sternum lies posteriorly (which may be associated with an increased thoracic kyphosis); or barrel chest, where the sternum lies forward and upwards (associated with emphysema) (Magee 1997). The clinician notes the movement of the ribcage during quiet respiration.

Observation of muscle form. The clinician observes the muscle bulk and muscle tone of the patient, comparing left and right sides. It must be remembered that handedness and level and frequency of physical activity may well produce differences in muscle bulk between sides. Some muscles are thought to shorten under stress, while other muscles weaken, producing movement or postural impairments (see Table 3.2).

Observation of soft tissues. The clinician observes the quality and colour of the patient's skin and any area of swelling or presence of scarring, and takes cues for further examination.

Observation of gait. The clinician observes the gait pattern if it is applicable to the patient's presenting symptoms.

Active physiological movements

For active physiological movements, the clinician notes the:

- quality of the movement
- range of the movement
- behaviour of the pain through the range of movement
- resistance through the range of movement and at the end of the range of movement
- provocation of any muscle spasm.

A movement diagram can be used to depict this information. The active movements with overpressure listed below (Figure 8.1) are tested with the patient in sitting. The clinician establishes the patient's symptoms at rest prior to each movement and corrects any movement deviation to determine its relevance to the patient's symptoms.

Active movements of the thoracic spine and possible modifications are shown in Table 8.1. It is worth mentioning the work of Robin McKenzie. If all movements are full and symptom-free on overpressure, but symptoms are aggravated by certain postures, and eased with postural correction, the condition is categorized as a postural syndrome (McKenzie & May 2006). If there are local, intermittent spinal symptoms with at least one movement and the restricted movement consistently produces concordant pain at end range with no reduction, abolition or peripheralisation of symptoms, the condition is categorized as a dysfunction syndrome (McKenzie & May 2006). If on repeated movement, centralization or abolition of symptoms occurs and are maintained over time, this is characterized as a reducible derangement syndrome. Two types of derangement are described (Table 8.2).

Numerous differentiation tests (Maitland et al. 2001) can be performed; the choice depends on the patient's signs and symptoms. For example, when turning the head around to the left reproduces the patient's left-sided infrascapular pain, differentiation between the cervical and thoracic spine may be required. The clinician can increase and decrease the rotation at the cervical and thoracic regions to find out what effect this has on the infrascapular pain. The patient turns the head and trunk around to the left; the clinician maintains the position of the cervical spine and derotates the thoracic spine, noting the pain response. If symptoms remain the same or increase, this might suggest the cervical spine is the source of the symptoms. The position

of cervical and thoracic rotation is then resumed and this time the clinician maintains the position of the thoracic spine and derotates the cervical spine to neutral, noting the pain response (Figure 8.2A). If the symptoms remain the same or increase, this implicates the thoracic spine. It may be necessary to examine other regions to determine their relevance to the patient's symptoms as they may be the source of the symptoms, or they may be contributing to the symptoms. The joints within these regions can be tested fully (see relevant chapter) or partially with the use of screening tests (see Chapter 3 for further details).

Observation of aggravating functional activities or positions. Depending on the irritability, severity and nature of the symptoms it is important to observe at least one key functional restriction of the patient as this may be contributing to ongoing

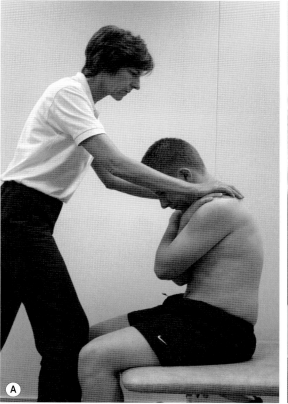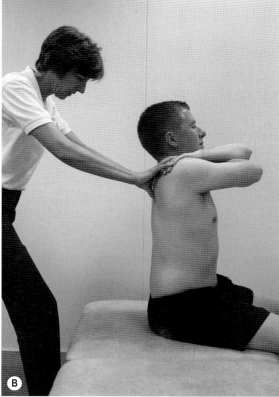

Figure 8.1 • Overpressures to the thoracic spine. These movements are all carried out with the patient's arms crossed. A Flexion. Both hands on top of the shoulders, angle pressure down and posteriorly through the mid-thoracic spine to increase thoracic flexion. B Extension. Both hands on top of shoulders, angle pressure down and anteriorly through the sternum. The pelvis may be positioned into a posterior rotation to isolate extension to the thoracic spine.

(Continued)

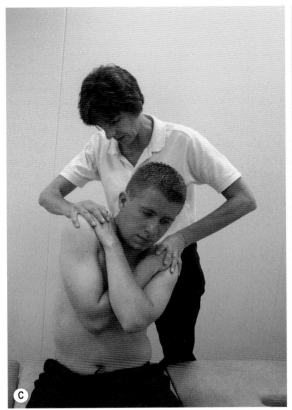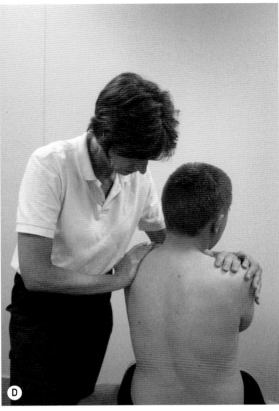

Figure 8.1—cont'd • C Lateral flexion. Both hands on top of the shoulders apply a force to increase thoracic lateral flexion. D Rotation. The right hand rests behind the patient's left shoulder and the left hand lies on the front of the right shoulder. Both hands then apply a force to increase right thoracic rotation.

(Continued)

symptoms; it also ensures that you maintain a patient-focused perspective. Altering any impairments and noting the response of the symptoms will guide further relevant testing.

Sustained natural apophyseal glides (SNAGs). Although these are largely treatment techniques they can serve as an important differential diagnostic tool. They are applied to the thoracic vertebra or ribs whilst the patient performs a painful active movement. For example, a glide can be performed either centrally or unilaterally on a thoracic vertebra in the direction of the facet joint plane. If there is a reduction in pain, this segment is implicated as a source of the pain. For further details on these techniques, see Chapter 3 and Mulligan (2006). Figure 8.2B demonstrates a left rotation SNAG on the T6 transverse process. In this example, the technique aims to facilitate the glide of the right inferior facet of T6 upwards on T7.

Passive physiological movements

These can take the form of passive physiological intervertebral movements (PPIVMs), which examine the movement at each segmental level. PPIVMs can be a useful adjunct to passive accessory intervertebral movements to identify segmental hypomobility and hypermobility. PPIVMs are usually performed in sitting for the mid-thoracic region. The clinician palpates between adjacent spinous processes or transverse processes to feel the range of intervertebral movement during thoracic flexion, extension, rotation and lateral flexion. Figure 8.3 demonstrates PPIVMs for flexion of the thoracic spine.

Muscle tests

The muscles that need to be tested will depend on the area of the signs and symptoms and may include

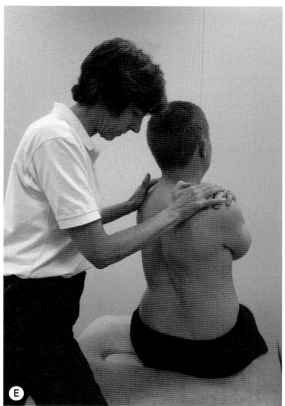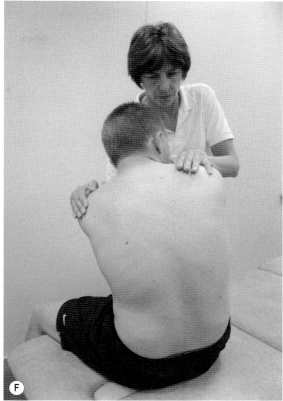

Figure 8.1—cont'd • E Combined right rotation/extension. This movement is a combination of right rotation and extension. Both hands are placed on top of the shoulders; the patient then actively rotates – note the symptoms produced – the clinician then passively extends the thoracic spine as for extension overpressure and notes any change in symptoms. **F** Combined flexion/right rotation. Both hands are placed on top of the shoulders and a flexion force is localised to the thoracic spine. Note the symptoms produced. Maintaining flexion, both hands apply a right rotation. Note change in symptoms.

muscles of the cervical spine and upper limbs or the lumbar spine and lower limbs. Muscle tests include examining muscle strength, control, and length.

Muscle strength

The clinician may test the trunk flexors, extensors, lateral flexors and rotators and other relevant muscle groups as necessary. For details of these general tests readers are directed to Cole et al. (1988), Hislop & Montgomery (1995) and Kendall et al. (1993).

Greater detail may be required to test the strength of muscles, in particular those thought prone to becoming weak (Table 3.2). Details of testing the strength of these muscles are given in Chapter 3.

Muscle control

The functional recruitment of muscles is considered to be more important than the overall strength of a muscle group (Janda 1994, 2002; Sahrmann 2002). This is assessed initially by observing posture and the quality of movement, noting any changes in muscle recruitment patterns and by palpating the relevant muscles.

Movement impairment around the scapula has been described by a number of workers (Jull & Janda 1987; Janda 1994; Sahrmann 2002) and may cause thoracic spine symptoms (Jull & Janda 1987; Janda 1994; Sahrmann 2002); these can be assessed by observation of upper-limb movements and specific muscle testing. Abdominal, thoracic and thoracolumbar extensor muscles attach to the ribcage and

Table 8.1 Active movements and possible modifications

Active physiological movements	Modifications
Thoracic spine	Repeated
Flexion	Speed altered
Extension	Combined (Edwards 1999)
Left lateral flexion	e.g.
Right lateral flexion	– flexion then rotation
Left rotation	– extension then rotation
Right rotation	Compression or distraction
Repetitive flexion (rep flex)	Sustained
Repetitive extension (rep ext)	Injuring movement
Repetitive rotation left (rep rot)	Differentiation tests
Repetitive rotation right (rep rot)	Function
?Cervical spine	
?Upper limb	
?Lumbar spine	
?Lower limbs	

Table 8.2 Derangement syndromes of the thoracic spine (McKenzie & May 2006)

Reducible Derangement

Centralisation: in response to therapeutic loading strategies pain is progressively abolished in a distal to proximal direction, and each progressive abolition is retained over time, until all symptoms are abolished.

If back pain only is present this moves from a widespread to a more central location and then is abolished.

Pain is decreased and then abolished during the application of therapeutic loading strategies.

The change in pain location, or decrease or abolition of pain remain better, and should be accompanied or preceded by improvements in the mechanical presentation (range of movement and/or deformity).

Irreducible Derangement

Peripheralisation of symptoms: increase or worsening of distal symptoms in response to therapeutic loading strategies, and/or no decrease, abolition, or centralisation of pain.

changes in their recruitment patterns may result in thoracic spine and ribcage dysfunction.

These recruitment patterns can vary from:

- overactivity, resulting in increased compression and reduced mobility of passive structures, to
- underactivity, resulting in lack of stability or control of segmental movement (O'Sullivan 2005).

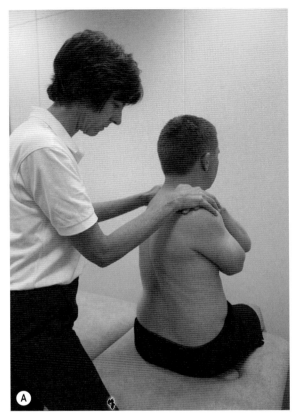

Figure 8.2 • Differentiation testing. A The clinician maintains right rotation of the thoracic spine while the patient returns the head to neutral.

(Continued)

Muscle length

The clinician tests the length of muscles, in particular those thought prone to shorten (Janda 1994). Details of testing the length of these muscles are given in Chapter 3.

Neurological tests

Neurological examination includes neurological integrity testing, neurodynamic tests and some other nerve tests.

Neurological integrity

The distribution of symptoms will determine the appropriate neurological examination to be carried out. Symptoms confined to the mid-thoracic region require dermatome/cutaneous nerve testing only,

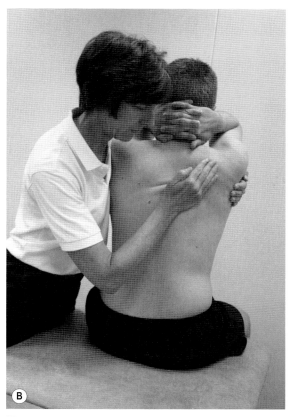

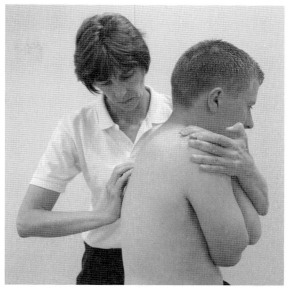

Figure 8.3 • Passive physiological intervertebral movements for flexion of the thoracic spine. The clinician's right middle or index finger is placed in the gap between adjacent spinous processes and the patient is passively flexed by grasping around the thorax with the left hand.

Figure 8.2—cont'd • B Using a sustained natural apophyseal glide on T6 with left rotation, the clinician applies a cephalad posteroanterior glide to the T6 right transverse process while the patient moves into left rotation. Any changes in symptoms are noted.

since there is no myotome or reflex that can be tested. If symptoms spread proximally or distally, a neurological examination of the upper or lower limbs respectively is indicated; see Chapter 3.

Dermatomes/peripheral nerves. Light touch and pain sensation of the thorax are tested using cotton wool and pinprick respectively, as described in Chapter 3. Knowledge of the cutaneous distribution of nerve roots (dermatomes) and peripheral nerves enables the clinician to distinguish the sensory loss due to a root lesion from that due to a peripheral nerve lesion. The cutaneous nerve distribution and dermatome areas are shown in Chapter 3.

Neurodynamic tests

The following neurodynamic tests may be carried out in order to ascertain the degree to which neural tissue

is responsible for the production of the patient's symptom(s):

- passive neck flexion
- upper-limb neurodynamic tests
- straight-leg raise
- passive knee bend
- slump.

These tests are described in detail in Chapter 3.

Central nervous system testing – upper motor nerve lesions

Plantar response – Babinski's sign (Walton 1989). Pressure applied from the heel along the lateral border of the plantar aspect of the foot produces flexion of the toes in the normal. Extension of the big toe with downward fanning of the other toes occurs with an upper motor neurone lesion.

Clonus. Dorsiflex the ankle briskly, maintain the foot in that position and a rhythmic contraction may be found. More than three beats is considered abnormal.

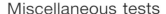

Miscellaneous tests

Respiratory tests

These tests are appropriate for patients whose spinal dysfunction is such that respiration is affected and may include conditions such as severe scoliosis and ankylosing spondylitis.

Auscultation and examination of the patient's sputum may be required, as well as measurement of the patient's exercise tolerance.

Vital capacity can be measured using a hand-held spirometer. Normal ranges are 2.5–6 litres for men and 2–5 litres for women (Johnson 1990).

Maximum inspiratory and expiratory pressures ($P_{I\,max}$/MIP, $P_{E\,max}$/MEP) reflect respiratory muscle strength and endurance. A maximum static inspiratory or expiratory effort can be measured by a hand-held mouth pressure monitor (Micromedical, Chatham, Kent, UK). Normal values (Wilson et al. 1984) are:

$$P_{I\,max} > 100 \text{ cmH}_2\text{O for males}$$
$$> 70 \text{ cmH}_2\text{O for females}$$
$$P_{E\,max} > 140 \text{ cmH}_2\text{O for males}$$
$$> 90 \text{ cmH}_2\text{O for females.}$$

Vascular tests

Tests for thoracic outlet syndrome are described in Chapter 9.

Palpation

The clinician palpates the thoracic spine and, if appropriate, the cervical/lumbar spine and upper/lower limbs. It is useful to record palpation findings on a body chart (see Figure 2.3) and/or palpation chart (see Figure 3.36).

The clinician should note the following:

- temperature, sweating and trophic skin changes (pitting oedema, shiny and inelastic skin) of the area and extremities
- any increase in skin moisture
- bony anomalies: increased or decreased prominence of bones; deviation of the spinous process from the centre; vertebral rotation – assessed by palpating the position of the transverse processes
- mobility and feel of superficial tissues, e.g. scarring

- reduced muscle tone or wasting
- the presence or elicitation of any muscle spasm
- tenderness of bone, ligaments, muscle, tendon, trigger points (shown in Figure 3.37) and nerves
- symptoms (usually pain) provoked or reduced on palpation.

Passive accessory intervertebral movements

It is useful to use the palpation chart and movement diagrams (or joint pictures) to record findings. These are explained in detail in Chapter 3.

The clinician should note the following:

- quality of movement
- range of movement
- resistance through the range and at the end of the range of movement
- behaviour of pain through the range
- any provocation of muscle spasm.

The thoracic spine (T1–T12) accessory movements and rib accessory movements are shown in Figures 8.4–8.6 and listed in Table 8.3. Accessory movements can then be tested in other regions suspected to be a source of, or contributing to, the patient's symptoms. Following accessory movements to the thoracic region, the clinician reassesses all the physical asterisks (movements or tests that have been found to reproduce the patient's symptoms) in order to establish the effect of the accessory movements on the patient's signs and symptoms.

Examination of the ribcage

The ribs are strongly attached to the thoracic spine via the costovertebral and costotransverse joints and their associated ligaments. It may therefore be necessary to test these joints for mobility and pain provocation. Very few studies have been done on the biomechanics of the intact thoracic spine and ribcage. However, a model proposed by Lee (2003) is useful for clinical assessment. Lee proposes that movements of the rib joints are influenced by the mechanics of the thoracic spine. For example, flexion results in the inferior facet joint of the upper vertebra and its same-numbered rib gliding/rolling in a superior, anterior direction – a rib's mobility into flexion could therefore be palpated by applying a cephalad glide to it near the costotransverse joint (Figure 8.5A). The reverse occurs with extension

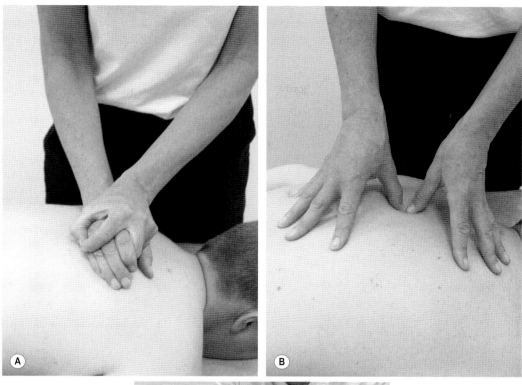

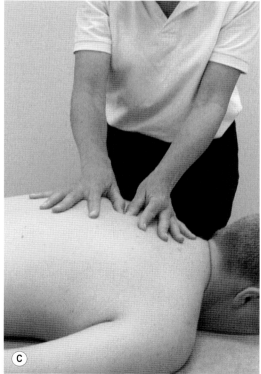

Figure 8.4 • Thoracic spine (T1–T12) accessory movements. A Central posteroanterior. A pisiform grip is used to apply pressure to the spinous process. B Unilateral posteroanterior. Thumb pressure is applied to the transverse process. C Transverse. Thumb pressure is applied to the lateral aspect of the spinous process.

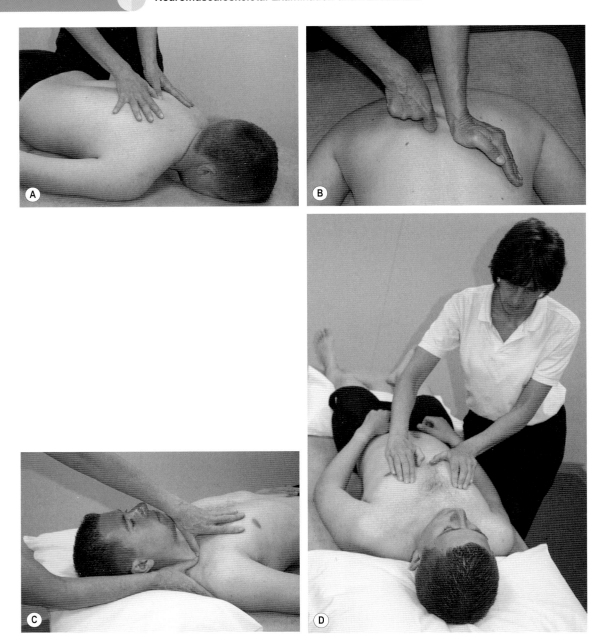

Figure 8.5 • Accessory movements to ribs. A Unilateral posteroanterior cephalad glide. Thumb pressure applied to the rib lateral to the costotransverse joint. B Posteroanterior glide. Thumb pressure is applied to the posterior aspect of the rib whilst the contralateral transverse processes of the vertebrae to which the rib is attached are fixed. C Longitudinal caudad glide first rib. Thumb pressure is applied to the superior aspect of the first rib and pressure is applied downwards towards the feet. Pressure can be applied anywhere along the superior aspect of the rib. The rib can also be motion-tested with respiration. D Motion testing of the sternal ribs (2–7) with respiration. Anteroposterior pressure can also be applied to the anterior aspect of the rib, testing for symptom reproduction and stiffness.

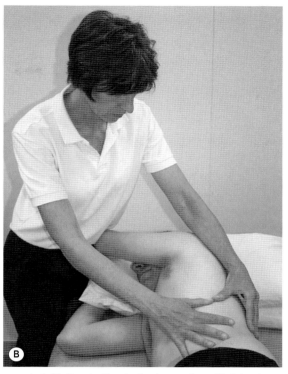

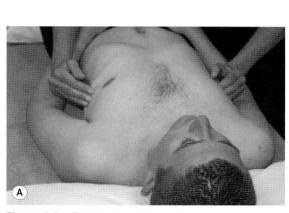

Figure 8.6 • Rib lateral motion testing and accessory movement. **A** Motion testing to the lower ribs with lateral costal breathing. **B** A caudad glide is applied to the lateral part of the rib with the patient in side-lying. The thumb is placed along the line of the rib.

and the glide direction applied to the rib would be caudad. This is particularly applicable to the ribs that attach to the sternum (ribs 2–7). The lower ribs are less strongly attached to the thoracic spine and are therefore less influenced by thoracic spine movements.

A posteroanterior glide applied to the rib angle will test the anatomical structures that resist anterior translation of the rib. First, fix the contralateral transverse processes of the two vertebrae to which the rib is attached. For example when applying a postero-anterior glide to the fourth rib on the right, fix T3 and T4 on the left (Figure 8.5B). If no movement is allowed to occur at the thoracic spine and symptoms are reproduced the costal joints and ligaments are implicated.

Respiration

During inspiration the first rib elevates, moving the manubrium into an anterior superior direction.

A common dysfunction of the first and second rib is when they remain in elevation. This can be caused by joint stiffness or scaleni overactivity. These ribs can be motion-tested by palpation with breathing and/or longitudinal caudad glides (Figure 8.5C).

The biomechanics of rib and thoracic spine during inspiration are largely the same as extension whilst expiration and flexion are similar. Rib dysfunctions can be assessed by palpating rib mobility with respiration. The mechanics of the costal joints of the ribs that attach to the sternum are oriented largely to facilitate upward and superior movement of the sternum during inspiration – pump-handle motion (Levangie & Norkin 2005). The reverse occurs during expiration. The mobility of individual ribs can be palpated over the anterior ribcage whilst asking the patient to breathe (Figure 8.5D); this is best done in supine-lying but can be assessed in functional positions. An anteroposterior glide will assess for pain provocation and mobility. Sternocostal and costochondral can be palpated for tenderness.

Table 8.3 Accessory movements, choice of application and reassessment of the patient's asterisks

Accessory movements	Choice of application	Identify any effect of accessory movements on patient's signs and symptoms
Thoracic spine	Start position e.g.	Reassess all asterisks
↕ Central posteroanterior	– in flexion	
⌐˙⌐ Unilateral posteroanterior	– in extension	
⇄ Transverse	– in lateral flexion	
Accessory movements to ribs 1–12	– in flexion and rotation	
↔ Caud/ceph	– in extension and rotation	
↕ Anteroposterior	Speed of force application	
↕ Posteroanterior	Direction of the applied force	
↦ Med Medial glide	Point of application of applied force	
Costochondral, interchondral and sternocostal joints		
↕ Anteroposterior		
?Cervical spine	As above	Reassess all asterisks
?Upper-limb joints	As above	Reassess all asterisks
?Lumbar spine	As above	Reassess all asterisks
?Lower-limb joints	As above	Reassess all asterisks

The lower ribs have a more upward and lateral motion and increase the transverse diameter of the lower thorax during inspiration – bucket-handle motion (Levangie & Norkin 2005). Individual rib movement can be motion-tested by the clinician palpating laterally whilst asking the patient to do lateral costal breathing (Figure 8.6A). A cephalad or caudad glide applied laterally along the rib will assess for mobility and pain provocation. This can be done with the patient in supine-lying where both sides can be compared, or a more detailed assessment of the ribs laterally can be done with the patient in side-lying (Figure 8.6B).

Completion of the examination

Having carried out the above tests, the examination of the thoracic spine is now complete. The subjective and physical examinations produce a large amount of information, which should be recorded accurately and quickly. It is vital at this stage to highlight with an asterisk (*) important findings from the examination. These findings must be reassessed at, and within, subsequent treatment sessions to evaluate the effects of treatment on the patient's condition.

The physical testing procedures which specifically indicate joint, nerve or muscle tissues, as a source of the patient's symptoms, are summarised in Table 3.10. The strongest evidence that a joint is the source of the patient's symptoms is that active and passive physiological movements, passive accessory movements and joint palpation all reproduce the patient's symptoms, and that, following a treatment dose, reassessment identifies an improvement in the patient's signs and symptoms. Weaker evidence includes an alteration in range, resistance or quality of physiological and/or accessory movements and tenderness over the joint, with no alteration in signs and symptoms after treatment.

The strongest evidence that a muscle is the source of a patient's symptoms is if active movements, an isometric contraction, passive lengthening and palpation of a muscle all reproduce the patient's symptoms, and that, following a treatment dose directed at the muscle, the reassessment identifies an improvement in the patient's signs and symptoms. Further evidence of muscle dysfunction may be suggested by reduced strength or poor-quality recruitment during the active physiological movement.

The strongest evidence that a nerve is the source of the patient's symptoms is when active and/or passive physiological movements reproduce the symptoms, which are then increased or decreased with an additional sensitising movement, at a distance from the patient's symptoms. In addition, there is reproduction of the patient's symptoms on palpation of the nerve, and following neurodynamic testing.

On completion of the physical examination the clinician should:

- explain the findings of the physical examination and how these findings relate to the subjective assessment. An attempt should be made to clear up any misconceptions patients may have regarding their illness or injury
- collaborate with the patient and via problem-solving together devise a treatment plan and discuss the prognosis
- warn the patient of possible exacerbation up to 24–48 hours following the examination

- request the patient to report details on the behaviour of the symptoms following examination at the next attendance
- evaluate the findings, formulate a clinical diagnosis and write up a problem list
- determine the objectives of treatment
- devise an initial treatment plan.

In this way, the clinician will have developed the following hypotheses categories (adapted from Jones & Rivett 2004):

- function: abilities and restrictions
- patient's perspective on his/her experience
- source of symptoms. This includes the structure or tissue that is thought to be producing the patient's symptoms, the nature of the structure or tissues in relation to the healing process and the pain mechanisms
- contributing factors to the development and maintenance of the problem. There may be environmental, psychosocial, behavioural, physical or heredity factors
- precautions/contraindications to treatment and management. This includes the severity and irritability of the patient's symptoms and the nature of the patient's condition
- management strategy and treatment plan
- prognosis – this can be affected by factors such as the stage and extent of the injury as well as the patient's expectation, personality and lifestyle.

For guidance on treatment and management principles, the reader is directed to the companion textbook (Petty 2011).

References

Bogduk, N., Marsland, A., 1988. The cervical zygapophyseal joints as a source of neck pain. Spine 13 (6), 610–617.

Clinical Standards Advisory Report, 1994. Report of a CSAG committee on back pain. HMSO, London.

Cloward, R.B., 1959. Cervical discography: a contribution to the aetiology and mechanism of neck, shoulder and arm pain. Ann. Surg. 150 (6), 1052–1064.

Cole, J.H., Furness, A.L., Twomey, L.T., 1988. Muscles in action, an approach to manual muscle testing. Churchill Livingstone, Edinburgh.

Edmondston, S.J., Singer, K.P., 1997. Thoracic spine: anatomical and biomechanical considerations for manual therapy. Man. Ther. 2 (3), 132–143.

Edwards, B.C., 1999. Manual of combined movements: their use in the examination and treatment of mechanical vertebral column disorders, second ed. Butterworth-Heinemann, Oxford.

Grieve, G.P., 1994. Counterfeit clinical presentations. Manipulative Physiotherapist 26, 17–19.

Hislop, H., Montgomery, J., 1995. Daniels and Worthingham's muscle

testing, techniques of manual examination, seventh ed. W B Saunders, Philadelphia.

Janda, V., 1994. Muscles and motor control in cervicogenic disorders: assessment and management. In: Grant, R. (Ed.), Physical therapy of the cervical and thoracic spine, second ed. Churchill Livingstone, New York, p. 195.

Janda, V., 2002. Muscles and motor control in cervicogenic disorders. In: Grant, R. (Ed.), Physical therapy of the cervical and thoracic spine, third ed. Churchill Livingstone, New York, p. 182.

Johnson, N.M., 1990. Respiratory medicine, second ed. Blackwell Scientific Publications, Oxford.

Jones, M.A., Rivett, D.A., 2004. Clinical reasoning for manual therapists. Butterworth-Heinemann, Edinburgh.

Jull, G.A., Janda, V., 1987. Muscles and motor control in low back pain: assessment and management. In: Twomey, L.T., Taylor, J.R. (Eds.), Physical therapy of the low back. Churchill Livingstone, New York, p. 253.

Kendall, F.P., McCreary, E.K., Provance, P.G., 1993. Muscles testing and function, fourth ed. Williams & Wilkins, Baltimore, MD.

Lee, D., 2003. The thorax: an integrated approach, second ed. Orthopedic Physical Therapy, White Rock, BC, Canada.

Levangie, P.K., Norkin, C.C., 2005. Joint structure and function. A comprehensive analysis, fourth ed.

F. A Davis, Philadelphia, pp. 198–200.

Magee, D.J., 1997. Orthopedic physical assessment, third ed. W B Saunders, Philadelphia.

Maitland, G.D., Hengeveld, E., Banks, K., et al., 2001. Maitland's vertebral manipulation, sixth ed. Butterworth-Heinemann, Oxford.

McKenzie, R.A., May, S.J., 2006. The Cervical and Thoracic Spine: Mechanical Diagnosis and Therapy. Spinal Publications New Zealand Ltd., Waikanae, New Zealand.

Mulligan, B.R., 2006. Manual therapy 'NAGs', 'SNAGs', 'MWMs' etc., fifth ed. Plane View Services, New Zealand.

Oda, I., Abumi, K., Cunningham, B.W., et al., 2002. An in vitro human cadaveric study investigating the biomechanical properties of the thoracic spine. Spine 27 (3), E64–E70.

O'Sullivan, P., 2005. Diagnosis and classification of chronic low back pain: maladaptive movement and motor control impairments as underlying mechanisms. Man. Ther. 10 (4), 242–255.

Petty, N.J., 2011. Principles of neuromusculoskeletal treatment and management: a guide for therapists, second ed. Churchill Livingstone, Edinburgh.

Sahrmann, S.A., 2002. Diagnosis and treatment of movement impairment syndromes. Mosby, St Louis.

Waddell, G., 2004. The back pain revolution, second ed. Churchill Livingstone, Edinburgh.

Walton, J.H., 1989. Essentials of neurology, sixth ed. Churchill Livingstone, Edinburgh.

Wilson, S.H., Cooke, N.T., Edwards, R.H.T., et al., 1984. Predicted normal values for maximal respiratory pressures in Caucasian adults and children. Thorax 39, 535–538.

Examination of the shoulder region

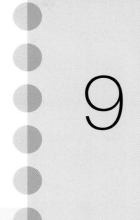

9

Chris Mercer Colette Ridehalgh

CHAPTER CONTENTS

Possible causes of pain and/or limitation of movement

This region includes the sternoclavicular, acromioclavicular and glenohumeral joints and their surrounding soft tissues.

- Trauma:
  - ○ fracture of the clavicle, humerus or scapula
  - ○ dislocation of one of the above joints
  - ○ ligamentous sprain
  - ○ muscular strain
- Tendinopathy, particularly of the rotator cuff or long head of biceps
- Spontaneous conditions, e.g. adhesive capsulitis and rupture of the long head of biceps
- Osteoarthritis
- Inflammatory disorders, e.g rheumatoid arthritis
- Infection, e.g. tuberculosis
- Bursitis
- Muscle imbalance-related problems, e.g. winged scapula due to weakness of serratus anterior
- Snapping scapula (grinding sensation beneath the scapula on movement due to rib prominence)
- Neoplasm
- Thoracic outlet syndrome
- Hypermobility and instability syndromes
- Referral of symptoms from:
  - ○ viscera, e.g. lungs, heart, diaphragm, gallbladder and spleen (Brown 1983)
  - ○ joints, e.g. cervical spine, thoracic spine, elbow, wrist or hand.

Further details of the questions asked during the subjective examination and the tests carried out in the physical examination can be found in Chapters 2 and 3, respectively.

The order of the subjective questioning and the physical tests described below can be altered as appropriate for the patient being examined.

Subjective examination

Body chart

The following information concerning the type and area of current symptoms can be recorded on a body chart (see Figure 2.3).

Area of current symptoms

Be exact when mapping out the area of the symptoms. Symptoms from the glenohumeral joint are commonly felt at the insertion of deltoid but may be referred proximally to the low cervical spine and/or distally to the forearm and hand. Acromioclavicular and sternoclavicular joint lesions are often felt locally around the joint, although it is not uncommon for the acromioclavicular joint to refer pain proximally over the area of the upper trapezius. Ascertain which is the worst symptom and record where the patient feels the symptoms are coming from.

Areas relevant to the region being examined

All other relevant areas are checked for symptoms; it is important to ask about pain or even stiffness, as this may be relevant to the patient's main symptom. Mark unaffected areas with ticks (✓) on the body chart. Check for symptoms in the cervical spine, thoracic spine, elbow, wrist and hand.

Quality of pain

Establish the quality of the pain. Catching pain or arcs of pain are typical of impingement-related problems around the shoulder. Clunking felt within the shoulder joint may indicate labral pathology or instability.

Intensity of pain

The intensity of pain can be measured using, for example, a visual analogue scale, as shown in Chapter 2.

Abnormal sensation

Check for any altered sensation locally around the shoulder region as well as over the spine and distally in the arm.

Constant or intermittent symptoms

Ascertain the frequency of the symptoms, whether they are constant or intermittent. If symptoms are constant, check whether there is variation in the intensity of the symptoms, as constant unremitting pain may be indicative of more serious pathology.

Relationship of symptoms

Determine the relationship between symptomatic areas – do they come together or separately? For example, the patient may have shoulder pain without neck pain, or the pains may always be present together.

Behaviour of symptoms

Aggravating factors

For each symptomatic area a series of questions can be asked:

- What movements, activities or positions bring on or make the patient's symptoms worse?
- How long does it take before symptoms are aggravated?
- Is the patient able to maintain this position or movement?
- What happens to other symptoms when this symptom is produced or made worse?
- How do the symptoms affect function, e.g. reaching, dressing, overhead activities, sport and social activities?
- Does the patient have a feeling of instability in the shoulder?

The clinician also asks the patient about theoretically known aggravating factors for structures that could be a source of the symptoms. Common aggravating factors for the shoulder are hand behind back, above-head activities, lifting and lying on the shoulder. Aggravating factors for other regions, which may need to be queried if they are suspected to be a source of the symptoms, are shown in Table 2.3.

Detailed information on each of the aggravating activities is useful in order to help determine the structures at fault and identify functional restrictions. This information can be used to determine the aims of treatment and any advice that may be required. The most notable functional restrictions are highlighted with asterisks (*), explored in the physical examination and reassessed at subsequent treatment sessions to evaluate treatment intervention.

Easing factors

For each symptomatic area a series of questions can be asked to help determine what eases the symptoms:

- What movements and/or positions ease the patient's symptoms?
- How long does it take before symptoms are eased? If symptoms are constant but variable it is important to know what the baseline is and how long it takes for the symptoms to reduce to that level.
- What happens to other symptoms when this symptom is eased?

Twenty-four-hour behaviour of symptoms

The clinician determines the 24-hour behaviour of symptoms by asking questions about night, morning and evening symptoms.

Night symptoms. The following questions may be asked:

- Do you have any difficulty getting to sleep?
- What position is most comfortable/ uncomfortable?
- What is your normal sleeping position?
- What is your present sleeping position?
- Can you lie on the affected shoulder?
- Do your symptoms wake you at night? If so,
  - ○ Which symptom(s)?
  - ○ How many times in the past week?
  - ○ How many times in a night?
  - ○ How long does it take to get back to sleep?
- How many and what type of pillows are used?

Morning and evening symptoms. The clinician determines the pattern of the symptoms first thing in the morning, through the day and at the end of the day. Morning stiffness that lasts more than 2 hours is suggestive of an inflammatory condition such as rheumatoid arthritis. Stiffness lasting only 30 minutes or less is likely to be mechanical or degenerative in nature.

Stage of the condition

In order to determine the stage of the condition, the clinician asks whether the symptoms are getting better, getting worse or remaining unchanged.

Special questions

Special questions must always be asked, as they may identify certain precautions or contraindications to the physical examination and/or treatment (Table 2.4). As mentioned in Chapter 2, the clinician must differentiate between conditions that are suitable for conservative management and systemic, neoplastic and other non-neuromusculoskeletal conditions, which require referral to a medical practitioner. The reader is referred to Appendix 2.3 for details of serious pathological processes that can mimic neuromusculoskeletal conditions (Grieve 1994a).

Previous shoulder dislocation. If the patient has a history of previous dislocation, care must be taken during the physical examination, e.g. for anterior dislocation the clinician should take care when positioning the shoulder in lateral rotation and abduction.

Neurological symptoms. Has the patient experienced symptoms of spinal cord compression, which are bilateral tingling in the hands or feet and/or disturbance of gait? Does the patient complain of gross weakness or altered sensation in the arm? This may indicate more than one level of nerve root compression at the cervical spine. Does the patient complain of altered sensation in the arm during abduction and lateral rotation, e.g. throwing activities? This may indicate anterior shoulder instability (Hill et al. 2008).

Vascular symptoms. Does the patient complain of coldness, change in colour or loss of sensation in the arm or hands? Does the patient get symptoms when the arms are raised or if working with the arms overhead? This may indicate a vascular problem and will need further testing.

Vertebrobasilar insufficiency. This is relevant where there are symptoms of pain, discomfort and/or altered sensation emanating from the cervical spine, where vertebrobasilar insufficiency may be provoked. Further questions about dizziness and testing for vertebrobasilar insufficiency are described more fully in Chapter 6.

History of the present condition

For each symptomatic area the clinician needs to know how long the symptom has been present, whether there was a sudden or slow onset and whether there was a known cause that provoked the onset of the symptom. If the onset was slow, the clinician finds out if there has been any change in the patient's life-style, e.g. a new job or hobby or a change in sporting activity; this may have contributed to the patient's condition. To confirm the relationship of the symptoms, the clinician asks what happened to other symptoms when each symptom began.

The clinician should ask whether the patient has a history of spontaneous dislocation/subluxation or a history of voluntary dislocation/subluxation (party trick movements).

Has the patient taken any medication for the pain, and if so what was its effect?

Past medical history

The following information is obtained from the patient and/or the medical notes:

- The details of any relevant medical history.
- The history of any previous attacks: how many episodes? when were they? what was the cause? what was the duration of each episode? and did the patient fully recover between episodes? If there have been no previous attacks, has the patient had any episodes of stiffness in the cervical spine, thoracic spine, shoulder or any other relevant region? Check for a history of trauma or recurrent minor trauma.
- Ascertain the results of any past treatment for the same or similar problem. Past treatment records may be obtained for further information

General health. The clinician ascertains the state of the patient's general health, and finds out if the patient suffers from any cough, breathlessness, chest pain, malaise, fatigue, fever, nausea or vomiting, stress, anxiety or depression. Symptoms in the shoulder may be referred from the lungs, pleura, heart, diaphragm, gallbladder and spleen (Brown 1983).

Weight loss. Has the patient noticed any recent unexplained weight loss?

Rheumatoid arthritis. Has the patient (or a member of his/her family) been diagnosed as having rheumatoid arthritis?

Drug therapy. What drugs are being taken by the patient? Has the patient been prescribed long-term (6 months or more) medication/steroids? Has the patient been taking anticoagulants?

Further investigations. Has the patient been X-rayed or had any other medical tests recently? The medical tests may include blood tests, magnetic resonance imaging, diagnostic ultrasound, arthroscopy and arthrogram.

Social and family history

Social and family history that is relevant to the onset and progression of the patient's problem is recorded. This includes the patient's perspectives, experience and expectations, age, employment, home situation and details of any leisure/sporting activities. The age, gender and ethnicity of patients and their cultural, occupational and social backgrounds may all affect their attitudes and feelings towards themselves, their condition and the clinician. The clinician needs to be aware of, and sensitive to, these attitudes, and to empathise and communicate appropriately so as to develop a rapport with the patient and thereby enhance the patient's compliance with the treatment.

Factors from this information may indicate direct or indirect mechanical influences on the shoulder. In order to treat the patient appropriately, it is important that the condition is managed within the context of the patient's social and work environment.

The clinician may ask the following types of questions to elucidate psychosocial factors:

- Have you had time off work in the past with your pain?
- What do you understand to be the cause of your pain?
- What are you expecting will help you?
- How is your employer/co-workers/family responding to your pain?
- What are you doing to cope with your pain?
- Do you think you will return to work? When?

Although these questions are described in relation to psychosocial risk factors for poor outcomes for patients with low-back pain (Waddell 2004), they may be relevant to patients with shoulder pain.

Plan of the physical examination

When all this information has been collected, the subjective examination is complete. It is useful at this stage to highlight with asterisks (*), for ease of reference, important findings and particularly one or more functional restrictions. These can then be re-examined at subsequent treatment sessions to evaluate treatment intervention.

In order to plan the physical examination, the following hypotheses need to be developed from the subjective examination:

- The regions and structures that should be examined as a possible source of the symptoms, e.g. rotator cuff, glenohumeral joint, cervical spine. Often it is not possible to examine fully at the first attendance and so examination of the structures must be prioritised over subsequent treatment sessions.

- Other contributing factors that should be examined, e.g. instability, posture, muscle imbalances and sporting technique, such as service and strokes for tennis.
- In what way should the physical tests be carried out? Will it be easy or hard to reproduce each symptom? Will it be necessary to use combined movements or repetitive movements to reproduce the patient's symptoms?
- Are symptoms severe and/or irritable? If symptoms are severe, physical tests may be carried out to just before the onset of symptom production or just to the onset of symptom production; no overpressures will be carried out, as the patient would be unable to tolerate this. If symptoms are irritable, physical tests may be examined to just before symptom production or just to the onset of provocation with fewer physical tests being examined to allow for a rest period between tests.
- Are there any precautions or contraindications to elements of the physical examination that need to be explored further, e.g. vertebrobasilar insufficiency, neurological involvement, cardiac problems?

A physical planning form can be useful for clinicians to help guide them through the clinical reasoning process (see Figure 2.10).

Physical examination

The information from the subjective examination helps the clinician to plan an appropriate physical examination. The severity, irritability and nature of the condition are the major factors that will influence the choice and priority of physical testing procedures. The first and overarching question the clinician might ask is: 'Is this patient's condition suitable for me to manage as a therapist?' The second question the clinician might ask is: 'Does this patient have a neuromusculoskeletal dysfunction that I may be able to help?' To answer that, the clinician needs to carry out a full physical examination; however, this may not be possible if the

symptoms are severe and/or irritable. If the patient's symptoms are severe and/or irritable, the clinician aims to explore movements as much as possible, within a symptom-free range. If the patient has constant and severe and/or irritable symptoms, then the clinician aims to find physical tests that ease the symptoms. If the patient's symptoms are non-severe and non-irritable, then the clinician aims to find physical tests that reproduce each of the patient's symptoms.

Each significant physical test that either provokes or eases the patient's symptoms is highlighted in the patient's notes by an asterisk (*) for easy reference. The highlighted tests are often referred to as 'asterisks' or 'markers'.

The order and detail of the physical tests described below need to be appropriate to the patient being examined. It is important that readers understand that the techniques shown in this chapter are only some of many examination techniques available. They represent some of the most commonly used techniques. The clinician is encouraged to consider the validity and reliability of all tests used. A brief mention of these issues follows the description of each test in the following text.

Observation

Informal observation

The clinician needs to observe the patient in dynamic and static situations; the quality of movement is noted, as are the postural characteristics and facial expression. Informal observation will have begun from the moment the clinician begins the subjective examination and will continue to the end of the physical examination.

Formal observation

Observation. The clinician examines the posture of the patient in sitting and standing, noting the posture of the shoulders, head and neck, thoracic spine and upper limbs. The clinician also notes bony and soft-tissue contours around the region. The clinician examines the muscle bulk and muscle tone of the patient, comparing left and right sides. It must be remembered that handedness and level and frequency of physical activity may well produce differences in muscle bulk between sides. Some muscles are thought to shorten under stress, while other muscles weaken, producing muscle imbalance (Table 3.2). The clinician may check the alignment of the head of the humerus with the acromion as this can give clues about possible mechanical insufficiencies. The clinician pinch-grips the anterior and posterior edges of the acromion with one hand and with the other hand pinch-grips the anterior and posterior aspects of the humerus. It is generally thought that, normally, no more than one-third of the humeral head lies anterior to the acromion. The clinician passively corrects any asymmetry to determine its relevance to the patient's problem.

It is worth noting that pure postural dysfunction rarely influences one region of the body in isolation and it may be necessary to observe the patient more fully for a full postural examination.

Joint integrity tests

Anterior shoulder instability

Anterior shoulder drawer test (Gerber & Ganz 1984) (Figure 9.1). With the patient supine and the shoulder in abduction (80–120°), forward flexion (0–20°) and lateral rotation (0–30°), the clinician stabilises the scapula and glides the humerus anteriorly. Excessive movement, a click and/or patient apprehension suggest that there is anterior shoulder instability.

Apprehension test (Figure 9.2). With the patient supine, the clinician takes the shoulder into 90° abduction and adds lateral rotation. The test is considered positive – indicating anterior instability – if the patient becomes apprehensive. Further confirmation can be achieved by using the relocation test

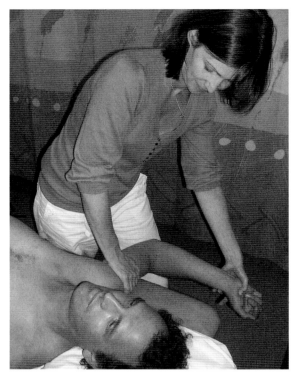

Figure 9.2 • Apprehension/relocation test.

(Jobe et al. 1989) where an anteroposterior force is applied to the head of the humerus (using the heel of the hand); apprehension is lessened and the clinician is able to take the shoulder further into lateral rotation. It has been proposed by Lo et al. (2004) that an additional component can be added to the test – a quick release of the posteriorly directed force. This so-called surprise test, taken with the findings of the apprehension and relocation test, has been shown to have a positive predictive value of 93.6% and negative predictive value of 71.9% (Lo et al. 2004).

Load and shift test (Hawkins & McCormack 1988) (Figure 9.3). With the patient in sitting or supine the clinician stabilises the scapula and applies a posteroanterior force to the humeral head whilst palpating the joint line to assess the amount of movement. This test can be graded from 0 to 3, with 0 being no movement and 3 being full dislocation. This can also be used as a test for posterior instability with the direction of force applied in a posterior direction. The test has been found to have a specificity of 100% and a sensitivity of 50% (Tzannes & Murrell 2002).

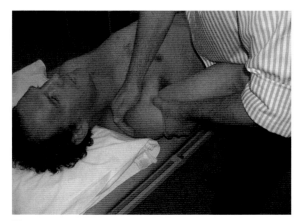

Figure 9.1 • Anterior shoulder drawer test.

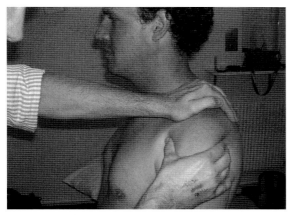

Figure 9.3 • Load and shift test.

Posterior shoulder instability

Jerk test (Figure 9.4). With the patient sitting and the shoulder abducted to 90° and medially rotated, the clinician applies an axial load to the humerus and moves the arm into horizontal flexion (Matsen et al. 1990). A positive test is indicated if there is a sudden jerk as the arm is moved into horizontal flexion and as it is returned to the start position.

Inferior shoulder instability

Sulcus sign (Matsen et al. 1990) (Figure 9.5). The clinician applies a longitudinal caudad force to the humerus with the patient sitting. A positive test is indicated if a sulcus appears distal to the acromion, suggesting inferior instability of the shoulder. The glenohumeral joint can then be externally rotated and the test repeated. It is thought that, if the test

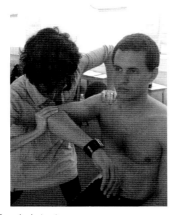

Figure 9.4 • Jerk test.

remains positive, multidirectional instability is likely, whereas a negative test upon application of the external rotation suggests a localised superior glenohumeral ligament or coracohumeral ligament dysfunction. The specificity of this test has been found to be 72% and the sensitivity 85% for positive tests greater than 1 cm (Tzannes & Murrell 2002).

Active physiological movements

For active physiological movements, the clinician notes:

- quality of movement
- range of movement
- behaviour of pain through the range of movement
- resistance through the range of movement and at the end of the range of movement
- provocation of any muscle spasm.

A movement diagram can be used to depict this information. The active movements with overpressure listed below are shown in Figure 9.6 and can be tested with the patient in standing and/or sitting. Movements are carried out on the left and right sides. The clinician establishes the patient's symptoms at rest, prior to each movement and corrects any movement deviation to determine its relevance to the patient's symptoms.

Active movements of the shoulder girdle and glenohumeral joint and possible modifications are shown in Table 9.1. Various differentiation tests (Maitland 1991) can be performed; the choice depends on the patient's signs and symptoms. For example, when shoulder abduction reproduces the patient's shoulder pain, differentiation between the glenohumeral joint, acromioclavicular joint and subacromial region may be required. The clinician can differentiate between the glenohumeral joint and the subacromial region by adding compression to the glenohumeral joint during the abduction movement; an increase in symptoms implicates the glenohumeral joint. Similarly, a longitudinal cephalad force can be applied to the humerus (to compress the subacromial structures) during the abduction movement; an increase in pain will implicate the subacromial structures. The clinician can implicate the acromioclavicular joint by applying a compression force to the acromioclavicular joint during the abduction movement; if the pain is increased this suggests the acromioclavicular joint may be the source of pain.

It may be necessary to examine other regions to determine their relevance to the patient's symptoms;

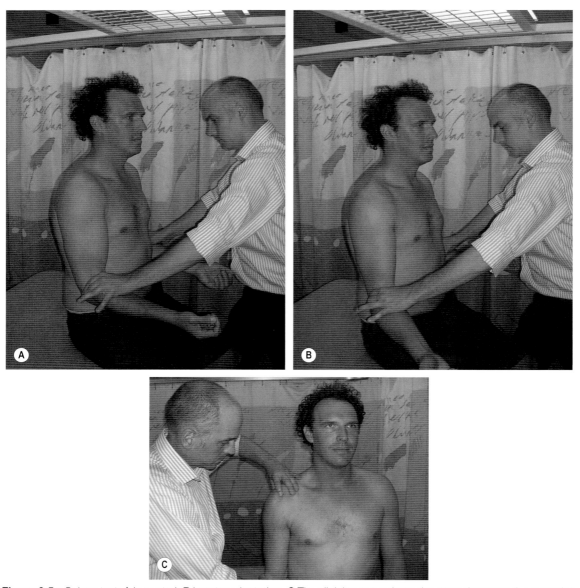

Figure 9.5 • Sulcus test: A in neutral; B in external rotation. C The clinician can palpate the space between the acromion and the head of the humerus whilst performing the sulcus test.

they may be the source of the symptoms, or they may be contributing to the symptoms. The most likely regions are the shoulder, sternoclavicular joint, cervical spine, thoracic spine, elbow, wrist and hand. The joints within these regions can be tested fully (see relevant chapter) or partially with the use of screening tests (see Chapter 3 for further details).

Some functional ability has already been tested by the general observation of the patient during the subjective and physical examinations, e.g. the postures adopted during the subjective examination and the ease or difficulty of undressing prior to the examination. Any further functional testing can be carried out at this point in the examination and may include various sitting postures or aggravating movements of the upper limb. Clues for appropriate tests can be obtained from the subjective examination findings, particularly aggravating factors.

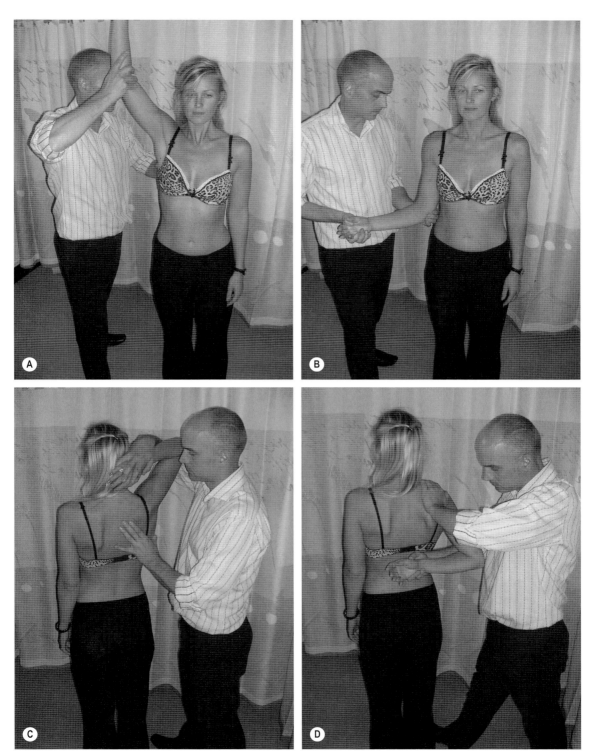

Figure 9.6 • Active movements with overpressure. **A** Flexion: apply pressure on the humerus into flexion whilst stabilising the scapula. **B** Lateral rotation: keeping the elbow close to the patient's side, apply pressure into lateral rotation. **C** Hand behind head (HBH): with the patient's arm in HBH position, apply further pressure into lateral rotation, adduction and flexion individually to test each component of the movement. **D** Hand behind back (HBB): with the patient's arm in HBB, apply further pressure into medial rotation, adduction and extension individually to test each component of the movement.

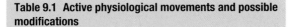

Table 9.1 Active physiological movements and possible modifications

Active physiological movements	Modifications
Shoulder girdle	
Elevation	Repeated
Depression	Speed altered
Protraction	Combined, e.g.
Retraction	– abduction with medial
Glenohumeral joint	or lateral rotation
Flexion	– medial/lateral rotation
Extension	with flexion
Abduction	Compression or
Adduction	distraction
Medial rotation	to scapulothoracic,
Lateral rotation	glenohumeral or
Hand behind neck (HBN)	acromioclavicular joints
Hand behind back (HBB)	Sustained
Horizontal flexion	Injuring movement
Horizontal extension	Differentiation tests
?Sternoclavicular joint	Functional ability
?Cervical spine	
?Thoracic spine	
?Elbow	
?Wrist and hand	

Capsular pattern. The capsular pattern for the glenohumeral joint is limitation of lateral rotation, abduction and medial rotation (Cyriax 1982).

Passive physiological movements

All the active movements described above can usually be examined passively with the patient in the supine position, comparing left and right sides. In addition, medial and lateral rotation of the scapula can be examined. A comparison of the response of symptoms to the active and passive movements can help to determine whether the structure at fault is non-contractile (articular) or contractile (extra-articular) (Cyriax 1982). If the lesion is non-contractile, such as ligament, then active and passive movements will be painful and/or restricted in the same direction. If the lesion is in a contractile tissue (i.e. muscle), active and passive movements are painful and/or restricted in opposite directions.

Muscle tests

Muscle strength

The clinician may choose to test the shoulder girdle elevators, depressors, protractors and retractors as well as the shoulder joint flexors, extensors, abductors, adductors, medial rotators and lateral rotators. For details of these general tests readers are directed to Cole et al. (1988), Hislop & Montgomery (1995) and Kendall et al. (1993). Greater detail may be required to test the strength of muscles, in particular those thought prone to become weak (Table 3.2); that is, serratus anterior, middle and lower fibres of trapezius and the deep neck flexors (Janda 1994). Testing the strength of these muscles is described in Chapter 3.

Isometric muscle testing for assessing muscle as a source of symptoms

The therapist may choose to test the shoulder girdle elevators, depressors, protractors and retractors, as well as the shoulder joint flexors, extensors, abductors, adductors, medial rotators and lateral rotators in the resting position and, if indicated, in different parts of the physiological range. In addition, the clinician observes the quality of the muscle contraction to hold this position (this can be done with the patient's eyes shut). The patient may, for example, be unable to prevent the joint from moving or may hold with excessive muscle activity; either of these circumstances may suggest a neuromuscular dysfunction.

Muscle control

There is good evidence to suggest that muscle control around the shoulder can be altered when pathology is present and that these changes may alter movement patterns at the shoulder (Ludewig & Cook 2000; Mell et al. 2005; Eckenode & Kelley 2008). Some of these changes will be obvious to the clinician, but more subtle changes may be difficult to interpret, and indeed the reliability of such observation has been shown to be low (Kibler et al. 2002). There is also known to be a wide range of muscle recruitment strategies both in people with no pain and more so in those with pain and pathology, and this makes visual assessment more complex (David et al. 2000; Shumway-Cook & Woollacott 2001; Magarey & Jones 2003). However, the clinician should observe the resting position of the scapula and note any abnormalities, such as excessive medial rotation, anterior tipping or superior migration. Abnormal scapular movement is a common problem with shoulder dysfunction. Common patterns of scapular movement in patients with pain or pathology are the loss of normal protraction and posterior tilt during glenohumeral elevation which can lead to the glenoid and humeral head congruency being lost. This can alter the optimal length–tension relationships of the scapular–humeral muscles and lead to altered dynamic control of the humeral head through range (Sahrmann 2002). Early or excessive scapular movement may occur with pathology, and the scapula may also fail to rotate fully laterally through range of elevation (Eckenode & Kelley 2008). This may be due to poor control of the scapulothoracic muscles, in particular the serratus anterior and trapezius. Overactivity in pectoralis minor may result in anterior tipping of the scapula. Excessive activity in the latissimus dorsi or the pectoralis major muscles may lead to muscle patterning problems and possible impingement or instability (Gibson 2005). Injury to the supraspinatus or the inferior cuff may lead to excessive superior translation of the humeral head and possible impingement problems (Eckenode & Kelley 2008). The clinician should be aware that optimal shoulder function is dependent not only on normal shoulder muscle activity, but also on normal muscle activity further down the kinetic chain, through the trunk and lower limbs (Kibler 1998).

Muscle length

The clinician mat choose to test the length of muscles, in particular those thought prone to shorten (Janda 1994); that is, latissimus dorsi, pectoralis major and minor, upper trapezius, levator scapulae and sternocleidomastoid. Testing the length of these muscles is described in Chapter 3.

Rotator cuff and biceps tests

Speed's test for bicipital tendinopathy (Figure 9.7). Tenderness in the bicipital groove when shoulder forward flexion is resisted (with forearm supination and elbow joint extension) suggests bicipital tendinopathy.

Yergason's test (Figure 9.8). The patient has the elbow flexed to 90° and forearm in full pronation. The clinician resists supination whilst palpating in the bicipital groove. Pain or subluxation of the tendon in the groove constitutes a positive test. Holtby & Razmjou (2004) found specificity of 79% and sensitivity of 43%.

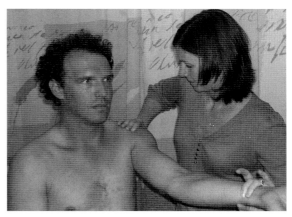

Figure 9.7 • Speed's test.

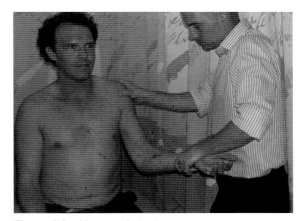

Figure 9.8 • Yergason's test.

Empty can test for supraspinatus tear (Figure 9.9). The patient abducts the arm to 90° in the scapular plane and then fully medially rotates the glenohumeral joint. The clinician then applies a force downwards towards the floor and the patient is asked to hold this position. The test is positive if there is reproduction of the patient's pain or there is weakness (Itoi et al. 1999). Muscle weakness is the greatest predictive indicator (Itoi et al. 1999).

Full can test for supraspinatus tear (Figure 9.10). This follows the same procedure as the empty can test but the shoulder is held in lateral rotation rather than medial rotation. This test is thought to be less pain-provoking than the empty can test. Weakness is a positive test and specificity has been found to be 77% and sensitivity 66% (Itoi et al. 1999).

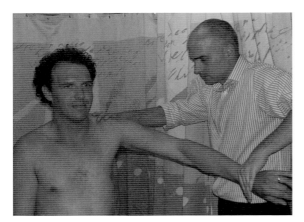

Figure 9.9 • Empty can test.

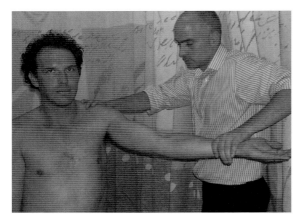

Figure 9.10 • Full can test.

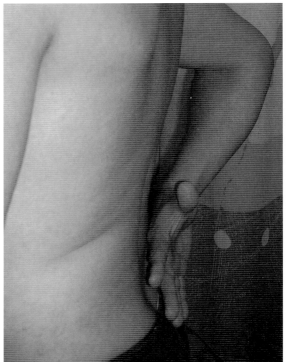

Figure 9.11 • Lift-off test.

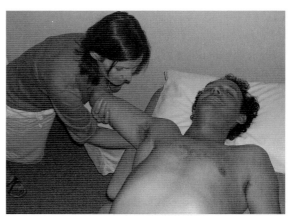

Figure 9.12 • Crank test.

Lift-off test (Gerber's test) (Figure 9.11). The patient puts the hand behind the back, with the dorsum of the hand resting on the mid-lumbar spine. The patient is asked to lift the hand away from the spine, to increase the internal rotation and extension at the glenohumeral joint. If the patient is unable to achieve this, then disruption of subscapularis is suspected.

Labral tests

Crank test (Figure 9.12). With the patient's shoulder in 160° of abduction in the scapular plane, the clinician applies an axial load through the glenohumeral joint, and then internally and externally rotates the arm. A positive test is indicated by pain with or without a click. Specificity has been found to vary from 56% to 93% and sensitivity from 46% to 91% (Liu et al. 1996; Stetson & Tenplin 2002).

Biceps load tests I and II (Figure 9.13)

- Biceps load test I: in 90° of abduction, with the patient's elbow in 90° flexion and the forearm supinated, the clinician resists elbow flexion. Pain reproduction indicates a positive test for a superior labral anterior posterior (SLAP) lesion.

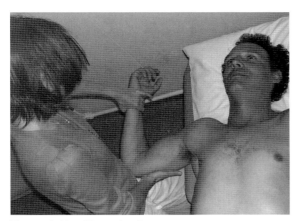

Figure 9.13 • Biceps load test.

Improvement in pain or apprehension indicates the absence of a SLAP lesion.

- Biceps load test II is the same as test I, performed at 120° of abduction. The choice of test should be guided by the range of abduction that is most provocative. Kim et al. (2001) found specificity to be 96.9% and sensitivity to be 89.7%.

Impingement tests

Neer test (Neer 1983) (Figure 9.14). With the patient in sitting the clinician forcibly elevates the shoulder in medial rotation. A pain response is positive for subacromial impingement. The specificity has been shown to be 30.5% and sensitivity 88.7% (Calis et al. 2000).

    Hawkins–Kennedy test (Hawkins & Bokor 1990) (Figure 9.15). With the patient in sitting with the shoulder and elbow flexed to 90°, the clinician fully internally rotates the patient's arm. Pain reproduction indicates a positive test. The arm can also be adducted if the initial test is negative. Specificity has been shown to be between 25% and 44% and sensitivity between 87% and 92% (Calis et al. 2000; Macdonald et al. 2000).

Neurological tests

Neurological examination includes neurological integrity testing and neurodynamic tests. These are not routinely examined, and are only indicated if the patient complains of neurological symptoms, or has pain in a distribution that may indicate neurological involvement, e.g. in a dermatomal pattern. Readers

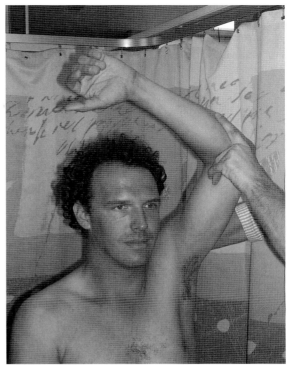

Figure 9.14 • Neer test.

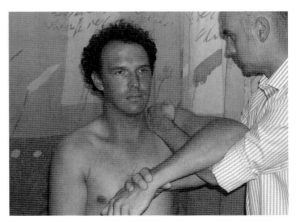

Figure 9.15 • Hawkins–Kennedy test.

are referred to Chapter 3 for neural integrity testing of the upper limb.

Neurodynamic tests

The upper-limb neurodynamic tests (ULNTs) may be carried out in order to ascertain the degree to which neural tissue is responsible for producing the patient's symptoms. The choice of tests should be influenced by the distribution of the patient's symptoms, e.g. if the patient has posterior upper-arm and lateral elbow pain, then ULNTs with a radial nerve bias may be indicated. These tests are described in detail in Chapter 3.

Vascular tests

Allen test. With the patient sitting and the arm abducted to 90°, the clinician horizontally extends and laterally rotates the arm (Magee 1997). Disappearance of the radial pulse on contralateral cervical rotation is indicative of thoracic outlet syndrome.

Adson's manoeuvre. In sitting, the patient's head is rotated towards the tested arm (Magee 1997). The patient then extends the head while the clinician extends and laterally rotates the shoulder. The patient then takes a deep breath and disappearance of the radial pulse indicates a positive test. It should be noted that disappearance of the pulse has been found to occur in a large percentage of asymptomatic subjects (Young & Hardy 1983; Swift & Nichols 1984).

Palpation of pulses

If it is suspected that the circulation is compromised, the brachial pulse is palpated on the medial aspect of the humerus in the axilla.

Palpation

The shoulder region is palpated, as well as the cervical spine and thoracic spine and upper limbs as appropriate. It is useful to record palpation findings on a body chart (see Figure 2.3) and/or palpation chart (see Figure 3.36).

The clinician notes the following:

- the temperature of the area
- localised increased skin moisture
- the presence of oedema or effusion
- mobility and feel of superficial tissues, e.g. ganglions, nodules and scar tissue
- the presence or elicitation of any muscle spasm
- tenderness of bone, bursae (subacromial and subdeltoid), ligaments, muscle, tendon (long head of biceps, subscapularis, infraspinatus, teres minor, supraspinatus, pectoralis major and long head of triceps), tendon sheath, trigger points

(shown in Figure 3.37) and nerve. Palpable nerves in the upper limb are as follows:

- ○ The suprascapular nerve can be palpated along the superior border of the scapula in the suprascapular notch.
- ○ The dorsal scapular nerve can be palpated medial to the medial border of the scapula.
- ○ The brachial plexus can be palpated in the posterior triangle of the neck; it emerges at the lower third of sternocleidomastoid.
- ○ The median nerve can be palpated over the anterior elbow joint crease, medial to the biceps tendon, also at the wrist between palmaris longus and flexor carpi radialis.
- ○ The radial nerve can be palpated around the spiral groove of the humerus, between brachioradialis and flexor carpi radialis, in the forearm and also at the wrist in the snuffbox.
- increased or decreased prominence of bones
- pain provoked or reduced on palpation.

Accessory movements

It is useful to use the palpation chart and movement diagrams (or joint pictures) to record findings. These are explained in detail in Chapter 3.

The clinician notes the:

- quality of movement
- range of movement
- resistance through the range and at the end of the range of movement
- behaviour of pain through the range
- provocation of any muscle spasm.

Glenohumeral, acromioclavicular and sternoclavicular joint accessory movements should be tested in provocative positions/ranges when the patient is non-severe and non-irritable, as this is most likely to reproduce symptoms and guide treatment. Some accessory movements to the glenohumeral joint are shown in Figure 9.16. A list of accessory movements with possible modifications is provided in Table 9.2. The neutral position can be useful in severe and irritable patients, or as an initial testing procedure to familiarise the patient with handling techniques. Following accessory movements to the shoulder region, the clinician reassesses all the physical

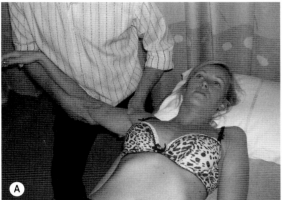

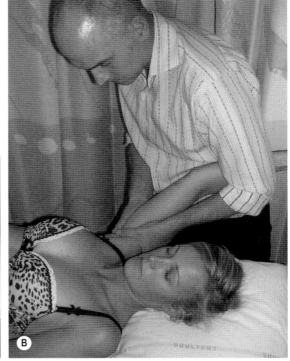

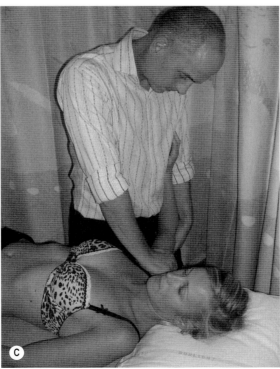

Figure 9.16 • A Longitudinal caudad in abduction: apply a force towards the patient's feet, pushing through the humeral head. This technique can be applied in different ranges of movement depending on the patient presentation.
B Posteroanterior glenohumeral joint in elevation: apply a posteroanterior pressure through the head of humerus. Lateral or longitudinal glides may also be used in this position depending on the patient presentation and movement restriction.
C Anteroposterior glenohumeral joint in abduction: support the patient's elbow with one hand and apply an anteroposterior force through the head of humerus with the other hand. This technique can be applied in different ranges of movement depending on the patient presentation.

Table 9.2 Accessory movements, choice of application and reassessment of the patient's asterisks

Accessory movements	Choice of application	Identify any effect of accessory movements on patient's signs and symptoms
Glenohumeral joint ↕ Anteroposterior ↕ Posteroanterior ←•• Caud Longitudinal caudad ←•• Ceph Longitudinal cephalad •→ Lat Lateral •→ Med Medial	Start position, e.g. — glenohumeral joint in flexion, abduction — acromioclavicular joint accessory movements carried out with glenohumeral joint in horizontal flexion Speed of force application Direction of the applied force Point of application of applied force	Reassess all asterisks
Acromioclavicular joint ↕ Anteroposterior ↕ Posteroanterior ←•• Caud Longitudinal caudad		
Sternoclavicular joint ↕ Anteroposterior ↕ Posteroanterior ←•• Caud Longitudinal caudad ←•• Ceph Longitudinal cephalad		
Cervical spine	As above	Reassess all asterisks
Thoracic spine	As above	Reassess all asterisks
Elbow	As above	Reassess all asterisks
Wrist and hand	As above	Reassess all asterisks

asterisks in order to establish the effect of the accessory movements on the patient's signs and symptoms. Accessory movements can then be tested for other regions suspected to be a source of, or contributing to, the patient's symptoms. Again, following accessory movements to any one region, the clinician reassesses all the asterisks. Regions that may be examined are the cervical spine, thoracic spine, elbow, wrist and hand.

Completion of the examination

Having carried out the above tests, the examination of the shoulder region is now complete. The subjective and physical examinations produce a large amount of information, which must be recorded accurately and quickly. It is vital at this stage to highlight with an asterisk (*) important findings from the examination.

These findings must be reassessed at, and within, subsequent treatment sessions to evaluate the effects of treatment on the patient's condition.

The physical testing procedures which specifically indicate joint, nerve or muscle tissues as a source of the patient's symptoms are summarised in Table 3.10. The strongest evidence that a joint is the source of the patient's symptoms is that active and passive physiological movements, passive accessory movements and joint palpation all reproduce the patient's symptoms, and that, following a treatment dose, reassessment identifies an improvement in the patient's signs and symptoms. Weaker evidence includes an alteration in range, resistance or quality of physiological and/ or accessory movements and tenderness over the joint, with no alteration in signs and symptoms after treatment. One or more of these findings may indicate a dysfunction of a joint, which may or may not be contributing to the patient's condition.

The strongest evidence that a muscle is the source of a patient's symptoms is if active movements, an isometric contraction, passive lengthening and palpation of a muscle all reproduce the patient's symptoms, and that, following a treatment dose, reassessment identifies an improvement in the patient's signs and symptoms. Further evidence of muscle dysfunction may be suggested by reduced strength or poor quality during the active physiological movement and the isometric contraction, reduced range, and/or increased/decreased resistance, during the passive lengthening of the muscle, and tenderness on palpation, with no alteration in signs and symptoms after treatment. One or more of these findings may indicate a dysfunction of a muscle, which may or may not be contributing to the patient's condition.

The strongest evidence that a nerve is the source of the patient's symptoms is when active and/or passive physiological movements reproduce the symptoms, which are then increased or decreased with an additional sensitising movement, at a distance from the symptoms. In addition, there is reproduction of the patient's symptoms on palpation of the nerve and following neurodynamic testing, and, following a treatment dose, reassessment identifies an improvement in the patient's signs and symptoms. Further evidence of nerve dysfunction may be suggested by reduced range (compared with the asymptomatic side) and/or increased resistance to the various arm movements, and tenderness on nerve palpation.

On completion of the physical examination the clinician will:

- explain the findings of the physical examination and how these findings relate to the subjective assessment. An attempt should be made to clear up any misconceptions patients may have regarding their illness or injury
- collaborate with the patient and via problem-solving together devise a treatment plan and discuss the prognosis

- warn the patient of possible exacerbation up to 24–48 hours following the examination
- request the patient to report details on the behaviour of the symptoms following examination at the next attendance
- explain the findings of the physical examination and how these findings relate to the subjective assessment. It is helpful to clear up any misconceptions patients may have regarding their illness or injury
- evaluate the findings, formulate a clinical hypothesis and write up a problem list
- determine the objectives of treatment
- devise an initial treatment plan.

In this way, the clinician will have developed the following hypotheses categories (adapted from Jones & Rivett 2004):

- function: abilities and restrictions
- patient's perspective on his/her experience
- source of symptoms, including the structure or tissue that is thought to be producing the patient's symptoms, the nature of the structure or tissues in relation to the healing process and the pain mechanisms
- contributing factors to the development and maintenance of the problem. There may be environmental, psychosocial, behavioural, physical or heredity factors
- precautions/contraindications to treatment and management. This includes the severity and irritability of the patient's symptoms and the nature of the patient's condition
- management strategy and treatment plan
- prognosis – this can be affected by factors such as the stage and extent of the injury as well as the patient's expectation, personality and lifestyle.

For guidance on treatment and management principles, the reader is directed to the companion textbook (Petty 2011).

References

Brown, C., 1983. Compressive, invasive referred pain to the shoulder. Clin. Orthop. Relat. Res. 173, 55–62.

Calis, M., Akgün, K., Birtane, M., et al., 2000. Diagnostic values of clinical diagnostic tests in subacromial impingement syndrome. Ann. Rheum. Dis. 59, 44–47.

Cole, J.H., Furness, A.L., Twomey, L.T., 1988. Muscles in action, an approach to manual muscle testing. Churchill Livingstone, Edinburgh.

Cyriax, J., 1982. Textbook of orthopaedic medicine – diagnosis of soft tissue lesions, eighth ed. Baillière Tindall, London.

David, G., Magarey, M., Jones, M., et al., 2000. EMG and strength correlates of selected shoulder muscles during rotations of the glenohumeral joint. J. Clin. Biomech. 2, 95–102.

Eckenode, B.J., Kelley, M.J., 2008. Clinical biomechanics of the shoulder. In: Wilk, K.E., Reinold, M.M.,

Andrew, J.R. (Eds.), The athlete's shoulder, second ed. Churchill Livingstone, London, pp. 16–35.

Gerber, C., Ganz, R., 1984. Clinical assessment of instability of the shoulder. J. Bone Joint Surg. 66B (4), 551–556.

Gibson, J., 2005. Muscle patterning instability. In: Proceedings from Kinetic Control and MACP 2nd International Conference on Movement Dysfunction, Edinburgh.

Grieve, G.P., 1994a. Counterfeit clinical presentations. Manipulative Physiotherapist 26, 17–19.

Grieve, G.P., 1994b. Thoracic musculoskeletal problems. In: Grieve, G.P. (Ed.), Modern manual therapy of the vertebral column. Churchill Livingstone, Edinburgh, ch 29, pp. 401–428.

Hawkins, R.J., Bokor, D.J., 1990. Clinical evaluation of shoulder problems. In: Rockwood, C.A., Matsen, F.A. (Eds.), The shoulder. W B Saunders, Philadelphia, p. 149.

Hawkins, R.J., McCormack, R.G., 1988. Posterior shoulder instability. Orthopedics 11 (2), 101–107.

Hill, A.M., Bull, A.M.J., Richardson, J., et al., 2008. The clinical assessment and classification of shoulder instability. Curr. Orthop. 22, 208–225.

Hislop, H., Montgomery, J., 1995. Daniels and Worthingham's muscle testing, techniques of manual examination, seventh ed. W B Saunders, Philadelphia.

Holtby, R., Razmjou, H., 2004. Accuracy of the Speeds and Yergasons tests in detecting biceps pathology and SLAP lesions; comparison with arthroscopic findings. Arthroscopy 20 (3), 231–236.

Itoi, E., Kido, T., Sano, A., et al., 1999. Which test is more useful, the full can test or the empty can test, in detecting a torn supraspinatus tendon? Am. J. Sports Med. 27 (1), 65–68.

Janda, V., 1994. Muscles and motor control in cervicogenic disorders: assessment and management. In: Grant, R. (Ed.), Physical therapy of the cervical and thoracic spine, second ed. Churchill Livingstone, New York, p. 195.

Janda, V., 2002. Muscles and motor control in cervicogenic disorders. In: Grant, R. (Ed.), Physical therapy of the cervical and thoracic spine, third ed. Churchill Livingstone, New York, p. 182.

Jobe, F.W., Kvitne, R.S., Giangarra, C.E., 1989. Shoulder pain in the overhand or throwing athlete: the relationship of anterior instability and rotator cuff impingement. Orthop. Rev. 18, 963–975.

Jones, M.A., Rivett, D.A., 2004. Clinical reasoning for manual therapists. Butterworth-Heinemann, Edinburgh.

Kendall, F.P., McCreary, E.K., Provance, P.G., 1993. Muscles testing and function, fourth ed. Williams & Wilkins, Baltimore.

Kibler, W.B., 1998. The role of the scapula in athletic shoulder function. Am. J. Sports Med. 26 (2), 335–339.

Kibler, W.B., Uhl, T.L., Maddin, J.W., 2002. Qualitative clinical evaluation of scapular dysfunction: a reliability study. J. Shoulder Elbow Surg. 11, 550–556.

Kim, S.H., Ha, K.I., Ahn, J.H., et al., 2001. Biceps load test II: a clinical test for SLAP lesions of the shoulder. Arthroscopy 17 (2), 160–164.

Liu, S.H., Henry, M.H., Nuccion, S.L., 1996. A prospective evaluation of a new physical examination in predicting labral tears. Am. J. Sports Med. 24 (6), 721–725.

Lo, I.K., Nonweiler, B., Woolfrey, M., et al., 2004. An evaluation of the apprehension, relocation and surprise tests for anterior shoulder instability. Am. J. Sports Med. 32 (2), 301–307.

Ludewig, P.M., Cook, T.M., 2000. Alterations in shoulder kinematics and associated muscle activity in people with symptoms of shoulder impingement. Phys. Ther. 80, 276–291.

Macdonald, P.B., Clark, P., Sutherland, K., 2000. An analysis of the diagnostic accuracy of the Hawkins and Neer subacromial impingement signs. J. Shoulder Elbow Surg. 9 (4), 299–301.

Magarey, M., Jones, M., 2003. Dynamic evaluation and early management of altered motor control around the shoulder complex. Man. Ther. 8 (4), 195–206.

Magee, D.J., 1997. Orthopedic physical assessment, third ed. W B Saunders, Philadelphia.

Maitland, G.D., 1991. Peripheral manipulation, third ed. Butterworth-Heinemann, London.

Matsen, F.A., Thomas, S.C., Rockwood, C.A., 1990. Anterior glenohumeral instability. In: Rockwood, C.A., Matsen, F.A. (Eds.), The shoulder. W B Saunders, Philadelphia, p. 526.

Mell, A.R., Lascalza, S., Goffey, P., 2005. Effect of rotator cuff pathology on shoulder rhythm. J. Shoulder Elbow Surg. 14, 58S–64S.

Neer, C.S., 1983. Impingement lesions. Clin. Orthop. Relat. Res. 173, 70–77.

Petty, N.J., 2011. Principles of neuromusculoskeletal treatment and management: a guide for therapists, second ed. Churchill Livingstone, Edinburgh.

Sahrmann, S.A., 2002. Diagnosis and treatment of movement impairment syndromes. Mosby, St Louis.

Shumway-Cook, A., Woollacott, M.J., 2001. Motor control: theory and practical applications. Lippincott Williams and Wilkins, Philadelphia.

Stetson, W.B., Tenplin, K., 2002. The Crank test, the Obrien test and routine magnetic resonance imaging scans in the diagnosis of labral tears. Am. J. Sports Med. 30 (6), 806–809.

Swift, T.R., Nichols, F.T., 1984. The droopy shoulder syndrome. Neurology 34, 212–215.

Tzannes, A., Murrell, G.A.C., 2002. Clinical examination of the unstable shoulder. Sports Med. 32 (7), 447–457.

Waddell, G., 2004. The back pain revolution, second ed. Churchill Livingstone, Edinburgh.

Young, H.A., Hardy, D.G., 1983. Thoracic outlet syndrome. Br. J. Hosp. Med. 29, 459–461.

Examination of the elbow region

Dionne Ryder

CHAPTER CONTENTS

Possible causes of pain and/or limitation of movement

This region includes the humeroulnar joint, the radiohumeral joint and the superior radioulnar joints with their surrounding soft tissues.

- Trauma:
  - ○ fracture of humerus, radius or ulna
  - ○ dislocation of the head of the radius (most commonly seen in young children)
  - ○ ligamentous sprain
  - ○ muscular strain
  - ○ Volkmann's ischaemic contracture
- Common flexor origin dysfunction/lateral epicondylalgia/tennis elbow
- Common extensor origin dysfunction/medial epicondylalgia/golfer's elbow
- Degenerative conditions: osteoarthrosis
- Calcification of tendons or muscles, e.g. myositis ossificans
- Inflammatory disorders: rheumatoid arthritis
- Infection, e.g. tuberculosis
- Compression of, or injury to, the ulnar nerve
- Bursitis (of subcutaneous olecranon, subtendinous olecranon, radioulnar or bicipitoradial bursa)
- Cubital varus or cubital valgus
- Neoplasm: rare
- Hypermobility syndrome
- Referral of symptoms from the cervical spine, thoracic spine, shoulder, wrist or hand.

Further details of the questions asked during the subjective examination and the tests carried out in the physical examination can be found in Chapters 2 and 3 respectively.

The order of the subjective questioning and the physical tests described below should be justified through sound clinical reasoning and appropriate for the patient being examined.

Subjective examination

Body chart

The following information concerning the type and area of current symptoms can be recorded on a body chart (see Figure 2.3).

Area of current symptoms

Be precise when mapping out the area of the symptoms. A lesion in the elbow joint complex may refer symptoms distally to the forearm and hand, particularly if the common flexor or extensor tendons of the forearm are affected at the elbow. Ascertain which is the worst symptom and record where the patient feels the symptoms are coming from.

Areas relevant to the region being examined

It is important to check for any symptoms, for example pain and/or stiffness, in the cervical spine, thoracic spine and shoulder, as these are areas capable of referring symptoms into the elbow and so may be relevant to the patient's main symptoms. Mark unaffected areas with ticks (✓) on the body chart.

Quality of pain

Establish the quality of the pain in order to assist in determining possible pain mechanisms, e.g. sharp, burning.

Intensity of pain

The intensity of pain can be measured using, for example, a visual analogue scale, as shown in Chapter 2.

Depth of pain

Establish the depth of the pain. Does the patient feel it is on the surface or deep inside?

Abnormal sensation

Check for any altered sensation (such as paraesthesia or numbness) locally around the elbow region as well as over the shoulder and spine and distally in the wrist and hand.

Constant or intermittent symptoms

Ascertain the frequency of the symptoms, whether they are constant or intermittent. If symptoms are constant, check whether there is variation in the intensity of the symptoms, as constant unremitting pain may be indicative of a serious pathology.

Relationship of symptoms

Through careful questioning of the patient determine the relationship between the symptomatic areas, e.g. do the symptoms come together or separately? Can the patient experience elbow pain without shoulder or neck pain or are the pains always present together? Which symptom comes on first?

Behaviour of symptoms

Aggravating factors

In order to determine the impact that symptoms in the upper limb may have on normal function the clinician must find out if the patient is left- or right-handed as there may be increased stress on the dominant side. For each symptomatic area, discover what movements and/or positions aggravate the patient's symptoms, i.e. what brings them on (or makes them worse)? is the patient able to maintain this position or movement (severity)? what happens to other symptoms when this symptom is produced (or is made worse)? and how long does it take for symptoms to ease once the position or movement is stopped (irritability)? These questions help to confirm the relationship between the symptoms.

The clinician also asks the patient about theoretically known aggravating factors for structures that could be a source of the symptoms. Common aggravating factors for the elbow are gripping, pronation and supination of the forearm. The clinician ascertains how the symptoms affect function, e.g. leaning on the forearm or hand, writing, turning a key in a lock, opening a bottle, typing, gripping, lifting, carrying, work, sport and leisure activities. Ask about the training regimen for any sporting activities.

Aggravating factors for other regions, which may need to be queried if they are suspected to be a source of the symptoms, are shown in Table 2.3.

Easing factors

For each symptomatic area, the clinician asks what movements and/or positions ease the patient's symptoms, how long it takes to ease them and what happens to other symptoms when this symptom is relieved. These questions help to confirm the relationship between the symptoms and determine their irritability.

The clinician asks the patient about theoretically known easing factors for structures that could be a source of the symptoms. For example, symptoms from the elbow joint may be relieved by pulling the forearm away from the upper arm and a semiflexed posture out of close pack extension will be a position of comfort. Symptoms from neural tissues may be relieved by shoulder girdle elevation, which reduces tension on the brachial plexus. Find out what happens to other symptoms when one symptom is relieved; this helps confirm the relationship of symptoms.

Using clinical reasoning skills the clinician can then analyse the positions or movements that aggravate or ease the symptoms to help determine the structure(s) at fault. This information can be used to determine the irritability of the condition, the appropriate vigour/extent of the physical examination, the aims of treatment and any advice that may be required.

The most notable functional restrictions are highlighted with asterisks (*), explored in the physical examination and reassessed at subsequent treatment sessions to evaluate treatment intervention.

Twenty-four-hour behaviour of symptoms

The clinician determines the 24-hour behaviour of symptoms by asking questions about night, morning and evening symptoms.

Night symptoms. Suggested questions to establish behavior of symptoms at night are detailed in Chapter 2. Elbow dysfunction may have an impact on sleep positions, as the patient may not be able to lie on the affected side.

Morning and evening symptoms. The clinician determines the pattern of the symptoms first thing in the morning, through the day and at the end of the day.

Stage of the condition

In order to determine the stage of the condition the clinician asks whether the symptoms are getting better, getting worse or remaining unchanged.

Special questions

Special questions must always be asked, as they may identify certain precautions or contraindications to the physical examination and/or treatment (see

Table 2.4). As mentioned in Chapter 2, the clinician must differentiate between neuromusculoskeletal conditions that are suitable for treatment and management and systemic, neoplastic and other non-neuromusculoskeletal conditions which require referral to a medical practitioner.

The following information is routinely obtained from patients.

General health. The clinician ascertains the state of the patient's general health and finds out if the patient suffers from any malaise, fatigue, fever, nausea or vomiting, stress, anxiety or depression.

Weight loss. Has the patient noticed any recent unexplained weight loss?

Serious illness. Does the patient have a history of serious pathology such as cancer, human immunodeficiency virus (HIV), tuberculosis?

Inflammatory arthritis. Has the patient (or a member of his/her family) been diagnosed as having an inflammatory condition such as rheumatoid arthritis or reactive arthritis such as ankylosing spondylitis?

Cardiovascular disease. Does the patient have a history of cardiovascular disease, e.g. angina, previous myocardial infarction, stroke? Does the patient have a pacemaker fitted?

Respiratory disease. Does the patient have any condition which affects breathing? If so, how is it managed?

Epilepsy. Is the patient epileptic? What type of seizures does s/he have and when was the last seizure?

Thyroid disease. Does the patient have a history of thyroid disease? How well is it managed? Thyroid dysfunction is associated with a higher incidence of neuromusculoskeletal conditions (Cakir et al. 2003).

Diabetes mellitus. Has the patient been diagnosed as having diabetes? How long since diagnosis? How is the diabetes managed? How well controlled is the condition? Diabetes mellitus is associated with delayed tissue healing and peripheral neuropathy.

Osteoporosis. Has the patient been diagnosed with osteoporosis? Patients who present with a history of fractures following falls should be considered at risk. Have they been investigated with a dual-energy X-ray absorptiometry (DXA) scan? If so, when? and what was the result?

Neurological symptoms. Has the patient experienced any neural tissue symptoms such as tingling, pins and needles, pain or hypersensitivity in the upper limb and/or hand? Consider whether symptoms are likely to be peripheral or spinal nerve in origin. Are these symptoms unilateral or bilateral?

Has the patient noticed any weakness in the hand? or has s/he experienced symptoms of spinal cord compression, which are bilateral tingling in the hands or feet and/or disturbance of gait?

Drug history. Has the patient been on long-term steroids? Has the patient been taking anticoagulants? Has the patient been taking medication for the current symptoms, either prescribed or over the counter? If so, what is s/he taking? How long has s/he been taking it? Is it effective? It is useful to ascertain when the patient took the last dose because medication prior to the assessment may mask symptoms during the physical examination (Chapter 2).

Radiograph and medical imaging. Has the patient been X-rayed or had any other medical tests recently? These results will provide information that will help guide rehabilitation and indicate likely prognosis. Other medical tests may include blood tests, magnetic resonance imaging or a bone scan. For further information on these tests, the reader is referred to Refshauge & Gass (2004).

History of the present condition

For each symptomatic area, the clinician needs to know how long the symptoms have been present. Did these symptoms develop suddenly or gradually? Was there a known cause that provoked the onset of the symptoms? If the onset of symptoms was associated with trauma, e.g. a fall, the clinician may ask why and how the patient fell. Did the patient fall on the outstretched hand, possibly fracturing the radial head, or on the tip of the elbow, injuring the olecranon? If associated with a throwing action did the patient feel a 'pop', which may indicate a ligamentous injury (Cain et al. 2003)? If the onset was gradual, can the development of symptoms be associated with a change in the patient's lifestyle, e.g. a new job or leisure activity or a change in sporting activity? To confirm the relationship of symptoms, the clinician asks what happened when symptoms first began and how over time symptoms have developed or changed. In addition the clinician needs to identify what treatment, if any, the patient has sought so far and its outcome. Is this the first episode or is there a history of elbow problems? If so, how many episodes? when were they? was there a cause? what was the duration of each episode? and did the patient fully recover between episodes? If there have been no previous episodes, has the patient had any episodes of stiffness in the cervical spine,

thoracic spine, shoulder, elbow, wrist, hand or any other relevant region?

Past medical history

The following information is obtained from the patient and/or medical notes:

- details of any medical history such as major or long-standing illnesses, accidents or surgery that are relevant to the patient's condition.

Social history

In order to treat the patient appropriately, it is important that the condition is managed within the context of the patient's social and work environment. Social history that is relevant to the onset and progression of the patient's problem is recorded. This includes age, employment, home situation and details of any leisure activities. Does the patient's job involve sustained positions of wrist flexion or extension, so implicating the common flexor/extensor origins at the elbow? Alternatively does the patient undertake repetitive activities, e.g. typing, pipetting, production line work? This information may indicate direct and/or indirect mechanical influences on the elbow. In cases of trauma, ask specifically about any potential compensation claims.

Family history

Family history that is relevant to the onset and progression of the patient's problem is recorded.

Expectations and goals

An appreciation of the possible influences of psychosocial risk factors highlights the importance of ascertaining the patient's perspective on the presenting condition. It is important to discuss with patients their experience and expectations they may have of therapy so that the clinician can use this to identify patient concerns and manage them appropriately (see Chapter 2).

Plan of the physical examination

When all this information has been collected, the subjective examination is complete. It is useful at this stage to reconfirm briefly with patients the clinician's understanding of their main complaint and offer them the opportunity to add anything that they may not have raised so far before explaining the purpose and plan for the physical examination. For ease of reference highlight with asterisks (*) important subjective findings and particularly one or more functional restrictions. These can be re-examined at subsequent treatment sessions to evaluate treatment intervention.

In order to plan the physical examination, the following hypotheses should be developed from the subjective examination:

- Are there any precautions and/or contraindications to elements of the physical examination that need to be explored further, such as neurological involvement, recent fracture, trauma, steroid therapy or rheumatoid arthritis? There may also be certain contraindications to further examination and treatment, e.g. symptoms of cord compression.

- Clinically reasoning throughout the subjective examination, using distribution of symptoms, pain mechanisms described, behaviour of symptoms as well as the history of onset, the clinician must decide on structures that could be the cause of the patient's symptoms. The clinician should have a prioritised list of working hypotheses based on the most likely causes of the patient's symptoms. These may include the structures underneath the symptomatic area, e.g. joints, muscles, nerves and fascia, as well as the regions referring into the area. These possible referring regions will need to be examined as a possible cause of symptoms, e.g. cervical spine, thoracic spine, shoulder and wrist and hand. In complex cases it is not always possible to examine fully at the first attendance and so, using clinical reasoning skills, the clinician will need to prioritise and justify what 'must' be examined in the first assessment session and what 'should' or 'could' be followed up at subsequent sessions.

- What are the pain mechanisms driving the patient's symptoms? and what impact will this information have on an understanding of the patient's problem and subsequent management decisions? For example, pain associated with repetitive activities may indicate inflammatory or neurogenic nociception. This would indicate an early assessment of activities and advice to the patient to pace activities. Patients' acceptance and willingness to be an active participant in their management will depend on their perspective and subsequent behavioural response to their symptoms. If patients are demonstrating fear avoidance behaviours, then the clinician's ability to explain and teach them about their condition will be pivotal to achieving a successful outcome.

- Once the clinician has decided on the tests to include in the physical examination the next consideration should be how the physical tests should be carried out? Are symptoms severe and/or irritable? Will it be easy or hard to reproduce each symptom? If symptoms are severe, physical tests may be carried out to just before the onset of symptom production or just to the onset of symptom production; no overpressures will be carried out, as the patient would be unable to tolerate this. If symptoms are irritable, physical tests may be examined to just before symptom production or just to the onset of provocation, with fewer physical tests being examined to allow for a rest period between tests. Alternatively, will it be necessary to use combined movements and repetitive movements in order to reproduce the patient's symptoms?

A physical planning form can be useful for clinicians to help guide them through the clinical reasoning process (see Figure 2.10).

Physical examination

The information from the subjective examination helps the clinician to plan an appropriate physical examination. The severity, irritability and nature of the condition are the major factors that will influence the choice and priority of physical testing procedures. The first and overarching question the clinician might ask is: 'Does this patient have a neuromusculoskeletal dysfunction?' If the answer is yes then the second question the clinician might ask is: 'Is this neuromusculoskeletal dysfunction suitable for me to manage?' To answer that, the clinician needs to carry out an appropriate physical examination; however, this may not be possible if the symptoms are severe and/or irritable. If the patient's symptoms are severe and/or irritable, the clinician aims to explore movements as much as possible within a symptom-free range. If the patient has constant and severe and/or irritable symptoms, then the clinician aims to find physical tests that ease the symptoms. If the patient's symptoms are non-severe and non-irritable, then the clinician aims to find physical tests that reproduce each of the patient's symptoms.

Each significant physical test that either provokes or eases the patient's symptoms is highlighted in the patient's notes by an asterisk (*) for easy reference. The highlighted tests are often referred to as 'asterisks' or 'markers'.

The order and detail of the physical tests described below will need to be modified for the patient being examined; some tests will be irrelevant, some tests will be carried out briefly, while it will be necessary to investigate others more fully. It is important that readers understand that the techniques shown in this chapter are some of many; technique selection will depend on the patient's complaint, the relative size of the clinician and patient, as well as the clinician's preference.

Observation

Informal observation

Informal observation will begin from the moment the clinician meets the patient to walk him or her through to the treatment area and continue to the end of the physical examination. The clinician should note the patient's ability and willingness to move the upper limb as well as their general posture.

Formal observation

Observation of posture. The patient should be suitably undressed so that the clinician can observe the bony landmarks and soft-tissue contours of the elbow region, as well as the patient's posture in sitting and standing, noting the posture of the head and neck, thoracic spine and upper limbs. Right and left sides should be compared. Poor posture of the neck, trunk and upper limbs, e.g. tight pectoralis minor and weak lower trapezius, have been identified in sports people with elbow pathology (Wilke et al. 2002). If the patient's posture is corrected, does this change the patient's symptoms? The clinician can assess the carrying angle of the elbow by placing the patient's arm in the anatomical position. The normal carrying angle is 5–10° in males and 10–15° in females; greater than 15° is cubital valgus and less than 5–10° is cubital varus (Magee 2006). If there is swelling at the elbow then the joint may be held in a semiflexed position out of close pack position. If the patient demonstrates elbow hyperextension then more generalised hypermobility should be assessed (Simmonds & Keer 2007).

Observation of muscle form. The clinician examines the muscle bulk and muscle tone of the patient, comparing left and right sides. It must be remembered that handedness and level and frequency of physical activity may well produce differences in muscle bulk between sides.

Observation of soft tissues. The clinician observes the colour of the patient's skin and notes any swelling over the elbow region, e.g. olecranon bursitis will be evident by swelling over the olecranon process or related areas.

Observation of the patient's attitudes and feelings. The age, gender and ethnicity of patients and their cultural, occupational and social backgrounds may affect their attitudes and feelings towards themselves, their condition and the clinician. The clinician needs to be aware of and sensitive to these attitudes, and to empathise and communicate appropriately so as to develop a rapport with the patient and thereby enhance the patient's compliance with the treatment.

Joint integrity tests

The clinician observes the relative position of the olecranon and the medial and lateral epicondyles. They should form a straight line with the elbow in extension and an isosceles triangle with the elbow in 90° flexion (Figure 10.1) (Magee 2006). Alteration in this positioning may indicate a fracture or dislocation.

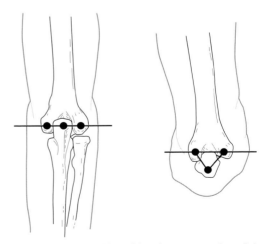

Figure 10.1 • The position of the olecranon and medial and lateral epicondyles should form a straight line with the elbow in extension and an isosceles triangle with the elbow flexed to 90°. (From Magee 2006, with permission.)

Ligamentous instability test

The medial (ulnar) collateral ligament is tested by applying an abduction force to the forearm with the elbow in 20–30° flexion. The lateral (radial) collateral ligament is tested by applying an adduction force to the forearm with the elbow in 20–30° flexion. These tests are shown in Figure 10.2A and B. Quality of end-feel, excessive movement or reproduction of the patient's symptoms is a positive test and suggests instability of the elbow joint (Volz & Morrey 1993).

Posterolateral pivot shift apprehension test (O'Driscoll et al. 1991)

Recurrent posteroloateral instability of the elbow can be difficult to diagnose. To test for the presence of instability the patient lies supine with the arm raised above the head whilst the clinician grasps the patient's wrist and elbow. A supination force is applied through the wrist. The elbow is then flexed with valgus stress and axial compression applied at the elbow. Increasing patient apprehension with increasing flexion indicates a positive test. It is thought that the cause of posterolateral instability is due to laxity of the ulnar portion of the ulnohumeral collateral ligament resulting in rotatory subluxation of the ulnohumeral joint and secondary dislocation of the radiohumeral joint.

Functional testing

Some functional ability has already been assessed through general observation of the patient during the subjective and physical examinations, e.g. the postures adopted during the subjective examination

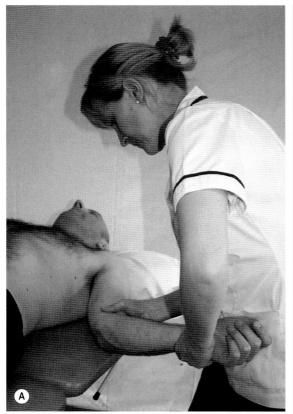
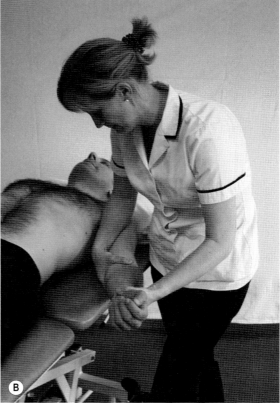

Figure 10.2 • Passive physiological movements to the elbow complex. **A** Abduction. The right hand stabilises the humerus while the left hand abducts the forearm. **B** Adduction. The right hand stabilises the humerus while the left hand adducts the forearm.

(Continued)

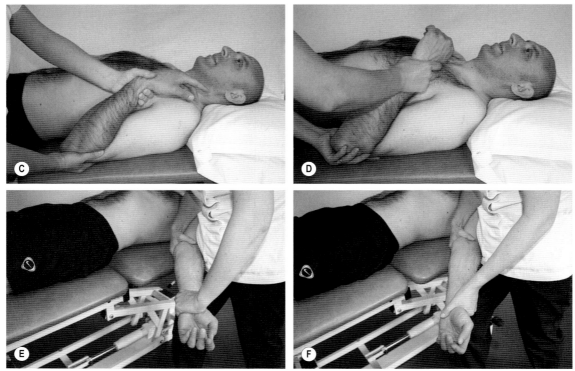

Figure 10.2—cont'd • **C** Flexion/abduction. The right hand supports underneath the upper arm while the left hand takes the arm into flexion and abduction. **D** Flexion/adduction. The left hand supports underneath the upper arm while the right hand takes the arm into flexion and adduction. **E** Extension/abduction. The right hand supports underneath the upper arm while the left hand takes the arm into extension and abduction. **F** Extension/adduction. The right hand supports underneath the upper arm while the left hand takes the forearm into extension and adduction.

and the ease or difficulty of undressing prior to the examination. Clues for assessment of suitable functional movements can be obtained from the subjective examination findings, particularly aggravating factors. The American Shoulder and Elbow Surgeons have adopted a standardised form for assessment of the elbow, including functional components to standardised elbow assessment (King et al. 1999). Does the patient have a functional range into flexion? The major role of the elbow is to allow the hand to be brought towards the mouth for drinking and eating tasks. For this the patient will need to have 90° flexion mid-position between pronation and supination.

Active physiological movements

For active physiological movements of the elbow complex, the clinician makes a note of the following:

• range of movement
• quality of movement

• behaviour of pain through the range of movement
• resistance through the range of movement and at the end of the range of movement
• provocation of any muscle spasm.

A movement diagram can be used to depict this information. The active movements with overpressure listed below and shown in Figure 10.3 are tested with the patient lying supine or sitting. Movements are carried out on the left and right sides. The clinician establishes symptoms at rest prior to each movement, and corrects any movement deviation to determine its relevance to the patient's symptoms. Active physiological movements of the elbow and forearm and possible modifications are shown in Table 10.1.

Various differentiation tests (Maitland et al. 2005) can be performed; the choice depends on the patient's signs and symptoms. For example, when elbow flexion reproduces the patient's elbow pain, differentiation between the radiohumeral and

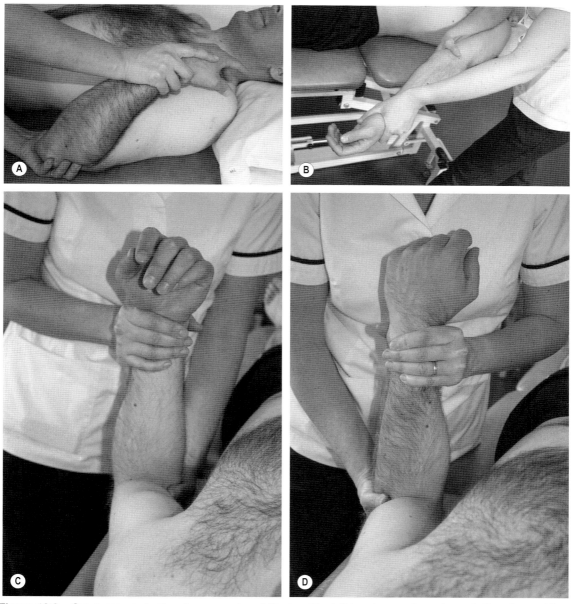

Figure 10.3 • Overpressures to the elbow complex. **A** Flexion. The left hand supports underneath the elbow while the right hand flexes the elbow. **B** Extension. The right hand supports underneath the elbow while the left hand extends the elbow. **C** Supination. **D** Pronation.

humeroulnar joint may be required. In this case, the clinician takes the elbow into flexion to produce the symptoms and then in turn adds a compression force through the radius and then through the ulna by radial and ulnar deviation of the wrist and compares the pain response in each case (Figure 10.4). If symptoms are from the radioulnar joint, for example, then the patient may feel an increase in pain when compression is applied to the radiohumeral joint but not when compression is applied to the humero-ulnar joint. The converse would occur for the humer-oulnar joint.

Table 10.1 Active physiological movements and possible modifications

Active physiological movements	Modifications
Elbow flexion	Repeated
Elbow extension	Speed altered
Forearm pronation	Combined, e.g.
Forearm supination	— flexion with pronation or
?Shoulder	supination
?Cervical spine	— pronation with elbow flexion or
?Thoracic spine	Extension
?Wrist and hand	Compression or distraction, e.g.
	— compression to humeroulnar
	joint in flexion
	Sustained
	Injuring movement
	Differentiation tests
	Function

Capsular pattern. The capsular pattern for the elbow joint is greater limitation of flexion than extension, and the pattern for the inferior radioulnar joint is full range with pain at extremes of range (Cyriax 1982).

It may be necessary to examine other regions to determine their relevance to the patient's symptoms; they may be the source of the symptoms, or they may be contributing to the symptoms. The regions most likely are the shoulder, cervical spine, thoracic spine, wrist and hand. The joints within these regions can be tested fully (see relevant chapter) or partially with the use of screening tests provided in Chapter 3.

Mobilisations with movement (MWMs). (Mulligan 1999). MWMs are sustained accessory glides applied to a joint during active or passive movement. Although largely seen as treatment techniques, MWMs can serve as a useful diagnostic tool.

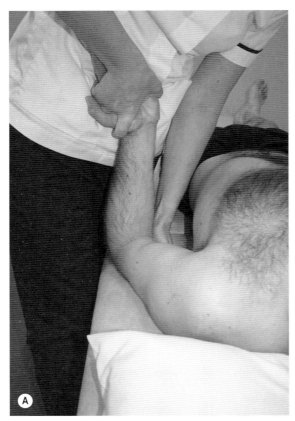 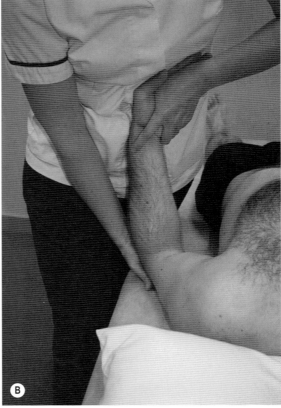

Figure 10.4 • Differentiation test between the radiohumeral and humeroulnar joint. The clinician takes the elbow into flexion to produce the symptoms and then in turn adds a compression force through the radius (**A**) and then the ulna (**B**) by taking the wrist into radial and ulnar deviation respectively.

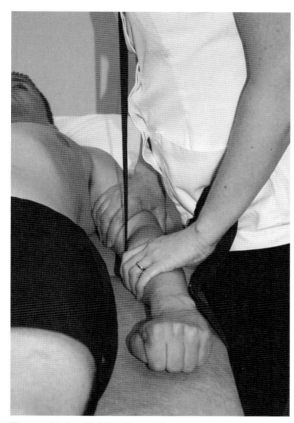

Figure 10.5 • Mobilisations with movement for lateral elbow pain on wrist extension and finger flexion. The right hand supports the upper arm while the left hand applies a lateral glide and the patient actively extends the wrist and/or flexes the fingers.

The patient is positioned supine with the upper limb fully supported in internal rotation and forearm pronation. Using a seatbelt the clinician applies a lateral glide to the ulna as the patient actively extends the wrist and/or flexes the fingers (Figure 10.5). For patients with suspected tennis elbow, pain relief is a positive finding, indicating a tracking or positional fault at the elbow that is contributing to the soft-tissue lesion (Vicenzino 2003). These techniques can be used to confirm and refute hypotheses.

Passive physiological movements

All the active movements described above can be examined passively with the patient usually in supine, comparing left and right sides. A comparison of the response of symptoms to the active and passive movements can help to determine whether the structure at fault is non-contractile (articular) or contractile (extra-articular) (Cyriax 1982). If the lesion due to dysfunction is non-contractile, such as would occur in ligaments, then active and passive movements will be painful and/or restricted in the same direction. If the lesion is in a contractile tissue (i.e. muscle), then active and passive movements are painful and/or restricted in opposite directions.

Additional movement (Figure 10.2) can be tested passively (Maitland et al. 2005), including:

- abduction
- adduction
- flexion/abduction
- flexion/adduction
- extension/abduction
- extension/adduction.

Muscle tests

Muscle tests include examining muscle strength, length and isometric muscle testing.

Muscle strength

The clinician tests the elbow flexors, extensors, forearm pronators, supinators and wrist flexors, extensors, radial deviators and ulnar deviators and any other relevant muscle groups. For details of these general tests, readers are directed to Cole et al. (1988), Hislop & Montgomery (1995) or Kendall et al. (1993). Greater detail may be required to test the strength of muscles, in particular those thought prone to weakness (Janda 1994, 2002). These muscles and a description of the tests for muscle strength are given in Chapter 3. Pain and weakness on gripping is a sign of lateral epicondylalgia (Haker 1993).

Muscle length

The clinician tests for lateral epicondylalgia by stretching the extensor muscles of the wrist and hand. This is done by extending the elbow, pronating the forearm and then flexing the wrist and fingers (Mills test). A positive test (i.e. muscle shortening) is indicated if the patient's symptoms are reproduced or if range of movement is limited compared with the other side. The clinician must be clear that this position will also stress the radial nerve and so if positive will need to consider a neural component and look at the addition of neural sensitisers (Butler 2000).

The clinician tests for medial epicondylalgia by stretching the flexor muscles of the wrist and hand. This is done by extending the elbow, supinating the forearm and then extending the wrist and fingers. A positive test is indicated if the patient's symptoms are reproduced or if the range of movement is limited compared with the other side. The clinician must be clear that this position will also stress the median nerve and so if positive will need to consider a neural component and look at the addition of neural sensitisers (Butler 2000).

The clinician may test the length of other muscles in the upper quadrant (Janda 1994, 2002). Descriptions of the tests for muscle length are given in Chapter 3.'

Isometric muscle testing

The clinician tests the elbow flexors, extensors, forearm pronators, supinators and wrist flexors, extensors, radial deviators and ulnar deviators (and any other relevant muscle group) in resting position in different parts of the physiological range and, if indicated, in subjectively reported symptomatic postures. In addition the clinician observes the quality of the muscle contraction to hold this position (this can be done with the patient's eyes shut). The patient may, for example, be unable to prevent the joint from moving or may hold with excessive muscle activity; either of these circumstances would suggest a neuromuscular dysfunction.

Repeated microtrauma to the common flexor and extensor origins produces degenerative changes within the tendon, resulting in persistent symptoms. An additional test for common extensor dysfunction is an isometric contraction of extension of the third digit distal to the proximal interphalangeal joint activating extensor carpi radialis brevis – reproduction of pain or weakness over the lateral epicondyle indicates a positive test. In the same way, isometric contraction of the flexor muscles of the wrist and hand can be examined for flexor origin pain.

Neurological tests

Neurological examination includes neurological integrity testing, neurodynamic tests and some other nerve tests.

Integrity of the nervous system

The integrity of the nervous system is tested if the clinician suspects that the symptoms are emanating from the spine or from a peripheral nerve.

Dermatomes/peripheral nerves. Light touch and pain sensation of the upper limb are tested using cotton wool and pinprick respectively, as described in Chapter 3. Following trauma or compression to peripheral nerves, it is vital to assess the cutaneous sensation, examining temperature sense, vibration, protective sensation, deep pressure to light touch, proprioception and stereognosis. The use of monofilaments and other tests is described in Chapter 3. Knowledge of the cutaneous distribution of nerve roots (dermatomes) and peripheral nerves (radial, median and ulnar) enables the clinician to distinguish the sensory loss due to a root lesion from that due to a peripheral nerve lesion. The cutaneous nerve distribution and dermatome areas are shown in Chapter 3.

Myotomes/peripheral nerves. The following myotomes are tested (see Chapter 3 for further details):

- C4: shoulder girdle elevation
- C5: shoulder abduction
- C6: elbow flexion
- C7: elbow extension
- C8: thumb extension
- T1: finger adduction.

A working knowledge of the muscular distribution of nerve roots (myotomes) and peripheral nerves enables the clinician to distinguish the motor loss due to a root lesion from that due to a peripheral nerve lesion. The peripheral nerve distributions are shown in Chapter 3.

Reflex testing. The following deep tendon reflexes are tested (see Chapter 3 for further details):

- C5–C6: biceps
- C7: triceps and brachioradialis.

Neurodynamic tests

The upper-limb neurodynamic tests (1, 2a, 2b and 3) may be carried out in order to ascertain the degree to which neural tissue is responsible for the production of the patient's elbow symptom(s). These tests are described in detail in Chapter 3.

Other nerve tests

Ulnar nerve

Tinel's sign at the elbow. This is used to determine the distal point of sensory nerve regeneration. The clinician taps the ulnar nerve where it lies in the groove between the olecranon and the medial epicondyle and the most distal point that produces tingling sensation in the distribution of the ulnar nerve indicates the point of recovery of the sensory nerve (Magee 2006).

Test for cubital tunnel syndrome. The ulnar nerve may be injured or compressed as a result of trauma or degenerative disease. Sustained elbow flexion for 3–5 minutes producing paraesthesia in the distribution of the ulnar nerve is a positive test for cubital tunnel syndrome (Buehler & Thayer 1988).

Median nerve

Pinch-grip test. This tests for anterior interosseous nerve entrapment (anterior interosseous syndrome) between the two heads of pronator teres muscle (Magee 2006). The test is considered positive if the patient is unable to pinch tip to tip the index finger and thumb.

Test for pronator syndrome. With the elbow flexed to 90°, the clinician resists pronation as the elbow is extended. Tingling in the distribution of the median nerve is a positive test. This involves compression of the median nerve just proximal to the formation of the anterior interosseous nerve (Magee 2006). In addition to the anterior interosseous syndrome described above, the flexor carpi radialis, palmaris longus and flexor digitorum muscles are affected, thus weakening grip strength; there is also sensory loss in the distribution of the median nerve.

Test for humerus supracondylar process syndrome. This test involves compression of the median nerve as it passes under the ligament of Struthers (found in 0.6–2% of the population) running from the shaft of the humerus to the medial epicondyle. Pain is reproduced on elbow extension and supination and in addition there is pinch and grip weakness (Ay et al. 2002). As the brachial artery accompanies the nerve there may also be associated vascular symptoms.

Radial nerve. The radial nerve may be injured at the elbow as a complication of a humeral shaft fracture.

Test for radial tunnel syndrome. This involves compression of the posterior interosseous nerve between the two supinator heads in the canal of Frohse (found in 30% of the population) (Magee 2006). Forearm extensor muscles are affected, weakening the strength of wrist and finger extension; there are no sensory symptoms. This syndrome can mimic lateral epicondylalgia.

Tests for circulation

Thoracic outlet syndrome. This test is described in Chapter 9.

Palpation of pulses. If circulation is suspected of being compromised, the brachial artery pulse is palpated on the medial aspect of humerus in the axilla and the radial artery at the wrist.

Palpation

The elbow region is palpated, as well as the cervical spine and thoracic spine, shoulder, wrist and hand as appropriate. It is useful to record palpation findings on a body chart (see Figure 2.3) and/or palpation chart (see Figure 3.36).

The clinician notes the following:

- the temperature of the area
- localised increased skin moisture
- the presence of oedema or effusion; this can be measured using a tape measure and comparing left and right sides
- mobility and feel of superficial tissues, e.g. ganglions, nodules and scar tissue
- the presence or elicitation of any muscle spasm
- pain provoked or reduced on palpation
   ○ anteriorly: palpate the cubital fossa, biceps tendon, median nerve medial to the biceps tendon and brachial artery, coronoid process of ulna and head of the radius – location confirmed by pronation and supination of the forearm
   ○ medially: palpate wrist flexor pronator muscles, fan-shaped medial collateral ligament and the ulnar nerve posterior to medial epiconyle
   ○ laterally: palpate wrist extensors, brachioradialis and supinator, cordlike lateral collateral ligament and annular ligament
   ○ posteriorly – palpate the olecranon process in 90° flexion: triceps tendon insertion.

Accessory movements

It is useful to use the palpation chart and movement diagrams (or joint pictures) to record findings. These are explained in detail in Chapter 3.

The clinician notes the:

- quality of movement
- range of movement
- resistance through the range and at the end of the range of movement
- behaviour of pain through the range
- provocation of any muscle spasm.

Humeroulnar joint (Figure 10.6), radiohumeral joint (Figure 10.7), superior radioulnar joint (Figure 10.8) and inferior radioulnar (Figure 10.9) joint accessory movements are listed in Table 10.2. Note that each of these accessory movements will move more than one of the joints in the elbow complex – a medial glide on the olecranon, for example, will cause movement at the superior radioulnar joint as well as the humeroulnar joint.

Following accessory movements to the elbow region, the clinician reassesses all the physical asterisks (movements or tests that have been found to reproduce the patient's symptoms) in order to establish the effect of the accessory movements on the patient's signs and symptoms. Accessory movements can then be tested for other regions suspected to be a source of or contributing to the patient's symptoms. Again, following accessory movements to any one region the clinician reassesses all the asterisks. Regions likely to be examined are the cervical spine, thoracic spine, shoulder, wrist and hand (Table 10.2).

Completion of the examination

Having carried out the above tests, the examination of the elbow region is now complete. The subjective and physical examinations produce a large amount of information, which should be recorded accurately and quickly. It is vital at this stage to highlight with an asterisk (*) important findings from the examination. These findings must be reassessed at, and within, subsequent treatment sessions to evaluate the effects of treatment on the patient's condition.

The physical testing procedures which specifically indicate joint, nerve or muscle tissues, as a source of the patient's symptoms, are summarised in Table 3.10. The strongest evidence that a joint is the source of the patient's symptoms is that active and passive physiological movements, passive accessory movements and joint palpation all reproduce the patient's symptoms, and that, following a treatment dose, reassessment identifies an improvement in the patient's signs and symptoms. Weaker evidence includes an alteration in range, resistance or quality of physiological and/or accessory movements and tenderness over the joint, with no alteration in signs and symptoms after treatment. One or more of these findings may indicate a dysfunction of a joint which may, or may not, be contributing to the patient's condition.

The strongest evidence that a muscle is the source of a patient's symptoms is if active movements, an

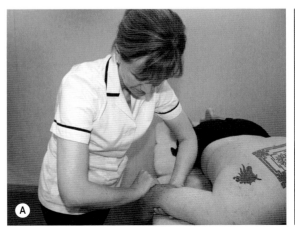
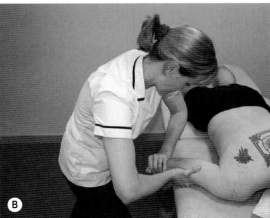

Figure 10.6 • Humeroulnar accessory movements. A Medial glide on the olecranon. The left hand supports underneath the upper arm and the right heel of the hand applies a medial glide to the olecranon. B Lateral glide on the olecranon. The right hand supports the forearm while the left hand applies a lateral glide to the olecranon.

(Continued)

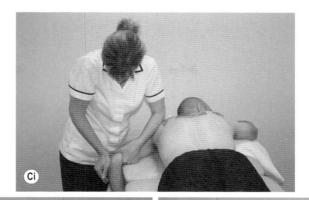

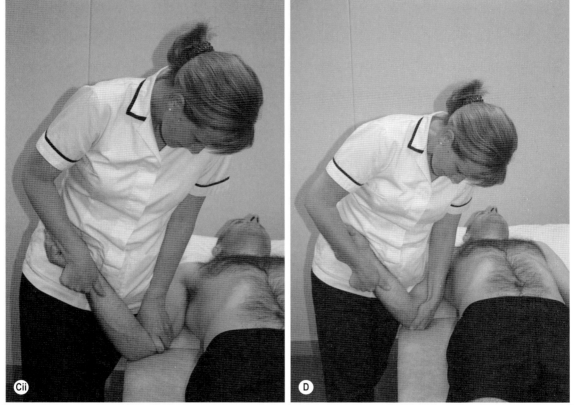

Figure 10.6—cont'd • C Longitudinal caudad. Longitudinal caudad can be applied directly on the olecranon; (i) the left hand supports underneath the upper arm and the right heel of the hand applies a longitudinal caudad glide to the olecranon or (ii) the left hand stabilises the upper arm and the right hand grips the shaft of the ulna and pulls the ulna upwards to produce a longitudinal caudad movement at the humeroulnar joint. **D** Compression. The left hand supports underneath the elbow while the right hand pushes down through the shaft of the ulna.

isometric contraction, passive lengthening and palpation of a muscle all reproduce the patient's symptoms, and that, following a treatment dose, reassessment identifies an improvement in the patient's signs and symptoms. Further evidence of muscle dysfunction may be suggested by reduced strength or poor quality during the active physiological movement and the isometric contraction, reduced range and/or increased/ decreased resistance, during the passive lengthening of the muscle and tenderness on palpation, with no

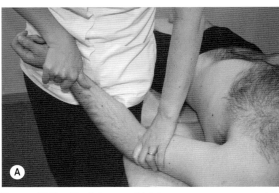
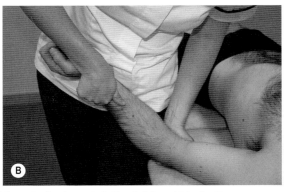

Figure 10.7 • Radiohumeral joint accessory movements. **A** Longitudinal caudad. The left hand blocks the upper arm movement and the right hand pulls the radial side of the forearm. **B** Longitudinal cephalad. The left hand supports underneath the elbow and the right hand pushes down through the radial side of the forearm.

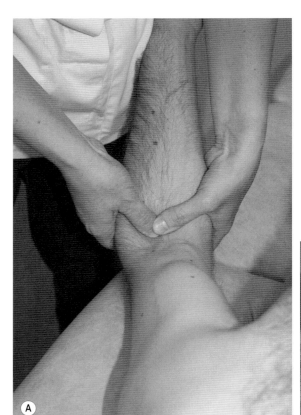
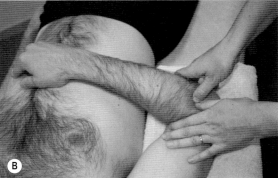

Figure 10.8 • Superior radioulnar joint accessory movements. **A** Anteroposterior. Thumb pressure is applied slowly through the soft tissue to the anterior aspect of the head of the radius. **B** Posteroanterior. Thumb pressure is applied to the posterior aspect of the head of the radius.

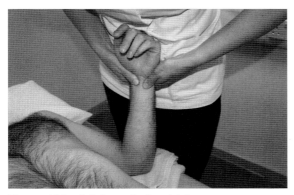

Figure 10.9 • Inferior radioulnar joint accessory movements: anteroposterior/posteroanterior glide. The left and right hands each grasp the anterior and posterior aspect of the radius and ulna. The hands then apply a force in opposite directions to produce an anteroposterior/posteroanterior glide.

alteration in signs and symptoms after treatment. One or more of these findings may indicate a dysfunction of a muscle which may, or may not, be contributing to the patient's condition.

The strongest evidence that a nerve is the source of the patient's symptoms is when active and/or passive physiological movements reproduce the patient's symptoms, which are then increased or decreased with an additional sensitising movement, at a distance from the patient's symptoms. In addition, there is reproduction of the patient's symptoms on palpation of the nerve and neurodynamic testing, sufficient to be considered a treatment dose, results in an improvement in the above signs and symptoms. Further evidence of nerve dysfunction may be suggested by reduced range (compared with the asymptomatic side) and/or increased resistance to the various arm movements, and tenderness on nerve palpation.

Table 10.2 Accessory movements, choice of application and reassessment of the patient's asterisks

Accessory movements	Choice of application	Identify any effect of accessory movements on patient's signs and symptoms
Humeroulnar joint	Start position, e.g.	Reassess all asterisks
←← Med Medial glide on olecranon or coronoid ←← Lat Lateral glide on olecranon or coronoid ←←← Caud Longitudinal caudad Comp Compression	— in flexion — in extension — in pronation — in supination	
Radiohumeral joint	— in flexion and supination	
←←← Caud Longitudinal caudad ←←← Ceph Longitudinal cephalad	— in flexion and pronation — in extension and supination	
Superior radioulnar joint	— in extension and pronation	
↕ Anteroposterior ↕ Posteroanterior	Speed of force application Direction of the applied force	
Inferior radioulnar joint	Point of application of applied force	
↕ Anteroposterior ↕ Posteroanterior		
?Cervical spine	As above	Reassess all asterisks
?Thoracic spine	As above	Reassess all asterisks
?Shoulder	As above	Reassess all asterisks
?Wrist and hand	As above	Reassess all asterisks

On completion of the physical examination, the clinician:

- explains the findings of the physical examination and how these findings relate to the subjective assessment. Any misconceptions patients may have regarding their symptoms should be cleared up here
- warns the patient of possible exacerbation up to 24–48 hours following the examination
- requests the patient to report details on the behaviour of the symptoms following examination at the next attendance
- evaluates the findings, formulates a clinical diagnosis and writes up a problem list
- discusses with the patient the objectives of treatment
- through discussion with the patient devises an initial treatment plan.

In this way, the clinician will have sufficient information to develop the following hypotheses categories (adapted from Jones & Rivett 2004):

- activity capability/restriction/participant capability/restriction
- patient's perspectives on his/her experience
- pathobiological mechanisms. This includes the structure or tissue that is thought to be producing the patient's symptoms, the nature of the structure or tissues in relation to both the healing process and the pain mechanisms
- physical impairments and associated structures/tissue sources
- contributing factors to the development and maintenance of the problem. There may be environmental, psychosocial, behavioural, physical or heredity factors
- precautions/contraindications to treatment and management. This includes the severity and irritability of the patient's symptoms and the nature of the patient's condition
- management strategy and treatment plan
- prognosis – this can be affected by factors such as the stage and extent of the injury as well as the patient's expectation, personality and lifestyle.

For guidance on treatment and management principles, the reader is directed to the companion textbook (Petty 2011).

References

Ay, S., Bektas, U., Yilmaz, C., et al., 2002. An unusual supracondylar process syndrome. J. Hand Surg. 27 (5), 913–915.

Buehler, M.J., Thayer, D.T., 1988. The elbow flexion test; a clinical test for cubital tunnel syndrome. Clin. Orthop. 233, 213–216.

Butler, D., 2000. The sensitive nervous system. Neuro Orthopaedic Institute, Adelaide, p. 327.

Cain, L., Dugas, J., Wolf, R., et al., 2003. Elbow injuries in throwing athletes: a current concept review. Am. J. Sports Med. 31 (4), 621–635.

Cakir, M., Samanci, N., Balci, N., et al., 2003. Musculoskeletal manifestations in patients with thyroid disease. Clin. Endocrinol. (Oxf.) 59 (2), 162–167.

Cole, J.H., Furness, A.L., Twomey, L.T., 1988. Muscles in action, an approach to manual muscle testing. Churchill Livingstone, Edinburgh.

Cyriax, J., 1982. Textbook of orthopaedic medicine – diagnosis of soft tissue lesions, eighth ed. Baillière Tindall, London.

Haker, E., 1993. Lateral epicondylalgia: diagnosis, treatment and evaluation. Crit. Rev. Phys. Rehabil. Med. 5, 129–154.

Hislop, H., Montgomery, J., 1995. Daniels and Worthingham's muscle testing, techniques of manual examination, seventh ed. W B Saunders, Philadelphia.

Janda, V., 1994. Muscles and motor control in cervicogenic disorders: assessment and management. In: Grant, R. (Ed.), Physical therapy of the cervical and thoracic spine, second ed. Churchill Livingstone, New York, p. 195.

Janda, V., 2002. Muscles and motor control in cervicogenic disorders. In: Grant, R. (Ed.), Physical therapy of the cervical and thoracic spine, third ed. Churchill Livingstone, New York, p. 182.

Jones, M.A., Rivett, D.A., 2004. Clinical reasoning for manual therapists. Butterworth-Heinemann, Edinburgh.

Kendall, F.P., McCreary, E.K., Provance, P.G., 1993. Muscles testing and function, fourth ed. Williams & Wilkins, Baltimore.

King, G., Richards, R., Zuckerman, J., et al., 1999. A standardized method for assessment of elbow function. J. Shoulder Elbow Surg. 8, 351–354.

Magee, D.J., 2006. Orthopedic physical assessment, fourth ed. Elsevier, Philadelphia.

Maitland, G.D., Hengeveld, E., Banks, K., et al., 2005. Maitland's peripheral manipulation, fourth ed. Butterworth-Heinemann, London.

Mulligan, B.R., 1999. Manual therapy 'NAGs', 'SNAGs', 'MWMs' etc., fourth ed. Plane View Services, New Zealand.

O'Driscoll, S.W., Bell, D.F., Morrey, B.F., 1991. Posteroloateral rotary instability of the elbow. J. Bone Joint Surg. Am. 73, 441.

Petty, N.J., 2011. Principles of neuromusculoskeletal treatment and management: a guide for therapists, second ed. Churchill Livingstone, Edinburgh.

Refshauge, K., Gass, E. (Eds.), 2004. Musculoskeletal physiotherapy clinical science and evidence-based practice. Butterworth-Heinemann, Oxford.

Simmonds, J., Keer, R., 2007.
Hypermobility and the hypermobility
syndrome. Man. Ther. 12, 298–309.

Vicenzino, B., 2003. Lateral
epicondylalgia: a musculoskeletal
perspective. Man. Ther. 8 (2), 66–79.

Volz, R.C., Morrey, B.F., 1993. The
physical examination of the elbow. In:
Morrey, B.F. (Ed.), The elbow and its
disorders, second ed. W B Saunders,
Philadelphia, p. 73.

Wilke, K.E., Meister, K., Andrews, J.R.,
2002. Current concepts in the
rehabilitation of the overhead
throwing athlete. Am. J. Sports Med.
30 (1), 136–151.

Examination of the wrist and hand

Dionne Ryder

CHAPTER CONTENTS

Possible causes of pain and/or limitation of movement

This region includes the superior and inferior radio-ulnar, radiocarpal, mid-carpal, intercarpal, carpometacarpal, intermetacarpal, metacarpophalangeal and interphalangeal joints and their surrounding soft tissues:

- Trauma:
  - ○ fracture of the radius, ulna (e.g. Colles or Smith fracture), carpal or metacarpal bones or phalanges
  - ○ dislocation of interphalangeal joints
  - ○ crush injuries to the hand
  - ○ ligamentous sprain
  - ○ muscular strain
  - ○ tendon and tendon sheath injuries
  - ○ digital amputations
  - ○ peripheral nerve injuries
- Degenerative conditions: osteoarthrosis
- Inflammatory conditions: rheumatoid arthritis
- Tenosynovitis, e.g. de Quervain's disease
- Carpal tunnel syndrome
- Guyon's canal compression
- Infections, e.g. animal or human bites
- Dupuytren's disease
- Raynaud's disease
- Complex regional pain syndrome includes reflex sympathetic dystrophy and causalgia
- Neoplasm (rare)
- Hypermobility syndrome
- Referral of symptoms from the cervical spine, thoracic spine, shoulder or elbow.

Further details of the questions asked during the subjective examination and the tests carried out in the physical examination can be found in Chapters 2 and 3 respectively.

The order of the subjective questioning and the physical tests described below should be justified through sound clinical reasoning and altered as appropriate for the patient being examined.

Subjective examination

Body chart

The following information concerning the type and area of current symptoms can be recorded on a body chart (see Figure 2.3). In order to be specific, it may be necessary to use an enlarged chart of the hand and wrist.

Area of current symptoms

Be precise when mapping out the area of the symptoms. Lesions of the joints in the wrist and hand region usually produce localised symptoms over the affected joint. Ascertain which is the worst symptom and record where the patient feels the symptoms are coming from.

Areas relevant to the region being examined

It is important to check for any symptoms, for example pain and/or stiffness in the cervical spine, thoracic spine, shoulder and elbow, as these are areas capable of referring symptoms into the wrist and hand and so may be relevant to the patient's main symptoms. Mark unaffected areas with ticks (✓) on the body chart.

Quality of pain

Establish the quality of the pain in order to assist in determining possible pain mechanisms, e.g. sharp, burning.

Intensity of pain

The intensity of pain can be measured using, for example, a visual analogue scale, as shown in Chapter 2.

Depth of pain

Establish the depth of the pain. Does the patient feel it is on the surface or deep inside?

Abnormal sensation

Check for any altered sensation (such as paraesthesia or numbness) locally around the wrist and hand, as well as proximally over the elbow, shoulder and spine as appropriate. For a brief assessment, where this is

appropriate, sensation testing can be limited to: index finger and thumb, for median nerve; little finger and hypothenar eminence for ulnar nerve; and first and second metacarpal for radial nerve (dorsal branch).

Constant or intermittent symptoms

Ascertain the frequency of the symptoms; whether they are constant or intermittent. If symptoms are constant, check whether there is variation in the intensity of the symptoms, as constant unremitting pain may be indicative of a serious pathology.

Relationship of symptoms

Through careful questioning of the patient determine the relationship between the symptomatic areas, e.g. do the symptoms come together or separately? Can the patient experience wrist pain without the elbow pain, or are the pains always present together? Which symptom comes on first?

Behaviour of symptoms

Aggravating factors

In order to determine the impact that symptoms in the upper limb may have on normal function the clinician must find out if the patient is left- or right-handed as there may be increased stress on the dominant side. For each symptomatic area, discover what movements and/or positions aggravate the patient's symptoms, i.e. what brings them on (or makes them worse)? is the patient able to maintain this position or movement (severity) or does s/he have to stop or change position? what happens to other symptoms when this symptom is produced (or is made worse)? and how long does it take for symptoms to ease once the position or movement (irritability) is stopped? These questions are crucial in helping to confirm the relationship between the symptoms, the possible structures that may be at fault and the severity and irritability of the symptoms, and so how searching the physical examination will need to be.

Common aggravating factors for the wrist and hand are flexion and extension of the wrist, resisted grips (both pinch and power) and grips with pronation and supination, e.g. opening doors, writing, turning a key in a lock, as well as weight-bearing activities, e.g. leaning on the forearm or hand. It is useful to ask specifically about activities associated with work, sport and leisure activities. Cold intolerance commonly occurs after nerve injury, causing pain and vascular changes in cold weather. There are a number of functional screening forms that can be used to measure impact on function and patient perceptions of their dysfunction, e.g. Michigan Hand Outcomes Questionnaire (Chung et al. 1998) and Carpal Tunnel Function Disability Form (Levine et al. 1993).

Aggravating factors for other regions, which may need to be queried if they are suspected to be a source of the symptoms, are shown in Table 2.3.

Easing factors

For each symptomatic area, the clinician asks what movements and/or positions ease the patient's symptoms, how long it takes to ease them, whether they subside completely and what happens to other symptoms when this symptom is relieved. These questions help to confirm the relationship between the symptoms and determine their irritability.

The clinician asks the patient about theoretically known easing factors for structures that could be a source of the symptoms. For example, symptoms from the wrist that are articular in nature may be relieved by holding the wrist in a semiflexed posture out of close pack extension, whereas symptoms originating from neural tissue may be eased by certain cervical and upper-limb out-of-tension positions, e.g. ipsilateral cervical side flexion or shoulder girdle elevation.

Using clinical reasoning skills the clinician can then analyse the positions or movements that aggravate or ease the symptoms to help determine the structure(s) at fault. This information can be used to determine the irritability of the condition, the appropriate vigour of the physical examination, the aims of treatment and any advice that may be required. The most notable functional restrictions are highlighted with asterisks (*), explored in the physical examination and reassessed at subsequent treatment sessions to evaluate treatment intervention.

Twenty-four-hour behaviour of symptoms

The clinician determines the 24-hour behaviour of symptoms by asking questions about night, morning and evening symptoms.

Night symptoms. Suggested questions to establish behaviour of symptoms at night are detailed in Chapter 2. Symptoms of neural origin such as carpal tunnel syndrome are often worse at night as blood pressure drops and neural tissue becomes more ischaemic (Bland 2000).

Morning and evening symptoms. The clinician determines the pattern of the symptoms first thing in the morning, through the day and at the end of the day (Chapter 2).

Special questions

Special questions must always be asked, to identify if there are any precautions or contraindications to the physical examination and/or treatment (see Table 2.4). As mentioned in Chapter 2, the clinician must differentiate between neuromusculoskeletal conditions that are suitable for treatment and management and systemic, neoplastic and other non-neuromusculoskeletal conditions, which require referral to a medical practitioner.

The following information is routinely obtained from patients.

General health. The clinician ascertains the state of the patient's general health, and finds out if the patient suffers from malaise, fatigue, fever, nausea or vomiting, stress, anxiety or depression.

Weight loss. Has the patient noticed any recent unexplained weight loss?

Serious illness. Does the patient have a history of serious pathology such as cancer, human immunodeficiency virus (HIV) or tuberculosis?

Inflammatory arthritis. Has the patient (or a member of his/her family) been diagnosed as having an inflammatory condition such as rheumatoid arthritis?

Cardiovascular disease. Does the patient have a history of cardiovascular disease, e.g. angina, previous myocardial infarction, stroke? Does the patient have a pacemaker fitted?

Respiratory disease. Does the patient have any condition which affects breathing? If so, how is it managed?

Epilepsy. Is the patient epileptic? What type of seizures does s/he have and when was the last seizure?

Thyroid disease. Does the patient have a history of thyroid disease? How well is it managed? Thyroid dysfunction is associated with a higher incidence of neuromusculoskeletal conditions such as Dupuytren's contracture, trigger finger and carpal tunnel syndrome (Cakir et al. 2003).

Diabetes mellitus. Has the patient been diagnosed as having diabetes? How long since diagnosis? How is the diabetes managed? How well controlled is the condition? Healing of tissues is likely to be slower in the presence of this disease. Diabetic neuropathic involvement of the hands may present with a glove distribution of thermal sensitivity deficits (Guy et al. 1985).

Osteoporosis. Patients who present with a history of fractures following falls should be considered at risk: Colles fracture has been shown to be associated with an increased risk of hip fracture (Earnshaw et al. 1998). Have they been investigated with a dual-energy X-ray absorptiometry (DEXA) scan? If so, when? and what was the result?

Dupuytren's disease. Has the patient or anyone in the patient's family been diagnosed with Dupuytren's disease? Increased incidence of the disease with a positive family history has not been confirmed and there are stronger correlations with smoking and manual occupations (Gudmundsson et al. 2000).

Neurological symptoms. Has the patient experienced any neural tissue symptoms such as tingling, pins and needles, pain or hypersensitivity in the upper limb and/or hand? Consider whether symptoms are likely to be peripheral or spinal nerve in origin. Are these symptoms unilateral or bilateral? Has the patient noticed any weakness in the hand? or has s/he experienced symptoms of spinal cord compression, which are bilateral tingling in the hands or feet and/or disturbance of gait?

Drug history. Has the patient been on long-term steroids? Has the patient been taking anticoagulants? Has the patient been taking medication for current symptoms, either prescribed or over the counter? If so, what is s/he taking? How long has s/he been taking it? Is it effective? It is useful to ascertain when the patient took the last dose because medication prior to the assessment may mask symptoms during their physical examination (Chapter 2).

Radiograph and medical imaging. Has the patient been radiographed or had any other medical tests recently? Radiographs are vital in hand or joint fractures, dislocations and joint disease. Bone position, i.e. the width of the scapholunate gap, or radiographs called stress tests, whereby joints are imaged in positions of stress, can be useful in revealing instabilities that would not be apparent in neutral resting positions of the joint (Lichtman et al. 1981). These results will provide information that will help guide rehabilitation and indicate likely prognosis. Other medical tests may include blood tests, magnetic resonance imaging or a bone scan. For further information on these tests, the reader is referred to Refshauge & Gass (2004).

History of the present condition

For each symptomatic area, the clinician needs to know how long the symptoms have been present. Did these symptoms develop suddenly or gradually? Was there a known cause that provoked the onset of the symptoms? If the onset of symptoms was associated with trauma, e.g. a fall, the clinician may ask why and how the patient fell. Did the patient fall on the outstretched extended wrist, possibly fracturing distal radius or scaphoid? or was s/he injured as a result of an assault? was the injury accidental or self-inflicted with a knife or glass? If the onset was gradual, can the development of symptoms be associated with a change in the patient's lifestyle, e.g. a new job or leisure activity or a change in sporting activity? To confirm the relationship of symptoms, the clinician asks what happened when symptoms first began and how over time symptoms have developed or changed. In addition the clinician needs to identify what treatment, if any, the patient has sought so far and its outcome. Is this the first episode or is there a history of wrist and hand problems? If so, how many episodes? when were they? was there a cause? what was the duration of each episode? and did the patient fully recover between episodes? If there have been no previous episodes, has the patient had any episodes of stiffness in the cervical spine, thoracic spine, shoulder, elbow, wrist, hand or any other relevant region?

Past medical history

The following information is obtained from the patient and/or medical notes:

- details of any past medical history such as major or long-standing illnesses, accidents or surgery that are relevant to the patient's condition.

Social history

In order to treat the patient appropriately, it is important that the condition is managed within the context of the patient's social and work environment. Social history that is relevant to the onset and progression of the patient's problem is recorded. This includes age, home situation, employment and details of any leisure activities. Does the patient/s job involve sustained positions of wrist flexion or extension? Alternatively, does the patient undertake repetitive activities, e.g. typing, playing musical instruments?

This information may indicate direct and/or indirect mechanical influences on the wrist and hand.

In cases of trauma ask specifically about any potential compensation claims.

Family history

Family history that is relevant to the onset and progression of the patient's problem is recorded.

Expectation and goals

An appreciation of the possible influences of psychosocial risk factors highlights the importance of ascertaining the patient's perspective on the presenting condition. It is important to discuss with patients their experience and expectations of therapy so that the clinician can use this to identify and manage patient concerns (Chapter 2). The hand is a visual part of the body, an important tool to communication, for example through gesturing or sign language, and so deformity or dysfunction can have a significant psychological impact.

Plan of the physical examination

When all this information has been collected, the subjective examination is complete. It is useful at this stage to reconfirm briefly with patients the clinician understanding of their main complaint, and offer them the opportunity to add anything that they may not have raised so far before explaining to them the purpose and plan for the physical examination. For ease of reference highlight with asterisks (*) important subjective findings and particularly one or more functional restrictions. These can then be re-examined at subsequent treatment sessions to evaluate treatment intervention.

In order to plan the physical examination, the following need to be developed from the subjective examination:

- Are there any precautions and/or contraindications to elements of the physical examination that need to be explored further, such as neurological involvement, recent fracture, trauma, steroid therapy or rheumatoid arthritis? There may also be certain contraindications to further examination and treatment, e.g. symptoms of cord compression.

- Clinically reasoning throughout the subjective examination, the clinician should have a prioritised list of working hypotheses based on the most likely causes of the patient's symptoms. These include the structures underneath the symptomatic area, e.g. joints, muscles, nerves and fascia, as well as the regions referring into the area. All will need to be examined as a possible cause of symptoms, e.g. cervical spine, thoracic spine, shoulder and elbow. In complex cases it is not always possible to examine fully at the first attendance and so, using clinical reasoning skills, the clinician will need to prioritise and justify what 'must' be examined in the first assessment session and what 'should' or 'could' be followed up at subsequent sessions.

- What are the pain mechanisms driving the patient's symptoms and how will this information impact on an understanding of the problem and subsequent management decisions? For example, pain associated with sustained wrist and hand positions when typing may indicate ischaemic nociception. This would indicate an early assessment of workstation ergonomics and advice to the patient to pace the work and move regularly. Patients' acceptance and willingness to be an active participant in their management will depend on their perspective and subsequent behavioural response to their symptoms. If patients are demonstrating fear avoidance behaviours then the clinician's ability to explain and teach them about their condition will be pivotal to achieving a successful outcome.

- Once the clinician has decided on the tests to include in the physical examination the next consideration should be how the physical tests should be carried out? If symptoms are severe, physical tests may be carried out to just before the onset of symptom production or just to the onset of symptom production; no overpressures will be carried out, as the patient would be unable to tolerate this. If symptoms are irritable, physical tests may be examined to just before symptom production or just to the onset of provocation with fewer physical tests being examined to allow for rest period between tests. Alternatively will it be necessary to use combined movements and repetitive movements in order to reproduce the patient's symptoms?

A physical planning form can be useful for clinicians to help guide them through the clinical reasoning process (see Figure 2.10).

Physical examination

The information from the subjective examination helps the clinician to plan an appropriate physical examination. The severity, irritability and nature of the condition are the major factors that will influence the choice and priority of physical testing procedures. The first and overarching question the clinician might ask is: 'Does this patient have a neuromusculoskeletal dysfunction?' If the answer is yes, then the second question the clinician might ask is: 'Is this neuromusculoskeletal dysfunction suitable for me to manage?' To answer that, the clinician needs to carry out an appropriate physical examination; however, this may not be possible if the symptoms are severe and/or irritable. If the patient's symptoms are severe and/or irritable, the clinician aims to explore movements as much as possible, within a symptom-free range. If the patient has constant and severe and/or irritable symptoms, then the clinician aims to find physical tests that ease the symptoms. If the patient's symptoms are non-severe and non-irritable, then the clinician aims to find physical tests that reproduce each of the patient's symptoms.

Each significant physical test that either provokes or eases the patient's symptoms is highlighted in the patient's notes by an asterisk (*) for easy reference. The highlighted tests are often referred to as 'asterisks' or 'markers'.

The order and detail of the physical tests described below need to be modified for the patient being examined; some tests will be irrelevant, some tests will be carried out briefly, while it will be necessary to investigate others more fully. It is important that readers understand that the techniques shown in this chapter are some of many; technique selection will depend on the patient's complaint, the relative size of the clinician and patient, as well as the clinician's preference.

Observation

Informal observation

Informal observation will begin from the moment the clinician meets the patient to walk him or her through to the treatment area and will continue to the end of the physical examination. The clinician should note the patient's ability and willingness to move the upper limb as well as their general posture.

Formal observation

Observation of posture. The patient should be suitably undressed so that the clinician can observe the bony and soft-tissue contours of the elbow, wrist and hand, as well as the patient's posture in sitting and standing, noting the posture of the head and neck, thoracic spine and upper limbs. Right and left sides should be compared. Look for abnormal posture of the hand such as dropped wrist and fingers indicative of a radial nerve palsy, clawing of the ring and little fingers in ulnar nerve palsy or adducted thumb in median nerve palsy.

Observation of muscle form. The clinician examines the muscle bulk and muscle tone of the patient, comparing left and right sides. It must be remembered that handedness and level and frequency of physical activity may well produce differences in muscle bulk between sides. Check for wasting of specific muscles such as the first dorsal interosseous muscle supplied by the ulnar nerve, or opponens pollicis supplied by the median nerve.

Observation of soft tissues. The clinician observes the colour of the patient's skin, any swelling, increased hair growth on the hand, brittle fingernails, infection of the nail bed, sweating or dry palm, shiny skin, scars and bony deformities, and takes cues for further examination. These changes could be indicative of a peripheral nerve injury, peripheral vascular disease, diabetes mellitus, Raynaud's disease, complex regional pain syndrome (previously reflex sympathetic dystrophy) or shoulder–hand syndrome (Magee 2006).

Common deformities of the hand include the following:

- Swan-neck deformity of fingers or thumb: the proximal interphalangeal joint (PIPJ) is hyperextended and the distal interphalangeal joint (DIPJ) is flexed (Figure 11.1). It has a variety of causes; see Eckhaus (1993) for further details.
- Boutonnière deformity of fingers or thumb: the PIPJ is flexed and the DIPJ is hyperextended (Figure 11.2). The central slip of the extensor tendon is damaged and the lateral bands displace volarly (Eddington 1993).
- Claw hand: the little and ring fingers are hyperextended at the metacarpophalangeal joint (MCPJ) and flexed at the interphalangeal joints. This condition is due to ulnar nerve palsy.

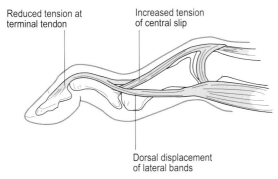

Reduced tension at
terminal tendon

Increased tension
of central slip

Dorsal displacement
of lateral bands

Figure 11.1 • Swan-neck deformity. (From Eckhaus
1993, with permission.)

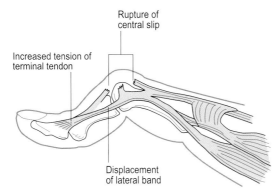

Rupture of
central slip

Increased tension of
terminal tendon

Displacement
of lateral band

Figure 11.2 • Boutonnière deformity. (From Eddington
1993, with permission.)

- Dupuytren's contracture: fixed flexion deformity
  of the MCPJ and PIPJ, particularly affecting
  the ring or little finger.
- Mallet finger: rupture of the terminal extensor
  tendon at the DIPJ.
- Clinodactyly: congenital radial deviation of the
  distal joints of the fingers, most commonly seen in
  the little finger.
- Camptodactyly: congenital flexion contracture at
  the PIPJ and DIPJ, commonly seen in the little
  finger.
- Heberden's nodes over the dorsum of the DIPJs
  are indicative of osteoarthritis.
- Bouchard's nodes over the dorsum of the PIPJs are
  indicative of rheumatoid arthritis.
- Club nails, where there is excessive soft tissue
  under the nail, are indicative of respiratory or
  cardiac disorders.

Observation of the patient's attitudes and feelings.
The age, gender and ethnicity of patients and their
cultural, occupational and social backgrounds may
affect their attitudes and feelings towards themselves, their condition and the clinician. It must be
remembered that hands are particularly visual and
are used regularly to show feelings in conversation,
as well as for function. The clinician needs to be
aware of, and sensitive to, the patient's feelings
and empathise and communicate appropriately so
as to develop a rapport with the patient.

Joint integrity tests

At the wrist, ligamentous instability can occur most
commonly between the scaphoid and lunate (dorsal
intercalated segment instability), and between the
lunate and triquetrum (volar intercalated segment
instability). These instabilities need to be diagnosed
by passive movement tests as routine radiographs
may appear normal (Taleisnik 1988; Trail et al.
2007).

Watson's (scaphoid shift) test. The clinician
applies a posterior glide to the distal pole of the scaphoid while passively moving the wrist from a position
of ulnar deviation and slight extension to radial deviation and slight flexion (Figure 11.3). Posterior subluxation of the scaphoid and/or reproduction of the
patient's pain indicate instability of the scaphoid
(Watson et al. 1988).

Lunotriquetral ballottement (Reagan's) test.
This tests for instability at the joint between the
lunate and triquetral bones occurring due to a loss
of integrity of the lunotriquetral ligament. Excessive
movement, crepitus or pain with anterior and posterior glide of the lunate on the triquetrum indicates
a positive test (Magee 2006).

Mid-carpal shift test. With the patient's wrist in
neutral and forearm pronated, a palmar force is
applied to the distal portion of capitate and the wrist
is axially loaded and deviated ulnarly. The test is positive if a painful 'clunk' is felt and the manoeuvre
reproduces the patient's symptoms (Lichtman &
Wroten 2006).

**Ligamentous instability test for the joints of the
thumb and fingers.** Excessive movement when an
abduction or adduction force is applied to the joint
is indicative of joint instability as a result of laxity
of the collateral ligaments. To test the thumb ulnar
collateral ligament, test with the MCPJ positioned in
extension. When an incomplete rupture is present

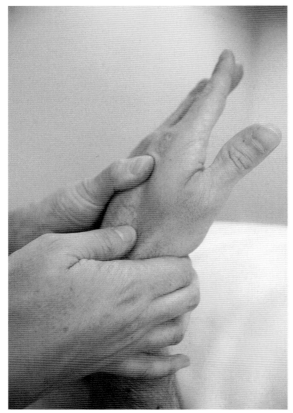

Figure 11.3 • Watson scaphoid shift test. Anterior to posterior glide applied to scaphoid moving whilst moving the wrist from ulnar deviation and extension to flexion and radial deviation.

valgus stress testing reveals minimal or no instability (less than 30° of laxity or less than 15° more laxity than in the non-injured thumb). When a complete rupture is present, valgus stress testing with the MCPJ positioned in extension reveals marked laxity (more than 30° or more than 15° more laxity than in the non-injured thumb (Heyman 1997).

Functional testing

Some functional ability has already been tested by the general observation of the patient during the subjective and physical examinations, e.g. the postures adopted during the subjective examination and the ease or difficulty of undressing prior to the physical examination. Any further functional testing can be carried out at this point in the examination and may include various activities of the upper limb such as using a computer, handling tools and writing. Clues for appropriate tests can be obtained from the subjective examination findings, particularly aggravating factors. Functional testing of the hand is very important and can include the ability to perform various power and precision (or pinch) grips, as well as more general activities, such as fastening a button, tying a shoelace and writing.

Common documented dexterity tests are as follows.

The Purdue pegboard test (Blair et al. 1987). A timed test measuring fine coordination of the hand with a series of unilateral and bilateral standardised tests using pegs and washers.

Nine-hole peg test (Totten & Flinn-Wagner 1992). A simple timed test, placing nine pegs in nine holes. Excellent for children or those with cognitive difficulties.

Minnesota rate of manipulation test (Totten & Flinn-Wagner 1992). Measures gross coordination and dexterity. Used in work assessment for arm–hand dexterity.

Moberg pick-up test (Moberg 1958). This test uses nine standardised everyday objects. Each is picked up as quickly as possible and placed in a pot, first with the eyes open and then with eyes closed. This tests both dexterity and functional sensation.

Jebson–Taylor hand function test (Jebson et al. 1969). There are seven functional subtests to this test, such as turning over a card, writing and simulated eating, designed to test prehension and manipulative skills.

Active physiological movements

For active physiological movements of the wrist and hand, the clinician notes the following:

- range of movement
- quality of movement
- behaviour of pain through the range of movement
- resistance through the range of movement and at the end of the range of movement
- provocation of any muscle spasm.

A movement diagram can be used to depict this information. The active movements with overpressure shown in Figure 11.4 are tested with the patient in supine or sitting. Movements are carried out on the left and right sides and compared. The clinician establishes the patient's symptoms at rest, prior to each

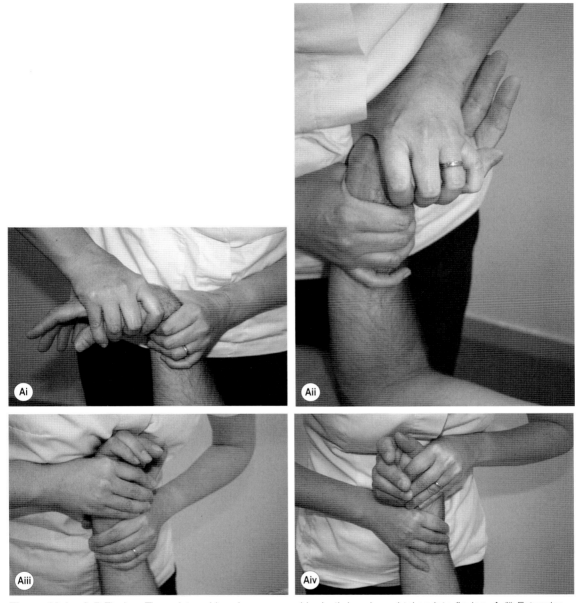

Figure 11.4 • A (i) Flexion. The wrist and hand are grasped by both hands and taken into flexion. A (ii) Extension. The right hand supports the patient's forearm and the left hand takes the wrist and hand into extension. Overpressures to the wrist and hand. A (iii) Radial deviation. The left hand supports just proximal to the wrist joint while the right hand moves the wrist into radial deviation. A (iv) Ulnar deviation. The right hand supports just proximal to the wrist joint while the left hand moves the wrist into ulnar deviation.

(Continued)

movement, and corrects any movement deviation to determine its relevance to the patient's symptoms.

The active physiological movements of the forearm, wrist and hand, and possible modifications, are shown in Table 11.1. Figure 11.5 shows the movement available at the carpometacarpal joint of the thumb. Various differentiation tests (Maitland et al. 2005) can be performed; the choice depends

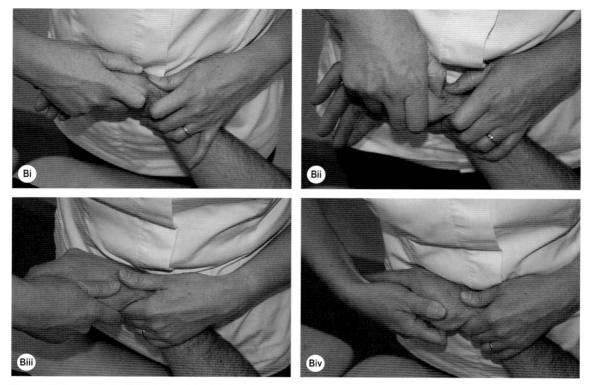

Figure 11.4—cont'd • B (i) Flexion. The left hand supports the carpus while the right hand takes the metacarpal into flexion. B (ii) Extension. The left hand supports the carpus while the right hand takes the metacarpal into extension. B Carpometacarpal joint of thumb. For all these movements, the hands are placed immediately proximal and distal to the joint line. B (iii) Abduction and adduction. The left hand supports the carpus while the right hand takes the metacarpal into abduction and adduction. B (iv) Opposition. The right hand supports the carpus while the left hand takes the metacarpal across the palm into opposition.

(Continued)

on the patient's signs and symptoms. For example, when supination reproduces the patient's wrist symptoms, differentiation between the inferior radioulnar joint and the radiocarpal joint may be required. The patient actively moves the forearm into supination just to the point where symptoms are produced. The clinician applies a supination force to the radius and ulna; if the symptoms are coming from the inferior radioulnar joint, then pain may increase. The radiocarpal joint is then isolated: a supination force around the scaphoid and lunate is applied, while maintaining the supination position of the forearm; if the symptoms are coming from the radiocarpal joint, then pain may increase. A pronation force to the scaphoid and lunate might then be expected to reduce symptoms (Figure 11.6).

Capsular pattern. Capsular patterns for these joints (Cyriax 1982) are as follows:

- inferior radioulnar joint: full range but pain at extremes of range
- wrist: flexion and extension equally limited
- carpometacarpal joint of the thumb: full flexion, more limited abduction than extension
- thumb and finger joints: more limitation of flexion than of extension.

It may be necessary to examine other regions to determine their relevance to the patient's symptoms; they may be the source of the symptoms, or they may be contributing to the symptoms. The regions most likely are the cervical spine, thoracic spine, shoulder and elbow. The joints within these regions can be tested fully (see relevant chapter) or partially with the use of screening tests (in Chapter 3).

Mobilisations with movement (MWMs) (Mulligan 1999). MWMs are sustained accessory glides

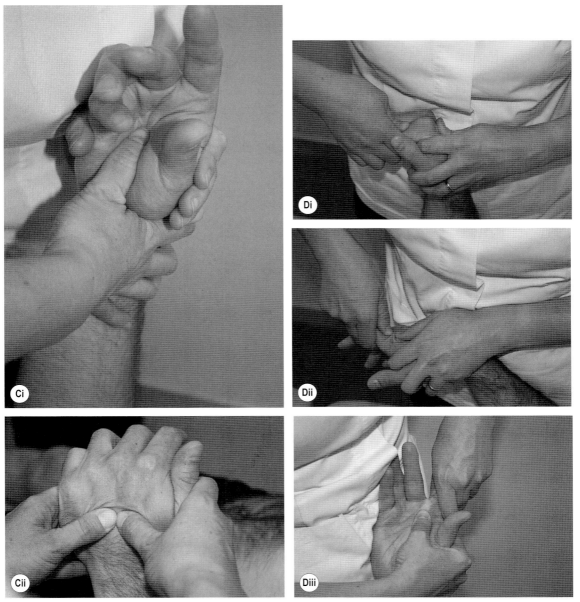

Figure 11.4—cont'd • **C** Distal intermetacarpal joints. **C** (i) Horizontal flexion. The right thumb is placed in the centre of the palm at the level of the metacarpal heads. The left hand cups around the back of the metacarpal heads and moves them into horizontal flexion. **C** (ii) Horizontal extension. The thumbs are placed in the centre of the dorsum of the palm at the level of the metacarpal heads. The fingers wrap around the anterior aspect of the hand and pull the metacarpal heads into horizontal extension. **D** Metacarpophalangeal joints. **D** (i) Flexion. The left hand supports the metacarpal while the right hand takes the proximal phalanx into flexion. **D** (ii) Extension. The right hand supports the metacarpal while the left hand takes the proximal phalanx into extension. **D** (iii) Abduction and adduction. The right hand supports the metacarpal while the left hand takes the proximal phalanx into abduction and adduction.

(Continued)

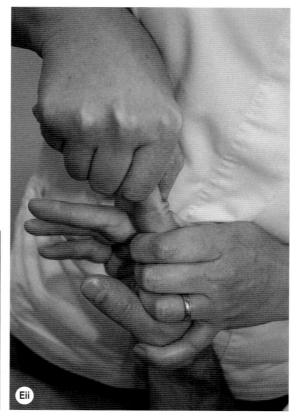

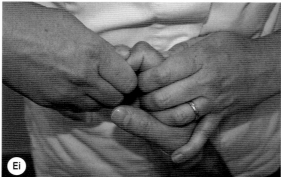

Figure 11.4—cont'd • E Proximal and distal interphalangeal joints. E (i) Flexion. The left hand supports the metacarpophalangeal joint in extension while the right hand takes the proximal interphalangeal joint into flexion. E (ii) Extension. The left hand supports the metacarpophalangeal joint in extension while the right hand takes the proximal interphalangeal joint into extension.

Table 11.1 Active physiological movements and possible modifications

Active physiological movements	Modifications
Forearm pronation	Repeated
Forearm supination	Speed altered
Wrist flexion	Combined, e.g.
Wrist extension	– wrist flexion in supination
Radial deviation	– wrist ulnar deviation with flexion
Ulnar deviation	Compression or distraction, e.g.
Carpometacarpal and metacarpophalangeal joints of thumb	– wrist extension with distraction
– flexion	– metacarpophalangeal joint flexion with compression
– extension	Sustained
– abduction	Injuring movement
– adduction	Differentiation tests
– opposition	Function includes:
	– power grips: hook, cylinder, fist and spherical span

(Continued)

Table 11.1 Active physiological movements and possible modifications—cont'd

Active physiological movements	Modifications

Distal intermetacarpal joints
– horizontal flexion
– horizontal extension
Metacarpophalangeal joints (of the fingers)
– flexion
– extension
– adduction
– abduction
Proximal and distal interphalangeal joints
– flexion
– extension
?Cervical spine
?Thoracic spine
?Shoulder
?Elbow
	– precision (or pinch) grips: pulp pinch, tip-to-tip pinch,
	  tripod pinch and lateral key grip, fastening a button,
	  tying a shoelace, writing
	– Purdue pegboard test
	– nine-hole peg test
	– Minnesota rate of manipulation test
	– Moberg pick-up test
	– Jebson–Taylor hand function test

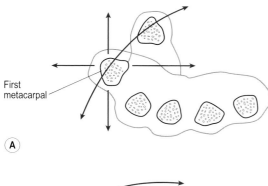

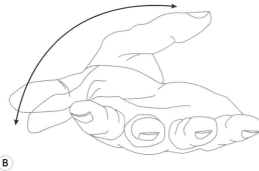

Figure 11.5 • Movement at the carpometacarpal joint of the thumb. (From Fess & Philips 1987, with permission). A The arrows illustrate the multiple planes of movement that occur at the carpometacarpal joint of the thumb. B The arrow illustrates the movement of the thumb from a position of adduction against the second metacarpal to a position of extension and abduction away from the hand and fingers. It can then be rotated into positions of opposition and flexion.

applied to a joint during active or passive movement. Although largely seen as treatment techniques MWMs can serve as a useful diagnostic tool.

Forearm pronation and supination. The patient actively supinates or pronates the forearm while the clinician applies a sustained anterior or posterior force to the distal end of the ulna at the wrist. Figure 11.7 demonstrates a posteroanterior force to distal ulna as the patient actively supinates. An increase in painfree range or reduced pain on active supination or pronation is a positive examination finding, indicating a mechanical joint problem.

Wrist. The patient actively flexes or extends the wrist while the clinician applies a sustained medial or lateral glide to the carpal bones. Figure 11.8 demonstrates a lateral glide to the carpal bones as the patient actively extends the wrist. An increase in painfree range or reduced pain is a positive examination finding.

Interphalangeal joints. The patient actively flexes or extends the finger while the clinician applies a sustained medial or lateral glide just distal to the affected joint. Figure 11.9 demonstrates a medial glide to the DIPJ as the patient actively extends the joint. An increase in painfree range or reduced pain is a positive examination finding.

Passive physiological movements

All the active movements described above can be examined passively with the patient usually in sitting or supine, comparing left and right sides.

A comparison of the response of symptoms to the active and passive movements can help to determine whether the structure at fault is non-contractile (articular) or contractile (extra-articular) (Cyriax 1982). If the lesion due to dysfunction is non-contractile, such as would occur in ligaments, then active and passive movements will be painful and/or restricted in the same direction. If the lesion is in a contractile tissue (i.e. muscle), active and passive movements are painful and/or restricted in opposite directions.

Muscle tests

Muscle tests include examining muscle strength, length, isometric muscle testing and some other muscle tests.

Muscle strength

Grip strength, comparing left and right sides, can be measured using a dynamometer. The second handle position is recommended and three trials are carried out recording the mean value (American Society for Surgery of the Hand 1990) with the wrist between 0° and 15° of extension (Pryce 1980). Pinch strength can be measured using a pinch meter, again repeating the test three times and taking the mean value. Measure and record pure pinch, lateral key pinch and tripod grip separately.

Manual muscle testing may be carried out for the following muscle groups:

* elbow: flexors and extensors
* forearm: pronators and supinators
* wrist joint: flexors, extensors, radial deviators and ulnar deviators

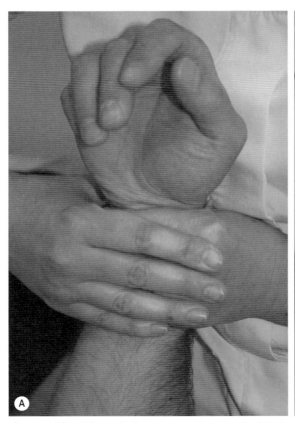
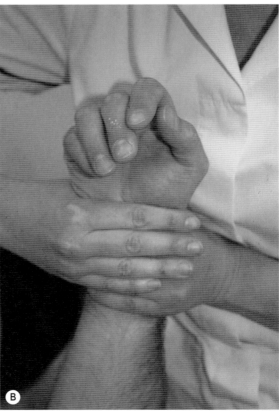

Figure 11.6 • Differentiation between the superior/inferior radioulnar joint with radiocarpal joint and mid-carpal joints. The patient supinates the forearm to the onset of symptoms. The clinician then: **A** applies a supination force to the radius and ulna; **B** holds the radius and ulna and applies a supination force around the proximal row of carpal bones to affect the radiocarpal joint;

(Continued)

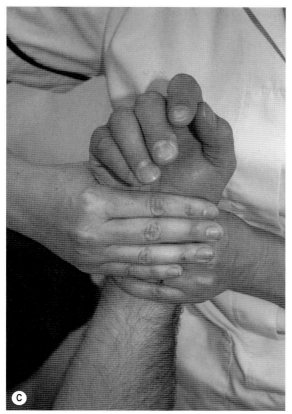

Figure 11.6—cont'd • C fixes the proximal row of carpal bones and applies a supination force of the distal carpal bones. The clinician determines the effect of each overpressure on the symptoms. The symptoms would be expected to increase when the supination force is applied to the symptomatic level; further examination of accessory movements of individual bones may then identify a symptomatic joint. This is a somewhat crude attempt to differentiate between joints and so it may be a helpful test on only some patients.

- thenar eminence: flexors, extensors, adductors, abductors and opposition
- hypothenar eminence: flexors, extensors, adductors, abductors and opposition
- finger: flexors, extensors, abductors and adductors.

For details of these general tests the reader is directed to Cole et al. (1988), Hislop & Montgomery (1995) or Kendall et al. (1993).

Greater detail may be required to test the strength of muscles, in particular those thought prone to

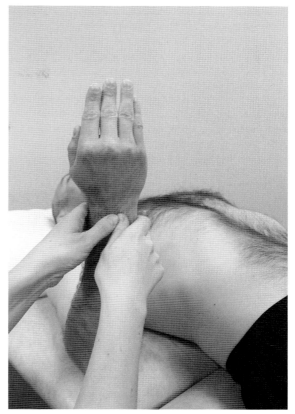

Figure 11.7 • Mobilisation with movement for supination. A posteroanterior force is applied to the ulna as the patient actively supinates.

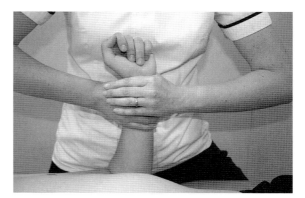

Figure 11.8 • Mobilisation with movement for wrist extension. The right hand supports the forearm while the left hand cups around the ulnar aspect of the wrist and applies a lateral glide as the patient actively extends the wrist.

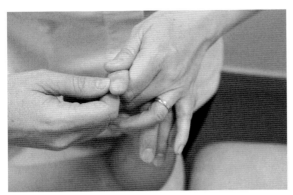

Figure 11.9 • Mobilisation with movement for finger extension. The left hand supports the finger joint. The right hand applies a medial glide just distal to the distal interphalangeal joint as the patient actively extends the joint.

become weak (Janda 1994, 2002). These muscles and a description of the test for muscle strength are given in Chapter 3.

Muscle length

Tenodesis action. Tests the balance in the extrinsic flexor and extensor muscle length. With the wrist flexed, the fingers and thumb will extend; with the wrist extended, the fingers will flex towards the palm and the thumb oppose towards the index finger (Neumann 2002).

Intrinsic muscle tightness. In a normal hand, the clinician is able to maintain MCPJ passively in extension and then passively flex the interphalangeal joints. Intrinsic muscle tightness is where there is increased range of passive interphalangeal joint flexion when the MCPJs are positioned in flexion. Further details on intrinsic muscle tightness can be found in Aulicino (1995).

Extrinsic muscle tightness. The clinician compares the range of passive interphalangeal joint movement with the MCPJs positioned in flexion and then in extension. Extensor tightness is when there is a greater range of interphalangeal joint flexion with the MCPJs in extension. Conversely, flexor tightness is where there is a greater range of interphalangeal joint extension with the MCPJs in flexion.

The clinician may test the length of other muscles, in particular those thought prone to shorten (Janda 1994, 2002). Descriptions of the tests for muscle length are given in Chapter 3.

Isometric muscle testing

Test forearm pronation and supination, wrist flexion, extension, radial and ulnar deviation, finger and thumb flexion, extension, abduction and adduction and thumb opposition in resting position and, if indicated, in different parts of the physiological range depending on subjective clues to provoking activities. The clinician observes the quality of the muscle contraction to hold this position (this can be done with the patient's eyes shut). The patient may, for example, be unable to prevent the joint from moving or may hold with excessive muscle activity, i.e. adopt substitution or compensatory strategies; either of these circumstances would suggest a neuromuscular dysfunction. In addition manual muscle testing can be useful in differential diagnosis of nerve compression trauma. For example, following carpal tunnel compression, damage to the median nerve can be checked by testing the isometric strength of opponens pollicis and abductor pollicis brevis.

Other muscle/tendon tests

Sweater finger sign test. Loss of DIPJ flexion when a fist is made is a positive test indicating a ruptured flexor digitorum profundus (FDP) tendon. The ring finger is most commonly affected (Magee 2006).

Finkelstein test for de Quervain's disease. The clinician grasps the patient's thumb and deviates the hand towards the ulna. A positive test will reproduce the patient's pain over the tip of the ulnar styloid (Figure 11.10) (Elliott 1992, Magee 2006). Reproduction of the patient's pain is indicative of de Quervain's disease – intrinsic degenerative

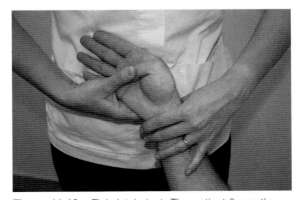

Figure 11.10 • Finkelstein test. The patient flexes the thumb and the clinician guides the patient into ulnar deviation of the wrist.

changes of the abductor pollicis longus and extensor pollicis brevis tendons in the first dorsal compartment (Clarke et al. 1998).

Linburg's sign. This tests for tendinitis at the interconnection between flexor pollicis longus and the flexor indices (Magee 2006). The thumb is flexed on to the hypothenar eminence and the index finger is extended. Limited range of index finger extension is a positive test.

Test for flexor digitorum superficialis (FDS). The clinician holds all of any three fingers in extension and asks the patient actively to flex the MCPJ and PIPJ of the remaining finger. The DIPJ should be flail as the FDP has been immobilised. If the FDS is inactive, the finger will flex strongly at the DIPJ as well as at the PIPJ and MCPJ, indicating activity of FDP. If the finger does not flex at all, neither flexor is active. Be aware that a proportion of the population does not have an effective FDS to the little finger, so the test is then invalidated for this digit (Austin et al. 1989).

Tennis/golfer's elbow. Repeated microtrauma to the common flexor and extensor origins produces degenerative changes within the tendon, resulting in persistent symptoms. An additional test for common extensor dysfunction is an isometric contraction of extension of the third digit distal to the PIPJ activating extensor carpi radialis brevis – reproduction of pain or weakness over the lateral epicondyle indicates a positive test. In the same way, isometric contraction of the flexor muscles of the wrist and hand can be examined for flexor origin pain.

Neurological tests

Neurological examination includes neurological integrity testing, neurodynamic tests and some other nerve tests.

Integrity of the nervous system

The integrity of the nervous system is tested if the clinician suspects that the symptoms are emanating from the spine or from a peripheral nerve.

Dermatomes/peripheral nerves. Light touch and pain sensation of the upper limb are tested using cotton wool and pinprick respectively, as described in Chapter 3. Following trauma or compression to peripheral nerves, it is vital to assess the cutaneous sensation, examining temperature sense, vibration, protective sensation, deep pressure to light touch, proprioception and stereognosis. The use of monofilaments and other tests is described in

Chapter 3. Knowledge of the cutaneous distribution of nerve roots (dermatomes) and peripheral nerves (radial, median and ulnar) enables the clinician to distinguish the sensory loss due to a root lesion from that due to a peripheral nerve lesion. The cutaneous nerve distribution and dermatome areas are shown in Chapter 3.

Myotomes/peripheral nerves. The following myotomes are tested (see Chapter 3 for further details):

- C5: shoulder abduction
- C6: elbow flexion
- C7: elbow extension
- C8: thumb extension
- T1: finger adduction.

A working knowledge of the muscular distribution of nerve roots (myotomes) and peripheral nerves enables the clinician to distinguish the motor loss due to a root lesion from that due to a peripheral nerve lesion. The peripheral nerve distributions are shown in Chapter 3.

Reflex testing. The following deep tendon reflexes are tested (see Chapter 3):

- C5–C6: biceps
- C7: triceps and brachioradialis.

Deep tendon reflexes are not usually tested in the forearm, wrist and hand. The Hoffman's reflex can be tested if an upper motor neurone dysfunction is suspected. The clinician 'flicks' the terminal phalanx of the index, middle or ring fingers and, in a positive test, the reflex flexion of other distal phalanx will be seen (Magee 2006).

Neurodynamic tests

The upper-limb neurodynamic tests (1, 2a, 2b and 3) may be carried out in order to ascertain the degree to which neural tissue is responsible for the production of the patient's symptom(s). These tests are described in detail in Chapter 3.

Other nerve tests

Median nerve

Carpal tunnel syndrome is the commonest peripheral nerve compression neuropathy.

Tinel's sign (Tubiana et al. 1998). This test is used to determine the first detectable sign of nerve regeneration or of nerve damage as in the case of nerve compression. The clinician taps from distal to proximal along the line of the nerve, until the patient feels a 'pins and needles' sensation peripherally in the nerve distribution. The most distal point of pins and needles sensation indicates the furthest point of axonal regeneration, or, in the case of compression of the median nerve, will produce tingling into median nerve innervated digits. Tinel's sign is not always accurate (Tubiana et al. 1998) and so needs to be used in conjunction with other tests, such as pain, temperature, vibration and, at a later stage of regeneration, monofilaments, electromyogram and two-point discrimination.

Phalen's wrist flexion test (American Society for Surgery of the Hand 1990). One-minute sustained bilateral wrist flexion producing paraesthesia in the distribution of the median nerve indicates a positive test.

Reverse Phalen's test (Linscheid & Dobyns 1987). The patient makes a fist with the wrist in extension and the clinician applies pressure over the carpal tunnel for 1 minute. Paraesthesia in the distribution of the median nerve indicates a positive test.

Carpal compression test (Durkan 1991). The clinician exerts even pressure with both thumbs over the median nerve in the carpal tunnel for up to 30 seconds. The time taken from the start of compression to the onset of symptoms in the median nerve is noted. This is a useful alternative test to Phalen's test whereby range of movement at the wrist may be restricted or painful (González del Pino et al. 1997).

Ulnar nerve

Froment's sign for ulnar nerve paralysis (Magee 2006). The patient holds a piece of paper between the index finger and thumb in a lateral key grip, and the clinician attempts to pull it away. In ulnar nerve paralysis, flexion at the interphalangeal joint of the thumb due to paralysis of adductor pollicis (Froment's sign) and clawing of the little and ring fingers are apparent as a result of paralysis of the interossei and lumbrical muscles and the unopposed action of the extrinsic extensors and flexors.

Tests for circulation and swelling

If it is suspected that the circulation is compromised, the pulses of the radial and ulnar arteries are palpated at the wrist.

Allen test for the radial and ulnar arteries at the wrist (American Society for Surgery of the Hand 1990). The clinician applies pressure to the radial

and ulnar arteries at the wrist and the patient is then asked to open and close the hand a few times and then to keep it open. The patency of each artery is tested by releasing the pressure over the radial and then the ulnar arteries. The hand should flush within 5 seconds on release of the pressure.

Tests for thoracic outlet syndrome. These have been described in Chapter 9.

Hand volume test (Blair et al. 1987). This can be used to measure swelling of the hand. A volumeter is used and a difference of 30–50 ml (there is often a 10-ml difference between right and left and dominant and non-dominant hands) between one measurement and the next indicates significant hand swelling (Bell-Krotoski et al. 1995).

Palpation

The wrist and hand region is palpated, as well as the cervical spine and thoracic spine, shoulder, and elbow as appropriate. It is useful to record palpation findings on a body chart (see Figure 2.3) and/or palpation chart (see Figure 3.36).

The clinician notes the following:

- the temperature of the area
- localised increased skin moisture
- the presence of oedema or effusion. This can be measured with a tape measure comparing left and right sides
- mobility and feel of superficial tissues, e.g. ganglions, nodules and scar tissue
- the presence or elicitation of any muscle spasm
- tenderness of bone, ligaments, muscle, tendon (forearm flexors and extensors and superficial tendons around the wrist), tendon sheath, trigger points (shown in Figure 3.37) and nerve
- palpable nerves in the upper limb are as follows:
  - ○ The median nerve can be palpated over the anterior elbow joint crease, medial to the brachial artery, as well as indirectly at the wrist between palmaris longus medially and flexor carpi radialis laterally
  - ○ The radial nerve can be palpated at the spiral groove of the humerus. The deep/motor branch may be palpated through anteroposterior pressure of radial head, as it enters the arcade of Frohse – approximately 2.5 cm distal to elbow crease and 2 cm medial to biceps tendon. The superficial/sensory branch of the radial nerve is palpable between the brachioradialis

tendon and extensor carpi radialis longus in the forearm. The terminal parts of the radial sensory nerve are palpable in the anatomical snuffbox at the wrist (Butler 2000)

○ The ulnar nerve can be palpated in the condylar groove of the humerus. The ulnar nerve is superficial at the wrist in Guyon's (pisohamate) canal between pisiform and the hook of hamate. The nerve can be injured following falls on the outstretched hand, compression through cycling or associated with typing (Baker et al. 2007)

• increased or decreased prominence of bones
• pain provoked or reduced on palpation, i.e. tenderness of scaphoid in the 'anatomical snuffbox'.

Accessory movements

It is useful to use the palpation chart and movement diagrams (or joint pictures) to record findings. These are explained in detail in Chapter 3. The clinician notes the following:

• the quality of movement
• the range of movement
• the resistance through the range and at the end of the range of movement
• the behaviour of pain through the range
• any provocation of muscle spasm.

Wrist and hand (Figure 11.11) accessory movements are listed in Table 11.2. Following accessory movements to the wrist and hand, the clinician reassesses

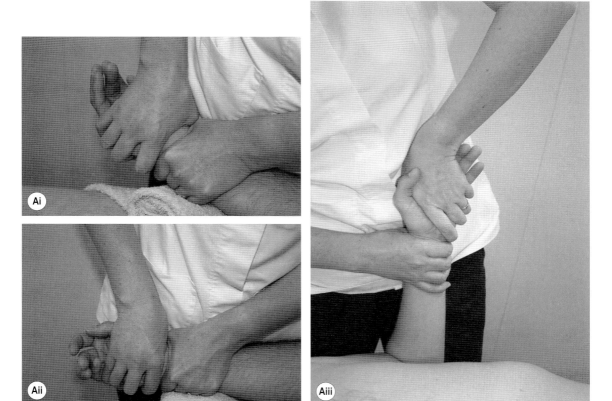

Figure 11.11 • Wrist and hand accessory movements. A (i) Anteroposterior and posteroanterior. Anteroposterior shown: the left hand grasps around the distal end of the radius and ulna and the right grasps the hand at the level of the proximal carpal row. The right hand then glides the patient's hand anteriorly to posteriorly. A (ii) Medial and lateral transverse. Medial shown: the left hand grasps around the distal radius and ulna and the right hand grasps the proximal carpal row, then glides the patient's hand medially. A (iii) Longitudinal cephalad. The right hand grasps around the distal radius and ulna and the left hand applies a longitudinal force to the wrist through the heel of the hand.

(Continued)

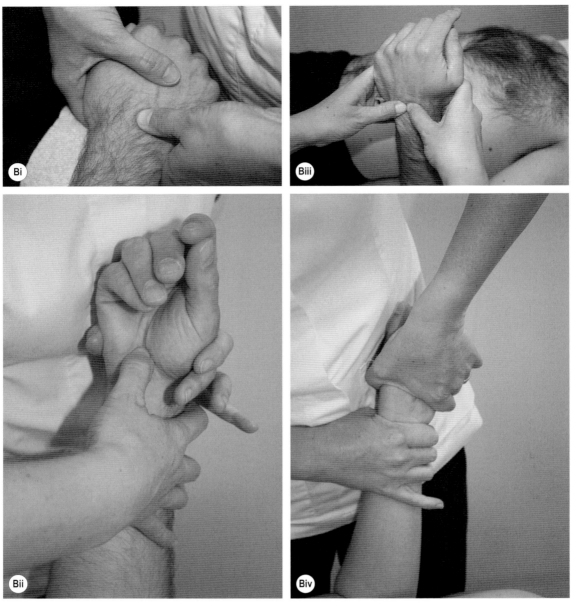

Figure 11.11 • B Intercarpal joints. B (i) Anteroposterior and posteroanterior. Thumb pressure can be applied to the anterior or posterior aspect of each carpal bone to produce an anteroposterior or posteroanterior movement respectively. A posteroanterior pressure to the lunate is shown here. B (ii) Horizontal flexion. The right thumb is placed in the centre of the anterior aspect of the wrist and the left hand cups around the carpus to produce horizontal flexion. B (iii) Horizontal extension. The thumbs are placed in the centre of the posterior aspect of the wrist and the fingers wrap around the anterior aspect of the carpus to produce horizontal extension. B (iv) Longitudinal cephalad and caudad. The right hand grasps around the distal end of the radius and ulna and the left grasps the hand at the level of the proximal end of the metacarpals. The right hand then pushes the hand towards the wrist (longitudinal cephalad) and away from the wrist (longitudinal caudad).

(Continued)

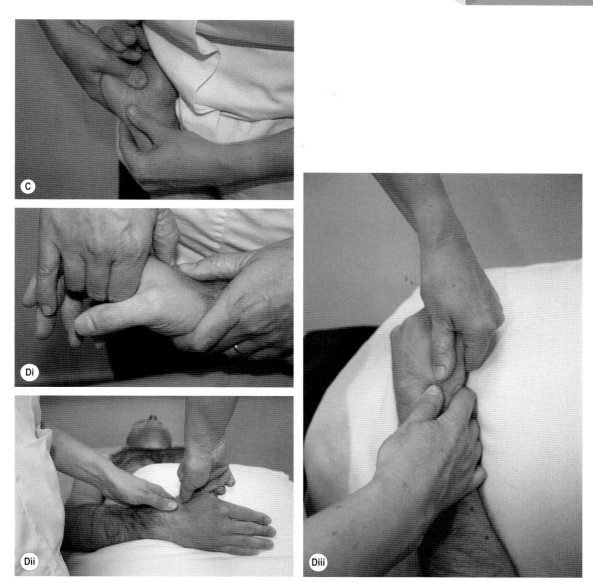

Figure 11.11—cont'd • C Pisotriquetral joint. Medial and lateral transverse, longitudinal caudad and cephalad and distraction. Shown here, the right hand stabilises the hand and the left hand grasps the triquetral bone and applies a medial and lateral transverse force to the bone. **D** Carpometacarpal joints. Fingers – the left hand grasps around the relevant distal carpal bone while the right hand grasps the proximal end of the metacarpal. **D** (i) Anteroposterior and posteroanterior. Posteroanterior shown: the right hand glides the metacarpal anteriorly. **D** (ii) Anteroposterior and posteroanterior. The left hand glides the thumb metacarpal anteriorly and posteriorly. **D** (iii) Medial and lateral rotation. The left hand rotates the thumb metacarpal medially and laterally.

(Continued)

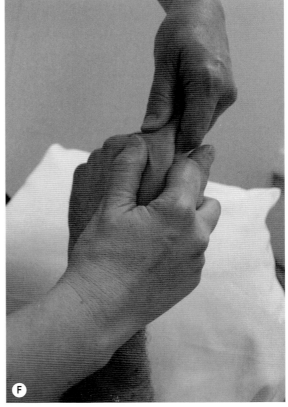

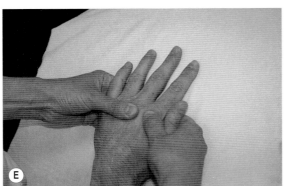

Figure 11.11—cont'd • E Proximal and distal intermetacarpal joints of the fingers – anteroposterior and posteroanterior. The finger and thumb of each hand gently pinch the anterior and posterior aspects of adjacent metacarpal heads and apply a force in opposite directions to glide the heads anteriorly and posteriorly. F Anteroposterior and posteroanterior. The left hand glides the proximal phalanx anteriorly and posteriorly.

all the physical asterisks (movements or tests that have been found to reproduce the patient's symptoms) in order to establish the effect of the accessory movements on the patient's signs and symptoms. Accessory movements can then be tested for other regions suspected to be a source of, or contributing to, the patient's symptoms. Again, following accessory movements to any one region, the clinician reassesses all the asterisks. Regions likely to be examined are the cervical spine, thoracic spine, shoulder and elbow (Table 11.2).

Completion of the examination

Having carried out the above tests, the examination of the wrist and hand is now complete. The subjective and physical examinations produce a large amount

of information, which needs to be recorded accurately and quickly. It is vital at this stage to highlight important findings from the examination with an asterisk (*). These findings must be reassessed at, and within, subsequent treatment sessions to evaluate the effects of treatment on the patient's condition.

The physical testing procedures which specifically indicate joint, nerve or muscle tissues, as a source of the patient's symptoms, are summarised in Table 3.10. The strongest evidence that a joint is the source of the patient's symptoms is that active and passive physiological movements, passive accessory movements and joint palpation all reproduce the patient's symptoms, and that, following a treatment dose, reassessment identifies an improvement in the patient's signs and symptoms. Weaker evidence includes an alteration in range, resistance or quality of physiological and/or accessory movements and

Table 11.2 Accessory movements, choice of application and reassessment of the patient's asterisks

Accessory movements	Choice of application	Identify any effect of accessory movements on patient's signs and symptoms
Radiocarpal joint		
↕ Anteroposterior ↕ Posteroanterior ↤ Med Medial transverse ↦ Lat Lateral transverse ↤ Ceph Longitudinal cephalad ↦ Caud Longitudinal caudad	Start position, e.g. in wrist flexion, extension, radial or ulnar deviation fingers or thumb in flexion, extension, abduction Direction of the applied force Point of application of applied force	Reassess all asterisks
Intercarpal joints		
↕ Anteroposterior ↕ Posteroanterior ↕↕ Anteroposterior/posteroanterior gliding HF Horizontal flexion HE Horizontal extension ↦ Ceph Longitudinal cephalad ↦ Caud Longitudinal caudad		
Pisotriquetral joint		
↤ Med Medial transverse ↦ Lat Lateral transverse ↦ Ceph Longitudinal cephalad ↦ Caud Longitudinal caudad Dist Distraction		
Carpometacarpal joints		
Fingers ↕ Anteroposterior ↕ Posteroanterior ↤ Med Medial transverse ↦ Lat Lateral transverse ↷ Medial rotation ↶ Lateral rotation		
Thumb		
↕ Anteroposterior ↕ Posteroanterior ↦ Med Medial transverse ↦ Lat Lateral transverse ↦ Ceph Longitudinal cephalad ↦ Caud Longitudinal caudad ↷ Med Medial rotation ↶ Lat Lateral rotation		

(Continued)

Table 11.2 Accessory movements, choice of application and reassessment of the patient's asterisks—cont'd

Accessory movements	Choice of application	Identify any effect of accessory movements on patient's signs and symptoms

Proximal and distal intermetacarpal joints

↕   Anteroposterior
↕   Posteroanterior
HF Horizontal flexion
HE Horizontal extension

MCP, proximal and distal interphalangeal joints of fingers and thumb

↕   Anteroposterior
↕   Posteroanterior
←•— Med Medial transverse
—•→ Lat   Lateral transverse
←•→ Ceph Longitudinal cephalad
←•→ Caud Longitudinal caudad
⤻ Med Medial rotation
⤸ Lat Lateral rotation

Ten movement test for the carpal bones (Kaltenborn 2002)

Movements around the capitate
– fix the capitate and move the trapezoid
– fix the capitate and move the scaphoid
– fix the capitate and move the lunate
– fix the capitate and move the hamate
Movement on the radial side of the wrist
– fix the scaphoid and move the trapezoid and
  trapezium
Movements in the radiocarpal joint
– fix the radius and move the scaphoid
– fix the radius and move the lunate
– fix the ulna and move the triquetrum
Movements on the ulnar side of the wrist
– fix the triquetrum and move the hamate
– fix the triquetrum and move the pisiform

?Cervical spine	As above	Reassess all asterisks
?Thoracic spine	As above	Reassess all asterisks
?Shoulder	As above	Reassess all asterisks
?Elbow	As above	Reassess all asterisks

MCP, metacarpophalangeal.

tenderness over the joint, with no alteration in signs and symptoms after treatment. One or more of these findings may indicate a dysfunction of a joint, which may or may not be contributing to the patient's condition.

The strongest evidence that a muscle is the source of a patient's symptoms is if active movements, an isometric contraction, passive lengthening and palpation of a muscle all reproduce the patient's symptoms, and that, following a treatment dose, reassessment identifies an improvement in the patient's signs and symptoms. Further evidence of muscle dysfunction may be suggested by reduced strength or poor quality during the active physiological movement and the isometric contraction, reduced range and/or increased/decreased resistance, during the passive lengthening of the muscle, and tenderness on palpation, with no alteration in signs and symptoms after treatment. One or more of these findings may indicate a dysfunction of a muscle which may, or may not, be contributing to the patient's condition.

The strongest evidence that a nerve is the source of the patient's symptoms is when active and/or passive physiological movements reproduce the patient's symptoms, which are then increased or decreased with an additional sensitising movement, at a distance from the patient's symptoms. In addition, there is reproduction of the patient's symptoms on palpation of the nerve, and neurodynamic testing, sufficient to be considered a treatment dose, results in an improvement in the above signs and symptoms. Further evidence of nerve dysfunction may be suggested by reduced range (compared with the asymptomatic side) and/or increased resistance to the various arm movements, and tenderness on nerve palpation.

On completion of the physical examination, the clinician:

- explains to the patient the findings of the physical examination and how these findings relate to the subjective assessment. Any misconceptions patients may have regarding their symptoms should be cleared up here
- warns the patient of possible exacerbation up to 24–48 hours following the examination
- requests the patient to report details on the behaviour of the symptoms following examination at the next attendance

- evaluates the findings, formulates a clinical diagnosis and writes up a problem list
- determines the objectives of treatment
- through discussion with the patient devises an initial treatment plan.

In this way, the clinician will have developed the following hypotheses categories (adapted from Jones & Rivett 2004):

- activity capability/restriction/participant capability/restriction
- patient's perspective on his/her experience
- pathobiological mechanisms. This includes the structure or tissue that is thought to be producing the patient's symptoms, the nature of the structure or tissues in relation to both the healing process and the pain mechanisms
- physical impairments and associated structures/ tissue sources
- contributing factors to the development and maintenance of the problem. There may be environmental, psychosocial, behavioural, physical or heredity factors
- precautions/contraindications to treatment and management. This includes the severity and irritability of the patient's symptoms and the nature of the patient's condition
- management strategy and treatment plan
- prognosis – this can be affected by factors such as the stage and extent of the injury as well as the patient's expectation, personality and lifestyle.

For guidance on treatment and management principles, the reader is directed to the companion textbook (Petty 2011).

References

American Society for Surgery of the Hand, 1990. The hand – examination and diagnosis, third ed. Churchill Livingstone, New York.

Aulicino, P., 1995. Clinical examination of the hand. In: Hunter, J.M., Mackin, E.J., Callahan, A.D. (Eds.), Rehabilitation of the hand: surgery and therapy, fourth ed. Mosby, St Louis, MO, p. 53.

Austin, G.J., Leslie, B.M., Ruby, L.K., 1989. Variations of the flexor digitorum superficialis of the small finger. J. Hand Surg. 14A, 262.

Baker, N., Cham, R., Cidboy, E., et al., 2007. Kinematics of the fingers and hands during computer keyboard use. Clin. Biomech. 22, 34–43.

Bell-Krotoski, J.A., Breger-Lee, D.E., Beach, R.B., 1995. Biomechanics and evaluation of the hand. In: Hunter, J.M., Mackin, E.J., Callahan, A.D. (Eds.), Rehabilitation of the hand: surgery and therapy, fourth ed. Mosby, St Louis, MO, p. 153.

Blair, S.J., McCormick, E., Bear-Lehman, J., et al., 1987. Evaluation of impairment of the upper extremity. Clin. Orthop. Relat. Res. 221, 42–58.

Bland, J.D., 2000. The value of the history in the diagnosis of carpal tunnel syndrome. J. Hand Surg. (British and European Volume) 25 (5), 445–450.

Butler, D., 2000. The sensitive nervous system. Neuro Orthopaedic Institute, Adelaide.

Cakir, M., Samanci, N., Balci, N., et al., 2003. Musculoskeletal manifestations in patients with thyroid disease. Clin. Endocrinol. (Oxf.) 59 (2), 162–167.

Chung, K.C., Pillsbury, M.S., Walter, M.R., et al., 1998. Reliability and validity testing of the Michigan hand outcomes questionnaire. J. Hand Surg. [Am.] 23, 584–587.

Clarke, M.T., Lyall, H.A., Grant, J.W., et al., 1998. The histopathology of De Quervain's disease. J. Hand Surg. (British and European) 23B (6), 732–734.

Cole, J.H., Furness, A.L., Twomey, L.T., 1988. Muscles in action, an approach to manual muscle testing. Churchill Livingstone, Edinburgh.

Cyriax, J., 1982. Textbook of orthopaedic medicine – diagnosis of soft tissue lesions, eighth ed. Baillière Tindall, London.

Durkan, J., 1991. A new diagnostic test for carpal tunnel syndrome. J. Bone Joint Surg. 73 (4), 535–538.

Earnshaw, S.A., Cawte, S.A., Worley, A., et al., 1998. Colles' fracture of the wrist as an indicator of underlying osteoporosis in post menopausal women: a prospective study of bone mineral density and bone turnover rate. Osteoporos. Int. 8 (1), 53–60.

Eckhaus, D., 1993. Swan-neck deformity. In: Clark, G.L., Wilgis, E.F.S., Aiello, B. (Eds.), Hand rehabilitation, a practical guide. Churchill Livingstone, Edinburgh, ch 16.

Eddington, L.V., 1993. Boutonnière deformity. In: Clark, G.L., Wilgis, E.F.S., Aiello, B. (Eds.), Hand rehabilitation, a practical guide. Churchill Livingstone, Edinburgh, ch 17.

Elliott, B.G., 1992. Finkelstein's test: a descriptive error that can produce a false positive. J. Hand Surg. 17B (4), 481–482.

Fess, E., Philips, C., 1987. Hand splinting, principles and methods. C V Mosby, St Louis, MO.

González del Pino, J., Delgado-Martínez, A.D., González González, I., et al., 1997. Value of the carpal compression test in the diagnosis of carpal tunnel syndrome. J. Hand Surg. [Br.] 22 (1), 38–41.

Gudmundsson, K.G., Arngrimsson, R., Sigfusson, N., et al., 2000. Epidemiology of Dupuytren's disease. Clinical, serological, and social assessment: the Reykjavik Study. J. Clin. Epidemiol. 53 (3), 291–296.

Guy, R.J., Clark, C.A., Malcolm, P.N., et al., 1985. Evaluation of thermal and vibration sensation in diabetic neuropathy. Diabetologia 28, 131–137.

Heyman, P., 1997. Injuries to the ulnar collateral ligament of the thumb metacarpophalangeal joint. J. Am. Acad. Orthop. Surg. 5 (224), 229.

Hislop, H., Montgomery, J., 1995. Daniels and Worthingham's muscle testing, techniques of manual examination, seventh ed. W B Saunders, Philadelphia.

Janda, V., 1994. Muscles and motor control in cervicogenic disorders: assessment and management. In: Grant, R. (Ed.), Physical therapy of the cervical and thoracic spine, second ed. Churchill Livingstone, New York, p. 195.

Janda, V., 2002. Muscles and motor control in cervicogenic disorders. In: Grant, R. (Ed.), Physical therapy of the cervical and thoracic spine, third ed. Churchill Livingstone, New York, p. 182.

Jebson, R.H., Taylor, N., Trieschmann, R.B., et al., 1969. An objective and standardized test of hand function. Arch. Phys. Med. Rehabil. 50, 311–319.

Jones, M.A., Rivett, D.A., 2004. Clinical reasoning for manual therapists. Butterworth-Heinemann, Edinburgh.

Kaltenborn, F.M., 2002. Manual mobilization of the joints, vol I, The extremities, sixth ed. Norli, Oslo.

Kendall, F.P., McCreary, E.K., Provance, P.G., 1993. Muscles, testing and function, fourth ed. Williams & Wilkins, Baltimore, MD.

Levine, D.W., Simmons, B.P., Koris, M.J., et al., 1993. A self administered questionnaire for the assessment of severity of symptoms and functional status in carpal tunnel syndrome. J. Bone Joint Surg. 75 (11), 1585–1592.

Lichtman, D.M., Wroten, E.S., 2006. Understanding midcarpal instability. J. Hand Surg. 31A (3), 491–498.

Lichtman, D.M., Schneider, J.R., Swafford, A.R., et al., 1981. Ulnar midcarpal instability – clinical and laboratory analysis. J. Hand Surg. 6A, 515–523.

Linscheid, R.L., Dobyns, J.H., 1987. Physical examination of the wrist. In: Post, M. (Ed.), Physical examination of the musculoskeletal system. Year Book Medical, Chicago, p. 80.

Magee, D.J., 2006. Orthopedic physical assessment, fourth ed. Saunders Elsevier, Philadelphia.

Maitland, G.D., Hengeveld, E., Banks, K., et al., 2005. Maitland's peripheral manipulation, fourth ed. Butterworth-Heinemann Elsevier, London.

Moberg, E., 1958. Objective methods for determining the functional value of sensibility in the hand. J. Bone Joint Surg. 40B (3), 454–476.

Mulligan, B.R., 1999. Manual therapy 'NAGs', 'SNAGs', 'MWMs' etc., fourth ed. Plane View Services, New Zealand.

Neumann, D., 2002. Kinesiology of the musculoskeletal system, foundations for physical rehabilitation. Mosby, St Louis, MO, p. 219.

Petty, N.J., 2011. Principles of neuromusculoskeletal treatment and management: a guide for therapists, second ed. Churchill Livingstone, Edinburgh.

Pryce, J.C., 1980. The wrist position between neutral and ulnar deviation that facilitates the maximum power grip strength. J. Biomech. 13, 505–511.

Refshauge, K., Gass, E. (Eds.), 2004. Musculoskeletal physiotherapy clinical science and evidence-based practice. Butterworth-Heinemann, Oxford.

Taleisnik, J., 1988. Carpal instability. J. Bone Joint Surg. 70A (8), 1262–1268.

Totten, P., Flinn-Wagner, S., 1992. Functional evaluation of the hand. In: Stanely, B., Tribuzi, S. (Eds.), Concepts in hand rehabilitation. F A Davies, New York, p. 128.

Trail, I.A., Stanley, J.K., Hayton, M.J., 2007. Twenty questions on carpal instability. J. Hand Surg. 32, 240–255.

Tubiana, R., Thomine, J.M., Mackin, E., 1998. Examination of the hand and wrist. Martin Dunitz, Boston, MA.

Watson, H.K., Ashmead, D.I.V., Makhlouf, M.V., 1988. Examination of the scaphoid. J. Hand Surg. 13A (5), 657–660.

Examination of the lumbar region

Laura Finucane   Chris Mercer

Possible causes of pain and/or limitation of movement

This region includes T12 to the sacrum and coccyx.

- Trauma and degeneration:
    - fracture of spinous process, transverse process, vertebral arch or vertebral body; fracture dislocation
    - spondylolysis and spondylolisthesis
    - ankylosing vertebral hyperostosis
    - Scheuermann's disease
    - syndromes: arthrosis of the zygapophyseal joints, spondylosis (intervertebral disc degeneration), intervertebral disc lesions, prolapsed intervertebral disc, osteitis condensans ilii, coccydynia, hypermobility
    - ligamentous sprain
    - muscular strain
    - congenital and acquired scoliosis
- Inflammatory:
    - ankylosing spondylitis
    - rheumatoid arthritis
- Metabolic:
    - osteoporosis
    - Paget's disease
    - osteomalacia
- Infections:
    - tuberculosis of the spine
    - pyogenic osteitis of the spine
- Discitus
- Tumours, benign and malignant
- Postural low-back pain
- Piriformis syndrome.

Further details of the questions asked during the subjective examination and the tests carried out in the physical examination can be found in Chapters 2 and 3 respectively.

The order of the subjective questioning and the physical tests described below can be altered as appropriate for the patient being examined.

Subjective examination

Body chart

The following information concerning the type and area of the current symptoms can be recorded on a body chart (see chapter 2 Figure 2.3).

Area of current symptoms

Be exact when mapping out the area of the symptoms. Lesions in the lumbar spine can refer symptoms over a large area – symptoms are commonly felt around the spine, abdomen, groin and lower limbs. Occasionally, symptoms may be felt in the head, cervical and thoracic spine. Ascertain which is the worst symptom and record the patient's interpretation of where s/he feels the symptom(s) are coming from.

The area of symptoms may, alongside other signs and symptoms, indicate illness behaviour (Table 12.1).

Areas relevant to the region being examined

All other relevant areas are checked for symptoms; it is important to ask about pain or stiffness, as this may be relevant to the patient's main symptom. Mark unaffected areas with ticks (✓) on the body chart. Check for symptoms in the cervical spine, thoracic spine, abdomen, groin and lower limbs.

Table 12.1 Indications of possible illness behaviour (Waddell 2004)

Signs and symptoms	Illness behaviour	Physical disease
Pain		
Pain drawing	Non-anatomical, regional, magnified	Localised, anatomical
Pain adjectives	Emotional	Sensory
Symptoms		
Pain	Whole-leg pain Pain at the tip of the coccyx	Musculoskeletal or neurological distribution
Numbness	Whole-leg numbness	Dermatomal
Weakness	Whole-leg giving way	Myotomal
Behaviour of pain	Constant pain	Varies with time and activity
Response to treatment	Intolerance of treatments Emergency hospitalisation	Variable benefit
Signs		
Tenderness	Superficial, non-anatomical	Musculoskeletal distribution
Axial loading	Low-back pain	Neck pain
Simulated rotation	Low-back pain	Nerve root pain
Straight-leg raise	Marked improvement with distraction	Limited on formal examination No improvement with distraction
Motor	Regional jerky, giving way	Myotomal
Sensory	Regional	Dermatomal

Quality of pain

Establish the quality of the pain.

Intensity of pain

The intensity of pain can be measured using, for example a visual analogue scale, as shown in Chapter 2. A pain diary may be useful for patients with chronic low-back pain to determine the pain patterns and triggering factors over a period of time.

Abnormal sensation

Check for any altered sensation over the lumbar spine and other relevant areas. Common abnormalities are paraesthesia and numbness.

Constant or intermittent symptoms

Establish the frequency of the symptoms and whether they are constant or intermittent. If symptoms are constant, check whether there is variation in the intensity of the symptoms, as constant unremitting pain may be indicative of sinister pathology.

Relationship of symptoms

If there is more than one area of symptoms, determine the relationship between symptomatic areas – do they come together or separately? For example, the patient could have thigh pain without lumbar spine pain, or the pains may always be present together. It is possible that there may be two separate sources of symptoms.

Behaviour of symptoms

Aggravating factors

For each symptomatic area a series of questions can be asked:

- What movements and/or positions bring on or make the patient's symptoms worse?
- How long does it take before symptoms are aggravated?
- Is the patient able to maintain this position or movement?
- What happens to other symptoms when this symptom is produced or made worse?
- How do the symptoms affect function, e.g. sitting, standing, lying, bending, walking, running, walking on uneven ground and up and down stairs,

washing, driving, lifting and digging, work, sport and social activities? Further detail about these activities may needs to be gathered. For example, the patient may complain that driving aggravates the symptoms. Finding out what particular aspect of driving worsens the symptoms will help to determine the structure at fault.

The clinician may ask the patient about theoretically known aggravating factors for structures that could be a source of the symptoms. However, this evidence is not conclusive as functional movements invariably stress other parts of the body. Common aggravating factors for the lumbar spine are flexion (e.g. when putting shoes and socks on), sitting, standing, walking, standing up from the sitting position, driving and coughing/sneezing. These movements and positions can increase symptoms because they stress various structures in the lumbar spine (Table 12.2). Aggravating factors for other regions, which may need to be queried if they are suspected to be a source of the symptoms, are shown in Table 2.3 Chapter 2.

Easing factors

For each symptomatic area a series of questions can be asked to help determine what eases the symptoms:

- What movements and/or positions ease the patient's symptoms?
- How long does it take before symptoms are eased? If symptoms are constant but variable it is important to know what the baseline is and how long it takes for the symptoms to reduce to that level.
- What happens to other symptoms when this symptom is eased?

The clinician asks the patient about theoretically known easing factors for structures that could be a source of the symptoms. Commonly suggested aggravating and found easing factors for the lumbar spine are shown in Table 12.2. A recent review paper suggests that there is little difference in intradiscal pressure between sitting and standing, and this should be considered when looking at the table (Claus et al 2008). The clinician can then analyse the position or movement that eases the symptoms to help determine the structure at fault.

Aggravating and easing factors will help to determine the irritability of the patient's symptoms. These factors may help to determine the areas at fault and identify functional restrictions and also the relationship between symptoms. The severity can be determined by the intensity of the symptoms

Table 12.2 Effect of position and movement on pain-sensitive structures of the lumbar spine (Jull 1986)

Activity	Symptoms	Possible structural and pathological implications
Sitting		Compressive forces (White & Panjabi 1990) High intradiscal pressure (Nachemson 1992) Limited effect on intradiscal pressure (Claus et al 2008)
Sitting with extension	Decreased	Intradiscal pressure reduced Decreased paraspinal muscle activity (Andersson et al. 1977)
	Increased	Greater compromise of structures of lateral and central canals Compressive forces on lower zygapophyseal joints
Sitting with flexion	Decreased	Little compressive load on lower zygapophyseal joints Greater volume lateral and central canals Reduced disc bulge posteriorly
	Increased	Very high intradiscal pressure Increased compressive loads upper and mid-zygapophyseal joints
Prolonged sitting	Increased	Gradual creep of tissues (Kazarian 1975)
Sit to stand	Increased	Creep, time for reversal, difficulty in straightening up Extension of spine, increase in disc bulge posteriorly
Standing	Increased	Creep into extension
Walking	Increased	Shock loads greater than body weight Compressive load (vertical creep) (Kirkaldy-Willis & Farfan 1982) Compressive loads decrease disc height (Adams et al 2000; Kingma 2000; Hutton et al 2003) Leg pain – neurogenic claudication, intermittent claudication
Driving	Increased	Sitting: compressive forces Vibration: muscle fatigue, increased intradiscal pressure, creep (Pope & Hansson 1992) Increased dural tension sitting with legs extended Short hamstrings: pulls lumbar spine into greater flexion
Coughing/sneezing/straining	Increased	Increased pressure subarachnoid space Increased intradiscal pressure Mechanical 'jarring' of sudden uncontrolled movement

and whether the symptoms are interfering with normal activities of daily living, such as work and sleep. This information can be used to determine the direction of the physical examination as well as the aims of treatment and any advice that may be required. The most relevant subjective information should be highlighted with an asterisk (*), explored in the physical examination and reassessed at subsequent treatment sessions to evaluate treatment intervention.

Twenty-four-hour behaviour of symptoms

The clinician determines the 24-hour behaviour of symptoms by asking questions about night, morning and evening symptoms.

Night symptoms. Although night pain is a recognised red flag, it should be noted that night symptoms are common in back pain (Harding et al. 2004). It is necessary to establish whether the patient is being woken and kept awake by the symptoms. Patients complaining of needing to sleep upright or get up should raise some concern.

The following questions may be asked:

- Do you have any difficulty getting to sleep?
- Do your symptom(s) wake you at night? If so:
  ○ Which symptom(s)?
  ○ How many times in a night?
  ○ How many times in the past week?
  ○ What do you have to do to get back to sleep?

If sleep is an issue, further questioning may be useful to determine management.

Morning and evening symptoms. The clinician determines the pattern of the symptoms first thing in the morning, through the day and at the end of the day. Morning stiffness that lasts more than 2 hours is suggestive of an inflammatory condition such as ankylosing spondylitis. Stiffness lasting only 30 minutes or less is likely to be mechanical and degenerative in nature. Patients with these symptoms may also report increased symptoms at the end of the day and at night time. This may warrant further investigation. Patients reporting an increase in symptoms first thing may be indicative of a disc prolapse.

Stage of the condition

In order to determine the stage of the condition, the clinician asks whether the symptoms are getting better, getting worse or remaining unchanged.

Special questions

Special questions must always be asked, as they may identify certain precautions or contraindications to the physical examination and/or treatment (see Table 2.4). As mentioned in Chapter 2, the clinician must differentiate between conditions that are suitable for conservative management and systemic, neoplastic and other non-neuromusculoskeletal conditions, which require referral to a medical practitioner. The reader is referred to Appendix 2.3 for details of various serious pathological processes which can mimic neuromusculoskeletal conditions (Grieve 1994b).

Neurological symptoms. Neurological symptoms may include pins and needles, numbness and weakness. These symptoms need to be mapped out on the body chart.

Has the patient experienced symptoms of cauda equina compression (i.e. compression below L1), which are saddle anaesthesia/paraesthesia, sexual or erectile dysfunction, loss of vaginal sensation, bladder and/or bowel sphincter disturbance (loss of control, retention, hesitancy, urgency or a sense of incomplete evacuation) (Lavy et al. 2009) These symptoms may be due to interference of S3 and S4 (Grieve 1981). Prompt imaging and surgical attention are required to prevent permanent sphincter paralysis (Lavy et al. 2009).

Has the patient experienced symptoms of spinal cord compression (i.e. compression above the L1 level, which may include the cervical and thoracic cord and brain), such as bilateral tingling in hands or feet and/or disturbance of gait? Are there motor, sensory or tonal changes in all four limbs? Does the patient report coordination changes, including gait disturbance?

History of the present condition

For each symptomatic area, the clinician needs to know how long the symptom has been present, whether there was a sudden or slow onset and whether there was a known cause that provoked the onset of the symptom. If the onset was slow, the clinician finds out if there has been any change in the patient's lifestyle, e.g. a new job or hobby or a change in sporting activity. To confirm the relationship between the symptoms, the clinician asks what happened to other symptoms when each symptom began. Has the patient had previous similar episodes? if so did s/he have treatment for this? and what was the outcome?

Past medical history

The following information is obtained from the patient and/or the medical notes:

- The details of any relevant medical history. Visceral structures are capable of masquerading as musculoskeletal conditions, for example the pelvic organs, bowel and kidneys can refer to lumbar spine and sacral regions. Any relevant history related to these organs is important to help differentiate the cause of symptoms. For further information refer to the chapter on masqueraders by Grieve (1994b).

- The history of any previous episodes: how many? when were they? what was the cause? what was the duration of each episode? and did the patient fully recover between episodes? Does the patient perceive the current condition to be better, the same or worse in relation to other previous episodes? If there have been no previous attacks, has the patient had any episodes of stiffness in the lumbar spine, thoracic spine or any other relevant region? Check for a history of trauma or recurrent minor trauma.

- Ascertain the results of any past treatment for the same or similar problem. Past treatment records may be obtained for further information.

General health. Ascertain the general health of the patient – find out if the patient suffers from any malaise, fatigue, fever, nausea or vomiting, stress, anxiety or depression.

Weight loss. Has the patient noticed any recent unexplained weight loss?

Rheumatoid arthritis. Has the patient (or a member of his/her family) been diagnosed as having rheumatoid arthritis?

Serious pathology. Does the patient have a previous history of serious pathology such as tuberculosis or cancer?

Inflammatory arthritis. Has the patient (or a member of his/her family) been diagnosed as having an inflammatory condition such as rheumatoid arthritis)?

Cardiovascular disease. Is there a history of cardiac disease, e.g. angina?

Blood pressure. If the patient has raised blood pressure, is it controlled with medication?

Respiratory disease. Does the patient have a history of lung pathology, including asthma? How is it controlled?

Diabetes. Does the patient suffer from diabetes? If so, is it type 1 or type 2 diabetes? Is the patient's blood glucose controlled? How is the patient's blood glucose controlled? Through diet, tablet or injection? Patients with diabetes may develop peripheral neuropathy and vasculopathy, are at increased risk of infection and may take longer to heal than those without diabetes.

Epilepsy. Is the patient epileptic? When was the last seizure?

Thyroid disease. Does the patient have a history of thyroid disease? Thyroid dysfunction may cause musculoskeletal conditions such as adhesive capsulitis, Dupuytren's contracture, trigger finger and carpal tunnel syndrome (Cakir et al. 2003).

Osteoporosis. Has the patient had a dual-energy X-ray absorptiometry (DEXA) scan, been diagnosed with osteoporosis or sustained low impact fractures?

Previous surgery. Has the patient had previous surgery which may be of relevance to the presenting complaint?

Drug therapy. What drugs are being taken by the patient? Has the patient ever been prescribed long-term (6 months or more) medication/steroids? Has the patient been taking anticoagulants recently?

X-ray and medical imaging. Has the patient been X-rayed or had any other medical tests recently? Routine spinal X-rays are no longer considered necessary prior to conservative treatment as they identify only the normal age-related degenerative changes, which do not necessarily correlate with the symptoms experienced by the patient (Clinical Standards Advisory Report 1994). X-rays may be indicated in the younger patient (under 20 years) with conditions such as spondylolisthesis or ankylosing spondylitis and in the older patient (over 55 years) where management is difficult (Royal College of Radiologists 2007). In cases where there is a suspected fracture due to trauma or osteoporosis, X-rays are indicated in the first instance. The medical tests may include blood tests, magnetic resonance imaging, discography or a bone scan.

There are a number of patients whose pain may persist beyond the expected point of tissue healing. These patients will require a different approach to a traditional assessment. The following questions may be helpful in evaluating the psychosocial risk factors or 'yellow flags' for poor treatment outcome (Waddell 2004, Kendall et al. 1997):

- Have you had time off work in the past with back pain?
- What do you understand to be the cause of your back pain?
- What are you expecting will help you?
- How is your employer/co-workers/family responding to your back pain?
- What are you doing to cope with your back pain?
- Do you think you will return to work? When?

Readers are referred to the excellent text by Waddell (2004) for further details on the management of patients demonstrating psychosocial risk factors.

Social and family history

Social and family history that is relevant to the onset and progression of the patient's problem is recorded. This includes the patient's perspectives, experience and expectations, age, employment, home situation and details of any leisure activities. Factors from this information may indicate direct and/or indirect influences on the lumbar spine. In order to treat the patient appropriately, it is important to manage within the context of the patient's social and work environment.

Plan of the physical examination

When all this information has been collected, the subjective examination is complete. It is useful at this stage to highlight with asterisks (*), for ease of reference, important findings and particularly one or more functional restrictions. These can then be re-examined at subsequent treatment sessions to evaluate treatment intervention.

In order to plan the physical examination, the following hypotheses need to be developed from the subjective examination:

- The regions and structures that need to be examined as a possible cause of the symptoms, e.g. lumbar spine, thoracic spine, cervical spine, sacroiliac joint, pubic symphysis, hip, knee, ankle and foot, muscles and nerves. Often it is not possible to examine all of these areas fully at the first attendance and so examination of the structures must be prioritised over subsequent treatment sessions.

- In what way should the physical tests be carried out? Will it be easy or hard to reproduce each symptom? Will it be necessary to use combined movements and repetitive movements to reproduce the patient's symptoms? Are symptoms severe and/or irritable?

- If symptoms are severe, physical tests may be carried out to just before the onset of symptom production or just to the onset of symptom production; no overpressures will be carried out, as the patient would be unable to tolerate this.

- If symptoms are non-severe, physical tests will be carried out to reproduce symptoms fully and may include overpressures and combined movements.

- If symptoms are irritable, physical tests may be examined to just before symptom production or just to the onset of provocation with fewer physical tests being examined to allow for a rest period between tests.

- If symptoms are non-irritable physical tests will be carried out to reproduce symptoms fully and may include overpressures and combined movements.

Other factors that need to be examined include working and everyday postures, leg length and muscle weakness.

Are there any precautions and/or contraindications to elements of the physical examination that need to be explored further, such as significant neurological involvement, recent fracture, trauma, steroid therapy or rheumatoid arthritis? There may also be certain contraindications to further examination and treatment, e.g. symptoms of cord compression.

A physical planning form can be useful for clinicians to help guide them through the clinical reasoning process (see Figure 2.10).

Physical examination

The information from the subjective examination helps the clinician to plan an appropriate physical examination (Jones & Rivett 2004). The severity, irritability and nature of the condition are the major factors that will influence the choice and priority of physical testing procedures. The first and over-arching question the clinician might ask is: 'Is this patient's condition suitable for me to manage?' For example, a patient presenting with cauda equina compression symptoms may only need neurological integrity testing, prior to an urgent medical referral. The second question the clinician might ask is: 'Does this patient have a neuromusculoskeletal dysfunction that I may be able to help?' To answer that, the clinician needs to carry out a full physical examination; however, this may not be possible if the symptoms are severe and/or irritable. If the patient's symptoms are severe and/or irritable, the clinician aims to explore movements as much as possible, within a symptom-free range. If the patient has constant and severe and/or irritable symptoms, then the clinician aims to find physical tests that ease the symptoms. If the patient's symptoms are non-severe and non-irritable, then the clinician aims to find physical tests that reproduce each of the patient's symptoms.

Each significant physical test that either provokes or eases the patient's symptoms is highlighted in the patient's notes by an asterisk (*) for easy reference. The highlighted tests are often referred to as 'asterisks' or 'markers'.

The order and detail of the physical tests described below need to be appropriate to the patient being examined; some tests will be irrelevant, some tests will be carried out briefly, while it will be necessary to investigate others fully. It is important that readers understand that the techniques shown in this chapter are some of many; the choice depends mainly on the relative size of the clinician and patient, as well as the clinician's preference. For this reason, novice clinicians may initially want to try what is shown, but then quickly adapt to what is best for them.

Observation

Informal observation

This should begin as soon as the clinician sees the patient for the first time. This may be in the reception or waiting area, or as the patient enters the treatment room, and should continue throughout the subjective examination. The clinician should be aware of the patient's posture, demeanour, facial expressions, gait and interaction with the clinician, as these may all give valuable information regarding possible pain mechanisms and the severity and irritability of the problem.

Formal observation

The clinician observes the patient's spinal, pelvic and lower-limb posture in standing, from anterior, lateral and posterior views. The presence of a lateral shift, scoliosis, kyphosis or lordosis is noted. Any asymmetry in levels at the pelvis and shoulders is noted. Observation should include inspection of the muscle bulk, tone and symmetry. This may be related to the patient's handedness or physical activity, or may relate to the complaining symptom. Findings may lead the clinician to investigate muscle length/strength in the physical examination. Skin colour, areas of redness, swelling or sweating should be noted, as these may indicate areas of local pathology, or possibly a systemic or dermatological condition. The clinician should watch the patient performing simple functional tasks. Observation of gait, of sit-to-stand and dressing/undressing will help to give the clinician a good idea of how the patient is likely to move in the physical examination, and may help to highlight any problems such as hypervigilance and fear avoidance.

Active physiological movements

For active physiological movements, the clinician notes the:

- quality of movement
- range of movement
- behaviour of pain through the range of movement
- resistance through the range of movement and at the end of the range of movement
- provocation of any muscle spasm.

The active movements with overpressure listed are tested with the patient in standing and are shown in Figure 12.1. Active physiological movements of the lumbar spine and possible modifications are shown in Table 12.3. The clinician usually stands behind the patient to be able to see the quality and range of movement. Before starting the active movements, the clinician notes any deformity or deviation in the patient's spinal posture or any muscle

spasm. This may include scoliosis, a lateral shift, or a kyphotic or lordotic posture. Postural deformities can be corrected prior to starting the active movements to see if this changes the patient's symptoms. Symptom response through range is noted, and any deviation during movement can again be corrected to see if this changes symptoms. Changes in pain response may help to guide the treatment. Pain through range may result from a number of causes, including instability or lack of control of movement, a structural deformity or fear of movement. Activation of the postural control muscles may help to decrease through range pain, and this may suggest the use of muscle control exercises in the treatment programme. Equally, reassurance of the patient that movement is a good thing may also help to correct movement abnormalities.

Patients may exhibit a range of compensatory movement strategies, some of which may be a way to avoid pain (adaptive), but some of which are likely to be provocative (maladaptive). O'Sullivan (2006) describes typical movement patterns and related tests as part of a subclassification system for patients with low back pain.

Simple movements tested are:

- flexion
- extension
- lateral flexion to the right
- lateral flexion to the left
- lateral glide to the left
- lateral glide to the right
- left rotation
- right rotation.

At the end of range, if no symptoms have been produced and the problem is non-irritable, then overpressure may be applied in order to clear that single movement and to explore further for symptoms (Maitland et al. 2005). If this produces no symptoms and the clinician is still searching for the patient's pain, or is looking to screen the lumbar spine as a source of the pain, then these movements may be combined. The order in which the movements are combined will depend on the aggravating activities, and the patient's response to plane movements. An example of the combined movement of flexion, right lateral flexion and right rotation is shown in Figure 12.2.

Movements may also be repeated to see the effect this has on the patient's symptoms. McKenzie and May (2003) suggests a classification of low back pain based on presenting signs and symptoms, and the response of symptoms to movement (Table 12.4).

There is evidence to suggest that if peripheral pain centralises with repeated movements, then the prognosis for the patient is likely to be favourable. There is also evidence that patients respond well to treatment consisting of repeated movements in the direction that centralises their pain (Long et al. 2004; Hefford 2008).

Additional tests may also be useful to help to differentiate the lumbar spine from the hip and sacroiliac joint in standing. For example, when trunk rotation in standing on one leg (causing rotation in the lumbar spine and hip joint) reproduces the patient's buttock pain, differentiation between the lumbar spine and hip joint may be required. The clinician can increase and decrease the lumbar spine rotation and the pelvic rotation in turn, to find out what effect each has on the buttock pain. If the pain is emanating from the hip then the lumbar movements may have no effect, but pelvic movements may alter the pain; conversely, if the pain is emanating from the lumbar spine, then lumbar spine movements may alter the pain, but pelvic movement may have no effect. The hip can also be placed in a different position, in order to see how much it is contributing to the pain. It can be placed in a more or less provocative position, depending on the subjective aggravating factors and the irritability of the problem, and the pain response noted. Changes to symptom response may guide the clinician towards a more indepth hip assessment, or may equally focus the clinician on the lumbar spine. Compression or distraction of the sacroiliac joints can be added at the same time to see if this helps to change symptoms. Changes in pain may help guide the clinician towards a more indepth assessment of the sacroiliac joints (see Chapter 13).

Some functional ability has already been tested by the general observation of the patient during the subjective and physical examinations, e.g. the posture adopted during the subjective examination and the ease or difficulty of undressing and changing position prior to the examination. Any further functional testing can be carried out at this point in the examination and may include lifting, sitting postures and dressing.

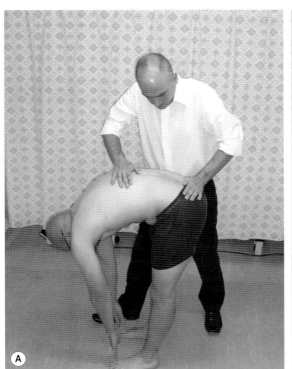 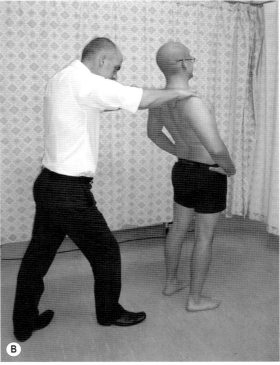

Figure 12.1 • Overpressures to the lumbar spine. **A** Flexion. The hands are placed proximally over the lower thoracic spine and distally over the sacrum. Pressure is then applied through both hands to increase lumbar spine flexion. **B** Extension. Both hands are placed over the shoulders, which are then pulled down in order to increase lumbar spine extension. The clinician observes the spinal movement.

(Continued)

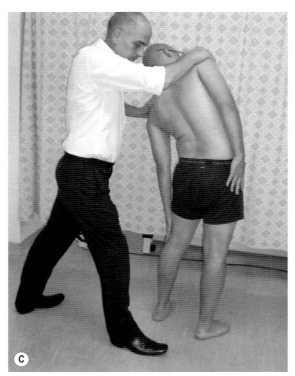

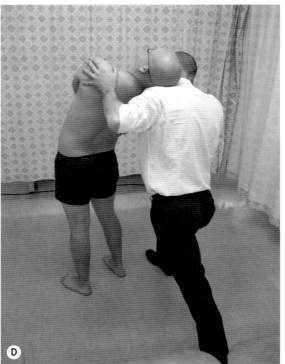

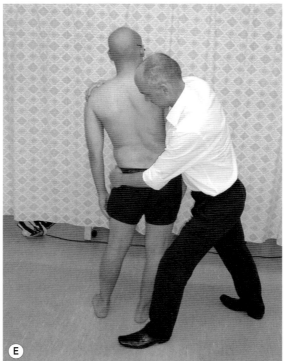

Figure 12.1—cont'd • C Lateral flexion. Both hands are placed over the shoulders and a force is applied that increases lumbar lateral flexion. **D** Right extension quadrant. This movement is a combination of extension, right rotation and right lateral flexion. The hand hold is the same as for extension. The patient actively extends and the clinician maintains this position and passively rotates the spine and then adds lateral flexion overpressure. **E** Right side gliding in standing. The clinician guides the movement, displacing the hips away from shoulders.

Table 12.3 Active physiological movements and possible modifications

Active physiological movements	Modifications
Lumbar spine	Repeated movements
Flexion	Speed altered
Extension	Combined movements (Edwards 1994, 1999), e.g.
Left lateral flexion	flexion then lateral flexion
Right lateral flexion	extension then lateral flexion
Left rotation	lateral flexion then flexion
Right rotation	lateral flexion then extension
Repetitive flexion in standing	Compression or distraction
Repetitive extension in standing	Sustained
Left side gliding in standing (SGIS)	Injuring movement
Left repetitive side gliding in standing (RSGIS)	Differentiation tests
Right SGIS	Function
Right RSGIS	
Flexion in lying	
Repetitive flexion in lying	
Extension in lying	
Repetitive extension in lying	
Sacroiliac joint Compression/distraction	
Hip medial/lateral rotation	
Knee Flexion/extension	

Clues for appropriate tests can be obtained from the subjective examination findings, particularly aggravating factors. These may be particularly helpful if the pain is proving difficult to reproduce with the other tests described.

Passive physiological movements

Passive physiological intervertebral movements (PPIVMs), which examine the movement at each segmental level may be a useful adjunct to passive

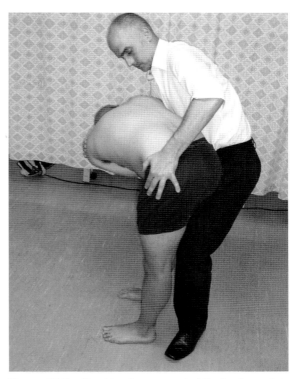

Figure 12.2 • Combined movement of the lumbar spine. The patient moves into lumbar spine flexion and the clinician then maintains this position and passively adds left lateral flexion.

accessory intervertebral movements (described later in this chapter) to identify segmental hypomobility and hypermobility (Grieve 1991). They can be performed with the patient in side-lying with the hips and knees flexed (Figure 12.3) or in standing. The clinician palpates the gap between adjacent spinous processes to feel the range of intervertebral movement during flexion, extension, lateral flexion and rotation. It is usually not necessary to examine all directions of movement, only the movement that has been most provocative or most positive during active movement tests, or the movement that most closely fits the patient's aggravating activities, e.g. if a patient says s/he has most pain when bending to tie shoelaces, then flexion would be the logical PPIVM choice.

It may be necessary to examine other regions to determine their relevance to the patient's symptoms; they may be the source of the symptoms, or they may be contributing to the symptoms. The regions most likely are the sacroiliac joint, hip, knee, foot and ankle.

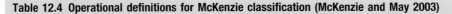

Table 12.4 Operational definitions for McKenzie classification (McKenzie and May 2003)

Reducible Derangement

Centralisation: in response to therapeutic loading strategies pain is progressively abolished in a distal to proximal direction, and each progressive abolition is retained over time, until all symptoms are abolished, and if back pain only is present this moves from a widespread to a more central location and then is abolished. Or pain is decreased and then abolished during the application of therapeutic loading strategies. The change in pain location, or decrease or abolition of pain remain better, and should be accompanied or preceded by improvements in the mechanical presentation (range of movement and/or deformity).

Irreducible Derangement

Peripheralisation of symptoms: increase or worsening of distal symptoms in response to therapeutic loading strategies, and/or no decrease, abolition, or centralisation of pain.

Dysfunction

Spinal pain only, and intermittent pain, and at least one movement is restricted, and the restricted movement consistently produces concordant pain at end-range, and there is no rapid reduction or abolition of symptoms, and no lasting production and no peripheralisation of symptoms.

ANR

History of radiculopathy or surgery in the last few months that has improved, but is now unchanging, and symptoms are intermittent, and symptoms in the limb, including 'tightness', and tension test is clearly restricted and consistently produces concordant pain or tightness at end-range, and there is no rapid reduction or abolition of symptoms, and no lasting production of distal symptoms.

Postural

Spinal pain only, and concordant pain only with static loading, and abolition of pain with postural correction, and no pain with repeated movements, and no loss of range of movement, and no pain during movement.

Joint integrity tests

In side-lying with the lumbar spine in extension and hips flexed to 90°, the clinician pushes along the femoral shafts while palpating the interspinous spaces between adjacent lumbar vertebrae to feel for any excessive movement (Figure 12.4). In the same position but with the lumbar spine in flexion, the clinician pulls along the shaft of the femur and again palpates the interspinous spaces to feel for any excessive movement. Observation of the quality of active flexion and extension can also indicate instability of the lumbar spine (see below). This test is described more fully by Maitland et al. (2005).

Muscle tests

The muscle tests may include examining muscle strength, control, length and isometric muscle testing. Depending on the patient presentation, these tests may not be a priority on day 1 of the examination, but they may well be part of the ongoing patient management and rehabilitation. Assessment should

be based on the subjective asterisks. If the clinician thinks that the muscle is the main source of symptoms, or a strong contributing factor to the patient's problem, then the muscle control component should be examined on day 1. Patients may complain of a feeling of weakness, of a lack of control of movement, or catches of pain through movement, and these types of descriptions should alert the clinician to the importance of the muscle component of the patient presentation. Muscle may be both a source of symptoms and a contributing factor.

Muscle strength

The clinician may test the trunk flexors, extensors, lateral flexors and rotators and any other relevant muscle groups, if these are indicated from the subjective examination. For details of these general tests readers are directed to Cole et al. (1988), Hislop & Montgomery (1995) or Kendall et al. (1993). There is good evidence to suggest that general exercise and strengthening exercises are likely to be of benefit for people with low-back pain (Van Tulder et al. 2005; Mercer et al. 2006; National Institute for Health and Clinical Excellence 2009).

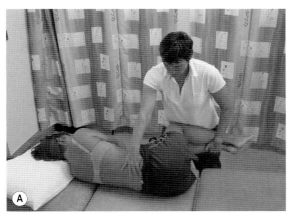
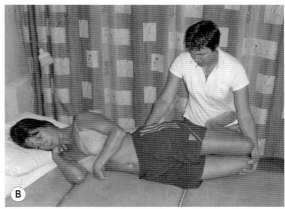

Figure 12.3 • Flexion/extension passive physiological intervertebral movements (PPIVMs) of the lumbar spine. **A** Flexion PPIVM: palpate the interspinous space of the spinal level being assessed. Flex the patient's hips and feel for gapping at the interspinous space. Assess the same movement at other lumbar levels to give an indication of the relative segmental motion. **B** Extension PPIVM: palpate the interspinous space of the spinal level being assessed. Extend the patient's hips and feel for the closing down or coming together of the spinous processes at the interspinous space. Assess the same movement at other lumbar levels to give an indication of the relative segmental motion. One leg may be used for this technique, depending on the relative size of the clinician and the patient.

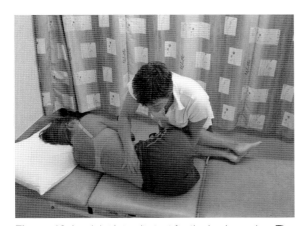

Figure 12.4 • Joint integrity test for the lumbar spine. The fingers are placed in the interspinous space to feel the relative movement of the spinous processes as the clinician passively pushes and then pulls along the femoral shafts.

Muscle control

There is good evidence to suggest that people with low-back pain have changes in their muscle activity (Hides et al. 1994, 2008; Hodges & Richardson 1999; O'Sullivan et al. 2002; Richardson et al. 2004; Dankaerts 2006). Whilst the evidence relating to effective rehabilitation of these muscles is limited to specific patient populations (O'Sullivan et al. 1997; Hides et al. 2001, 2008; Stevens et al. 2007), clearly the muscular control of trunk movement may

be relevant to the patient's pain and disability and should be considered in the assessment.

Specific testing of the trunk muscles includes assessment of the bulk and timing of onset of the deep trunk muscles. A method of measuring isometric muscle contraction of the lateral abdominal muscles has been described by Hodges & Richardson (1999). A pressure sensor (set at a baseline pressure of 70 mmHg) is placed between the lower abdomen and the couch with the patient in prone-lying. Abdominal hollowing is then attempted by the patient; this would normally cause a decrease in pressure of 6–10 mmHg. An increase in pressure of greater than 20 mmHg is purported to indicate the incorrect contraction of rectus abdominis. The clinician should also watch for excessive activity of the external oblique muscle. The evidence for these tests is limited.

Lumbar multifidus has also been found to atrophy in patients with low-back pain and so may provide some information to help the physical examination. (Hides et al. 1994). The patient lies prone and the clinician applies fairly deep pressure on either side of the lumbar spinous processes. The patient should be able to sustain a low-level contraction and continue to breathe normally. Normal function is described as the patient being able to sustain the correct contraction for 10 seconds and repeat the contraction 10 times.

More advanced testing of the deep muscles can be done in four-point kneeling, palpating the muscles whilst asking the patient to move either the trunk or individual limbs. These tests may transfer nicely into home exercise programmes if problems are identified. It is important to try to progress the patient to functional exercises as soon as possible in order to progress their treatment as quickly as possible.

Tests in standing and sitting, either on stable or unstable surfaces such as wobble boards or gym balls, may also be of use, with the clinician looking to see how the patient controls and moves the trunk, as well as the pain response to such tests. These tests may also help the clinician determine any degree of fear of movement on the part of the patient.

O'Sullivan (2006) describes a subclassification system for patients with low-back pain which explores functional movements and analyses the movement dysfunction. This system may help to determine aberrant movement patterns and altered muscular control of the spine, which can be addressed in treatment.

Vleeming et al. (1990a, b) describe anterior and posterior muscle sling systems across the trunk which may help to control trunk movement and support the spine These slings consists of large muscle groups that help to provide support, or 'force closure' across the trunk and pelvic joints, which are thought to help with control of movement.

Muscle length

The clinician may also choose to test the length of muscles which act on, or attach to, the trunk. Whilst shortened muscles may not necessarily be the source of symptoms, they may well contribute to movement dysfunction (Janda 1994). In the anterior and lateral muscle groups, the three hip flexor test may help to establish differences in muscle length. Ober's test may help with lateral muscle length and posteriorly the hamstrings and piriformis muscles may need to be assessed. Testing the length of these muscles is described in Chapter 3.

Neurological tests

Neurological examination includes neurological integrity testing, neurodynamic tests and other specific nerve tests.

Integrity of the nervous system

As a general guide, a neurological examination is indicated if the patient has symptoms below the level of the buttock crease, or if complaining of numbness, pins and needles, weakness or any neurological symptoms.

Dermatomes/peripheral nerves. Light touch and pain sensation of the lower limb are tested using cotton wool and pinprick respectively, as described in Chapter 3. It is always useful to quantify any variations from the normal, as this can then be used as an asterisk and retested at a later date. For example, if sensation to light touch is 4/10 at initial assessment, but then 7/10 following treatment, this identifies an important marker of change for the clinician and the patient. Knowledge of the cutaneous distribution of nerve roots (dermatomes) and peripheral nerves enables the clinician to distinguish the sensory loss due to a root lesion from that due to a peripheral nerve lesion. The cutaneous nerve distribution and dermatome areas are shown in Chapter 3. It should be remembered that these vary considerably from patient to patient, and also differ in textbooks, so they should be used only as a guide to the affected level or nerve.

It should be noted that sensation may be increased in certain conditions. The clinician should be aware of the possible different descriptions of these sensory variations, e.g. allodynia, hyperalgesia, analgesia and hyperpathia.

Myotomes/peripheral nerves. The following myotomes are tested in sitting or lying, or in a position of comfort for the patient. The clinician should take account of the patient's pain when testing the muscle power, as pain will often inhibit full cooperation from the patient, and may lead to a false-positive test.

- L2–3–4: hip flexion
- L2–3–4: knee extension
- L4–5–S1: foot dorsiflexion and inversion
- L4–5–S1: extension of the big toe
- L5–S1: eversion foot, contract buttock, knee flexion
- L5–S1: toe flexion
- S1–S2: knee flexion, plantarflexion
- S3–S4: muscles of the pelvic floor, bladder and genital function.

A working knowledge of the muscular distribution of nerve roots (myotomes) and peripheral nerves enables the clinician to distinguish the motor loss due to a root lesion from that due to a peripheral nerve lesion. The peripheral nerve distributions are shown in Chapter 3.

Reflex testing. The following deep tendon reflexes are tested with the patient relaxed, usually in sitting or lying (see Chapter 3 for further details):

- L3/4: knee jerk
- S1/2: ankle jerk.

Neurodynamic tests

The following neurodynamic tests may be carried out in order to ascertain the degree to which neural tissue is responsible for the production of the patient's symptoms. The choice of test should again be guided by the aggravating activities:

- passive neck flexion
- straight-leg raise
- femoral nerve tension test in side-lying
- slump.

Further tests may be added, in order to bias specific peripheral nerves, such as the sural nerve or common peroneal nerve, depending on the area of symptoms. These tests are described in detail in Chapter 3.

Other nerve tests

Plantar response to test for an upper motor neurone lesion (Walton 1989). Pressure applied from the heel along the lateral border of the plantar aspect of the foot produces flexion of the toes in the normal. Extension of the big toe with outward fanning of the other toes occurs with an upper motor neurone lesion.

Clonus. The patient's ankle is rapidly dorsiflexed by the clinician in order to elicit a stretch response in the calf. A normal response would be up to 2–4 beats of plantar flexion from the patient. More than this is suggestive of an upper motor neurone problem.

Coordination. Simple coordination tests can be used if the clinician suspects that there is an issue with control of movement. Finger–nose tests and heel–shin sliding tests done bilaterally may help to identify problems with coordination.

Cauda equina syndrome. Although there is no simple clinical test for this syndrome, any patient who complains of symptoms of cauda equina compression should have a full neurological examination. This should include neural integrity tests, as well as tests for saddle sensation and anal tone (Lavy et al. 2009). If the clinician is not trained to undertake these tests, then s/he should refer the patient immediately to a clinician who can check.

Miscellaneous tests

Vascular tests

If the patient's circulation is suspected of being compromised, the pulses of the femoral, popliteal and dorsalis pedis and posterior tibial arteries are palpated. The state of the vascular system can also be determined by the response of symptoms to dependence and elevation of the lower limbs. The clinician should be vigilant for male patients over the age of 65 who complain of diffuse low-back pain which is not mechanical in nature. Abdominal aortic aneurysms may present as low-back pain. The clinician should clearly ask about any vascular history when exploring the patient's past medical history.

Leg length

True leg length is measured from the anterior superior iliac spine to the medial or lateral malleolus. Apparent leg length is measured from the umbilicus to the medial or lateral malleolus. A difference in leg length of up to 1–1.3 cm is considered normal. If there is a leg length difference then test the length of individual bones, the tibia with knees bent and the femurs in standing. Ipsilateral posterior rotation of the ilium (on the sacrum) or contralateral anterior rotation of the ilium will result in a decrease in leg length (Magee 1997).

Palpation

The clinician palpates the lumbar spine and any other relevant areas. It is useful to record palpation findings on a body chart (see Figure 2.3) and/or palpation chart (see Figure 3.36).

The clinician notes the following:

- the temperature of the area
- localised increased skin moisture
- the presence of oedema or effusion
- mobility and feel of superficial tissues, e.g. ganglions, nodules and the lymph nodes in the femoral triangle
- the presence or elicitation of any muscle spasm
- tenderness of bone, trochanteric and psoas bursae (palpable if swollen), ligaments, muscle (Baer's point, for tenderness/spasm of iliacus, lies a third of the way down a line from the umbilicus to the anterior superior iliac spine), tendon, tendon sheath, trigger points (shown in Figure 3.37) and nerve. Nerves in the lower limb can be palpated at the following points:
  - the sciatic nerve two-thirds of the way along an imaginary line between the greater trochanter and the ischial tuberosity

○ the common peroneal nerve medial to the tendon of biceps femoris and also around the head of the fibula

○ the tibial nerve centrally over the posterior knee crease medial to the popliteal artery; it can also be felt behind the medial malleolus, which is more noticeable with the foot in dorsiflexion and eversion

○ the superficial peroneal nerve on the dorsum of the foot along an imaginary line over the fourth metatarsal; it is more noticeable with the foot in plantarflexion and inversion

○ the deep peroneal nerve between the first and second metatarsals, lateral to the extensor hallucis tendon

○ the sural nerve on the lateral aspect of the foot behind the lateral malleolus, lateral to the tendocalcaneus

• increased or decreased prominence of bones
• pain provoked or reduced on palpation. Widespread, superficial, non-anatomical tenderness suggests illness behaviour.

Passive accessory intervertebral movements

It is useful to use the palpation chart and movement diagrams (or joint pictures) to record findings. These are explained in detail in Chapter 3.

The clinician notes the:

• quality of movement
• range of movement
• resistance through the range and at the end of the range of movement
• behaviour of pain through the range
• provocation of any muscle spasm.

Lumbar spine (L1–L5) accessory movements are listed in Table 12.5. A central posteroanterior, unilateral posteroanterior and a transverse glide are shown in Figure 12.5. Lumbar spine accessory movements may need to be examined with the patient in flexion, extension, lateral flexion, rotation or a combination of these positions. Figure 12.6 shows right unilateral posteroanterior glide being performed in left lateral flexion. Following accessory movements to the

Table 12.5 Accessory movements, choice of application and reassessment of the patient's asterisks

Accessory movements	Choice of application	Identify any effect of accessory movements on patient's signs and symptoms
Lumbar spine (L1–L5) Central posteroanterior Unilateral posteroanterior Transverse Unilateral anteroposterior	Start position, e.g. – in flexion – in extension – in lateral flexion – in flexion and lateral flexion	Reassess all asterisks
Sacrum Posteroanterior pressure over base, body and apex Anterior gapping test Posterior gapping test	– in extension and lateral flexion Speed of force application Direction of the applied force Point of application of applied force	
Coccyx Posteroanterior		
?Sacroiliac joint	As above	Reassess all asterisks
?Hip	As above	Reassess all asterisks
?Knee	As above	Reassess all asterisks
?Foot and ankle	As above	Reassess all asterisks

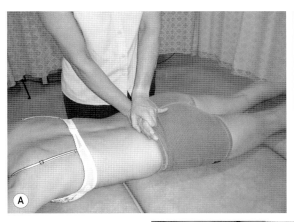
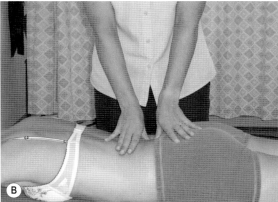
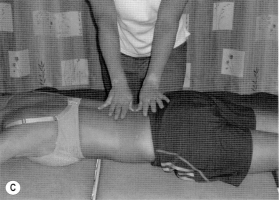

Figure 12.5 • Lumbar spine accessory movements. **A** Central posteroanterior. The pisiform grip is used to apply a posteroanterior pressure on the spinous process. **B** Unilateral posteroanterior. Thumb pressure is applied to the transverse process. **C** Transverse. Thumb pressure is applied to the lateral aspect of the spinous process.

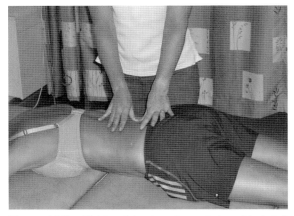

Figure 12.6 • Right unilateral posteroanterior glide in left lateral flexion.

lumbar region, the clinician reassesses all the physical asterisks (movements or tests that have been found to reproduce the patient's symptoms) in order to establish the effect of the accessory movements on the patient's signs and symptoms. Accessory movements can then be tested for other regions suspected to be a source of, or contributing to, the patient's symptoms. Again, following accessory movements to any one region, the clinician reassesses all the asterisks. Regions that may be examined are the sacroiliac, hip, knee, foot and ankle.

If the clinician feels that the symptoms may be difficult to reproduce, then s/he may choose to do the accessory movements in a more provocative position, which will be dependent on the aggravating active movements or provocative functional activities. Conversely, if the patient's condition is severe and irritable, the clinician may choose a non-provocative position for the accessory movements, or may chose to omit them completely from the initial examination.

Completion of the examination

This completes the examination of the lumbar spine. The subjective and physical examinations produce a large amount of information which needs to be recorded accurately and quickly. It is important, however, that the clinician does not examine in a rigid manner, simply following the suggested sequence outlined in the chart. Each patient presents differently and this needs to be reflected in the examination process. The therapist needs to be flexible in their approach depending on how the patient presents. It is vital at this stage to highlight important findings from the examination with an asterisk (*). These findings must be reassessed at, and within,

subsequent treatment sessions to evaluate the effects of treatment on the patient's condition.

On completion of the physical examination the clinician:

- explains the findings of the physical examination to the patient. Any questions patients may have regarding their illness or injury should be addressed at this stage
- evaluates the findings, formulates a clinical diagnosis and writes up a problem list
- in conjunction with the patient, determines the objectives of treatment, including clear, timed goals
- warns the patient of possible exacerbation up to 24–48 hours following the examination
- requests the patient to report details on the behaviour of the symptoms following examination at the next attendance.

For guidance on treatment and management principles, the reader is directed to the companion textbook (Petty 2011).

References

Adams, M.A., Freeman, B.J., Morrison, H.P., Nelson, I.W., Dolan, P., 2000. Mechanical initiation of intervertebral disc degeneration. Spine 25 (13), 1625–1636.

Andersson, G.B.J., Ortengren, R., Nachemson, A., 1977. Intradiskal pressure, intra-abdominal pressure and myoelectric back muscle activity related to posture and loading. Clin. Orthop. Relat. Res. 129, 156–164.

Cakir, M., Samanci, N., Balci, M.K., 2003. Musculoskeletal manifestations in patients with thyroid disease. Clin. Endocrinol. (Oxf.) 59 (2), 162–167.

Claus, A., Hides J., Moseley, G.L., Hodges, P., 2008. Sitting versus standing: Does intradiscal pressure cause disc degeneration or low back pain. Journal of Electromyography and Kinesiology 18 (2008) 550–558.

Clinical Standards Advisory Report, 1994. Report of a CSAG committee on back pain. HMSO, London.

Cole, J.H., Furness, A.L., Twomey, L.T., 1988. Muscles in action, an approach to manual muscle testing. Churchill Livingstone, Edinburgh.

Dankaerts, W., O'Sullivan, P., Burnett, A., et al., 2006. Altered patterns of superficial trunk muscle activation during sitting in non-specific chronic low back pain patients: importance of subclassification. Spine 31 (17), 2017–2023.

Edwards, B.C., 1994. Combined movements in the lumbar spine: their use in examination and treatment. In: Boyling, J.D., Palastanga, N. (Eds.), Grieve's modern manual therapy, second ed. Churchill Livingstone, Edinburgh, p. 745.

Edwards, B.C., 1999. Manual of combined movements: their use in the examination and treatment of mechanical vertebral column disorders, second ed. Butterworth-Heinemann, Oxford.

Grieve, G.P., 1981. Common vertebral joint problems. Churchill Livingstone, Edinburgh.

Grieve, G.P., 1991. Mobilisation of the spine, fifth ed. Churchill Livingstone, Edinburgh.

Grieve, G.P., 1994a. Counterfeit clinical presentations. Manipulative Physiotherapist 26, 17–19.

Grieve, G.P., 1994b. The masqueraders. In: Boyling, J.D., Palastanga, N. (Eds.), Grieve's modern manual therapy, second ed. Churchill Livingstone, Edinburgh, p. 745.

Harding, I., Davies, E., Buchannon, E., et al., 2004. Is the symptoms of night pain important in the diagnosis of serious spinal pathology in a back pain triage clinic? Spine J. 4 (5), S30.

Hefford, C., 2008. Mckenzie classification of mechanical spinal pain: profile of syndromes and directions of preference. Man. Ther. 13 (1), 75–81.

Hides, J.A., Stokes, M.J., Saide, M., et al., 1994. Evidence of lumbar multifidus muscle wasting ipsilateral to symptoms in patients with acute/subacute low back pain. Spine 19 (2), 165–172.

Hides, J., Jull, G., Richardson, C., 2001. Long-term effects of specific stabilizing exercises for first episode low back pain. Spine 26 (11), 243–248.

Hides, J., Gilmore, C., Stanton, W., et al., 2008. Multifidus size and symmetry among chronic LBP and healthy asymptomatic subjects. Man. Ther. 13 (1), 43–49.

Hislop, H., Montgomery, J., 1995. Daniels and Worthingham's muscle testing, techniques of manual examination, seventh ed. W B Saunders, Philadelphia.

Hodges, P.W., Richardson, C.A., 1999. Altered trunk muscle recruitment in people with low back pain with upper limb movement at different speeds. Arch. Phys. Med. Rehabil. 80, 1005–1012.

Hutton W.C., Malko J.A., Fajman W.A., 2003. Lumbar disc volume measured by MRI: effects of bed rest, horizontal exercise, and vertical loading. Aviation, Space Environ Med 74 (1), 73–78.

Janda, V., 1994. Muscles and motor control in cervicogenic disorders: assessment and management. In: Grant, R. (Ed.), Physical therapy of the cervical and thoracic spine, second ed. Churchill Livingstone, Edinburgh, p. 195.

Jones, M.A., Rivett, D.A., 2004. Clinical reasoning for manual therapists. Butterworth-Heinemann, Edinburgh.

Jull, G.A., 1986. Examination of the lumbar spine. In: Grieve, G.P. (Ed.), Modern manual therapy of the vertebral column. Churchill Livingstone, Edinburgh, p. 547.

Kazarian, L.E., 1975. Creep characteristics of the human spinal column. Orthop. Clin. North Am. 6 (1), 3–18.

Kendall, F.P., McCreary, E.K., Provance, P.G., 1993. Muscles: testing and function, fourth ed. Williams and Wilkins, Baltimore, MD.

Kendall, N., Linton, S., Main, C., 1997. Guide to assessing psychosocial yellow flags in acute low back pain: risk factors for long-term disability and work loss. Accident Rehabilitation & Compensation Insurance Corporation of New Zealand and the National Health Committee, Wellington, New Zealand, pp. 1–22.

Kirkaldy-Willis, W.H., Farfan, H.F., 1982. Instability of the lumbar spine. Clin. Orthop. Relat. Res. 165, 110–123.

Lavy, C., James, A., Wilson-Macdonald, J., et al., 2009. Cauda equina syndrome. Br. Med. J. 338, 881–884.

Long, A., Donelson, R., Fung, T., 2004. Does it matter which exercise? A randomized controlled trial of exercise for low back pain. Spine 29 (23), 2593–2602.

Magee, D.J., 1997. Orthopedic physical assessment, third ed. W B Saunders, Philadelphia.

Maitland, G.D., Hengeveld, E., Banks, K., et al., 2005. Maitland's vertebral manipulation, seventh ed. Butterworth-Heinemann, Edinburgh.

McKenzie, R.A., May, S.J., 2003. The Lumbar Spine: Mechanical Diagnosis and Therapy. Spinal Publications New Zealand Ltd, Waikanae, New Zealand.

Mercer, C., Jackson, A., Hettinga, D., et al., 2006. Clinical guidelines for the physiotherapy management of persistent low back pain. Chartered Society of Physiotherapy, London.

Nachemson, A., 1992. Lumbar mechanics as revealed by lumbar intradiscal pressure measurements. In: Jayson, M. I.V. (Ed.), The lumbar spine and back pain, fourth ed. Churchill Livingstone, Edinburgh, p. 157.

National Institute for Health and Clinical Excellence, 2009. Guidelines for the early management of persistent non specific low back pain. Available online at: www.nice.org.wk/CG88.

O'Sullivan, P.O., 2006. Classification of lumbopelvic disorders – why is it essential for management? Man. Ther. 11 (3), 169–170.

O'Sullivan, P.B., Twomey, L., Allison, G.T., 1997. Evaluation of specific stabilizing exercise in the treatment of chroninc low back pain with radiologic diagnosis of spondylolysis or spondylolisthesis. Spine 22 (24), 2959–2967.

O'Sullivan, P., Grahamslaw, K.M., Kendell, M., et al., 2002. The effect of different standing and sitting postures on trunk muscle activity in a pain-free population. Spine 27 (11), 1238–1244.

Petty, N.J., 2011. Principles of neuromusculoskeletal treatment and management: a guide for therapists, second ed. Churchill Livingstone, Edinburgh.

Pope, M.H., Hansson, T.H., 1992. Vibration of the spine and low back pain. Clin. Orthop. Relat. Res. 279, 49–59.

Richardson, C., Hodges, P.W., Hides, J., 2004. Therapeutic exercise for lumbopelvic stabilization. A motor control approach for the treatment and prevention of low back pain, second ed. Churchill Livingstone, Edinburgh.

Royal College of Radiologists, 2007. Making the best use of a department of clinical radiology. Guidelines for doctors, sixth ed. Royal College of Radiologists, London.

Stevens, V.K., Pascal, L., Coorevits, K.G., et al., 2007. The influence of specific training on trunk muscle recruitment patterns in healthy subjects during stabilisation exercises. Man. Ther. 12 (3), 271–279.

Van Tulder, M., Becker, A., Beckering, T., et al., 2005. Back Pain Europe European Guidelines on the management of persistent low back pain. Available online at: http//www.backpaineurope.org.

Vleeming, A., Stoeckart, R., Volkers, A.C., et al., 1990a. Relation between form and function in the sacroiliac joint. Part 1. Clinical anatomical aspects. Spine 15 (2), 130–132.

Vleeming, A., Stoeckart, R., Volkers, A.C., et al., 1990b. Relation between form and function in the sacroiliac joint. Part II. Biomechanical aspects. Spine 15 (2), 133–136.

Waddell, G., 2004. The back pain revolution, second ed. Churchill Livingstone, Edinburgh.

Walton, J.H., 1989. Essentials of neurology, sixth ed. Churchill Livingstone, Edinburgh.

White, A.A., Panjabi, M.M., 1990. Clinical biomechanics of the spine, second ed. J B Lippincott, Philadelphia.

Wilke, H., Neef, P., Hinz, B., Seidel, H., Claes, L., 1990. Intradiscal pressure together with anthropometric data–a data set for the validation of models. Clin Biomech. 16 (Suppl. 1), S111–S126.

Examination of the pelvis

13

Chris Mercer   Laura Finucane

Possible causes of pain and/or limitation of movement

This region includes the sacroiliac joint, sacrococcygeal joint and pubic symphysis with their surrounding soft tissues.

- Trauma and degeneration:
  - fracture of the pelvis
  - syndromes: arthrosis of the sacroiliac joint or pubic symphysis, osteitis condensans ilii, coccydynia, hypermobility, ilium on sacrum dysfunctions, sacrum on ilium dysfunctions
  - ligamentous sprain
  - muscular strain
- Inflammatory:
  - ankylosing spondylitis
  - rheumatoid arthritis
- Metabolic:
  - osteoporosis
  - Paget's disease
- Infections
- Tumours, benign and malignant
- Piriformis syndrome
- Referral of symptoms from the lumbar spine
- Pregnancy is very often associated with low-back pain – 88% of women studied by Bullock et al. (1987) and 96% of those studied by Moore et al. (1990).

The wealth of examination procedures documented for the sacroiliac joint and the frequency of isolated sacroiliac joint problems justifies a chapter on the examination of the pelvis. The examination of the pelvic region is normally preceded by a detailed examination of the lumbar spine (see Chapter 12). Examination of the hip joint may also be required.

Further details of the questions asked during the subjective examination and the tests carried out in the physical examination can be found in Chapters 2 and 3 respectively.

The order of the subjective questioning and the physical tests described below can be altered as appropriate for the patient being examined.

Subjective examination

Body chart

The following information concerning the type and area of current symptoms can be recorded on a body chart (see Figure 2.3).

Area of current symptoms

Be exact when mapping out the area of the symptoms. Pain localised over the sacral sulcus is indicative of sacroiliac joint dysfunction (Fortin et al. 1994). Common areas of referral from the sacroiliac joint are to the groin, buttock, anterior and posterior thigh. Ascertain which is the worst symptom and record where the patient feels the symptoms are coming from. Pain is often unilateral with sacroiliac joint problems, though it is classically bilateral in ankylosing spondylitis.

Areas relevant to the region being examined

All other relevant areas are checked for symptoms; it is important to ask about pain or even stiffness, as this may be relevant to the patient's main symptom. Mark unaffected areas with ticks (✓) on the body chart. Check for symptoms in the thoracic spine, lumbar spine, abdomen, groin and lower limbs.

Quality of pain

Establish the quality of the pain.

Intensity of pain

The intensity of pain can be measured using, for example, a visual analogue scale, as shown in Chapter 2. A pain diary may be useful for patients with chronic low-back pain, to determine the pain patterns and triggering factors over a period of time.

Abnormal sensation

Check for any altered sensation over the lumbar spine and sacroiliac joint and any other relevant areas. Common abnormalities are paraesthesia and numbness.

Constant or intermittent symptoms

Ascertain the frequency of the symptoms, whether they are constant or intermittent. If symptoms are constant, check whether there is variation in the intensity of the symptoms, as constant unremitting pain may be indicative of serious pathology.

Relationship of symptoms

If there is more than one area of symptom, determine the relationship between the symptomatic areas – do they come together or separately? For example, the patient could have buttock pain without back pain, or the pains may always be present together. It is possible that there may be two separate sources of symptoms.

Behaviour of symptoms

Aggravating factors

For each symptomatic area a series of questions may be asked:

- What movements and/or positions bring on or make the patient's symptoms worse?
- How long does it take before symptoms are aggravated?
- What happens to other symptoms when this symptom is produced or made worse?
- Is the patient able to maintain this position or movement?
- How do the symptoms affect function? e.g. sitting, standing, lying, bending, walking, running, walking on uneven ground and up and down stairs, washing, driving, lifting and digging, work, sport and social activities.

The clinician may ask the patient about theoretically known aggravating factors for structures that could be a source of the symptoms. However, this questioning does not provide conclusive evidence as functional movements invariably stress all parts of the body, and the activities listed below will also stress the lumbar spine and hips. Commonly cited aggravating factors for the sacroiliac joint are standing on one leg, turning over in bed, getting in or out of bed, sloppy standing with uneven weight distribution through the legs, habitual work stance, stepping up on the affected side and walking. Aggravating factors for other regions, which may need to be queried if they are suspected to be a source of the symptoms, are shown in Table 2.3.

Easing factors

For each symptomatic area a series of questions can be asked to help determine what eases the symptoms:

- What movements and/or positions ease the patient's symptoms?
- How long does it take before symptoms are eased? If symptoms are constant but variable it is important to know what the baseline is and how long it takes for the symptoms to reduce to that level.
- What happens to other symptoms when this symptom is eased?

The clinician asks the patient about theoretically known easing factors for structures that could be a source of the symptoms. For example, symptoms from the sacroiliac joint may be eased by crook-lying, sitting with the pelvis posteriorly tilted, stooping forwards in standing and/or applying a wide belt around the pelvis. One study has found that a pelvic support gave some relief of pain in 83% of pregnant women (Ostgaard et al. 1994). The clinician can then analyse the position or movement that eases the symptoms to help determine the structure at fault.

Aggravating and easing factors will help to determine the irritability of the patient's symptoms. These factors will help to determine the areas at fault and identify functional restrictions and also the relationship between symptoms. The severity can be determined by the intensity of the symptoms and whether the symptoms are interfering with normal activities of daily living, such as work and sleep. This information can be used to determine the direction of the physical examination as well as the aims of treatment and any advice that may be required. The most relevant subjective information should be highlighted with an asterisk (*), explored in the physical examination and reassessed at subsequent treatment sessions to evaluate treatment intervention.

Twenty-four-hour behaviour of symptoms

The clinician determines the 24-hour behaviour of symptoms by asking questions about night, morning and evening symptoms.

Night symptoms. Although night pain is a recognised red flag, it should be noted that night symptoms are common in back pain (Harding et al. 2004). It is necessary to establish whether the patient is being woken and kept awake by the symptoms. Patients complaining of needing to sleep upright or get up should raise some concern.

The following questions may be asked:

- Do you have any difficulty getting to sleep?
- Do your symptom(s) wake you at night? If so,

- Which symptom(s)?
- How many times in a night?
- How many times in the past week?
- What do you have to do to get back to sleep?
- If sleep is an issue, further questioning may be useful to determine management.

Morning and evening symptoms. The clinician determines the pattern of the symptoms first thing in the morning, through the day and at the end of the day. In ankylosing spondylitis, the cardinal and often earliest sign is erosion of the sacroiliac joints, which is often manifested by pain and stiffness around the sacroiliac joint and lumbar spine for the first few hours in the morning (Solomon et al. 2001). Stiffness lasting only 30 minutes or less is likely to be mechanical in nature.

Stage of the condition

In order to determine the stage of the condition, the clinician asks whether the symptoms are getting better, getting worse or remaining unchanged.

Special questions

Special questions must always be asked, as they may identify certain precautions or contraindications to the physical examination and/or treatment (Table 2.4). As mentioned in Chapter 2, the clinician must differentiate between conditions that are suitable for conservative management and systemic, neoplastic and other non-neuromusculoskeletal conditions, which require referral to a medical practitioner. The reader is referred to Appendix 2.3 for details of serious pathological processes that can mimic neuromusculoskeletal conditions (Grieve 1994).

Neurological symptoms. Neurological symptoms may include pins and needles, numbness and weakness. These symptoms need to be mapped out on the body chart.

Has the patient experienced symptoms of cauda equina compression (i.e. compression below L1), which are saddle anaesthesia/paraesthesia, sexual or erectile dysfunction, loss of vaginal sensation, bladder and/or bowel sphincter disturbance (loss of control, retention, hesitancy, urgency or a sense of incomplete evacuation) (Lavy et al. 2009)? These symptoms may be due to interference of S3 and S4 (Grieve 1981). Prompt imaging and surgical attention are required to prevent permanent sphincter paralysis (Lavy et al. 2009).

Has the patient experienced symptoms of spinal cord compression (i.e. compression above the L1 level, which may include the cervical and thoracic cord and brain), such as bilateral tingling in hands or feet and/or disturbance of gait? Are there motor and sensory tone changes in all four limbs? Does the patient report coordination changes, including gait disturbance?

General health. Ascertain the general health of the patient – find out if the patient suffers from any malaise, fatigue, fever, nausea or vomiting, stress, anxiety or depression. In addition, ask, if necessary, whether the patient is pregnant. It is common for low-back pain to be associated with pregnancy, although the underlying mechanism remains unclear. Research suggests that there may be a number of factors involved, including an increase in the load on the lumbar spine because of weight gain, hormonal changes causing hypermobility of the sacroiliac joint and pubic symphysis (Hagen 1974) and an increase in the abdominal sagittal diameter (Ostgaard et al. 1993). Little evidence supports the hypothesis that the pain is related to alteration in posture (Bullock et al. 1987; Ostgaard et al. 1993).

History of the present condition

For each symptomatic area, the clinician needs to know how long the symptom has been present, whether there was a sudden or slow onset and whether there was a known cause that provoked the onset of the symptom, such as a fall. If the onset was slow, the clinician finds out if there has been any change in the patient's lifestyle, e.g. a new job or hobby or a change in sporting activity. If the patient is pregnant, she may develop associated symptoms as early as week 18 and symptoms may persist following birth due to hormones (Bullock et al. 1987). Relaxin is not detectable after 3 months postpregnancy and unlikely to be the cause of symptoms (Sapsford et al. 1999). To confirm the relationship of symptoms, the clinician asks what happened to other symptoms when each symptom began.

Past medical history

The following information is obtained from the patient and/or the medical notes:

- The details of any relevant medical history, such as pelvic inflammatory disease or fractures of the lower limbs. Visceral structures are capable of masquerading as musculoskeletal conditions, for example the pelvic organs, including testes, ovaries and uterus, can refer to the sacral region. Any relevant history related to these organs is important to help differentiate the cause of symptoms.

- The history of any previous episodes: how many? when were they? what was the cause? what was the duration of each episode? and did the patient fully recover between episodes? Does the patient perceive the current condition to be better, the same or worse in relation to other episodes s/he may have experienced? If there have been no previous attacks, has the patient had any episodes of stiffness in the lumbar spine, thoracic spine or any other relevant region? Check for a history of trauma or recurrent minor trauma.

- Ascertain the results of any past treatment for the same or similar problem. Past treatment records may be obtained for further information.

Weight loss. Has the patient noticed any recent unexplained weight loss?

Rheumatoid arthritis. Has the patient (or a member of his/her family) been diagnosed as having rheumatoid arthritis?

Serious pathology. Does the patient have a previous history of serious pathology, such as tuberculosis or cancer?

Inflammatory arthritis. Has the patient (or a member of his/her family) been diagnosed as having an inflammatory condition such as rheumatoid arthritis?

Cardiovascular disease. Is there a history of cardiac disease, e.g. angina?

Blood pressure. If the patient has raised blood pressure, is it controlled with medication?

Respiratory disease. Does the patient have a history of lung pathology, including asthma? How is it controlled?

Diabetes. Does the patient suffer from diabetes? If so, is it type 1 or type 2 diabetes? Is the patient's blood glucose controlled? How is it controlled? Through diet, tablet or injection? Patients with diabetes may develop peripheral neuropathy and vasculopathy, are at increased risk of infection and may take longer to heal than those without diabetes.

Epilepsy. Is the patient epileptic? When was the last seizure?

Thyroid disease. Does the patient have a history of thyroid disease? Thyroid dysfunction may cause musculoskeletal conditions such as adhesive capsulitis, Dupuytren's contracture, trigger finger and carpal tunnel syndrome (Cakir et al. 2003).

Osteoporosis. Has the patient had a dual-energy X-ray absorptiometry (DEXA) scan, been diagnosed with osteoporosis or sustained frequent fractures?

Previous surgery. Has the patient had previous surgery which may be of relevance to the presenting complaint?

Drug therapy. What drugs is the patient taking? Has the patient ever been prescribed long-term (6 months or more) medication/steroids? Has the patient been taking anticoagulants recently?

Radiograph and medical imaging. Has the patient been radiographed or had any other medical tests recently? Routine spinal radiographs are no longer considered necessary prior to conservative treatment as they only identify the normal age-related degenerative changes, which do not necessarily correlate with the symptoms experienced by the patient (Clinical Standards Advisory Report 1994). Radiograph may be indicated in the younger patient (under 20 years) with conditions such as spondylolisthesis or ankylosing spondylitis and in the older patient (over 55 years) where management is difficult (Royal College of Radiologists 2007). In cases of suspected Ankylosing Spondylitis, radiographs of the sacro-iliac joints may not show significant changes until the patient has had AS for 6-9 years. In cases where there is a suspected fracture due to trauma or osteoporosis radiographs are indicated in the first instance. The medical tests may include blood tests, magnetic resonance imaging, myelography, discography or a bone scan.

There are a number of patients whose pain may persist beyond the expected point of tissue healing. These patients will require a different approach to a traditional assessment. The following questions may be helpful in evaluating the psychosocial risk factors, or 'yellow flags' for poor treatment outcome (Waddell 2004):

- Have you had time off work in the past with back pain?
- What do you understand to be the cause of your back pain?
- What are you expecting will help you?
- How is your employer/co-workers/family responding to your back pain?
- What are you doing to cope with your back pain?
- Do you think you will return to work? When?

Readers are referred to the excellent text by Waddell (2004) for further details on the management of patients demonstrating psychosocial risk factors.

Social and family history

Social and family history relevant to the onset and progression of the patient's condition is recorded. This includes the patient's perspectives, experience and expectations, age, employment, home situation and details of any leisure activities. Factors from this information may indicate direct and/or indirect mechanical influences on the sacroiliac joint. In order to treat the patient appropriately, it is important that the condition is managed within the context of the patient's social and work environment.

The clinician may ask the following types of question to elucidate psychosocial factors:

- Have you had time off work in the past with your pain?
- What do you understand to be the cause of your pain?
- What are you expecting will help you?
- How is your employer/co-workers/family responding to your pain?
- What are you doing to cope with your pain?
- Do you think you will return to work? When?

Although these questions are described in relation to psychosocial risk factors for poor outcomes for patients with low-back pain (Waddell 2004), they may be relevant to other patients.

Plan of the physical examination

When all this information has been collected, the subjective examination is complete. It is useful at this stage to highlight with asterisks (*), for ease of reference, important findings and particularly one or more functional restrictions. These can then be re-examined at subsequent treatment sessions to evaluate treatment intervention.

In order to plan the physical examination, the following hypotheses need to be developed from the subjective examination:

- The regions and structures that need to be examined as a possible cause of the symptoms, e.g. sacroiliac joint, pubic symphysis, lumbar spine, thoracic spine, hip, knee, ankle and foot, muscles and nerves. Often it is not possible to examine fully at the first attendance and so examination of the structures must be prioritised over subsequent treatment sessions.
- Other factors that need to be examined, e.g. working and everyday postures and leg length.

- In what way should the physical tests be carried out? Will it be easy or hard to reproduce each symptom? Will it be necessary to use combined movements or repetitive movements to reproduce the patient's symptoms? Are symptoms severe and/or irritable?
  - If symptoms are severe, physical tests may be carried out to just before the onset of symptom production or just to the onset of symptom production; no overpressures will be carried out, as the patient would be unable to tolerate this.
  - If symptoms are non-severe, physical tests will be carried out to reproduce symptoms fully and may include overpressures.
  - If symptoms are irritable, physical tests may be examined to just before symptom production or just to the onset of provocation with fewer physical tests being examined to allow for a rest period between tests.
  - If symptoms are non-irritable physical tests will be carried out to reproduce symptoms fully and may include overpressures.
- Are there any precautions and/or contraindications to elements of the physical examination that need to be explored further, such as neurological involvement, recent fracture, trauma, steroid therapy or rheumatoid arthritis? There may also be certain contraindications to further examination and treatment, e.g. symptoms of spinal cord or cauda equina compression.

A physical planning sheet can be useful for clinicians to help guide them through the clinical reasoning process (Figure 2.10).

Physical examination

The information from the subjective examination helps the clinician to plan an appropriate physical examination (Grieve 1991). The severity, irritability and nature of the condition are the major factors that will influence the choice and priority of physical testing procedures. The first and overarching question the clinician might ask is: 'Is this patient's condition suitable for me to manage as a therapist?' For example, a patient presenting with cauda equina compression symptoms may only need neurological integrity testing, prior to an urgent medical referral. The nature of the patient's condition has had a major impact on the physical examination. The second question the clinician might ask is: 'Does this patient

have a neuromusculoskeletal dysfunction that I may be able to help?' To answer that, the clinician needs to carry out a full physical examination; however, this may not be possible if the symptoms are severe and/or irritable. If the patient's symptoms are severe and/or irritable, the clinician aims to explore movements as much as possible, within a symptom-free range. If the patient has constant and severe and/or irritable symptoms, then the clinician aims to find physical tests that ease the symptoms. If the patient's symptoms are non-severe and non-irritable, then the clinician aims to find physical tests that reproduce each of the patient's symptoms.

Each significant physical test that either provokes or eases the patient's symptoms is highlighted in the patient's notes by an asterisk (*) for easy reference. The highlighted tests are often referred to as 'asterisks' or 'markers'.

The order and detail of the physical tests described below need to be appropriate to the patient being examined; some tests will be irrelevant, some tests will be carried out briefly, while others will need to be fully investigated. It is important that readers understand that the techniques shown in this chapter are some of many; the choice depends mainly on the relative size of the clinician and patient, as well as the clinician's preference. For this reason, novice clinicians may initially want to copy what is shown, but then quickly adapt to what is best for them and most appropriate to the individual patient.

Observation

Informal observation

This should begin as soon as the therapist sees the patient for the first time. This may be in the reception or waiting area, or as the patient enters the treatment room, and should continue throughout the subjective examination. The therapist should be aware of the patient's posture, demeanour, facial expressions, gait and interaction with the therapist, as these may all give valuable information regarding possible pain mechanisms and the severity and irritability of the problem.

Formal observation

The clinician observes the patient's spinal, pelvic and lower-limb posture in standing, from anterior, lateral and posterior views. The presence of any deformity of the spine is noted. Any asymmetry in levels at the pelvis, particularly of the iliac crests, the posterior and anterior superior iliac spine (ASIS), is noted. Any anomalies may guide the therapist into testing particular joint movements, or may help the therapist in deciding which of the tests described below are the most appropriate to use. Observation should also include inspection of the muscle bulk, tone and symmetry. This may be related to the patient's handedness or physical activity, or may relate to the complaining symptom. Findings may lead the clinician to investigate muscle length and strength in the physical examination. Skin colour, areas of redness, swelling or sweating should be noted, as these may indicate areas of local pathology, or possibly a systemic or dermatological condition. The clinician should watch the patient performing simple functional tasks. Observation of gait, of sit-to-stand and dressing/undressing will help to give the clinician a good idea of how the patient is likely to move in the physical examination, and may help to highlight any problems such as hypervigilance and fear avoidance.

Pain provocation tests

These tests for the sacroiliac joints have been shown to be reliable and valid when used as a raft of tests in combination. Various authors have proposed different combinations of tests (Laslett & Williams 1994; Vleeming 2003; Laslett et al 2005; Robinson et al. 2007; Stuber 2007). On their own, these tests have poor reliability, but there is some evidence to suggest that, when used together, the distraction, compression, posterior shear, pelvic torsion test, resisted abduction and sacral thrust tests may be reliable indicators of sacroiliac joint dysfunction (Laslett & Williams 1994; Laslett et al 2005; Stuber 2007). Positive tests should help to guide the therapist into treatment directed at the sacroiliac joint as a source of symptoms.

Posterior shear test (Figure 13.1) (Porterfield & DeRosa 1998)**.** With the patient in supine with the hip slightly flexed, the clinician applies a longitudinal cephalad force through the femur to produce an anteroposterior shear at the sacroiliac joint. Reproduction of the patient's symptoms may suggest a sacroiliac joint problem, although this test also stresses the hip joint.

Posterior gapping/compression test (Figure 13.2) (Laslett & Williams 1994; Magee 1997; Edwards 1999; Maitland et al. 2001). With the patient in supine or side-lying, the clinician applies a force that attempts to push the left and right ASIS towards each other. Reproduction of the patient's

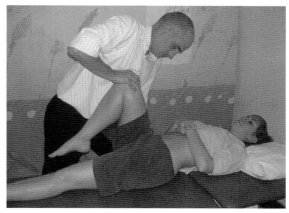

Figure 13.1 • Posterior shear test.

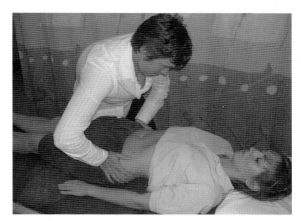

Figure 13.2 • Posterior gapping.

symptom(s) indicates a possible sprain of the posterior superior iliac joint (PSIS) or ligaments.

Anterior gapping/distraction test (Figure 13.3) (Laslett & Williams 1994; Magee 1997; Edwards 1999; Maitland et al. 2001). With the patient in supine, the clinician applies a force that attempts to push the left and right ASIS apart. Reproduction of the patient's symptoms may indicate a sprain of the anterior sacroiliac joint or ligaments

Flexion, abduction, external rotation (FABER) test (Figure 13.4) (Broadhurst & Bond 1998). With the patient in supine, the therapist places the patient's hip into full flexion, abduction and external rotation, noting the pain response.

Resisted abduction test (Broadhurst & Bond 1998) (Figure 13.5). With the patient supine, with the hip extended and abducted to 30°, the therapist

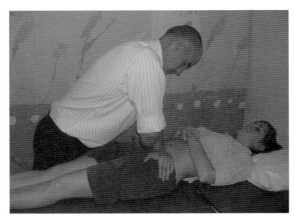

Figure 13.3 • Anterior gapping.

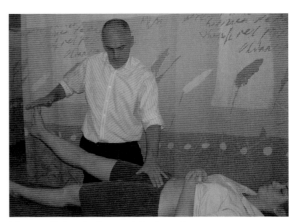

Figure 13.6 • Active straight-leg raise test.

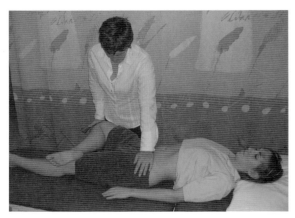

Figure 13.4 • Flexion, abduction, external rotation (FABER) test.

pushes the leg medially as the patient resists. Pain response is noted.

Active straight-leg raise test (Mens et al. 2001) (Figure 13.6). In supine, the patient is asked to lift one leg to around 30°. The pain response is noted, as is any trunk rotation, or excessive effort in lifting the leg. The therapist then compresses the sacroiliac joints by applying pressure medially over both ilia. The patient repeats the test. A positive test is indicated by a decrease in pain, or an easing of the effort in lifting the leg.

Pelvic torsion test (Gaenslen test) (Figure 13.7). In supine with the patient close to the edge of the plinth, the leg nearest the edge of the bed is extended whilst the opposite hip is fully flexed and overpressure is applied. This test is repeated on the other side of the plinth with the opposite leg. Pain response is noted.

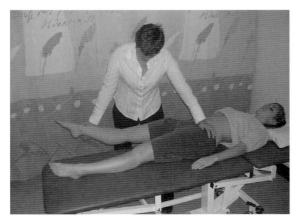

Figure 13.5 • Resisted abduction.

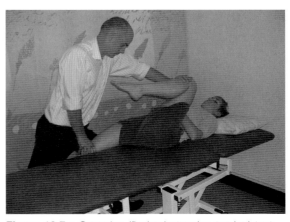

Figure 13.7 • Gaenslen (flexion/extension torsion) test.

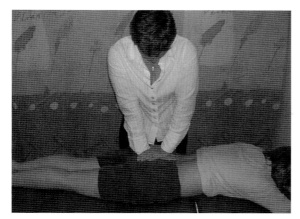

Figure 13.8 • Sacral thrust.

Sacral thrust test (Laslett & Williams 1994; Laslett et al 2005) (Figure 13.8). In prone, a posteroanterior thrust is applied to the sacrum by the therapist. Pain response is noted. This test has been shown to be less reliable than others.

Cranial shear test (Laslett & Williams 1994; Laslett et al 2005) (Figure 13.9). In prone, a cephalad glide is applied to the inferior aspect of the sacrum and the pain response is noted. This test has been shown to be less reliable than others.

Movement tests

Active physiological movements

There are no active physiological movements at the sacroiliac joint. The movements of the sacroiliac joint are nutation (anterior rotation of the sacrum) and counternutation (posterior rotation of the sacrum),

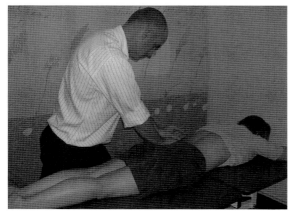

Figure 13.9 • Cranial shear.

which occur during movement of the spine and hip joints. Sacroiliac joint movements are therefore tested using active physiological movements of the lumbar spine and hip joints, while the sacroiliac joint is palpated by the clinician.

Numerous differentiation tests (Maitland et al. 2001) can be performed; the choice depends on the patient's signs and symptoms. For example, when the hip flexion/adduction test reproduces the patient's groin pain, it may be necessary to differentiate between the sacroiliac joint and the hip joint as a source of the symptoms. The position of the sacroiliac joint is altered by placing a towel between the sacrum and the couch, and the test is then repeated. If the pain response is affected by this alteration, the sacroiliac joint may be implicated as a source of the groin pain, as this test is thought to increase the stress on the sacroiliac joint and not the hip.

Some functional ability has already been tested by the general observation of the patient during the subjective and physical examinations, e.g. the postures adopted during the subjective examination and the ease or difficulty of undressing prior to the examination. Any further functional testing can be carried out at this point in the examination and may include functional activities such as turning over in bed, sitting to standing, lifting or sport-specific activities. Clues for appropriate tests can be obtained from the subjective examination findings, particularly aggravating factors.

Passive physiological movements

The sitting flexion test, standing flexion test and standing hip flexion test are often referred to as kinetic tests. These movement tests are purported to be indicators of movement at the sacroiliac joint (Lee 1999), but the majority of the evidence does not support this view (Levangie 1999; Vincent-Smith & Gibbons 1999; van de Wurff et al. 2000a, b; Freiberger & Riddle 2001; Riddle & Freburger 2002; Mousavi 2003; O'Sullivan & Beales 2007). The reliability and validity of these tests are yet to be established, and it is strongly recommended that the reader considers this when deciding whether or not to use these tests. They are presented here for information, as they are commonly used in clinical practice.

Sitting flexion (Piedallu's test). In sitting, the patient flexes the trunk and the clinician palpates movement of the left and right PSIS. The left and right PSIS should normally move equally in a superior direction. If the PSIS rises more on one side during lumbar spine flexion, it is thought to indicate hypomobility of the sacroiliac joint on that side.

Standing flexion. In standing the patient flexes the trunk and the clinician palpates the movement of the left and right PSIS. The left and right PSIS will normally move equally in a superior direction. If the PSIS rises more on one side during lumbar spine flexion, it is thought to indicate hypomobility of the sacroiliac joint on that side.

Standing hip flexion (Gillet test). In standing, the patient flexes the hip and knee and the clinician palpates the inferior aspect of the PSIS and the sacrum (at the same horizontal level) on the same side as the movement – ipsilateral test. If the PSIS does not move downwards and medially on the side of hip flexion, it may indicate hypomobility of the sacroiliac joint on that side. Abnormal findings may include hip hitching or movement of the PSIS in a superior direction.

For the contralateral test the patient flexes the hip and knee and the clinician palpates the inferior aspect of the PSIS and the sacrum (at the same horizontal level) on the opposite side to the movement; the test is repeated and compared with the opposite side. It tests the ability of the sacrum to move on the ilium. Abnormal findings may be no movement or superior movement of the sacrum relative to the PSIS.

Prone trunk extension test (Greenman 1996). In prone the depth of the sacral base and inferior lateral angle of the sacrum are palpated and compared left to right sides. A sacral base and inferior lateral angle that are both deep on the same side may suggest a sacral torsion. The prone extension test is used to differentiate between an anterior and posterior sacral torsion. The patient is asked to extend the lumbar spine while the clinician palpates the left and right sacral bases. If the asymmetry increases on lumbar extension it may indicate a posterior sacral torsion; if the asymmetry reduces, this may indicate an anterior sacral torsion.

Ilium on sacrum dysfunctions

Anterior rotation. The ilium is excessively anteriorly rotated relative to the sacrum; the ASIS is palpated inferior to the PSIS on the affected side.

Posterior rotation. The ilium is excessively posteriorly rotated relative to the sacrum; the ASIS is palpated superior to the PSIS on the affected side.

Upslip. This is where the pelvis on one side has 'slipped upwards' relative to the sacrum. The iliac crest and ischial tuberosity are palpated superior to the corresponding bony prominences on the opposite side. The height of the ASIS may vary as upslip dysfunctions can occur in conjunction with anterior or posterior rotation dysfunctions.

Sacrum on ilium dysfunctions

Torsion dysfunction. The depth of the sacral base and the inferior lateral angle on one side compared with the same prominences on the other side will be relatively superficial (posterior torsion) or relatively deep (anterior torsion). This is thought to be due to a rotation of the sacrum about an oblique axis (Greenman 1996).

Side-bent sacrum. The sacral base and inferior lateral angles are compared one side with the other. A side-bent sacrum is where the sacral base is deep and the inferior lateral angle inferior on one side, so for a left side-bent sacrum the left sacral base would be deep and the left inferior lateral angle would be inferior, compared with the right sacral base, which would be superficial, and the right inferior lateral angle, which would be superior (Greenman 1996).

Lumbar spine passive physiological intervertebral movements (PPIVMs). It may be necessary to examine lumbar spine PPIVMs, particularly for the L5/S1 level, as it is so closely associated with the pelvis (see Chapter 12 for further details).

Muscle tests

Muscle control

The clinician may test the trunk muscles; readers are referred to Chapters 3 and 12 for further details.

Muscle length

The clinician tests the length of muscles, in particular those thought prone to shorten (Janda 1994, 2002; Sahrmann 2002). A description of muscle length tests is given in Chapter 3.

Neurological tests

The neurological tests are the same as those for the lumbar spine (see Chapter 12).

Miscellaneous tests

The vascular and leg length tests are the same as those for the lumbar spine in Chapter 12.

Palpation

The clinician palpates over the pelvis, including the sacrum, sacroiliac joints, pubic symphysis and any other relevant areas. It is useful to record palpation findings on a body chart (see Figure 2.3) and/or palpation chart (Figure 3.36).

The clinician notes the following:

- the temperature of the area
- localised increased skin moisture
- the presence of oedema or effusion
- mobility and feel of superficial tissues, e.g. ganglions, nodules and lymph nodes in the femoral triangle
- the presence or elicitation of any muscle spasm
- tenderness of bone, trochanteric and psoas bursae (palpable if swollen), ligament, muscle (Baer's point, for tenderness/spasm of iliacus, lies a third of the way down a line from the umbilicus to the ASIS), tendon, tendon sheath, trigger points (shown in Figure 3.37) and nerve. Nerves in the lower limb can be palpated at the following points:
  - the sciatic nerve two-thirds of the way along an imaginary line between the greater trochanter and the ischial tuberosity with the patient in prone
  - the common peroneal nerve medial to the tendon of biceps femoris and also around the head of the fibula
  - the tibial nerve centrally over the posterior knee crease medial to the popliteal artery; it can also be felt behind the medial malleolus, which is more noticeable with the foot in dorsiflexion and eversion
  - the superficial peroneal nerve on the dorsum of the foot along an imaginary line over the fourth metatarsal; it is more noticeable with the foot in plantarflexion and inversion
  - the deep peroneal nerve between the first and second metatarsals, lateral to the extensor hallucis tendon
  - the sural nerve on the lateral aspect of the foot behind the lateral malleolus, lateral to the tendocalcaneus
- increased or decreased prominence of bones
- pain provoked or reduced on palpation.

Accessory movements

Accessory movements to the pubic symphysis, coccyx and sacroiliac joints may be examined. Accessory movements to the sacroiliac joint are shown in Figure 13.10.

Completion of the examination

Having carried out the above tests, examination of the sacroiliac joint is now complete. The subjective and physical examinations produce a large amount of information, which needs to be recorded accurately and quickly. It is vital at this stage to highlight important findings from the examination with an asterisk (*). These findings must be reassessed at, and within, subsequent treatment sessions to evaluate the effects of treatment on the patient's condition.

The strongest evidence that a joint is the source of the patient's symptoms is that active and passive physiological movements, passive accessory movements and joint palpation all reproduce the patient's symptoms, and that, following a treatment dose, reassessment identifies an improvement in the patient's signs and symptoms. Weaker evidence includes an alteration in range, resistance or quality of physiological and/or accessory movements and tenderness over the joint, with no alteration in signs and symptoms after treatment. One or more of these findings may indicate a dysfunction of a joint which may or may not be contributing to the patient's condition.

The strongest evidence that a muscle is the source of a patient's symptoms is if active movements, an isometric contraction, passive lengthening and palpation of a muscle all reproduce the patient's symptoms, and that, following a treatment dose, reassessment identifies an improvement in the patient's signs and symptoms. Further evidence of muscle dysfunction may be suggested by reduced strength or poor quality during the active physiological movement and the isometric contraction, reduced range and/or increased/decreased resistance, during the passive lengthening of the muscle, and tenderness on palpation, with no alteration in signs and symptoms after treatment. One or more of these findings may indicate a dysfunction of a muscle which may or may not be contributing to the patient's condition.

The strongest evidence that a nerve is the source of the patient's symptoms is when active and/or passive physiological movements reproduce the patient's symptoms, which are then increased or

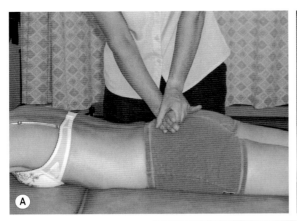
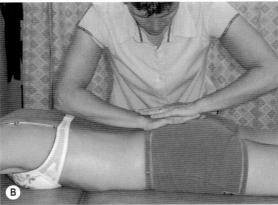
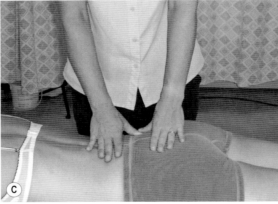

Figure 13.10 • Sacrum accessory movements. **A** Posteroanterior over the body of the sacrum. The heel of the hand is used to apply the pressure. **B** Sacral rock caudad. Pressure is applied to the base of the sacrum using the heel of the right hand in order to rotate the sacrum anteriorly in the sagittal plane, i.e. nutation. The left hand guides the movement. **C** Posteroanterior pressure over the posterior superior iliac spine. Thumb or pisiform can be used.

decreased with an additional neural sensitising movement, at a distance from the patient's symptoms. In addition, there is reproduction of the patient's symptoms on palpation of the nerve and neurodynamic testing. On completion of the physical examination the clinician:

- warns the patient of possible exacerbation up to 24–48 hours following the examination
- requests the patient to report details on the behaviour of the symptoms following examination at the next attendance
- explains the findings of the physical examination and how these findings relate to the subjective assessment. Any misconceptions patients may have regarding their illness or injury should be addressed
- evaluates the findings, formulates a clinical diagnosis and writes up a problem list

- determines the objectives of treatment
- devises an initial treatment plan.

In this way, the clinician will have developed the following hypotheses categories (adapted from Jones & Rivett 2004):

- function: abilities and restrictions
- patient's perspective on his/her experience
- source of symptoms. This includes the structure or tissue that is thought to be producing the patient's symptoms, the nature of the structure or tissues in relation to the healing process and the pain mechanisms.
- contributing factors to the development and maintenance of the problem. There may be environmental, psychosocial, behavioural, physical or heredity factors

- precautions/contraindications to treatment and management. This includes the severity and irritability of the patient's symptoms and the nature of the patient's condition
- management strategy and treatment plan

- prognosis – this can be affected by factors such as the stage and extent of the injury as well as the patient's expectation, personality and lifestyle.

For guidance on treatment and management principles, the reader is directed to the companion textbook (Petty 2011).

References

Broadhurst, N.A., Bond, M.J., 1998. Pain provocation tests for the assessment of sacroiliac joint dysfunction. J. Spinal Disord. 11 (4), 341–345.

Bullock, J.E., Jull, G.A., Bullock, M.I., 1987. The relationship of low back pain to postural changes during pregnancy. Aust. J. Physiother. 33 (1), 10–17.

Cakir, M., Samanci, N., Balci, M.K., 2003. Musculoskeletal manifestations in patients with thyroid disease. Clin. Endocrinol. (Oxf.) 59 (2), 162–167.

Clinical Standards Advisory Report, 1994. Report of a CSAG committee on back pain. HMSO, London.

Edwards, B.C., 1999. Manual of combined movements: their use in the examination and treatment of mechanical vertebral column disorders, second ed. Butterworth-Heinemann, Oxford.

Fortin, J.D., Aprill, C.N., Ponthieux, B., et al., 1994. Sacroiliac joint: pain referral maps upon applying a new injection technique. Part II. Clinical evaluation. Spine 19 (13), 1483–1489.

Freiberger, J.K., Riddle, D.L., 2001. Using published evidence to guide the examination of the sacroiliac joint region. Phys. Ther. 81, 1135–1143.

Greenman, P.E., 1996. Principles of manual medicine, second ed. Williams & Wilkins, Baltimore.

Grieve, G.P., 1981. Common vertebral joint problems. Churchill Livingstone, Edinburgh.

Grieve, G.P., 1991. Mobilisation of the spine, fifth ed. Churchill Livingstone, Edinburgh.

Grieve, G.P., 1994. Counterfeit clinical presentations. Manipulative Physiotherapist 26, 17–19.

Hagen, R., 1974. Pelvic girdle relaxation from an orthopaedic point of view. Acta Orthop. Scand. 45, 550–563.

Harding, I., Davies, E., Buchannon, E., et al., 2004. Is the symptoms of night pain important in the diagnosis of serious spinal pathology in a back pain triage clinic? Spine J. 4 (5), S30.

Janda, V., 1994. Muscles and motor control in cervicogenic disorders: assessment and management. In: Grant, R. (Ed.), Physical therapy of the cervical and thoracic spine, second ed. Churchill Livingstone, New York, p. 195.

Janda, V., 2002. Muscles and motor control in cervicogenic disorders. In: Grant, R. (Ed.), Physical therapy of the cervical and thoracic spine, third ed. Churchill Livingstone, New York, p. 182.

Jones, M.A., Rivett, D.A., 2004. Clinical reasoning for manual therapists. Butterworth-Heinemann, Edinburgh.

Laslett, M., Williams, M., 1994. The reliability of selected pain provocation tests for sacroiliac joint pathology. Spine 19 (11), 1243–1249.

Laslett M., Aprill C.N., McDonald B., Young SB., 2005. Diagnosis of sacroiliac joint pain: validity of individual provocation tests and composites of tests. Manual Therapy. 10 (3), 207–218.

Lavy, C., James, A., Wilson-MacDonald, J., et al., 2009. Cauda equina syndrome. Br. Med. J. 338, 881–884.

Lee, D., 1999. The pelvic girdle. An approach to the examination and treatment of the lumbo-pelvic-hip region, second ed. Churchill Livingstone, Edinburgh.

Levangie, P.K., 1999. Four clinical tests of sacroiliac joint dysfunction: the association of test results with innominate torsion among patients with and without low back pain. Phys. Ther. 79 (11), 1043–1057.

Magee, D.J., 1997. Orthopedic physical assessment, third ed. W B Saunders, Philadelphia.

Maitland, G.D., Hengeveld, E., Banks, K., et al., 2001. Maitland's vertebral manipulation, sixth ed. Butterworth-Heinemann, Oxford.

Mens, J.M.A., Vleming, A., Snijders, C., et al., 2001. Reliability and validity of the active straight leg raise test in posterior pelvic pain since pregnancy. Spine 26 (10), 1167–1171.

Moore, K., Dumas, G.A., Reid, J.G., 1990. Postural changes associated with pregnancy and their relationship with low-back pain. Clin. Biomech. 5 (3), 169–174.

Mousavi, S.J., 2003. Inter examiner and intra examiner reliability of eight sacroiliac joint static and dynamic tests. Phys. Ther. 13 (6), 225–232.

Ostgaard, H.C., Andersson, G.B.J., Schultz, A.B., et al., 1993. Influence of some biomechanical factors in low-back pain in pregnancy. Spine 18 (1), 61–65.

Ostgaard, H.C., Zetherstrom, G., Roos-Hansson, E., et al., 1994. Reduction of back and posterior pelvic pain in pregnancy. Spine 19 (8), 894–900.

O'Sullivan, P.B., Beales, 2007. Diagnosis and classification of pelvic girdle pain disorders – part 1: a mechanism based approach within a biopsychosocial framework. Man. Ther. 12 (2), 86–97.

Petty, N.J., 2011. Principles of neuromusculoskeletal treatment and management: a guide for therapists, second ed. Churchill Livingstone, Edinburgh.

Porterfield, J.A., DeRosa, C., 1998. Mechanical low back pain, perspectives in functional anatomy, second ed. W B Saunders, Philadelphia.

Riddle, D.L., Freburger, J.K., 2002. Evaluation of the presence of sacroiliac joint region dysfunction using a combination of tests: a multicenter intertester reliability study. Phys. Ther. 82 (8), 772–781.

Robinson, H.S., Brox, J.I., Robinson, R., et al., 2007. The reliability of selected motion and pain provocation tests for the sacroiliac joint. Man. Ther. 12 (1), 72–79.

Royal College of Radiologists, 2007. Making the best use of a department of clinical radiology. Guidelines for doctors, sixth ed. Royal College of Radiologists, London.

Sahrmann, S.A., 2002. Diagnosis and treatment of movement impairment syndromes. Mosby, St Louis.

Sapsford, R., Bullock-Saxton, J., Markwell, S., 1999. Women's health – a textbook for physiotherapists. W B Saunders, London.

Solomon, L., Warwick, D., Nayagam, S., 2001. Apley's system of orthopaedics and fractures, eighth ed. Arnold, London.

Stuber, K.J., 2007. Specificity, sensitivity and predictive values of clinical tests of the sacroiliac joint: a systematic review of the literature. J. Can. Chirop. Assoc. 51 (1), 30–41.

van de Wurff, P., Hagmeijer, R.H., Meyne, W., 2000a. Clinical tests of the sacroiliac joint. A systematic review. Part 1: reliability. Man. Ther. 5 (1), 30–36.

van de Wurff, P., Meyne, W., Hagmeijer, R.H., 2000b. Clinical tests of the sacroiliac joint. A systematic review. Part 2: validity. Man. Ther. 5 (2), 89–96.

Vincent-Smith, B., Gibbons, P., 1999. Inter examiner and intra examiner reliability of the standing flexion test. Man. Ther. 4 (2), 87–93.

Vleeming, A., 2003. European guidelines on the management of pelvic girdle pain. Available online at: http//www.backpaineurope.org.

Waddell, G., 2004. The back pain revolution, second ed. Churchill Livingstone, Edinburgh.

Examination of the hip region

14

Kieran Barnard

CHAPTER CONTENTS

Possible causes of pain and/or limitation of movement

- Trauma:
  - fracture of the neck or shaft of the femur
  - dislocation
  - contusion
  - ligamentous sprain
  - muscular strain
- Degenerative conditions: osteoarthrosis
- Femoroacetabular impingement
  - 'Cam' impingement
  - 'pincer' impingement
- Inflammatory disorders:
  - rheumatoid arthritis
  - acute pyogenic arthritis
  - ankylosing spondylitis
- Childhood disorders:
  - congenital dislocation of the hips
  - Perthes' disease
  - tuberculosis
- Adolescent disorders:
  - slipped femoral epiphysis
- Neoplasm: primary or secondary bone tumour
- Bursitis: subtrochanteric, ischiogluteal and iliopsoas
- Hypermobility
- Referral of symptoms from the lumbar spine, sacroiliac joint or pelvic organs.

Further details of the questions asked during the subjective examination and the tests carried out in the physical examination can be found in Chapters 2 and 3 respectively.

The order of the subjective questioning and the physical tests described below can be altered as appropriate for the patient being examined.

Subjective examination

Body chart

The following information concerning the type and area of current symptoms can be recorded on a body chart (see Figure 2.3).

Area of current symptoms

Be meticulous when mapping out the area of the symptoms. Lesions of the hip joint commonly refer symptoms into the groin, anterior thigh and knee. Ascertain which is the worst symptom and record where the patient feels the symptoms are coming from.

Areas relevant to the region being examined

Symptoms around the hip may be referred from more proximal anatomy, including arthrogenic, myogenic or neurogenic structures in the region of the lumbar spine or sacroiliac joints. Groin and medial thigh pain, for example, may be referred from the upper lumbar spine or may result from a peripheral neuropathy affecting the obturator nerve. Symptoms may also arise as a result of contributing factors such as weak hip lateral rotators or a compensated forefoot varus leading to medial femoral torsion. It is important therefore to include all areas of symptoms. Check all relevant areas including the lumbar spine, sacroiliac joint, knee and ankle joints for symptoms including pain or even stiffness, as this may be relevant to the patient's main symptom. Be sure to negate all possible areas that might refer or contribute to symptoms. The clinician marks unaffected areas with ticks (✓) on the body chart.

Quality of pain

Establish the quality of the pain, e.g. is the pain sharp, aching, throbbing?

Intensity of pain

The intensity of pain can be measured using, for example, a visual analogue scale, as shown in Chapter 2.

Depth of pain

Establish the depth of the pain. Does the patient feel it is on the surface or deep inside?

Abnormal sensation

Check for any altered sensation, such as paraesthesia or numbness, over the hip and other relevant areas.

Constant or intermittent symptoms

Ascertain the frequency of the symptoms, whether they are constant or intermittent. If symptoms are constant, check whether there is variation in the intensity of the symptoms, as constant unremitting pain may be indicative of serious pathology.

Relationship of symptoms

Determine the subjective relationship between symptomatic areas – do they come on together or separately? For example, the patient could have lateral thigh pain without back pain, or the pains may always be present together. Questions to clarify the relationship might include:

- Do you ever get your back pain without your thigh pain?
- Do you ever get your thigh pain without your back pain?
- If symptoms are constant: Does your thigh pain change when your back pain gets worse?

Behaviour of symptoms

Aggravating factors

For each symptomatic area, establish what movements and/or positions aggravate the patient's symptoms, i.e. what brings them on (or makes them worse)? is the patient able to maintain this position or movement (severity)? what happens to symptoms? and how long does it take for symptoms to ease once the position or movement is stopped (irritability)?

If a subjective relationship has already been established, it is helpful firstly to ask about the aggravating factors affecting the hypothesised source, e.g. lumbar spine, and follow up by establishing the aggravating factors affecting areas dependent on the source, e.g. the groin. If the aggravating factors for the two areas are the same or similar, this may further strengthen the hypothesis that there is a relationship between the two areas of symptoms.

Specific structures in the region of the hip may be implicated by correlating the area of symptoms with certain aggravating factors. For example, groin pain which is aggravated by putting on shoes (flexion) may be more indicative of an arthrogenic hip joint problem than, for example, a femoral nerve peripheral neuropathy.

It is important for the clinician to be as specific as possible when hunting for aggravating factors. Where possible, break the movement or activity down as this may provide clues for what to expect during the physical examination. 'What is it about . . .?' is a useful question to ask. Groin pain aggravated by 'gardening', for example, does not offer as much information as groin pain aggravated by 'weeding a flowerbed' (flexion) or 'pruning a high hedge' (extension).

The clinician ascertains how the symptoms affect function, such as static and active postures, e.g. sitting, standing, lying, bending, walking, running, walking on uneven ground and up and down stairs, driving, work, sport and social activities. Note details of the training regimen for any sports activities. The clinician finds out if the patient is left- or right-handed as there may be increased stress on the dominant side.

Detailed information on each of the above activities is useful in order to help determine the structure(s) at fault and identify functional restrictions. This information can be used to determine the aims of treatment and any advice that may be required. The most notable functional restrictions are highlighted with asterisks (*), explored in the physical examination and reassessed at subsequent treatment sessions to evaluate treatment intervention.

Easing factors

For each symptomatic area, the clinician asks what movements and/or positions ease the patient's symptoms, how long it takes for them to ease completely (if symptoms are intermittent) or back to the base level (if symptoms are constant) and what happens to other symptoms when this symptom is relieved. These questions help to confirm the relationship between the symptoms as well as determine the level of irritability.

Occasionally, particularly with symptoms that are irritable or with a patient who is catastrophising, it is difficult to establish clear and distinct aggravating factors. When this is the case it may be worth starting with the easing factors and working backwards. For example, if sitting down eases symptoms, it may be worth asking: 'Does that mean that standing makes your groin pain worse?'

At this point the clinician should be able to synthesise the information gained from the aggravating and easing factors and have a working hypothesis of the structure/s which might be at fault. Beware of, and do not dismiss, symptoms which do not conform to a mechanical pattern as this may be a sign of serious pathology.

Twenty-four-hour behaviour of symptoms

The clinician determines the 24-hour behaviour of symptoms by asking questions about night, morning and evening symptoms.

Night symptoms. It is important to establish whether the patient has pain at night. If so, does the patient have difficulty getting to sleep? How many times does the patient wake per night? How long does it take to get back to sleep?

It is crucial to establish whether the pain is position-dependent. The clinician may ask: 'Can you find a comfortable position in which to sleep?' or 'What is the most/least comfortable position for you?' Pain which is position-dependent is mechanical; pain which is not position-dependent and unremitting is non-mechanical and should arouse suspicion of more serious pathology.

Position-dependent pain may give clues as to the structure/s at fault; for example, patients with a trochanteric bursitis often have trouble sleeping and lying on the symptomatic side.

Morning and evening symptoms. The clinician determines the pattern of the symptoms first thing in the morning, through the day and at the end of the day. This information may provide clues as to the pain mechanisms driving the condition and the type of pathology present. For example, early-morning pain and stiffness lasting for more than half an hour may indicate inflammatory-driven pain.

Special questions

Hip-specific special questions may help in the generation of a clinical hypothesis. Such questions may include:

Squatting. Groin pain on squatting may implicate the hip joint as a source of symptoms.

Locking/catching. Locking and/or catching in the groin may be associated with femoroacetabular impingement (Zebala et al. 2007).

Crepitus. Crepitus with groin pain in the older patient may indicate degenerative change.

Neurological symptoms. During the subjective examination it is important to keep the hypothesis as open as possible. If, when questioning the patient and reviewing the body chart, a neurological lesion may be a possibility, establish with precision areas of pins and needles, numbness or weakness.

Has the patient experienced symptoms of spinal cord compression (compression of the spinal cord to L1 level), including bilateral tingling in hands or feet and/or disturbance of gait? Has the patient experienced symptoms of cauda equina compression (i.e. compression below L1)? Symptoms of cauda equina include perianal sensory loss and sphincter disturbance, with or without urinary retention. As well as retention, bladder symptoms may include reduced urine sensation, loss of desire to empty the bladder and a poor urine stream (Lavy et al. 2009). These symptoms may indicate compression of the sacral nerve roots and prompt surgical attention is required to prevent permanent disability.

History of the present condition

For each symptomatic area the clinician needs to know how long the symptom has been present, whether there was a sudden or slow onset and whether there was a known cause that provoked the onset of the symptom. If the onset was slow, the clinician finds out if there has been any change in the patient's lifestyle, e.g. a new job or hobby or a change in sporting activity or training schedule. The stage of the condition is established: are the symptoms getting better, staying the same or getting worse?

The clinician ascertains whether the patient has had this problem previously. If so, how many episodes has s/he had? when were they? what was the cause? what was the duration of each episode? and did the patient fully recover between episodes? If there is no previous history, has the patient had any episodes of pain and/or stiffness in the lumbar spine, knee, foot, ankle or any other relevant region?

To confirm the relationship between the symptoms, the clinician asks what happened to other symptoms when each symptom began. Symptoms which came on at the same time may indicate that the areas of symptoms are related. This evidence is further strengthened if there is a subjective relationship (symptoms come on at the same time or one is dependent on the other) and if the aggravating factors are the same or similar.

Has there been any treatment to date? The effectiveness of any previous treatment regime may help to guide patient management. Has the patient seen a specialist or had any investigations which may help with clinical diagnosis, such as blood tests, X-ray, arthroscopy, magnetic resonance imaging, myelography or a bone scan?

The mechanism of injury gives the clinician some important clues as to the injured structure around the hip, particularly in the acute stage, when a full physical examination may not be possible. For example, sudden buttock pain on sprinting may implicate the hamstring origin, whilst groin pain during extreme flexion activities such as hurdling or martial arts might implicate femoroacetabular impingement pathology (Laude et al. 2007).

Past medical history

A detailed medical history is vitally important to identify certain precautions or contraindications to the physical examination and/or treatment (see Table 2.4). As mentioned in Chapter 2, the clinician must differentiate between conditions that are suitable for conservative treatment and systemic, neoplastic and other non-neuromusculoskeletal conditions, which require referral to a medical practitioner.

The following information should be routinely obtained from patients.

General health. The clinician ascertains the state of the patient's general health and finds out if the patient suffers from any malaise, fatigue, fever, nausea or vomiting, stress, anxiety or depression.

Weight loss. Has the patient noticed any recent unexplained weight loss?

Serious pathology. Does the patient have a history of serious pathology, such as cancer, tuberculosis, osteomyelitis or human immunodeficiency virus (HIV)?

Inflammatory arthritis. Has the patient (or a member of his/her family) been diagnosed as having an inflammatory condition such as rheumatoid arthritis or polymyalgia rheumatica?

Cardiovascular disease. Is there a history of cardiac disease, e.g. angina? Does the patient have a pacemaker? If the patient has raised blood pressure, is it controlled with medication?

Respiratory disease. Does the patient have a history of lung pathology? How is it controlled?

Diabetes. Does the patient suffer from diabetes? If so, is it type 1 or type 2 diabetes? Is the patient's blood glucose controlled? How is it controlled? Is it through diet, tablet or injection? Patients with diabetes may develop peripheral neuropathy and vasculopathy, are at increased risk of infection and may take longer to heal than those without diabetes.

Epilepsy. Is the patient epileptic? When was the last seizure?

Thyroid disease. Does the patient have a history of thyroid disease? Thyroid dysfunction may cause musculoskeletal conditions such as adhesive capsulitis, Dupuytren's contracture, trigger finger and carpal tunnel syndrome (Cakir et al. 2003).

Osteoporosis. Has the patient had a dual-energy X-ray absorptiometry (DEXA) scan, been diagnosed with osteoporosis or sustained frequent fractures?

Previous surgery. Has the patient had previous surgery which may be of relevance to the presenting complaint?

Drug history

What medications are being taken by the patient? Has the patient ever been prescribed long-term (6 months or more) medication? Particular attention may need to be paid to the following:

Steroids. Long-term use of steroids for conditions such as polymyalgia rheumatica or chronic lung disease may lead to an increased risk of osteoporosis.

Anticoagulants. Anticoagulant medication such as warfarin prescribed for conditions such as atrial fibrillation may cause an increased risk of bleeding and therefore contraindicate certain therapeutic interventions such as high-velocity thrust techniques.

Non-steroidal anti-inflammatory drugs (NSAIDs). NSAIDs such as ibuprofen or diclofenac have systemic effects which may lead to gastrointestinal bleeding in some patients. Use of such medications should not be encouraged if they do not appear to be positively influencing the condition. Inflammatory nociceptive pain may however be relieved by NSAIDs.

Social and family history

Social and family history that is relevant to the onset and progression of the patient's problem is recorded. This includes the patient's perspectives, experience and expectations, age, employment, home situation and details of any leisure activities. Factors from this information may indicate direct and/or indirect mechanical influences on the hip. In order to treat the patient appropriately, it is important the condition is managed within the context of the patient's social and work environment.

The clinician may ask the following types of questions to elucidate psychosocial factors:

- Have you had time off work in the past with your pain?
- What do you understand to be the cause of your pain?
- What are you expecting will help you?
- How is your employer/co-workers/family responding to your pain?
- What are you doing to cope with your pain?
- Do you think you will return to work? When?

Although these questions are described in relation to psychosocial risk factors for poor outcomes for patients with low-back pain (Waddell 2004), they may be relevant to other patients.

Plan of the physical examination

When all this information has been collected, the subjective examination is complete. It is useful at this stage to highlight with asterisks (*), for ease of reference, important findings and particularly one or more functional restrictions. These can then be re-examined at subsequent treatment sessions to evaluate treatment intervention.

In order to plan the physical examination, the following hypotheses should be developed from the subjective examination:

- Is each area of symptoms severe and/or irritable? Will it be necessary to stop short of symptom reproduction, to reproduce symptoms partially or fully? If symptoms are severe, physical tests should be carried out to just short of symptom production or to the very first onset of symptoms; no overpressures will be carried out, as the patient would be unable to tolerate this. If symptoms are irritable, physical tests should be performed to just short of symptom production or just to the onset of symptoms with fewer physical tests being performed to allow for rest period between tests.

- What are the predominant pain mechanisms which might be driving the patient's symptoms? What are the active 'input mechanisms' (sensory pathways): are symptoms the product of a mechanical, inflammatory or ischaemic nociceptive process? What are the 'processing mechanisms': how has the patient processed this information? what are his or her thoughts and feelings about the pain? Finally, what are the 'output mechanisms': what is the patient's physiological, psychological and behavioural response to the pain? Clearly establishing which pain mechanisms may be causing and/or maintaining the condition will help the clinician manage both the condition and patient appropriately. The reader is directed to Gifford (1998) and Jones et al. (2002) for further reading.

- What are the possible arthrogenic, myogenic and neurogenic structures which could be causing the patient's symptoms: what structures could refer to the area of pain? and what structures are underneath the area of pain? For example, medial thigh pain could theoretically be referred from the lumbar spine or the sacroiliac joint. The structures directly under the medial thigh could also be implicated, for example the hip joint, the adductor muscles or the obturator nerve.

- In addition, are there any contributing factors which could be maintaining the condition? These could be:
  ○ physical, such as weak hip lateral rotators causing medial femoral torsion
  ○ environmental, for instance driving for a living
  ○ psychosocial, such as fear of serious pathology
  ○ behavioural, for instance excessive rest in an attempt to help the area heal.
- The clinician must decide, based on the evidence, which structures are most likely to be at fault and prioritise the physical examination accordingly. It is helpful to organise structures into ones that 'must', 'should' and 'could' be tested on day one and over subsequent sessions. This will develop the clinician's clinical reasoning and avoid a recipe-based hip assessment. Where possible it is advisable to clear an area fully. For example, if the clinician feels the lumbar spine needs to be excluded on day 1, s/he should fully assess this area, leaving no stone unturned, to implicate or negate this area as a source of symptoms. This approach will avoid juggling numerous potential sources of symptoms for several sessions, which may lead to confusion.
- Another way to develop the clinician's reasoning is to consider what to expect from each physical test. Will it be easy or hard to reproduce each symptom? Will it be necessary to use combined movements or repetitive movements? Will a particular test prove positive or negative? Will the pain be direction-specific? Synthesising evidence from the subjective examination and in particular the aggravating and easing factors should provide substantial evidence as to what to expect in the physical examination.
- Are there any precautions and/or contraindications to elements of the physical examination that need to be explored further, such as neurological involvement, recent fracture, trauma, steroid therapy or rheumatoid arthritis? There may also be certain contraindications to further examination and treatment, e.g. symptoms of spinal cord or cauda equina compression.

A physical planning form can be useful for clinicians to help guide them through the clinical reasoning process (see Figure 2.10).

Physical examination

The information from the subjective examination helps the clinician to plan an appropriate physical examination. The severity, irritability and nature of the condition are the major factors that will influence the choice and priority of physical testing procedures. The first and overarching question the clinician might ask is: 'Is this patient's condition suitable for me to manage as a therapist?' For example, a patient presenting with cauda equina compression symptoms may only need neurological integrity testing, prior to an urgent medical referral. The nature of the patient's condition has had a major impact on the physical examination. The second question the clinician might ask is: 'Does this patient have a neuromusculoskeletal dysfunction that I may be able to help?' To answer that, the clinician needs to carry out a full physical examination; however, this may not be possible if the symptoms are severe and/or irritable. If the patient's symptoms are severe and/or irritable, the clinician aims to explore movements as much as possible, within a symptom-free range. If the patient has constant and severe and/or irritable symptoms, then the clinician aims to find physical tests that ease the symptoms. If the patient's symptoms are non-severe and non-irritable, then the clinician aims to find physical tests that reproduce each of the patient's symptoms.

Each significant physical test that either provokes or eases the patient's symptoms is highlighted in the patient's notes by an asterisk (*) for easy reference. The highlighted tests are often referred to as 'asterisks' or 'markers'.

The order and detail of the physical tests described below need to be appropriate to the patient being examined; some tests will be irrelevant, some tests will be carried out briefly, while it will be necessary to investigate others fully. It is important that readers understand that the techniques shown in this chapter are some of many; the choice depends mainly on the relative size of the clinician and patient, as well as the clinician's preference. For this reason, novice clinicians may initially want to copy what is shown, but then quickly adapt to what is best for them.

Observation

Informal observation

The clinician needs to observe the patient in dynamic and static situations; the quality of lower-limb and general movement is noted, as are the postural characteristics and facial expression. Informal observation will have begun from the moment the clinician begins the subjective examination and will continue to the end of the physical examination.

Formal observation

Observation of posture. The clinician examines the patient's spinal and lower-limb posture from anterior, lateral and posterior views in standing. Specific observation of the pelvis involves noting its position in the sagittal, coronal and horizontal planes: in the sagittal plane, there may be excessive anterior or posterior pelvic tilt; in the coronal plane there may be a lateral pelvic tilt; and in the horizontal plane there may be rotation of the pelvis. These abnormalities will be identified by observing the relative position of the iliac crest, the anterior and posterior iliac spines, skin creases (particularly the gluteal creases), and the position of the pelvis relative to the lumbar spine and lower limbs. In addition, the clinician notes whether there is even weight-bearing through the left and right leg. The clinician passively corrects any asymmetry to determine its relevance to the patient's problem.

Observation of muscle form. The clinician observes the muscle bulk and muscle tone of the patient, comparing left and right sides. It must be remembered that the level and frequency of physical activity as well as the dominant side may well produce differences in muscle bulk between sides. Some muscles are thought to shorten under stress, while other muscles weaken, producing muscle imbalance (see Table 3.2). Patterns of muscle imbalance are thought to produce the postures mentioned above.

Observation of soft tissues. The clinician observes the quality and colour of the patient's skin and any area of swelling or presence of scarring, and takes cues for further examination.

Observation of balance. Balance is provided by vestibular, visual and proprioceptive information. This rather crude and non-specific test is conducted by asking the patient to stand on one leg with the eyes open and then closed. If the patient's balance is as poor with the eyes open as with the eyes closed, this suggests a vestibular or proprioceptive dysfunction (rather than a visual dysfunction). The test is carried out on the affected and unaffected sides; if there is greater difficulty maintaining balance on the affected side, this may indicate some proprioceptive dysfunction.

As well as monitoring the ability of the patient to balance on one leg, the clinician also pays close attention to the patient's pelvis. A pelvis that drops on the unsupported side indicates abductor weakness on the standing leg and is known as a positive Trendelenburg sign (Figure 14.1). A positive Trendelenburg sign is a common finding in patients who have undergone hip joint arthroplasty, and hip abductor function may be particularly compromised when the surgeon has employed a lateral approach to the hip (Baker & Bitounis 1989). A positive Trendelenburg sign invariably leads to a distinctive and inefficient gait (Hardcastle & Nade 1985).

Observation of gait. Analyse gait on even/uneven ground, slopes, stairs and running. Note the stride length and weight-bearing ability. Inspect the feet, shoes and any walking aids. The typical gait patterns that might be expected in patients with hip pain are the gluteus maximus gait, the Trendelenburg gait and the short-leg gait (see Chapter 3 for further details).

Observation of the patient's attitudes and feelings. The age, gender and ethnicity of patients and their cultural, occupational and social backgrounds will all affect their attitudes and feelings towards themselves, their condition and the clinician. The clinician needs to be aware of and sensitive to these attitudes, and to empathise and communicate appropriately so as to develop a rapport with the patient and thereby enhance the patient's compliance with the treatment.

Functional physical marker

It can be extremely useful to examine a functional physical marker specific to the patient's complaint. A functional marker which can be replicated in the clinical setting can often be identified when asking the patient about aggravating factors. It is recommended to examine a functional marker early in the assessment; this is for three reasons:

1. The marker will provide a useful initial snapshot of the patient's problem.
2. It may be possible to manipulate the marker to aid the clinical diagnosis and highlight possible treatment options (see below).
3. The marker will provide a useful physical marker (*).

An example of a functional marker may be sitting to standing causing groin and medial thigh pain, a movement which can be easily replicated in the clinic. How is the patient moving? Is the lumbar spine flexed or extended through the movement? Is the patient able to control the position of the pelvis? Is the foot pronating? Is the knee collapsing medially?

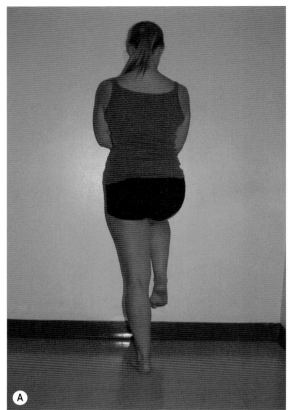 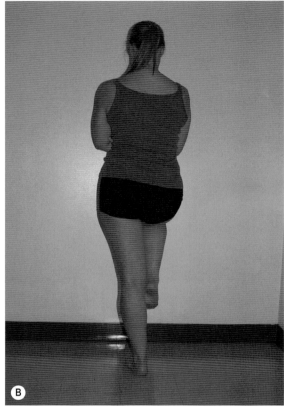

Figure 14.1 • Trendelenburg test. **A** The patient stands on the affected leg. **B** Positive test indicated by the pelvis dropping on the unsupported side.

Can the clinician change the patient's pain by manipulating the marker in some way? Does changing spinal posture during the movement or contracting the deep abdominal muscles alter the patient's pain? If the foot is pronating, does placing a block under the foot to prevent pronation make a difference to the pain and/or movement pattern? If the knee is collapsing medially, does it help to contract the gluteal muscles and instruct the patient to keep the patella in line with the foot when rising? Although tricky, the clinician may also attempt to add accessory glides to the hip as the patient rises or perhaps distract the hip using a seat belt to see if this alters symptoms.

By manipulating this marker in various ways, which need not be time-consuming, useful information may be gleaned as to the likely clinical diagnosis as well as the most appropriate way to manage the condition. Although this example highlights the art of clinical reasoning in practice, it is important to emphasise that functional markers are not standardised tests and will therefore lack a degree of validity

and reliability. The following section describes commonly performed orthopaedic tests for the examination of the hip.

Active physiological movements

Active physiological movements of the hip include flexion, extension, abduction, adduction, medial rotation and lateral rotation (Table 14.1). All movements may be performed bilaterally in supine, with the exception of extension, which may be more readily appreciated in prone. Movements are overpressed if symptoms allow (Figure 14.2).

The clinician establishes the patient's symptoms at rest, prior to each movement, and passively corrects any movement deviation to determine its relevance to the patient's symptoms. The following are noted:

- quality of movement
- range of movement

Table 14.1 Active physiological movements with possible modifications

Active physiological movements	Modifications
Flexion	Repeated
Extension	Speed altered
Abduction	Combined, e.g.
Adduction	– flexion with rotation
Medial rotation	– rotation with flexion
Lateral rotation	Compression or distraction, e.g.
?Lumbar spine	– through greater tuberosity
?Sacroiliac joint	with flexion
?Knee	Sustained
?Ankle and foot	Injuring movement
	Differentiation tests
	Functional ability

- behaviour of pain through the range of movement
- resistance through the range of movement and at the end of the range of movement
- provocation of any muscle spasm.

In a similar way to the manipulation of the functional physical marker, the thoughtful clinician may be able to manipulate physiological movements to help differentiation between tissues. For example, when trunk rotation with the patient standing on one leg (causing rotation in the lumbar spine and hip joint) reproduces the patient's buttock pain, differentiation between the lumbar spine and hip joint may be required. The clinician can increase and decrease the lumbar spine rotation and the pelvic rotation in turn, to find out what effect each movement has on the buttock pain. If the pain is coming from the hip then the lumbar spine movements will have no effect on the pain, but pelvic movements will alter the pain; conversely, if the pain is coming from the lumbar spine then lumbar spine movements will affect the pain but pelvic movement will have no effect.

It may be necessary to examine other regions to determine their relevance to the patient's symptoms; they may be the source of the symptoms, or they may be contributing to the symptoms. The most likely regions are the lumbar spine, sacroiliac joint, knee, foot and ankle. These regions can be quickly screened; see Chapter 3 for further details. Contrary to what their name might suggest, however, performing a clearing test on the lumbar spine for

example, does not fully negate this region as a source of symptoms and if there is any doubt the clinician is advised to assess the suspected area fully (see relevant chapter).

Capsular pattern. The capsular pattern for the hip joint (Cyriax 1982) is gross limitation of flexion, abduction and medial rotation, slight limitation of extension and no limitation of lateral rotation. This is one of the most useful capsular patterns to consider and may indicate osteoarthritis of the hip, particularly in the older patient.

Passive physiological movements

All the active movements described above can be examined passively with the patient usually in supine, comparing left and right sides. Comparison of the response of symptoms to the active and passive movements can help to determine whether the structure at fault is non-contractile (articular) or contractile (extra-articular) (Cyriax 1982). If the lesion is non-contractile, such as ligament, then active and passive movements will be painful and/or restricted in the same direction. If the lesion is in a contractile tissue (i.e. muscle) then active and passive movements are painful and/or restricted in opposite directions. For example, a hip adductor strain may be painful during active adduction and passive abduction. Such patterns are however theoretical and a muscle strain may be more readily assessed by contracting muscle isometrically where there will be little or no change in the length of non-contractile tissue.

To assess the patient's symptoms further passively it may be useful to explore the primary movements of flexion and adduction in the quadrant test.

Quadrant (flexion/adduction) test
(Maitland 1991)

The patient lies supine with one knee flexed. The clinician applies an adduction force to the hip and then moves the hip from just less than 90° flexion to full flexion (Figure 14.3). The quality, range and pain behaviour of the movement are noted. The movement can then be explored by arcing into abduction whilst maintaining end-of-range flexion and simultaneously adding a cephalad force through the shaft of the femur. If the clinician detects any areas of stiffness or resistance, or if the patient reports pain, pathology within the hip may be

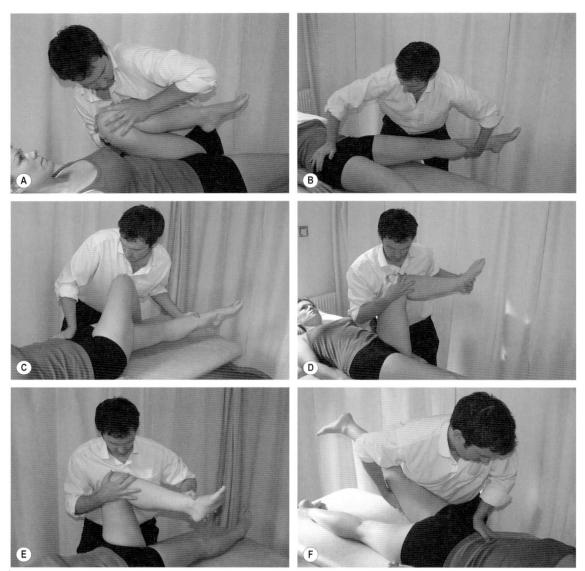

Figure 14.2 • Overpressures to the hip joint. **A** Flexion. Both hands rest over the knee and apply overpressure to hip flexion. **B** Abduction. The right hand stabilises the pelvis while the left hand takes the leg into abduction. **C** Adduction. With the right leg crossed over the left leg, the right hand stabilises the pelvis and the left hand takes the leg into adduction. **D** Medial rotation. The clinician's trunk and right hand support the leg. The left hand and trunk then move to rotate the hip medially. **E** Lateral rotation. The clinician's trunk and right hand support the leg. The left hand and trunk then move to rotate the hip laterally. **F** Extension. In prone, the left hand supports the pelvis whilst the right hand takes the leg into extension.

suspected, although the pelvis and lumbar spine will also be affected by this test.

Other regions may need to be examined to determine their relevance to the patient's symptoms; they may be the source of the symptoms, or they may be contributing to the symptoms. The most likely regions are the lumbar spine, sacroiliac joint, knee, ankle and foot. The joints within these regions can be tested fully (see relevant chapter) or partially with the use of clearing tests (Table 14.2).

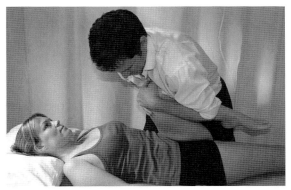

Figure 14.3 • Quadrant (flexion/adduction) test. The patient's thigh is fully supported by the clinician's arms and trunk. The clinician adds an adduction force into flexion and then arcs into abduction whilst simultaneously adding a cephalad force through the shaft of the femur.

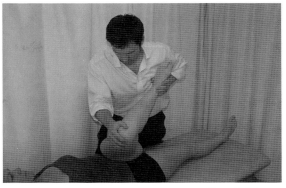

Figure 14.4 • Anterior impingement test. The clinician fully flexes the hip and then adducts and internally rotates the femur.

Anterior impingement test

The patient lies supine with one knee flexed. The clinician fully flexes the hip and then adducts and internally rotates the femur (Figure 14.4). This movement approximates the anterior aspect of the femoral neck with the acetabulum and is likely to reproduce pain in those suffering from femoroacetabular impingement syndrome (Klaue et al. 1991; Ganz et al. 2003; Philippon et al. 2007). Indeed, Philippon et al. (2007) found that, out of 301 patients treated arthroscopically for femoroacetabular impingement syndrome, this test was positive in 99% of patients.

FABER test

The FABER (flexion, abduction, external rotation) test has also been found to be a sensitive test in detecting femoroacetabular impingement syndrome. Philippon et al. (2007) found that 97% of patients with confirmed femoroacetabular impingement demonstrated a positive FABER test. With the

Table 14.2 Accessory movements, choice of application and reassessment of the patient's asterisks

Accessory movements	Modifications	Identify any effect of accessory movements on patient's signs and symptoms
Hip joint ↕ Anteroposterior ↕ Posteroanterior ↔ Caud Longitudinal caudad ↔ Lat Lateral transverse	Start position, e.g. – in flexion – in extension – in medial rotation – in lateral rotation (medial or lateral) – in flexion and medial rotation – in extension and lateral rotation Speed of force application Direction of the applied force Point of application of applied force	Reassess all asterisks
?Lumbar spine	As above	Reassess all asterisks
?Sacroiliac joint		
?Knee		
?Foot and ankle		

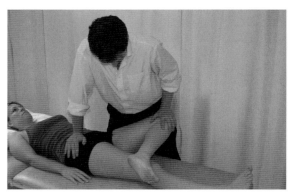

Figure 14.5 • Flexion, abduction, external rotation (FABER) test. The foot of the symptomatic leg is placed on the knee of the asymptomatic leg so the symptomatic leg lies in a flexed, abducted and externally rotated position. The clinician then stabilises the pelvis and adds some gentle downward pressure to the knee.

patient lying supine, the foot of the symptomatic leg is placed on the knee of the asymptomatic leg. The clinician then stabilises the pelvis and adds some gentle downward pressure to the knee (Figure 14.5). A positive test is indicated by the knee of the symptomatic leg resting further from the couch than the knee of the asymptomatic leg. As well as the presence of femoroacetabular impingement, a positive FABER test may indicate iliopsoas spasm or sacroiliac joint dysfunction (Magee 1997).

Muscle tests

Muscle tests include those examining muscle strength, control and length and isometric muscle testing.

Muscle strength

For a true appreciation of a muscle's strength, the clinician must test the muscle isotonically through the available range. During the physical examination of the hip, it may be appropriate to test the hip flexors, extensors, abductors, adductors, medial and lateral rotators and any other relevant muscle group. For details of these general tests readers are directed to Cole et al. (1988), Hislop & Montgomery (1995) or Kendall et al. (1993).

Greater detail may be required to test the strength of muscles, in particular those thought prone to become weak; that is, rectus abdominis, gluteus maximus, medius and minimus, vastus lateralis, medialis and intermedius, tibialis anterior and the peronei (Jull & Janda 1987; Sahrmann 2002). Testing the strength of these muscles is described in Chapter 3.

Muscle control

The relative strength of muscles is considered to be more important than the overall strength of a muscle group (Janda 1994, 2002; White & Sahrmann 1994; Sahrmann 2002). Relative strength is assessed indirectly by observing posture, as already mentioned, by the quality of active movement, noting any changes in muscle recruitment patterns and by palpating muscle activity in various positions.

Muscle length

The clinician may test the length of muscles, in particular those thought prone to shorten (Janda 1994); that is, erector spinae, quadratus lumborum, piriformis, iliopsoas, rectus femoris, tensor fasciae latae, hamstrings, tibialis posterior, gastrocnemius and soleus (Jull & Janda 1987; Sahrmann 2002). Testing the length of these muscles is described in Chapter 3.

Isometric muscle testing

Isometric muscle testing may help to differentiate whether symptoms are arising from contractile or non-contractile tissue. Isometric testing is described in detail in Chapter 3.

It may be appropriate to test the hip joint flexors, extensors, abductors, adductors, medial and lateral rotators (and other relevant muscle groups) in resting position and, if indicated, in different parts of the physiological range. The clinician notes the strength and quality of the contraction, as well as any reproduction of the patient's symptoms.

Neurological tests

Neurological examination includes neurological integrity testing and neurodynamic tests.

Integrity of the nervous system

The integrity of the nervous system is tested if the clinician suspects that the symptoms are emanating from the spine or from a peripheral nerve.

Dermatomes/peripheral nerves. Light touch and pain sensation of the lower limb are tested using cotton wool and pinprick respectively, as described in Chapter 3. Knowledge of the cutaneous distribution of nerve roots (dermatomes) and peripheral nerves enables the clinician to distinguish the sensory loss due to a root lesion from that due to a peripheral nerve lesion. The cutaneous nerve distribution and dermatome areas are shown in Chapter 3.

Myotomes/peripheral nerves. The following myotomes are tested (see Chapter 3 for further details):

- L2: hip flexion
- L3: knee extension
- L4: foot dorsiflexion and inversion
- L5: extension of the big toe
- S1: eversion of the foot, contract buttock, knee flexion
- S2: knee flexion, toe standing
- S3–S4: muscles of pelvic floor, bladder and genital function.

A working knowledge of the muscular distribution of nerve roots (myotomes) and peripheral nerves enables the clinician to distinguish the motor loss due to a root lesion from that due to a peripheral nerve lesion. The peripheral nerve distributions are shown in Chapter 3.

Reflex testing. The following deep tendon reflexes are tested (see Chapter 3):

- L3/4: knee jerk
- S1: ankle jerk.

Neurodynamic tests

The following neurodynamic tests may be carried out in order to ascertain the degree to which neural tissue is responsible for the production of the patient's symptom(s):

- passive neck flexion
- straight-leg raise
- passive knee bend
- slump.

These tests are described in detail in Chapter 3.

Miscellaneous tests

Vascular tests

If it is suspected that the circulation is compromised, the clinician palpates the pulses of the femoral, popliteal and dorsalis pedis arteries. The state of the vascular system can also be determined by the response of the symptoms to positions of dependency and elevation of the lower limbs.

Leg length

True leg length is measured from the anterior superior iliac spine to the medial or lateral malleolus. Apparent leg length is measured from the umbilicus to the medial or lateral malleolus. A difference in leg length of up to 1–1.3 cm is considered normal. If there is a leg length difference, test the length of individual bones: the tibia with knees bent and the femurs in standing. Ipsilateral posterior rotation of the ilium (on the sacrum) or contralateral anterior rotation of the ilium will result in a decrease in leg length (Magee 1997).

Ortolani's sign tests

This tests for congenital dislocation of the hips in infants. The clinician applies pressure against the greater trochanter and moves the hip joints into abduction and lateral rotation while applying some gentle traction (Magee 1997). A hard clunk followed by an increased range of movement is a positive test indicating dislocating hips.

Palpation

The clinician palpates the hip region and any other relevant area. It is useful to record palpation findings on a body chart (see Figure 2.3) and/or palpation chart (see Figure 3.36).

The clinician notes the following:

- the temperature of the area
- localised increased skin moisture
- the presence of oedema. This can be measured using a tape measure and comparing left and right sides
- mobility and feel of superficial tissues, e.g. ganglions, nodules, lymph nodes in the femoral triangle
- the presence or elicitation of any muscle spasm
- tenderness of bone (the greater trochanter may be tender because of trochanteric bursitis and the ischial tuberosity because of ischiogluteal bursitis); inguinal area tenderness may be due to iliopsoas bursitis (Wadsworth 1988), ligaments, muscle (Baer's point, for tenderness/spasm of

iliacus, lies a third of the way down a line from the umbilicus to the anterior superior iliac spine), tendon, tendon sheath, trigger points (shown in Figure 3.37) and nerve. Palpable nerves in the lower limb are as follows:

○ The sciatic nerve can be palpated two-thirds of the way along an imaginary line between the greater trochanter and the ischial tuberosity with the patient in prone.

○ The common peroneal nerve can be palpated medial to the tendon of biceps femoris and also around the head of the fibula.

○ The tibial nerve can be palpated centrally over the posterior knee crease medial to the popliteal artery; it can also be felt behind the medial malleolus, which is more noticeable with the foot in dorsiflexion and eversion.

○ The superficial peroneal nerve can be palpated on the dorsum of the foot along an imaginary line over the fourth metatarsal; it is more noticeable with the foot in plantarflexion and inversion.

○ The deep peroneal nerve can be palpated between the first and second metatarsals, lateral to the extensor hallucis tendon.

○ The sural nerve can be palpated on the lateral aspect of the foot behind the lateral malleolus, lateral to the tendocalcaneus.

• increased or decreased prominence of bones
• pain provoked or reduced on palpation.

Accessory movements

It is useful to use the palpation chart and movement diagrams (or joint pictures) to record findings. These are explained in detail in Chapter 3.

The clinician notes the following:

• quality of movement
• range of movement
• resistance through the range and at the end of the range of movement
• behaviour of pain through the range
• provocation of any muscle spasm.

Hip joint accessory movements are shown in Figure 14.6 and are listed in Table 14.2. Following accessory movements to the hip region, the clinician reassesses all the physical asterisks (movements or tests that have been found to reproduce the patient's symptoms) in order to establish the effect of the

accessory movements on the patient's signs and symptoms. Accessory movements can then be tested for other regions suspected to be a source of, or contributing to, the patient's symptoms. Again, following accessory movements to any one region, the clinician reassesses all the asterisks. Regions likely to be examined are the lumbar spine, sacroiliac joint, knee, foot and ankle (Table 14.2).

Mobilisations with movement (MWMs) (Mulligan 1999)

MWMs are sustained accessory glides applied to a joint during active or passive movement. They need not be prescriptive and the clinician is encouraged to experiment with different MWMs whilst closely monitoring the patient's symptomatic response. MWMs can be particularly helpful when exploring a functional physical marker.

Figure 14.7 illustrates an MWM for the hip which can be performed in supine. The clinician stabilises the pelvis and uses a seat belt to apply a lateral glide to the femur while the patient actively moves the hip into medial rotation or flexion. An increase in the range of movement and no pain or reduced pain on active medial rotation or flexion of the hip joint in the lateral glide position are positive examination findings, indicating a mechanical joint problem.

Completion of the examination

Having carried out all of the above tests, the examination of the hip region is now complete. The subjective and physical examinations produce a large amount of information, which needs to be recorded accurately and quickly. It is vital at this stage to highlight important findings from the examination with an asterisk (*). These findings must be reassessed at, and within, subsequent treatment sessions to evaluate the effects of treatment on the patient's condition.

The physical testing procedures which specifically indicate joint, nerve or muscle tissues, as a source of the patient's symptoms, are summarised in Table 3.10. The strongest evidence that a joint is the source of the patient's symptoms is that active and passive physiological movements, passive accessory movements and joint palpation all reproduce the patient's symptoms, and that, following a treatment dose, reassessment identifies an improvement in the patient's signs and symptoms. Weaker evidence includes an alteration

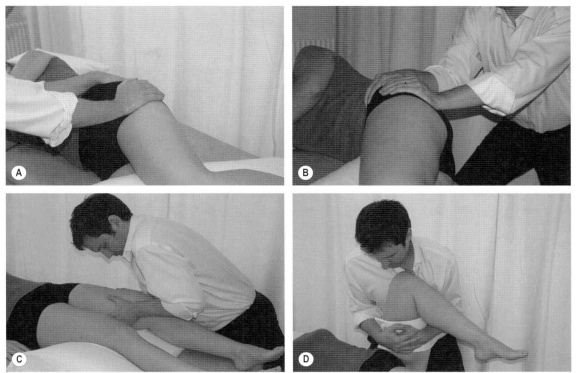

Figure 14.6 • Hip joint accessory movements. **A** Anteroposterior. With the patient in side-lying, pillows are placed between the patient's legs to position the hip joint in neutral. The left hand is then placed posterior on the iliac crest to stabilise the pelvis while the heel of the right hand applies an anteroposterior pressure over the anterior aspect of the greater trochanter. **B** Posteroanterior. With the patient in side-lying, pillows are placed between the patient's legs to position the hip joint in neutral. The right hand grips around the anterior aspect of the anterior superior iliac spine to stabilise the pelvis while the left hand applies a posteroanterior force to the posterior aspect of the greater trochanter. **C** Longitudinal caudad. The hands grip just proximal to the medial and lateral femoral epicondyles and pull the femur in a caudad direction. **D** Lateral transverse. The hip is flexed and a towel is placed around the upper thigh. The clinician clasps the hands together on the medial aspect of the thigh and pulls the leg laterally.

in range, resistance or quality of physiological and/or accessory movements and tenderness over the joint, with no alteration in signs and symptoms after treatment. One or more of these findings may indicate a dysfunction of a joint which may or may not be contributing to the patient's condition.

The strongest evidence that a muscle is the source of a patient's symptoms is if active movements, an isometric contraction, passive lengthening and palpation of a muscle all reproduce the patient's symptoms, and that, following a treatment dose, reassessment identifies an improvement in the patient's signs and symptoms. Further evidence of muscle dysfunction may be suggested by reduced strength or poor quality during the active physiological

movement and the isometric contraction, reduced range and/or increased/decreased resistance, during the passive lengthening of the muscle, and tenderness on palpation, with no alteration in signs and symptoms after treatment. One or more of these findings may indicate a dysfunction of a muscle which may or may not be contributing to the patient's condition.

The strongest evidence that a nerve is the source of the patient's symptoms is when active and/or passive physiological movements reproduce the patient's symptoms, which are then increased or decreased with an additional sensitising movement, at a distance from the patient's symptoms. In addition, there is reproduction of the patient's symptoms on palpation of the nerve and, following neurodynamic testing, sufficient

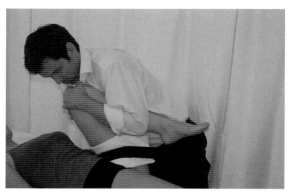

Figure 14.7 • Mobilisation with movement for hip flexion. The clinician stabilises the pelvis with the left hand and uses a seat belt to apply a lateral glide to the femur while the patient actively flexes the hip.

to be considered a treatment dose, results in an improvement in the above signs and symptoms. Further evidence of nerve dysfunction may be suggested by reduced range (compared with the asymptomatic side) and/or increased resistance to the various arm movements, and tenderness on nerve palpation.

On completion of the physical examination, the clinician:

- warns the patient of possible exacerbation up to 24–48 hours following the examination
- requests the patient to report details on the behaviour of the symptoms following examination at the next attendance
- explains the findings of the physical examination and how these findings relate to the subjective assessment. Any misconceptions patients may have regarding their illness or injury need to be addressed
- evaluates the findings, formulates a clinical diagnosis and writes up a problem list
- determines the objectives of treatment
- devises an initial treatment plan.

In this way, the clinician will have developed the following hypotheses categories (adapted from Jones & Rivett 2004):

- function: abilities and restrictions
- patient's perspective on his/her experience
- source of symptoms. This includes the structure or tissue that is thought to be producing the patient's symptoms, the nature of the structure or tissues in relation to the healing process and the pain mechanisms
- contributing factors to the development and maintenance of the problem. There may be environmental, psychosocial, behavioural, physical or heredity factors
- precautions/contraindications to treatment and management. This includes the severity and irritability of the patient's symptoms and the nature of the patient's condition
- management strategy and treatment plan
- prognosis – this can be affected by factors such as the stage and extent of the injury as well as the patient's expectation, personality and lifestyle.

For guidance on treatment and management principles, the reader is directed to the companion textbook (Petty 2011).

References

Baker, A.S., Bitounis, V.C., 1989. Abductor function after total hip replacement: an electromyographic and clinical review. J. Bone Joint Surg. Br. 71-B (1), 47–50.

Cakir, M., Samanci, N., Balci, N., et al., 2003. Musculoskeletal manifestations in patients with thyroid disease. Clin. Endocrinol. (Oxf.) 59 (2), 162–167.

Cole, J.H., Furness, A.L., Twomey, L.T., 1988. Muscles in action: an approach to manual muscle testing. Churchill Livingstone, Edinburgh.

Cyriax, J., 1982. Textbook of orthopaedic medicine – diagnosis of soft tissue lesions, eighth ed. Baillière Tindall, London.

Ganz, R., Parvizi, J., Beck, M., et al., 2003. Femoroacetabular impingement: a cause for osteoarthritis of the hip. Clin. Orthop. Relat. Res. 417, 112–120.

Gifford, L.S., 1998. Pain, the tissues and the nervous system: a conceptual model. Physiotherapy 84 (1), 27–36.

Hardcastle, P., Nade, S., 1985. The significance of the Trendelenburg test. J. Bone Joint Surg. Br. 67-B (5), 741–746.

Hislop, H., Montgomery, J., 1995. Daniels and Worthingham's muscle testing, techniques of manual examination, seventh ed. W B Saunders, Philadelphia.

Janda, V., 1994. Muscles and motor control in cervicogenic disorders: assessment and management. In: Grant, R. (Ed.), Physical therapy of the cervical and thoracic spine, second ed. Churchill Livingstone, New York, p. 195.

Janda, V., 2002. Muscles and motor control in cervicogenic disorders. In: Grant, R. (Ed.), Physical therapy of the cervical and thoracic spine, third ed. Churchill Livingstone, New York, p. 182.

Jones, M.A., Rivett, D.A., 2004. Clinical reasoning for manual therapists. Butterworth-Heinemann, Edinburgh.

Jones, M.A., Edwards, I., Gifford, L.S., 2002. Conceptual models for implementing biopsychosocial theory in clinical practice. Man. Ther. 7 (1), 2–9.

Jull, G.A., Janda, V., 1987. Muscles and motor control in low back pain: assessment and management. In: Twomey, L.T., Taylor, J.R. (Eds.), Physical therapy of the low back. Churchill Livingstone, New York, p. 253.

Kendall, F.P., McCreary, E.K., Provance, P.G., 1993. Muscles, testing and function, fourth ed. Williams & Wilkins, Baltimore.

Klaue, K., Durnin, C.W., Ganz, R., 1991. The acetabular rim syndrome. A clinical presentation of dysplasia of the hip. J. Bone Joint Surg. Br. 73 (3), 423–429.

Laude, F., Boyer, T., Nogier, A., 2007. Anterior femoroacetabular impingement. Joint Bone Spine 74, 127–132.

Lavy, C., James, A., Wilson-MacDonald, J., et al., 2009. Cauda equina syndrome. Br. Med. J. 338, 881–884.

Magee, D.J., 1997. Orthopedic physical assessment, third ed. W B Saunders, Philadelphia.

Maitland, G.D., 1991. Peripheral manipulation, third ed. Butterworth-Heinemann, London.

Mulligan, B.R., 1999. Manual therapy 'NAGs', 'SNAGs', 'MWMs' etc., fourth ed. Plane View Services, New Zealand.

Petty, N.J., 2011. Principles of neuromusculoskeletal treatment and management: a guide for therapists, second ed. Churchill Livingstone, Edinburgh.

Philippon, M.J., Maxwell, R.B., Johnston, T.L., et al., 2007. Clinical presentation of femoroacetabular impingement. Knee Surg. Sports Traumatol. Arthrosc. 15, 1041–1047.

Sahrmann, S.A., 2002. Diagnosis and treatment of movement impairment syndromes. Mosby, St Louis.

Waddell, G., 2004. The back pain revolution, second ed. Churchill Livingstone, Edinburgh.

Wadsworth, C.T., 1988. Manual examination and treatment of the spine and extremities. Williams & Wilkins, Baltimore.

White, S.G., Sahrmann, S.A., 1994. A movement system balance approach to musculoskeletal pain. In: Grant, R. (Ed.), Physical therapy of the cervical and thoracic spine, second ed. Churchill Livingstone, Edinburgh, p. 339.

Zebala, L.P., Schoenecker, P.L., Clohisy, J.C., 2007. Anterior femoroacetabular impingement: a diverse disease with evolving treatment options. Iowa Orthop. J. 27, 71–81.

Examination of the knee region

Kieran Barnard

CHAPTER CONTENTS

Possible causes of pain and/or limitation of movement

This region includes the tibiofemoral, patellofemoral and superior tibiofibular joints with their surrounding soft tissues.

- Trauma:
  - ○ fracture of the lower end of the femur, upper end of the tibia or patella
  - ○ dislocation of the patella
  - ○ haemarthrosis
  - ○ traumatic synovitis
  - ○ ligamentous sprain
  - ○ muscular strain
  - ○ meniscal tear
  - ○ meniscal cyst
  - ○ damage to fat pads
  - ○ Osgood–Schlatter disease
- Degenerative conditions:
  - ○ osteoarthrosis
  - ○ haemophilic arthritis
- Inflammatory conditions: rheumatoid arthritis
- Infection, e.g. acute septic arthritis (pyarthrosis), tuberculosis
- Chondromalacia patellae
- Osteochondritis desiccans
- Knee deformity: genu varum, genu valgum and genu recurvatum
- Popliteal cyst
- Bursitis: semimembranosus, pes anserine, prepatellar and infrapatellar
- Loose bodies
- Plica syndrome
- Hypermobility
- Tendinopathy, e.g. patella
- Iliotibial band friction syndrome
- Referral of symptoms from the lumbar spine, sacroiliac joint or hip joint regions.

Further details of the questions asked during the subjective examination and the tests carried out in the physical examination can be found in Chapters 2 and 3 respectively.

The order of the subjective questioning and the physical tests described below can be altered as appropriate for the patient being examined.

Subjective examination

Body chart

The following information concerning the type and area of the current symptoms can be recorded on a body chart (see Figure 2.3).

Area of current symptoms

Be meticulous when mapping out the area of the symptoms. A lesion in the knee joint complex may refer symptoms proximally to the thigh or distally to the foot and ankle. Ascertain which is the worst symptom and record where the patient feels the symptoms are coming from.

Areas relevant to the region being examined

Symptoms around the knee complex may be referred from more proximal anatomy, including arthrogenic, myogenic or neurogenic structures in the region of the lumbar spine, pelvis or hip. For example, anterior knee pain may be referred from the lumbar spine or may result from a peripheral neuropathy affecting the femoral nerve. Symptoms may also arise as a result of contributing factors affecting the foot and/or ankle complex. Using the same example, anterior knee pain may result from a compensated forefoot varus causing medial tibial torsion and a change in the angle of pull on the patella. It is important therefore to include all areas of symptoms. Check all relevant areas, including the lumbar spine, pelvis, hip, foot and ankle for symptoms including pain or even stiffness, as this may be relevant to the patient's main symptom. Be sure to negate all possible areas that might refer or contributing to the area of pain. Mark unaffected areas with ticks (✓) on the body chart.

Quality of pain

Establish the quality of the pain, e.g. is the pain sharp, aching, throbbing?

Intensity of pain

The intensity of pain can be measured using, for example, a visual analogue scale, as shown in Chapter 2.

Depth of pain

Establish the depth of the pain. Does the patient feel it is on the surface or deep inside? If appropriate, distinguish between pain felt underneath the patella and that felt in the tibiofemoral joint.

Abnormal sensation

Check for any altered sensation (such as paraesthesia or numbness) over the knee and other relevant areas.

Constant or intermittent symptoms

Ascertain the frequency of the symptoms, whether they are constant or intermittent. If symptoms are constant, check whether there is variation in the intensity of the symptoms, as constant unremitting pain may be indicative of serious pathology.

Relationship of symptoms

Determine the subjective relationship between symptomatic areas – do they come on together or separately? For example, the patient could have knee pain without back pain, or the pains may always be present together. Questions to clarify the relationship might include:

- Do you ever get your back pain without your knee pain?
- Do you ever get your knee pain without your back pain?
- If symptoms are constant: Does your knee pain change when your back pain gets worse?

Behaviour of symptoms

Aggravating factors

For each symptomatic area, establish what movements and/or positions aggravate the patient's symptoms, i.e. what brings them on (or makes them worse)? is the patient able to maintain this position or movement (severity)? what happens to and how long does it take for symptoms to ease once the position or movement is stopped (irritability)?

If a subjective relationship has already been established, it is helpful firstly to ask about the aggravating factors affecting the hypothesised source, e.g. lumbar spine, and follow up by establishing the aggravating factors affecting areas dependent on the source, e.g. the knee. If the aggravating factors for the two areas are the same or similar, this may further strengthen the hypothesis that there is a relationship between the two areas of symptoms.

If the knee is suspected, specific knee structures may be implicated by correlating the area of symptoms with certain aggravating factors. For example, anterior knee pain which is aggravated by stair climbing may implicate the patellofemoral joint (Brechter & Powers 2002), whereas posterior knee pain aggravated by squatting may implicate the menisci (McDermott 2006).

It is important for the clinician to be as specific as possible when hunting for aggravating factors. Where possible, break the movement or activity down as this may provide clues for what to expect during the physical examination. 'What is it about . . .?' is a useful question to ask. Knee pain aggravated by 'driving' does not offer as much information as knee pain aggravated by 'pushing the clutch' (extension), 'changing pedals' (twisting) or 'long distances on a motorway' (sustained flexion). Aggravating factors for other regions, which may need to be queried if they are suspected to be a source of the symptoms, are shown in Table 2.3.

The clinician ascertains how the symptoms affect function, such as: static and active postures, e.g. sitting, standing, lying, bending, walking, running, walking on uneven ground and up and down stairs, driving, work, sport and social activities. Note details of the training regimen for any sports activities. The clinician finds out if the patient is left- or right-handed as there may be increased stress on the dominant side.

Detailed information on each of the above activities is useful in order to help determine the structure(s) at fault and identify functional restrictions. This information can be used to determine the aims of treatment and any advice that may be required. The most notable functional restrictions are highlighted with asterisks (*), explored in the physical examination and reassessed at subsequent treatment sessions to evaluate treatment intervention.

Easing factors

For each symptomatic area, the clinician asks what movements and/or positions ease the patient's symptoms, how long it takes for them to ease completely (if symptoms are intermittent) or back to the base level (if symptoms are constant) and what happens to other symptoms when this symptom is relieved. These questions help to confirm the relationship between the symptoms as well as determine the level of irritability.

Occasionally, particularly with symptoms that are irritable or with a patient who is catastrophising, it is difficult to establish clear and distinct aggravating factors. When this is the case it may be worth starting with the easing factors and working backwards. For example, if knee extension eases symptoms, it may be worth asking: 'Does that mean that bending your knee makes your pain worse?'

At this point the clinician should be able to synthesise the information gained from the aggravating and easing factors and have a working hypothesis of the structure/s which might be at fault. Beware of, and do not dismiss, symptoms which do not conform to a mechanical pattern as this may be a sign of serious pathology.

Twenty-four-hour behaviour of symptoms

The clinician determines the 24-hour behaviour of symptoms by asking questions about night, morning and evening symptoms.

Night symptoms. It is important to establish whether the patient has pain at night. If so, does s/he have difficulty getting to sleep? How many times does s/he wake at night? How long does it take to get back to sleep?

It is crucial to establish whether the pain is position-dependent. The clinician may ask: 'Can you find a comfortable position in which to sleep?' or 'What is the most/least comfortable position for you?' Pain which is position-dependent is mechanical; pain which is not position-dependent and unremitting is non-mechanical and should arouse suspicion of more serious pathology.

Position-dependent pain may give clues as to the structure/s at fault; for example, patients with an injury to the medial meniscus often have trouble sleeping and lying with the symptomatic side uppermost as it compresses that side.

Morning and evening symptoms. The clinician determines the pattern of the symptoms first thing in the morning, through the day and at the end of the day. This information may provide clues as to the pain mechanisms driving the condition and the type of pathology present. For example, early-morning pain and stiffness lasting for more than half an hour may indicate inflammatory-driven pain.

Special questions

Knee-specific special questions may help in the generation of a clinical hypothesis. Such questions may include:

Swelling. Does the knee swell? If so, the clinician needs to establish whether the swelling occurred immediately after the injury or whether it took hours or days to form. Immediate swelling may indicate bleeding suggestive of significant trauma or rupture and is distinct from swelling occurring within hours of an injury, which is more suggestive of the build-up of inflammatory exudate.

Giving way. Giving way of the knee may be suggestive of either ligamentous instability or an inability of the surrounding musculature, particularly the quadriceps, to support the knee adequately. Ligamentous instability is normally the result of trauma, whilst giving way of muscular origin is more complex and may be due to weakness as a result of disuse, pain inhibition, joint effusion (Torry et al. 2000) or ligamentomuscular reflex inhibition (Solomonow 2009). Correlating giving way with the wider clinical picture may therefore provide useful information. For example, falling to the floor without warning and a history of trauma may represent mechanical instability whilst giving way without trauma and in the presence of pain and/or swelling may represent a muscular cause.

Locking. If locking is present, it is important to distinguish between true and 'pseudo'-locking. True locking might represent an intra-articular derangement such as a meniscal tear, whilst pseudo-locking may simply represent an unwillingness to move the knee due to pain. Qualifying locking by asking: 'Does your knee get stuck so you can't bend or straighten it?' may be helpful.

Crepitus. If crepitus is associated with pain it may help to build a clinical picture. For example, crepitus anteriorly when descending stairs may suggest chondromalacia patellae.

Neurological symptoms. During the subjective examination it is important to keep the hypothesis as open as possible. If, when questioning the patient and reviewing the body chart, a neurological lesion may be a possibility, establish with precision areas of pins and needles, numbness or weakness.

Has the patient experienced symptoms of spinal cord compression (compression of the spinal cord to L1 level), including bilateral tingling in hands or feet and/or disturbance of gait? Has the patient experienced symptoms of cauda equina compression (i.e. compression below L1)? Symptoms of cauda equina include perianal sensory loss and sphincter disturbance, with or without urinary retention. As well as retention, bladder symptoms may include reduced urine sensation, loss of desire to empty the bladder and a poor urine stream (Lavy et al. 2009). These symptoms may indicate compression of the sacral nerve roots and prompt surgical attention is required to prevent permanent disability.

History of the present condition

For each symptomatic area the clinician needs to know how long the symptom has been present, whether there was a sudden or slow onset and whether there was a known cause that provoked the onset of the symptom. If the onset was slow, the clinician finds out if there has been any change in the patient's lifestyle, e.g. a new job or hobby or a change in sporting activity or training schedule. The stage of the condition is established, by asking: are the symptoms getting better, staying the same or getting worse?

The clinician ascertains whether the patient has had this problem previously. If so, how many episodes has s/he had? when were they? what was the cause? what was the duration of each episode? and did the patient fully recover between episodes? If there is no previous history, has the patient had any episodes of pain and/or stiffness in the lumbar spine, hip, knee, foot, ankle or any other relevant region?

To confirm the relationship between the symptoms, the clinician asks what happened to other symptoms when each symptom began. Symptoms which came on at the same time may indicate that the areas of symptoms are related. This evidence is further strengthened if there is a subjective relationship (symptoms come on at the same time or one is dependent on the other) and if the aggravating factors are the same or similar.

Has there been any treatment to date? The effectiveness of any previous treatment regime may help to guide patient management. Has the patient seen a specialist or had any investigations which may help with clinical diagnosis, such as blood tests, radiograph, arthroscopy, magnetic resonance imaging, myelography or a bone scan?

The mechanism of injury gives the clinician some important clues as to the injured structure in the knee, particularly in the acute stage, when a full physical examination may not be possible. For example, pain on twisting or rising from a crouched position may indicate a meniscal injury (Drosos & Pozo

Table 15.1 The possible diagnoses suspected from the mechanism of injury (adapted from Magee 1997; Hayes et al. 2000)

Mechanism of injury	Possible structures injured	Comments
Hyperflexion	Posterior horn of medial and/or lateral meniscus ACL	May complain of locking
Prolonged flexion	Posterior horn of medial and/or lateral meniscus	Particularly in older patients May complain of locking
Hyperextension	Anterior tibial and/or femoral condyles PCL, ACL Posterior capsule Fat pad	Cruciate injury may result from tibial translation anteriorly (ACL) or posteriorly (PCL)
Valgus	Lateral tibial and/or femoral condyles MCL, ACL, PCL	Cruciate injury with severe force
Varus	Medial tibial and/or femoral condyles LCL, ITB	Uncommon
Flexion valgus without rotation	Lateral tibial and/or femoral condyles MCL Patellar subluxation/dislocation	
Flexion valgus with rotation	Lateral tibial and/or femoral condyles MCL, ACL Medial and/or lateral menisci Patellar subluxation/dislocation	Common injury. Immediate swelling (haemarthrosis) with a pop may suggest ACL rupture Meniscal injury may present with locking
Flexion varus without rotation	Medial tibial and/or femoral condyles ACL, posterolateral corner Medial and/or lateral menisci	Meniscal injury may present with locking
Extension with valgus	Anterolateral tibial and/or femoral condyles MCL, PCL Posteromedial corner	
Extension with varus	Anteromedial tibial and/or femoral condyles ACL Posterolateral corner Popliteal tendon	May lead to unstable posterolateral corner injury
Flexion with posterior tibial translation (dashboard injury)	PCL Posterior dislocation with severe force resulting in posterior instability ± patellar, proximal tibial and/or tibial plateau fracture	Most common mechanism for isolated PCL injury

ACL, anterior cruciate ligament; PCL, posterior cruciate ligament; MCL, medial collateral ligament; LCL, lateral collateral ligament; ITB, iliotibial band.

2004) whilst an anterior cruciate ligament (ACL) rupture may be suspected following an injury that involved rotation of the body on a fixed foot followed by immediate swelling (haemarthrosis). Such an injury may be (but not always) accompanied by a pop or cracking sound (Casteleyn et al. 1988). The possible diagnoses suspected from the mechanism of injury are given in Table 15.1.

Past medical history

A detailed medical history is vitally important to identify certain precautions or contraindications to the physical examination and/or treatment (see Table 2.4). As mentioned in Chapter 2, the clinician must differentiate between conditions that are suitable for conservative treatment and systemic, neoplastic and other non-neuromusculoskeletal conditions, which require referral to a medical practitioner.

The following information should be routinely obtained from patients.

General health. The clinician ascertains the state of the patient's general health and finds out if the patient suffers from any malaise, fatigue, fever, nausea or vomiting, stress, anxiety or depression.

Weight loss. Has the patient noticed any recent unexplained weight loss?

Serious pathology. Does the patient have a history of serious pathology such as cancer, tuberculosis, osteomyelitis or human immunodeficiency virus (HIV)?

Inflammatory arthritis. Has the patient (or a member of his/her family) been diagnosed as having an inflammatory condition such as rheumatoid arthritis or polymyalgia rheumatica?

Cardiovascular disease. Is there a history of cardiac disease, e.g. angina? Does the patient have a pacemaker? If the patient has raised blood pressure, is it controlled with medication?

Respiratory disease. Does the patient have a history of lung pathology? How is it controlled?

Diabetes. Does the patient suffer from diabetes? If so, is it type 1 or type 2 diabetes? Is the patient's blood glucose controlled? How is it controlled: through diet, tablet or injection? Patients with diabetes may develop peripheral neuropathy and vasculopathy, are at increased risk of infection and may take longer to heal than those without diabetes.

Epilepsy. Is the patient epileptic? When was the last seizure?

Thyroid disease. Does the patient have a history of thyroid disease? Thyroid dysfunction may cause musculoskeletal conditions such as adhesive capsulitis, Dupuytren's contracture, trigger finger and carpal tunnel syndrome (Cakir et al. 2003).

Osteoporosis. Has the patient had a dual-energy X-ray absorptiometry (DEXA) scan, been diagnosed with osteoporosis or sustained frequent fractures?

Previous surgery. Has the patient had previous surgery which may be of relevance to the presenting complaint?

Drug history

What medications are being taken by the patient? Has the patient ever been prescribed long-term (6 months or more) medication? Particular attention may need to be paid to the following:

Steroids. Long-term use of steroids for conditions such as polymyalgia rheumatica or chronic lung disease may lead to an increased risk of osteoporosis.

Anticoagulants. Anticoagulant medication such as warfarin prescribed for conditions such as atrial fibrillation may cause an increased risk of bleeding and therefore contraindicate certain therapeutic interventions such as high-velocity thrust techniques.

Non-steroidal anti-inflammatory drugs (NSAIDs). NSAIDs such as ibruprofen or diclofenac have systemic effects which may lead to gastrointestinal bleeding in some patients. Use of such medications should not be encouraged if they do not appear to be positively influencing the condition. Inflammatory nociceptive pain may however be relieved by NSAIDs.

Social and family history

Social and family history that is relevant to the onset and progression of the patient's problem is recorded. This includes the patient's perspectives, experience and expectations, age, employment, home situation and details of any leisure activities. Factors from this information may indicate direct and/or indirect mechanical influences on the knee. In order to treat the patient appropriately, it is important that the condition is managed within the context of the patient's social and work environment.

The clinician may ask the following types of questions to elucidate psychosocial factors:

- Have you had time off work in the past with your pain?
- What do you understand to be the cause of your pain?
- What are you expecting will help you?
- How is your employer/co-workers/family responding to your pain?
- What are you doing to cope with your pain?
- Do you think you will return to work? When?

Although these questions are described in relation to psychosocial risk factors for poor outcomes for patients with low-back pain (Waddell 2004), they may be relevant to other patients.

Plan of the physical examination

When all this information has been collected, the subjective examination is complete. It is useful at this stage to highlight with asterisks (*), for ease of reference, important findings and particularly one or more functional restrictions. These can then be re-examined at subsequent treatment sessions to evaluate treatment intervention.

In order to plan the physical examination, the following hypotheses should be developed from the subjective examination:

- Is each area of symptoms severe and/or irritable? Will it be necessary to stop short of symptom reproduction, to reproduce symptoms partially or fully? If symptoms are severe, physical tests should be carried out to just short of symptom production or to the very first onset of symptoms; no overpressures will be carried out, as the patient would be unable to tolerate this. If symptoms are irritable, physical tests should be performed to just short of symptom production or just to the onset of symptoms with fewer physical tests being performed to allow for a rest period between tests.

- What are the predominant pain mechanisms which might be driving the patient's symptoms? What are the active 'input mechanisms' (sensory pathways): are symptoms the product of a mechanical, inflammatory or ischaemic nociceptive process? What are the 'processing mechanisms': how has the patient processed this information, what are his or her thoughts and feelings about the pain? Finally, what are the 'output mechanisms': what is the patient's physiological, psychological and behavioural response to the pain? Clearly establishing which pain mechanisms may be causing and/or maintaining the condition will help the clinician manage both the condition and the patient appropriately. The reader is directed to Gifford (1998) and Jones et al. (2002) for further reading.

- What are the possible arthrogenic, myogenic and neurogenic structures which could be causing the patient's symptoms, i.e. what structures could refer to the area of pain and what structures are underneath the area of pain? For example, medial knee pain could theoretically be referred from the lumbar spine, the sacroiliac joint, the hip, the quadriceps and the hip adductors. The structures directly under the medial knee could also be implicated, for example the medial collateral ligament (MCL), the medial meniscus, the medial compartment joint surfaces, the medial facet of the patellofemoral joint, the pes anserine tendon and the saphenous nerve.

- In addition, are there any contributing factors which could be maintaining the condition? These could be:
  - physical, e.g. weak hip lateral rotators causing medial femoral torsion
  - environmental, e.g. driving for a living
  - psychosocial, e.g. fear of serious pathology
  - behavioural, e.g. excessive rest in an attempt to help the area heal.

- The clinician must decide, based on the evidence, which structures are most likely to be at fault and prioritise the physical examination accordingly. It is helpful to organise structures into ones that 'must', 'should' and 'could' be tested on day 1 and over subsequent sessions. This will develop the clinician's clinical reasoning and avoid a recipe-based knee assessment. It is advisable where possible to clear an area fully. For example, if the clinician feels the lumbar spine needs to be excluded on day 1, s/he should fully assess this area leaving no stone unturned to implicate or negate this area as a source of symptoms. This approach will avoid juggling numerous potential sources of symptoms for several sessions, which may lead to confusion.

- Another way to develop the clinician's reasoning is to consider what to expect from each physical test. Will it be easy or hard to reproduce each symptom? Will it be necessary to use combined movements or repetitive movements? Will a particular test prove positive or negative? Will the pain be direction-specific? Synthesising evidence from the subjective examination and in particular the aggravating and easing factors should provide substantial evidence as to what to expect in the physical examination.

- Are there any precautions and/or contraindications to elements of the physical examination that need to be explored further, such as neurological involvement, recent fracture, trauma, steroid therapy or rheumatoid arthritis? There may also be certain contraindications to further examination and treatment, e.g. symptoms of spinal cord or cauda equina compression.

A physical planning form can be useful for clinicians to help guide them through the clinical reasoning process (see Figure 2.10).

Physical examination

The information from the subjective examination helps the clinician to plan an appropriate physical examination. The severity, irritability and nature of the condition are the major factors that will influence the choice and priority of physical testing procedures. The first and overarching question the clinician might ask is: 'Is this patient's condition suitable for me to manage as a therapist?' For example, a patient presenting with cauda equina compression symptoms may only need neurological integrity testing prior to an urgent medical referral. The nature of the patient's condition has had a major impact on the physical examination. The second question the clinician might ask is: 'Does this patient have a neuromusculoskeletal dysfunction that I may be able to help?' To answer that, the clinician needs to carry out a full physical examination; however, this may not be possible if the symptoms are severe and/or irritable. If the patient's symptoms are severe and/or irritable, the clinician aims to explore movements as much as possible, within a symptom-free range. If the patient has constant and severe and/or irritable symptoms, then the clinician aims to find physical tests that ease the symptoms. If the patient's symptoms are non-severe and non-irritable, then the clinician aims to find physical tests that reproduce each of the patient's symptoms.

Each significant physical test that either provokes or eases the patient's symptoms is highlighted in the patient's notes by an asterisk (*) for easy reference. The highlighted tests are often referred to as 'asterisks' or 'markers'.

The order and detail of the physical tests described below need to be appropriate to the patient being examined; some tests will be irrelevant, some tests will be carried out briefly, while it will be necessary to investigate others fully. It is important that readers understand that the techniques shown in this chapter are some of many; the choice depends mainly on the relative size of the clinician and patient, as well as the clinician's preference. For this reason, novice clinicians may initially want to copy what is shown, but then quickly adapt to what is best for them.

Observation

Informal observation

The clinician needs to observe the patient in dynamic and static situations; the quality of movement is noted, as are the postural characteristics and facial expression. Informal observation will have begun from the moment the clinician begins the subjective examination and will continue to the end of the physical examination.

Formal observation

This is particularly useful in helping to determine the presence of intrinsic predisposing factors.

Observation of posture. The clinician examines the patient's lower-limb posture in standing and in sitting with the knee at 90°. Abnormalities include internal femoral rotation, enlarged tibial tubercle (seen in Osgood–Schlatter disease), genu varum/valgum/recurvatum, medial/lateral tibial torsion and excessive foot pronation. Genu valgum and genu varum are identified by measuring the distance between the ankles and the distance between the femoral medial epicondyles respectively. Normally, medial tibial torsion is associated with genu varum and lateral tibial torsion with genu valgum (Magee 1997).

Internal femoral rotation due to insufficient gluteal function is a common finding with patients with patellofemoral pain and can cause squinting of the patella and an increased Q angle. There may be abnormal positioning of the patella, such as a medial/lateral glide, a lateral tilt, an anteroposterior tilt, a medial/lateral rotation or any combination of these positions. An enlarged fat pad is usually associated with hyperextension of the knees and poor quadriceps control, particularly eccentric inner range (0–20° of flexion).

The clinician can palpate the talus medially and laterally; both aspects will normally be equally prominent in the mid-position of the subtalar joint. If the medial aspect of the talus is more prominent, this suggests that the subtalar joint is in pronation. The position of the calcaneus and talus can be examined: if the subtalar joint is pronated the calcaneus would be expected to be everted. Any abnormality will require further examination, as described in the section on palpation, below. In addition, the clinician notes whether there is even weight-bearing through the left and right legs. The clinician passively corrects any asymmetry to determine its relevance to the patient's problem.

It is worth remembering that pure postural dysfunction rarely influences one region of the body in isolation and it may be necessary to observe the patient more fully for a full postural examination.

The clinician examines dynamic postures such as gait, stair climbing and squatting. Observation of gait may reveal, for example, excessive pelvic rotation (about a horizontal plane) associated with anterior pelvic tilt. This may be due to hyperextension of the knees and limited extension and external rotation of the hip.

Observation of muscle form. The clinician observes the muscle bulk and muscle tone of the patient, comparing left and right sides. It must be remembered that the level and frequency of physical activity as well as the dominant side may well produce differences in muscle bulk between sides. Some muscles are thought to shorten under stress, while other muscles weaken, producing muscle imbalance (see Table 3.2).

Observation of soft tissues. The clinician observes the quality and colour of the patient's skin, any area of swelling, joint effusion or presence of scarring, and takes cues for further examination.

Observation of balance. Balance is provided by vestibular, visual and proprioceptive information. This rather crude and non-specific test is conducted by asking the patient to stand on one leg with the eyes open and then closed. If the patient's balance is as poor with the eyes open as with the eyes closed, this suggests a vestibular or proprioceptive dysfunction (rather than a visual dysfunction). The test is carried out on the affected and unaffected side; if there is greater difficulty maintaining balance on the affected side, this may indicate some proprioceptive dysfunction.

Observation of gait. Analyse gait on even/uneven ground, slopes, stairs and running. Note the stride length and weight-bearing ability. Inspect the feet, shoes and any walking aids.

Observation of the patient's attitudes and feelings. The age, gender and ethnicity of patients and their cultural, occupational and social backgrounds will all affect their attitudes and feelings towards themselves, their condition and the clinician. The clinician should be aware of and sensitive to these attitudes, and empathise and communicate appropriately so as to develop a rapport with the patient and thereby enhance the patient's compliance with the treatment.

Functional physical marker

It can be extremely useful to examine a functional physical marker specific to the patient's complaint. A functional marker which can be replicated in the clinical setting can often be identified when asking the patient about aggravating factors. It is recommended to examine a functional marker early in the assessment; this is for three reasons:

1. The marker will provide a useful initial snapshot of the patient's problem.
2. It may be possible to manipulate the marker to aid the clinical diagnosis and highlight possible treatment options (see below).
3. The marker will provide a useful physical marker (*).

An example of a functional marker would be descending stairs in a patient with anterior knee pain. The clinician can replicate this movement by asking the patient to step off a block and observe the movement. Does the movement reproduce the patient's pain? How is the patient moving? Is s/he able to control the position of the pelvis? Is the foot pronating? Is there any internal tibial torsion or medial patellar squinting?

Can the clinician change the patient's pain by manipulating the marker in some way? If the foot is pronating, does placing a block under the foot to prevent pronation change the patient's pain and/or movement pattern? Does contracting the deep abdominal muscles to control pelvic movement make a difference? If there is internal femoral torsion, does contracting the gluteal muscles and instructing the patient to keep the patella in line with the foot help? The clinician could also add accessory glides to the patella, the head of fibula, the tibia or the femur during the movement to see if these movements alter symptoms.

By manipulating this marker in various ways, which need not be time-consuming, useful information may be gleaned as to the likely clinical diagnosis as well as the most appropriate way to manage the condition. Although this example highlights the art of clinical reasoning in practice, it is important to emphasise that functional markers are not standardised tests and will therefore lack a degree of validity and reliability. The following section describes commonly performed orthopaedic tests for the examination of the knee. Although more standardised than the use of a functional physical marker, the validity underpinning some of these tests is more robust than the validity underpinning others. For an excellent review of the validity of common orthopaedic tests of the knee, the reader is referred to Malanga et al. (2003). As always, the clinician is encouraged to synthesise information from the whole subjective and physical examination to reach a reasoned view of the patient's condition, rather than placing too much emphasis on any one test.

Joint effusion tests

The clinician firstly checks for a knee joint effusion, which may not be necessary if a large effusion is obvious. It is important to distinguish between soft-tissue swelling, which may be localised and superficial, for example in the presence of a low-grade MCL sprain, and swelling within the joint, which may represent a more significant intra-articular injury, e.g. an ACL rupture.

Patellar tap test

With the patient lying supine, the clinician adds pressure across the suprapatellar pouch with one hand which will squeeze fluid under the patella. With the other hand the clinician applies a light downward force to the patella which, in the presence of an effusion, will feel as if it is 'floating' and may 'tap' against the underlying femoral condyles.

Sweep test

This test is also known as the brush or stroke test. With the patient lying supine, the clinician uses the palm of one hand to sweep fluid proximally up the medial side of the knee into the suprapatellar pouch. The other hand is then used to sweep distally down the lateral side of the knee. In the presence of an effusion a small bulge of fluid appears on the medial side of the knee.

Joint integrity tests

For all of the joint integrity tests below, a positive test is indicated by excessive movement relative to the unaffected side.

Valgus stress tests

With the patient supine, the clinician palpates the medial joint line of the knee and applies a valgus force to 'gap' the medial aspect of the knee. The clinician may perform this test with the knee in full extension and in 20–30° flexion (Figure 15.1); the clinician compares the left and right knee range of movement; excessive movement would be considered a positive test. If the test is positive in slight flexion but negative in full extension, a partial MCL tear is suspected, whilst a test which is positive in both flexion and extension may suggest a complete MCL rupture with possible posteromedial corner and anterior and/or posterior cruciate ligament injury (Kurzweil & Kelley 2006).

As well as the pure tests described above, it may be beneficial to explore valgus stress testing with and/or through varying degrees of flexion, extension and rotation. Although moving away from the more standardised tests may reduce the validity and reliability of the technique, in some patients, thinking outside the narrow confines of the tests as described may help the clinician reproduce mild symptoms or establish a physical marker. Such variations may even be helpful as treatment techniques.

Varus stress tests

With the patient supine, the clinician palpates the lateral joint line and applies a varus force to 'gap' the lateral aspect of the knee. The clinician may perform this test with the knee in full extension and in 20–30° flexion (Figure 15.2). The clinician compares the left and right knee range of movement; excessive movement would be considered a positive test. If the test is positive in slight flexion, as well as the lateral collateral ligament (LCL), the test may suggest injury to the posterolateral capsule, arcuate–popliteus complex, iliotibial band and biceps femoris tendon. A positive test in full extension may implicate the LCL, posterolateral capsule,

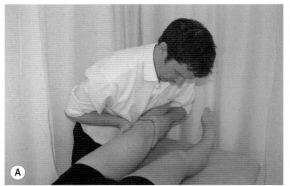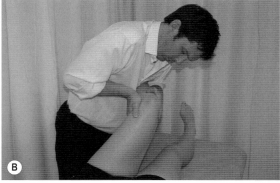

Figure 15.1 • Valgus stress test with the knee in (A) extension and (B) some flexion.

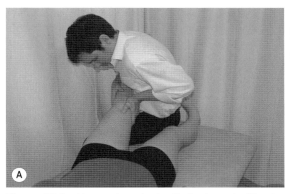
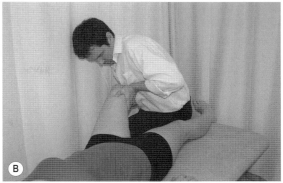

Figure 15.2 • Varus stress test with the knee in (A) extension and (B) some flexion.

the arcuate–popliteus complex, anterior and posterior cruciate ligaments and lateral gastrocnemius muscle (Magee 1997).

Again, as with the valgus stress test, in some patients it may be helpful to explore this test with and/or through varying degrees of flexion, extension and rotation.

Lachman test

The Lachman test is primarily a test for the integrity of the ACL, although the posterior oblique ligament and the arcuate–popliteus complex may also be stressed (Magee 1997). With the patient in supine and with the knee flexed (0–30°), the clinician stabilises the femur and applies a posteroanterior force to the tibia along the plane of the joint (Figure 15.3A). A positive test is indicated by a soft end-feel and excessive motion. A positive Lachman test has consistently been shown to be the strongest

physical indicator of ACL rupture (Jonsson et al. 1982; Katz & Fingeroth 1986; Mitsou & Vallianatos 1988; Ostrowski 2006). The test has its disadvantages, however, as it can be technically difficult, especially if the clinician has small hands or the patient has a particularly large leg. In such circumstances, one modification which may help is for the patient to rest the knee over the clinician's thigh, as shown in Figure 15.3B. This will stabilise the knee, take some of the leg's weight and allow the patient's muscles to relax fully.

Anterior drawer test

The anterior drawer test is similar to the Lachman test but is carried out with the knee flexed to 90°. This test is easier to perform than the Lachman test but is less specific to the ACL. The clinician applies the same posteroanterior force to the tibia along the plane of the joint, feeling the movement of the

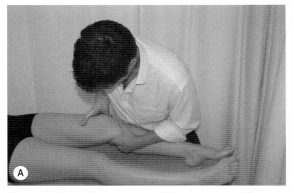
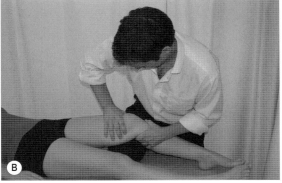

Figure 15.3 • A Lachman test. The clinician stabilises the femur with the right hand and with the left hand applies a posteroanterior force to the tibia. B Modified Lachman test. The patient's knee rests over the clinician's thigh and is stabilised by the right hand. The left hand applies a posteroanterior force to the tibia.

tibia anteriorly and any contraction of the hamstring muscle group, which may oppose the movement (Figure 15.4). Sitting on the patient's foot may help to stabilise the leg. A positive test, indicated by a soft end-feel and excessive motion, may indicate injury to the ACL, posterior oblique ligament, arcuate–popliteus complex, posteromedial and posterolateral joint capsules, MCL and the iliotibial band (Magee 1997). Again, exploring this test with other angles of knee flexion, and with internal or external tibial rotation, may be relevant and necessary for some patients. Varying the anterior drawer test to include internal and external tibial rotation is known as the Slocum test. With the addition of internal tibial rotation, excessive movement on the lateral aspect of the knee is thought to indicate anterolateral instability, whilst excessive movement of the medial aspect of the knee with the addition of lateral rotation may represent anteromedial instability.

Pivot shift test

A further test for anterolateral stability and ACL integrity is the pivot shift test. The patient lies supine with the hip slightly flexed and medially rotated and with the knee flexed. In the first part of the test, the lower leg is medially rotated at the knee and the clinician moves the knee into extension while applying a posteroanterior force to the fibula. The tibia subluxes anteriorly when there is anterolateral instability. In the second part of the test, the clinician applies an abduction stress to the lower leg and passively moves the knee from extension to flexion while maintaining the medial rotation of the lower leg (Figure 15.5). A positive test is indicated if at about 20–40° of knee flexion the tibia 'jogs' backward (reduction of the subluxation) and reproduces the patient's feeling of the knee 'giving way'.

Although a difficult test to master, in the diagnosis of ACL rupture in the anaesthetised patient, the pivot shift demonstrates excellent validity. Unfortunately this is not the case when the patient is awake as specificity values may drop to as low as 35% (Malanga et al. 2003). The pivot shift test should therefore only be used as an adjunct to, and not in place of, the Lachman and anterior drawer tests. Indeed, some may question the use of this test at all in the conscious patient.

Posterior drawer test

The posterior drawer test is typically carried out with the knee flexed to 90°. The clinician first inspects the knee to check the tibia is not sagging posteriorly and then applies an anteroposterior force to the tibia (Figure 15.6). A positive test is indicated by excessive motion due to injury of one or more of the following structures: posterior cruciate ligament, arcuate–popliteus complex, posterior oblique ligament and ACL (Magee 1997). If the clinician inadvertently performs the test on a tibia which is already sagging posteriorly, due to injury of the aforementioned structures, the test may appear falsely negative.

As mentioned in previous tests, exploring the posterior drawer test in different angles of knee

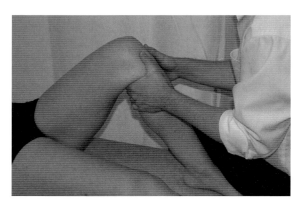

Figure 15.4 • Anterior drawer test. With the knee around 90° flexion the clinician sits lightly on the patient's foot to stabilise the leg. The fingers grasp around the posterior aspect of the calf to apply the posteroanterior force, while the thumbs rest over the anterior joint line to feel the movement.

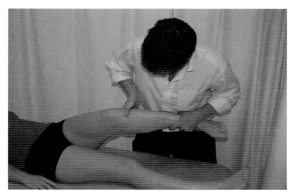

Figure 15.5 • Lateral pivot shift. The clinician applies an abduction stress to the lower leg with the right hand and the left hand passively moves the knee from extension to flexion, while maintaining the medial rotation of the lower leg.

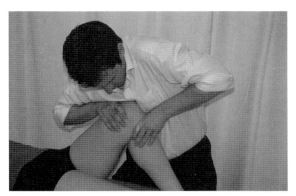

Figure 15.6 • Posterior drawer test. With the knee around 90° flexion, the right hand supports the knee and the web space of the left hand applies an anteroposterior force to the tibia.

flexion, and with internal or external tibial rotation, may be relevant and necessary for some patients. The addition of external tibial rotation during the posterior drawer test is particularly useful to check for posterolateral instability, which would be indicated by excessive movement at the lateral aspect of the tibia (Hughston & Norwood 1980).

Dial test

A further useful test to assess for posterolateral instability is the dial test (Figure 15.7). During this test the patient lies prone and the clinician externally rotates the tibia at both 30° and 90°. Increased rotation compared with the uninjured side at 30° but not 90° may indicate posterolateral corner instability, whilst increased rotation at 30° and 90° may indicate injury to both the posterolateral corner and ACL (Malone et al. 2006).

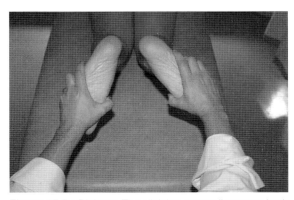

Figure 15.7 • Dial test. The clinician externally rotates both tibia at both 30° and 90°.

Meniscal tests

McMurray test

During the McMurray test, the medial meniscus is typically tested using a combination of knee flexion/extension with lateral rotation of the tibia whilst compressing the medial compartment. The clinician palpates the medial joint line and passively flexes and then laterally rotates the knee so that the posterior part of the medial meniscus is rotated with the tibia – a 'snap' of the joint may occur if the meniscus is torn. The knee is then moved from this fully flexed position to 90° flexion (to full extension for some patients), so the whole of the posterior part of the meniscus is tested (Figure 15.8). A positive test occurs if the clinician feels a click, which may be heard, indicating a tear of the medial meniscus (McMurray 1942). The test is then repeated to bias the lateral meniscus, this time using a combination of knee flexion/extension with medial rotation of the tibia whilst compressing the lateral compartment (Figure 15.9).

Clinicians vary in performing this test; they may, for example, internally and externally rotate the tibia while moving the knee from full flexion to extension. The key is to explore both the medial and lateral compartments fully. It is worth noting that tears most commonly occur at the posterior horns of the menisci. Most positive findings during the McMurray test therefore occur towards end-of-range flexion when the menisci are maximally loaded.

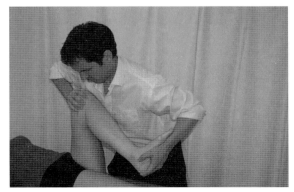

Figure 15.8 • Medial meniscus. The right hand supports the knee and palpates the medial joint line. The left hand laterally rotates the lower leg and moves the knee from full flexion to extension.

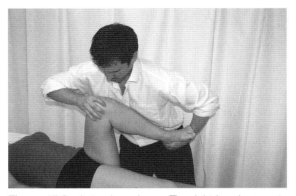

Figure 15.9 • Lateral meniscus. The right hand supports the knee and palpates the lateral joint line. The left hand medially rotates the lower leg and moves the knee from full flexion to extension.

Apley test

The menisci can also be tested with the patient in prone with the knee flexed to 90° (compression/distraction test; Apley 1947). The clinician medially and laterally rotates the tibia with distraction and then compression (Figure 15.10). If symptoms are worse on compression, this may suggest a meniscus injury; if symptoms are worse on distraction, this suggests a ligamentous injury (Apley 1947). Malanga et al. (2003) point out that the sensitivity values for the McMurray test are far superior to the Apley test and the clinician would be wise to opt for the McMurray test over the Apley test if s/he decides to choose between the two.

Joint line tenderness

Palpation of the medial and lateral joint lines should not be overlooked when suspicious of a meniscal tear. Although joint line palpation should be used as an adjunct to, and not a replacement for, the McMurray test, it is of note that joint line tenderness is likely to be present in those with meniscal tears (Malanga et al. 2003). Such tenderness could of course also be emanating from structures other than the meniscus, e.g. the MCL, but the index of suspicion may be heightened if, for example, valgus stress testing were negative and the MCL proximal and distal to the joint line was painfree.

Patellofemoral tests

Clarke test

Patellofemoral provocation tests typically are of limited benefit as these tests are often provocative to some degree in the asymptomatic population. Thankfully, patellofemoral pain usually offers the clinician strong subjective clues from which to build a clinical hypothesis such as pain descending stairs and provocation tests should be seen as the icing on the cake of the assessment.

The Clarke test is possibly the most widely used patellofemoral provocation test. With the patient lying supine or in long sitting and the knee in full extension, the clinician places the web space of one hand just superior to the patella and applies a gentle downward and caudad force (Figure 15.11). The patient is then instructed to contract the quadriceps by pushing the back of their knee into the bed.

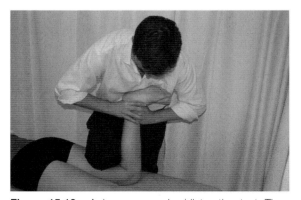

Figure 15.10 • Apley compression/distraction test. The clinician gently rests his/her leg over the back of the patient's thigh to stabilise and then grasps around the lower calf to rotate and distract the knee. No stabilisation is required for compression.

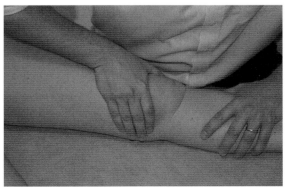

Figure 15.11 • Clarke test. The clinician places the web space of the right hand just superior to the patella and applies a gentle downward and caudad force. The patient then contracts the quadriceps.

The test is positive if pain is reproduced. As the test is often painful in the absence of patellofemoral dysfunction the clinician must beware of the falsely positive test and when positive it is helpful to ask the patient, 'Was that your pain?'

Fairbank's apprehension test

This is considered a test for patellar subluxation or dislocation. It is typically carried out with the patient's knee in 30° of flexion; the clinician passively moves the patella laterally and a positive test is indicated by apprehension of the patient and/or excessive movement (Eifert-Mangine & Bilbo 1995). There may also be a reflex contraction of the quadriceps in the presence of instability. It may be necessary and relevant for some patients to test the patellar glide with the knee in other angles of knee flexion.

Active physiological movements

Active physiological movements of the knee include flexion, extension, medial rotation of the tibia and lateral rotation of the tibia (Table 15.2). The primary movements of flexion and extension are tested bilaterally with the patient in supine. Movements of flexion and extension are overpressed if symptoms allow (Figure 15.12). Tibial rotation can be readily tested with the patient in sitting, although clinically it is unusual to find an isolated rotation dysfunction.

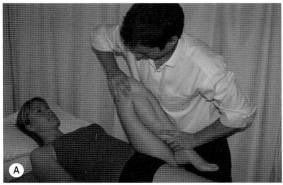

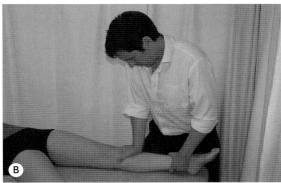

Figure 15.12 • Overpressures to the knee. **A** Flexion. One hand supports the knee while the other hand applies overpressure to flexion. **B** Extension. One hand stabilises the tibia while the other hand lifts the lower leg into extension.

The clinician establishes the patient's symptoms at rest, prior to each movement and passively corrects any movement deviation to determine its relevance to the patient's symptoms. The following are noted:

- quality of movement
- range of movement
- behaviour of pain through the range of movement
- resistance through the range of movement and at the end of the range of movement
- provocation of any muscle spasm

In a similar way to the manipulation of the functional physical marker, the thoughtful clinician may be able to manipulate physiological movements to help differentiate between tissues. For example, when knee flexion in prone reproduces the patient's anterior knee pain, differentiation between knee joint, anterior thigh muscles and neural tissues may be required. Adding a compression force through the lower leg will stress the knee joint without particularly altering the muscle length or neural tissue. If

Table 15.2 Active physiological movements with possible modifications

Active physiological movements	Modifications
Knee flexion	Repeated
Knee extension	Speed altered
Medial rotation of the knee	Combined, e.g.
Lateral rotation of the knee	– flexion with internal rotation
?Lumbar spine	Compression or distraction
?Sacroiliac joint	Sustained
?Hip	Injuring movement
?Foot and ankle	Differentiation tests
	Function

symptoms are increased, this would suggest that the knee joint (patellofemoral or tibiofemoral joint) may be the source of the symptoms.

It may be necessary to examine other regions to determine their relevance to the patient's symptoms; they may be the source of the symptoms, or they may be contributing to the symptoms. The most likely regions are the lumbar spine, sacroiliac joint, hip, foot and ankle. These regions can be quickly screened; see Chapter 3 for further details. Contrary to what their name might suggest, however, performing a clearing test on the lumbar spine, for example, does not fully negate this region as a source of symptoms and if there is any doubt the clinician is advised to assess the suspected area fully (see relevant chapter).

Passive physiological movements

All of the active movements described above can be examined passively with the patient in supine, comparing left and right sides. Comparison of the response of symptoms to the active and passive movements can help to determine whether the structure at fault is non-contractile (articular) or contractile (extra-articular) (Cyriax 1982). If the lesion is non-contractile, such as ligament, then active and passive movements will be painful and/or restricted in the same direction. If the lesion is in a contractile tissue (i.e. muscle) then active and passive movements are painful and/or restricted in opposite directions. For example, a quadriceps strain may be painful during active extension and passive flexion. Such patterns are however theoretical and a muscle strain may be more readily assessed by contracting muscle isometrically where there will be little or no change in the length of non-contractile tissue.

To assess the patient's symptoms passively it may be useful to explore the primary movements of flexion and/or extension with varying degrees of varus or valgus force (Figure 15.13). It is also possible to add a degree of medial or lateral tibial rotation when exploring these movements. The key is for the clinician to search for the patient's symptoms and not feel

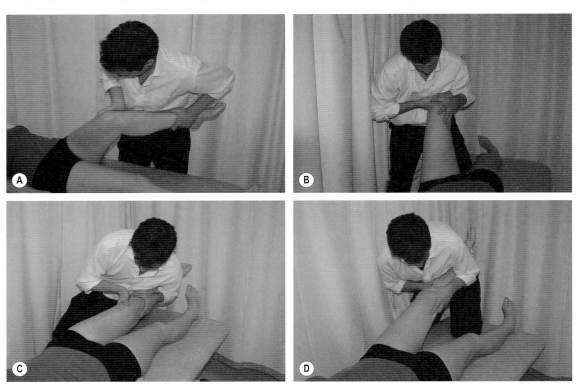

Figure 15.13 • Passive physiological joint movements to the knee. A Flexion/valgus. The patient's knee is flexed passively whilst a valgus force is applied. B Flexion/varus. The patient's knee is flexed passively whilst a varus force is applied. C Extension/valgus. The patient's knee is extended passively whilst a valgus force is applied. D Extension/varus. The patient's knee is extended passively whilst a varus force is applied.

constrained by a recipe-based knee assessment. Often it is helpful to refer back to the patient's aggravating factors for clues. For example, if the patient's pain is in knee flexion, the clinician may need to hunt in a similar range of flexion combining different movement components.

As with active physiological movements, it may be necessary to examine other regions such as the lumbar spine, sacroiliac joint, hip, foot and ankle, which may be the source or contributing to the patient's symptoms.

Muscle tests

Muscle tests include examining muscle strength, control, length and isometric muscle testing.

Muscle strength

For a true appreciation of a muscle's strength, the clinician must test the muscle isotonically through the available range. During the physical examination of the knee, it may be appropriate to test the knee flexors/extensors and the ankle dorsiflexors/plantarflexors and any other relevant muscle groups.

Strength tests for lower-limb muscles thought particularly prone to becoming weak – gluteus maximus, medius and minimus, vastus lateralis, medialis and intermedius, tibialis anterior and the peronei (Jull & Janda 1987; Sahrmann 2002) – are described in Chapter 3.

Muscle length

The clinician may test the length of muscles, in particular those thought prone to shorten (Janda 1994, 2002); that is, erector spinae, quadratus lumborum, piriformis, iliopsoas, rectus femoris, tensor fasciae latae, hamstrings, tibialis posterior, gastrocnemius and soleus (Jull & Janda 1987; Sahrmann 2002). Testing the length of these muscles is described in Chapter 3.

Isometric muscle testing

Isometric muscle testing may help to differentiate whether symptoms are arising from contractile or non-contractile tissue. Isometric testing is described in detail in Chapter 3.

It may be appropriate to test the isometric strength of the knee flexors (with tibia medially and laterally rotated to stress, in particular, the lateral and medial hamstrings, respectively), extensors and ankle dorsiflexors and plantarflexors in resting position and, if indicated, in different parts of the physiological range. The clinician notes the strength and quality of the contraction, as well as any reproduction of the patient's symptoms.

Muscle control

The single-leg squat is a particularly useful test of lower-limb dynamic alignment and muscle control. The phenomenon of 'medial collapse', where the whole knee is seen to deviate medially during the test, is a common finding in patients with patellofemoral pain (Powers 2003; Levinger et al. 2007). This seemingly simple task requires significant control of the pelvis, hip and knee, and may also be influenced by the position of the rear foot. If the test is performed poorly and reproduces the patient's symptoms, the clinician may attempt to correct the lower-limb alignment to see if this changes the patient's symptoms.

An imbalance of the vastus medialis obliquus (VMO) and the vastus lateralis has also been identified in patients with patellofemoral pain (Mariani & Caruso 1979; Voight & Wieder 1991). On quadriceps contraction, the patella may glide laterally as a result of weakness of VMO (McConnell 1996) and may contract after vastus lateralis (Voight & Wieder 1991). The timing of activation of VMO and vastus lateralis can be more objectively assessed using a dual-channel biofeedback machine. In addition, the inferior pole of the patella may be displaced posteriorly as the quadriceps contracts, which may result in fat pad irritation (McConnell 1996).

Neurological tests

Neurological examination includes neurological integrity testing and neurodynamic tests.

Integrity of the nervous system

The integrity of the nervous system is tested if the clinician suspects the symptoms are emanating from the spine or from a peripheral nerve.

Dermatomes/peripheral nerves. Light touch and pain sensation of the lower limb are tested using cotton wool and pinprick respectively, as described in Chapter 3. Knowledge of the cutaneous distribution of nerve roots (dermatomes) and peripheral nerves enables the clinician to distinguish the sensory loss due to a root lesion from that due to a peripheral nerve lesion. The cutaneous nerve distribution and dermatome areas are shown in Chapter 3.

Myotomes/peripheral nerves. The following myotomes are tested and are shown in Chapter 3.

- L2: hip flexion
- L3: knee extension
- L4: foot dorsiflexion and inversion
- L5: extension of the big toe
- S1: eversion of the foot, contract buttock, knee flexion
- S2: knee flexion, toe standing
- S3–S4: muscles of pelvic floor, bladder and genital function.

A working knowledge of the muscular distribution of nerve roots (myotomes) and peripheral nerves enables the clinician to distinguish the motor loss due to a root lesion from that due to a peripheral nerve lesion. The peripheral nerve distributions are shown in Chapter 3.

Reflex testing. The following deep tendon reflexes are tested and are shown in Chapter 3.

- L3/4: knee jerk
- S1: ankle jerk.

Neurodynamic tests

The following neurodynamic tests may be carried out in order to ascertain the degree to which neural tissue is responsible for the production of the patient's symptom(s):

- passive neck flexion
- straight-leg raise
- passive knee bend
- slump.

These tests are described in detail in Chapter 3.

Miscellaneous tests

Vascular tests

If the circulation is suspected of being compromised, the clinician palpates the pulses of the femoral, popliteal and dorsalis pedis arteries. The state of the vascular system can also be determined by the response of symptoms to positions of dependence and elevation of the lower limbs.

Leg length

True leg length is measured from the anterior superior iliac spine to the medial or lateral malleolus. Apparent leg length is measured from the umbilicus to the medial or lateral malleolus. A difference in leg length of up to 1–1.3 cm is considered normal. If there is a leg length difference, test the length of individual bones, the tibia with knees bent and the femurs in standing. Ipsilateral posterior rotation of the ilium (on the sacrum) or contralateral anterior rotation of the ilium will result in a decrease in leg length (Magee 1997).

Palpation

The clinician palpates the knee region and any other relevant areas. It is useful to record palpation findings on a body chart (see Figure 2.3) and/or palpation chart (see Figure 3.36).

The clinician notes the following:

- the temperature of the area
- localised increased skin moisture
- the presence of oedema or effusion – the clinician examines with the patellar tap and sweep test to assess if joint effusion is present. The circumference of the limb or joint can be measured with a tape measure and left and right sides compared
- mobility and feel of superficial tissues, e.g. ganglions, nodules, scar tissue
- the presence or elicitation of any muscle spasm
- tenderness of bone (the upper pole of the patella and the femoral condyle may be tender in plica syndrome, while the undersurface of the patella may be tender with patellofemoral joint problems), bursae (prepatellar, infrapatellar), ligaments, muscle, tendon, tendon sheath, trigger points (shown in Figure 3.37) and nerve. Palpable nerves in the lower limb are as follows:
  - The sciatic nerve can be palpated two-thirds of the way along an imaginary line between the greater trochanter and the ischial tuberosity with the patient in prone.
  - The common peroneal nerve can be palpated medial to the tendon of biceps femoris and also around the head of the fibula.
  - The tibial nerve can be palpated centrally over the posterior knee crease medial to the popliteal artery; it can also be felt behind the medial malleolus, which is more noticeable with the foot in dorsiflexion and eversion.
  - The superficial peroneal nerve can be palpated on the dorsum of the foot along an imaginary line over the fourth metatarsal; it is more noticeable with the foot in plantarflexion and inversion.

○ The deep peroneal nerve can be palpated between the first and second metatarsals, lateral to the extensor hallucis tendon.

○ The sural nerve can be palpated on the lateral aspect of the foot behind the lateral malleolus, lateral to the tendocalcaneus.

- Increased or decreased prominence of bones – observe the position of the patella in terms of glide, lateral tilt, anteroposterior tilt and rotation on the femoral condyles (see below) (McConnell 1996). The quadriceps (Q) angle can be measured. It is 'the angle formed by the intersection of the line of pull of the quadriceps muscle and the patellar tendon measured through the centre of the patella' (McConnell 1986). The normal outer value is considered to be in the region of 15°

- pain provoked or reduced on palpation.

Increased or decreased prominence of bones. The optimal position of the patella is one where the patella is parallel to the femur in the frontal and sagittal planes and the patella is midway between the two condyles of the femur when the knee is slightly flexed (Grelsamer & McConnell 1998). In terms of the position of the patella, the following may be noted:

- The base of the patella normally lies equidistant (±5 mm) from the medial and lateral femoral epicondyles when the knee is flexed 20°. If the patella lies closer to the medial or lateral femoral epicondyle, it is considered to have a medial or lateral glide respectively. The clinician also needs to test for any lateral glide of the patella on quadriceps contraction. The clinician palpates the left and right base of the patella and the VMO and vastus lateralis with thumbs and fingers respectively while the patient is asked to extend the knee. In some cases the patella is felt to glide laterally, indicating a dynamic problem, and VMO may be felt to contract after vastus lateralis; VMO is normally thought to be activated simultaneously with, or slightly earlier than, vastus lateralis. Quite a large difference will be needed to enable the clinician to feel a difference in the timing of muscle contraction.

- The lateral tilt is calculated by measuring the distance of the medial and lateral borders of the patella from the femur. The patella is considered to have a lateral tilt, for example, when the distance is decreased on the lateral aspect and increased on the medial aspect such that the patella faces laterally. A lateral tilt is considered to be due to a tight lateral retinaculum (superficial

and deep fibres) and iliotibial band. When a passive medial glide is first applied (see below), the patellar tilt may be accentuated, indicating a dynamic tilt problem implicating a tight lateral retinaculum (deep fibres).

- The anteroposterior tilt is calculated by measuring the distance from the inferior and superior poles of the patella to the femur. Posterior tilt of the patella occurs if the inferior pole lies more posteriorly than the superior pole and may lead to fat pad irritation and inferior patellar pain. Dynamic control of a posterior patellar tilt is tested by asking the patient to brace the knee back and observing the movement of the tibia. With a positive patellar tilt the foot moves away from the couch and the proximal end of the tibia is seen to move posteriorly; this movement is thought to pull the inferior pole of the patella into the fat pad.

- Rotation is the relative position of the long axis of patella to the femur, and is normally parallel. The patella is considered to be laterally rotated if the inferior pole of the patella is placed laterally to the long axis of the femur. A lateral or medial rotation of the patella is considered to be due to tightness of part of the retinaculum. The most common abnormality seen in patellofemoral pain is both a lateral tilt and a lateral rotation of the patella, which is thought to be due to an imbalance of the medial (weakness of VMO) and lateral structures (tightness of the lateral retinaculum and/or weakness of vastus lateralis) of the patella (McConnell 1996).

- Testing the length of the lateral retinaculum. With the patient in side-lying and the knee flexed approximately 20°, the clinician passively glides the patella in a medial direction. The patella will normally move sufficiently to expose the lateral femoral condyle; if this is not possible then tightness of the superficial retinaculum is suspected. The deep retinaculum is tested as above, but with the addition of an anteroposterior force to the medial border of the patella. The lateral border of the patella is normally able to move anteriorly away from the femur; inability may suggest tightness of the deep retinaculum.

Accessory movements

It is useful to use the palpation chart and movement diagrams (or joint pictures) to record findings. These are explained in detail in Chapter 3.

The clinician notes the following:

- quality of movement
- range of movement
- resistance through the range and at the end of the range of movement
- behaviour of pain through the range
- provocation of any muscle spasm.

Patellofemoral joint (Figure 15.14), tibiofemoral joint (Figure 15.15) and superior tibiofibular joint (Figure 15.16) accessory movements are listed in Table 15.3. All movements can be explored in various degrees of flexion/extension and medial/lateral tibial rotation. The clinician reassesses all the physical asterisks (movements or tests that have been found to reproduce the patient's symptoms)

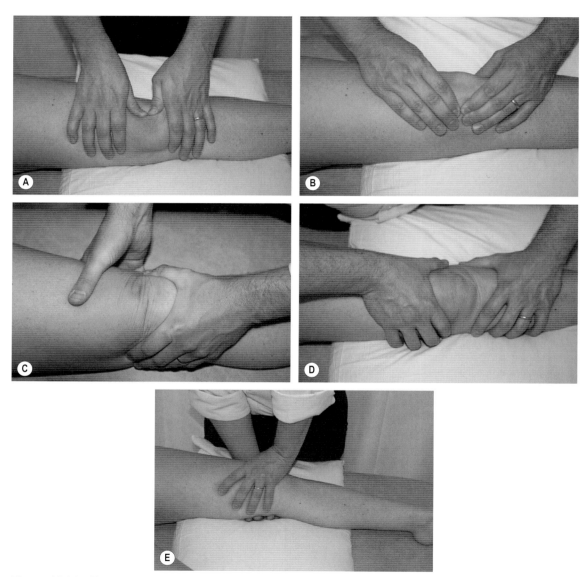

Figure 15.14 • Patellofemoral joint accessory movements. **A** Medial transverse. The thumbs move the patella medially. **B** Lateral transverse. The fingers move the patella laterally. **C** Longitudinal cephalad. The left hand pushes the patella in a cephalad direction. **D** Longitudinal caudad. The right hand pushes the patella in a caudad direction. **E** Compression. The left hand rests over the anterior aspect of the patella and pushes the patella towards the femur.

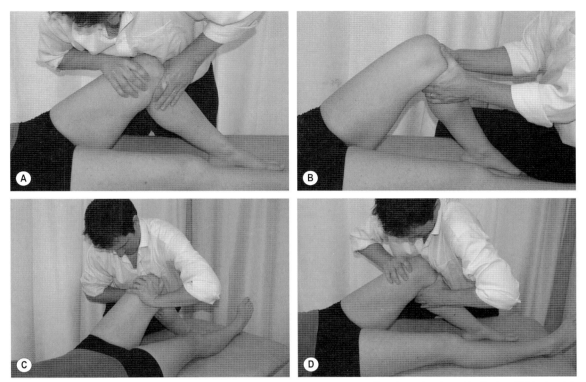

Figure 15.15 • Tibiofemoral joint accessory movements. **A** Anteroposterior. The knee is placed in flexion. With the right hand stabilising, the web space of the left hand is placed around the anterior aspect of the tibia and applies an anteroposterior force to the knee. **B** Posteroanterior. The knee is placed in flexion and the clinician lightly sits on the patient's foot to stabilise this position. The fingers grasp around the posterior aspect of the calf to apply the force, while the thumbs rest over the anterior joint line to feel the movement. **C** Medial transverse. The left hand stabilises the medial aspect of the thigh while the right hand applies a medial force to the tibia. **D** Lateral transverse. The right hand stabilises the lateral aspect to the thigh while the left hand applies a lateral force to the tibia.

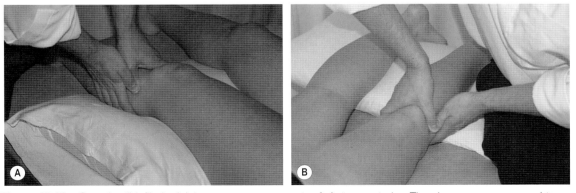

Figure 15.16 • Superior tibiofibular joint accessory movements. **A** Anteroposterior. Thumb pressures are used to apply an anteroposterior force to the anterior aspect of the head of the fibula. **B** Posteroanterior. Thumb pressures are used to apply a posteroanterior force to the posterior aspect of the head of the fibula.

Table 15.3 Accessory movements, choice of application and reassessment of the patient's asterisks

Accessory movements	Choice of application	Identify any effect of accessory movements on patient's signs and symptoms
Patellofemoral joint		
Med Medial transverse	Start position, e.g.	
Lat Lateral transverse	– in flexion	
Ceph Longitudinal cephalad	– in extension	
Medial rotation	– in medial rotation	
medial tilt	– in lateral rotation	Reassess all asterisks
Lateral rotation	– in flexion and lateral rotation	
Lateral tilt	– in extension and medial rotation	
Comp Compression	Speed of force application	
Distr Distraction	Direction of the applied force Point of application of applied force	
Tibiofemoral joint		
Anteroposterior		
Posteroanterior	As above	Reassess all asterisks
Med Medial transverse		
Lat Lateral transverse		
Superior tibiofibular joint		
Anteroposterior		
Posteroanterior		
Ceph Longitudinal cephalad by eversion of the foot	As above	Reassess all asterisks
Caud Longitudinal caudad by inversion of the foot		
Other Regions to consider		
?Lumbar spine		
?Sacroiliac joint	As above	Reassess all asterisks
?Hip		
?Foot and ankle		

following accessory movements, in order to establish the effect of the accessory movements on the patient's signs and symptoms. Accessory movements can then be tested for other regions suspected to be a source of, or contributing to, the patient's symptoms. Again, following accessory movements, the clinician reassesses all the asterisks. Regions likely to be examined are the lumbar spine, sacroiliac joint, hip, foot and ankle (Table 15.3).

Mobilisations with movement (MWMs)
(Mulligan 1999)

MWMs are sustained accessory glides applied to a joint during active or passive movement. They need not be prescriptive and the clinician is encouraged to experiment with different MWMs whilst closely monitoring the patient's symptomatic response. MWMs can be particularly helpful when exploring a functional physical marker. For example, if the patient complains of medial joint line pain when rising from sitting, it may be helpful to apply adapted versions of the tibiofemoral accessory movements described above (Figure 15.15) to the knee during standing to see if any glides change symptoms. Two further examples of MWMs are described below:

Tibiofemoral joint. A medial glide may be applied with medial joint pain and a lateral glide with lateral joint pain. The patient lies prone and the clinician stabilises the thigh and applies a glide to the tibia using a seat belt around the tibia (Figure 15.17). The glide is then maintained while the patient actively flexes or extends the knee. An increased range of movement which is painfree would indicate a mechanical joint problem.

Superior tibiofibular joint. This test is carried out if the patient has posterolateral knee pain. The patient in lying or standing actively flexes or extends the knee while the clinician applies a posteroanterior glide to the fibula head (Figure 15.18). Once again, increased range of movement that is painfree would indicate a mechanical joint problem.

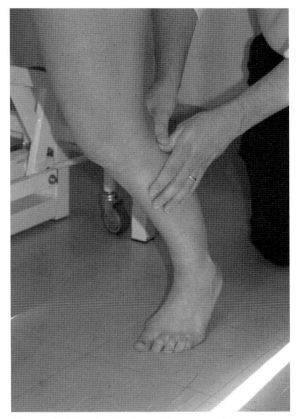

Figure 15.18 • Mobilisation with movement for the proximal tibiofibular joint. In standing the clinician applies a posteroanterior force to the fibula while the patient actively flexes the knee.

Completion of the examination

Having carried out all the above tests, the examination of the knee region is now complete. The subjective and physical examination produces a large amount of information, which needs to be recorded accurately and quickly. The outline subjective and physical examination charts in Chapters 2 and 3 may be useful for some clinicians. It is important, however, that the clinician does not examine in a rigid manner, simply following the suggested sequence outlined in the chart. Each patient presents differently and this needs to be reflected in the examination process. It is vital at this stage to highlight important findings from the examination with an asterisk (*). These findings must be reassessed at, and within, subsequent treatment sessions to evaluate the effects of treatment on the patient's condition.

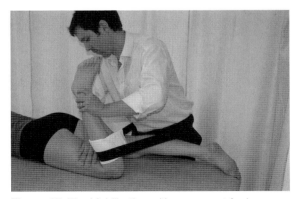

Figure 15.17 • Mobilisation with movement for knee flexion. The right hand stabilises the thigh and the seat belt is used to apply a medial glide to the tibia, while the patient actively flexes the knee.

The physical testing procedures which specifically indicate joint, nerve or muscle tissues, as a source of the patient's symptoms, are summarised in Table 3.10. The strongest evidence that a joint is the source of the patient's symptoms is that active and passive physiological movements, passive accessory movements and joint palpation all reproduce the patient's symptoms, and that, following a treatment dose, reassessment identifies an improvement in the patient's signs and symptoms. Weaker evidence includes an alteration in range, resistance or quality of physiological and/or accessory movements and tenderness over the joint, with no alteration in signs and symptoms after treatment. One or more of these findings may indicate a dysfunction of a joint which may, or may not, be contributing to the patient's condition.

The strongest evidence that a muscle is the source of a patient's symptoms is if active movements, an isometric contraction, passive lengthening and palpation of a muscle all reproduce the patient's symptoms, and that, following a treatment dose, reassessment identifies an improvement in the patient's signs and symptoms. Further evidence of muscle dysfunction may be suggested by reduced strength or poor quality during the active physiological movement and the isometric contraction, reduced range and/or increased/decreased resistance, during the passive lengthening of the muscle, and tenderness on palpation, with no alteration in signs and symptoms after treatment. One or more of these findings may indicate a dysfunction of a muscle which may or may not be contributing to the patient's condition.

The strongest evidence that a nerve is the source of the patient's symptoms is when active and/or passive physiological movements reproduce the patient's symptoms, which are then increased or decreased with an additional sensitising movement, at a distance from the patient's symptoms. In addition, there is reproduction of the patient's symptoms on palpation of the nerve and neurodynamic testing, sufficient to be considered a treatment dose, results in an improvement in the above signs and symptoms. Further evidence of nerve dysfunction may be suggested by reduced range (compared with the asymptomatic side) and/or increased resistance to the various arm movements, and tenderness on nerve palpation.

On completion of the physical examination the clinician:

- warns the patient of possible exacerbation up to 24–48 hours following the examination
- requests the patient to report details on the behaviour of the symptoms following examination at the next attendance
- explains the findings of the physical examination and how these findings relate to the subjective assessment. Any misconceptions patients may have regarding their illness or injury should be addressed
- evaluates the findings, formulates a clinical diagnosis and writes up a problem list
- determines the objectives of treatment
- devises an initial treatment plan.

In this way, the clinician will have developed the following hypotheses categories (adapted from Jones & Rivett 2004):

- function: abilities and restrictions
- patient's perspective on his/her experience
- source of symptoms. This includes the structure or tissue that is thought to be producing the patient's symptoms, the nature of the structure or tissues in relation to the healing process and the pain mechanisms
- contributing factors to the development and maintenance of the problem. There may be environmental, psychosocial, behavioural, physical or heredity factors
- precautions/contraindications to treatment and management. This includes the severity and irritability of the patient's symptoms and the nature of the patient's condition
- management strategy and treatment plan
- prognosis – this can be affected by factors such as the stage and extent of the injury as well as the patient's expectation, personality and lifestyle.

For guidance on treatment and management principles, the reader is directed to the companion textbook (Petty 2011).

References

Apley, A.G., 1947. The diagnosis of meniscus injuries: some new clinical methods. J. Bone Joint Surg. 29B, 78–84.

Brechter, J.H., Powers, C.M., 2002. Patellofemoral joint stress during stair ascent and descent in persons with and without patellofemoral pain. Gait Posture 16 (2), 115–123.

Cakir, M., Samanci, N., Balci, N., et al., 2003. Musculoskeletal manifestations in patients with thyroid disease. Clin. Endocrinol. (Oxf.) 59 (2), 162–167.

Casteleyn, P.P., Handelberg, F., Opdecam, P., 1988. Traumatic haemarthrosis of the knee. J. Bone Joint Surg. Br. 70B (3), 404–406.

Cyriax, J., 1982. Textbook of orthopaedic medicine – diagnosis of soft tissue lesions, eighth ed. Baillière Tindall, London.

Drosos, G.I., Pozo, J.L., 2004. The causes and mechanisms of meniscal injuries in the sporting and non-sporting environment in an unselected population. Knee 11 (2), 143–149.

Eifert-Mangine, M.A., Bilbo, J.T., 1995. Conservative management of patellofemoral chondrosis. In: Mangine, R.E. (Ed.), Physical therapy of the knee, second ed. Churchill Livingstone, New York, p. 113.

Gifford, L.S., 1998. Pain, the tissues and the nervous system: a conceptual model. Physiotherapy 84 (1), 27–36.

Grelsamer, R., McConnell, J., 1998. The patella in a team approach. Aspen, Gaithersburg.

Hayes, C.W., Brigido, M.K., Jamadar, D.A., et al., 2000. Mechanism-based pattern approach to classification of complex injuries of the knee depicted at MR imaging. Radiographics 20, S121–S134.

Hughston, J.C., Norwood, L.A., 1980. The posterolateral drawer test and external rotational recurvatum test for posterolateral rotary instability of the knee. Clin. Orthop. Relat. Res. 147, 82–87.

Janda, V., 1994. Muscles and motor control in cervicogenic disorders: assessment and management. In: Grant, R. (Ed.), Physical therapy of the cervical and thoracic spine, second ed. Churchill Livingstone, New York, p. 195.

Janda, V., 2002. Muscles and motor control in cervicogenic disorders. In: Grant, R. (Ed.), Physical therapy of the cervical and thoracic spine, third ed. Churchill Livingstone, New York, p. 182.

Jones, M.A., Rivett, D.A., 2004. Clinical reasoning for manual therapists. Butterworth-Heinemann, Edinburgh.

Jones, M.A., Edwards, I., Gifford, L.S., 2002. Conceptual models for implementing biopsychosocial theory in clinical practice. Man. Ther. 7 (1), 2–9.

Jonsson, T., Althoff, B., Peterson, L., et al., 1982. Clinical diagnosis of ruptures of the anterior cruciate ligament: a comparative study of the Lachman test and anterior drawer sign. Am. J. Sports Med. 10, 100–102.

Jull, G.A., Janda, V., 1987. Muscles and motor control in low back pain: assessment and management. In: Twomey, L.T., Taylor, J.R. (Eds.), Physical therapy of the low back. Churchill Livingstone, New York, p. 253.

Katz, J.W., Fingeroth, R.J., 1986. The diagnostic accuracy of ruptures of the anterior cruciate ligament comparing the Lachman test, the anterior drawer sign, and the pivot shift test in acute and chronic knee injuries. Am. J. Sports Med. 14 (1), 88–91.

Kurzweil, P.R., Kelley, S.T., 2006. Physical examination and imaging of the medial collateral ligament and posteromedial corner of the knee. Sports Med. Arthrosc. 14 (2), 67–73.

Lavy, C., James, A., Wilson-MacDonald, J., et al., 2009. Cauda equina syndrome. Br. Med. J. 338, 881–884.

Levinger, P., Gilleard, W., Coleman, C., 2007. Femoral medial deviation angle during a one-leg squat test in individuals with patellofemoral pain syndrome. Phys. Ther. Sport 8, 163–168.

Magee, D.J., 1997. Orthopedic physical assessment, third ed. W B Saunders, Philadelphia.

Malanga, G.A., Andrus, S., Nadler, S.F., et al., 2003. Physical examination of the knee: a review of the original test description and scientific validity of common orthopedic tests. Arch. Phys. Med. Rehabil. 84, 592–603.

Malone, A.A., Dowd, G.S.E., Saifuddin, A., 2006. Injuries of the posterior cruciate ligament and posterolateral corner of the knee. Injury 37, 485–501.

Mariani, P.P., Caruso, I., 1979. An electromyographic investigation of subluxation of the patella. J. Bone Joint Surg. 61-B (2), 169–171.

McConnell, J., 1986. The management of chondromalacia patellae: a long term solution. Aust. J. Physiother. 32 (4), 215–223.

McConnell, J., 1996. Management of patellofemoral problems. Man. Ther. 1 (2), 60–66.

McDermott, I.D., 2006. Meniscal tears. Curr. Orthop. 20 (2), 85–94.

McMurray, T.P., 1942. The semilunar cartilages. Br. J. Surg. 29 (116), 407–414.

Mitsou, A., Vallianatos, P., 1988. Clinical diagnosis of ruptures of the anterior cruciate ligament: a comparison between the Lachman test and the anterior drawer sign. Injury 19, 427–428.

Mulligan, B.R., 1999. Manual therapy 'NAGs', 'SNAGs', 'MWMs' etc., fourth ed. Plane View Services, New Zealand.

Ostrowski, J.A., 2006. Accuracy of 3 diagnostic tests for anterior cruciate ligament tears. J. Athl. Train. 41 (1), 120–121.

Petty, N.J., 2011. Principles of neuromusculoskeletal treatment and management: a guide for therapists, second ed. Churchill Livingstone, Edinburgh.

Powers, C.M., 2003. The influence of altered lower extremity kinematics on patellofemoral joint dysfunction: a theoretical perspective. J. Orthop. Sports Phys. Ther. 3, 639–646.

Sahrmann, S.A., 2002. Diagnosis and treatment of movement impairment syndromes. Mosby, St Louis.

Solomonow, M., 2009. Ligaments: a source of musculoskeletal disorders. J. Bodyw. Mov. Ther. 13 (2), 136–154.

Torry, M.R., Decker, M.J., Viola, R.M., et al., 2000. Intra-articular knee effusion induces quadriceps avoidance gait patterns. Clin. Biomech. 15, 147–159.

Voight, M.L., Wieder, D.L., 1991. Comparative reflex response times of vastus medialis obliquus and vastus lateralis in normal subjects and subjects with extensor mechanism dysfunction. Am. J. Sports Med. 19 (2), 131–137.

Waddell, G., 2004. The back pain revolution, second ed. Churchill Livingstone, Edinburgh.

Examination of the foot and ankle

16

Chris Murphy

CHAPTER CONTENTS

Possible causes of pain and/or limitation of movement

This region includes the inferior tibiofibular, talo-crural, subtalar, mid-tarsal, tarsometatarsal, inter-metatarsal, metatarsophalangeal, first and fifth rays and interphalangeal joints with their surrounding soft tissues. A ray is a functional unit formed by a metatarsal and its associated cuneiform; for the fourth and fifth rays it refers to the metatarsal alone (Norkin & Levangie 1992). Most commonly in clinical practice podiatrists and physiotherapists consider function of the range of movement and function of the first ray (Christensen & Jennings 2009).

Ankle

- Trauma:
  - fracture of the tibia, fibula, e.g. Pott's fracture
  - ligamentous sprain, e.g. medial or lateral ligament of the ankle and inferior tibiofibular ligaments
  - muscular strain, e.g. peritendinitis of tendocalcaneus and rupture of the tendocalcaneus
  - tarsal tunnel syndrome
  - tenosynovitis
- Osteochondritis dissecans of the talus
- Degenerative conditions: osteoarthrosis
- Inflammatory conditions: rheumatoid arthritis
- Infection, e.g. tuberculosis
- Endocrine diseases: diabetes.

Foot

Childhood foot

- Congenital talipes equinovarus (idiopathic club foot)
- Talipes calcaneovalgus
- In- and out-toeing (adducted and abducted stance respectively)

- Overpronated foot
- Pes cavus and planus
- Köhler's disease (osteochondritis of the navicular)
- Freiberg's disease of lesser metatarsal heads (commonly second)
- Sever's disease causing a painful heel
- Retrocalcaneal bump (soft-tissue or bony)
- Malignancy.

Adolescent foot

- Hallux valgus
- Exostoses
- Retrocalcaneal heel bumps (soft-tissue or bony).

Adult foot

- Rheumatoid arthritis
- Gout
- Diabetic foot
- Paralysed foot, e.g. upper or lower motor neurone lesion, peripheral nerve injury
- Overuse syndrome and foot strain.

Rear foot

- Retrocalcaneal heel bumps (soft-tissue or bony)
- Soft-tissue conditions, e.g. bursitis, tendinitis, tendinosis, fat pad bruising.

Forefoot

- Brailsford's disease (osteochondritis of the navicular)
- Forefoot varus and valgus, forefoot supinatus, forefoot adduction and abduction
- Pes cavus and planus
- Plantar fasciosis
- Anterior metatarsalgia
- Stress fracture (e.g. metatarsals, navicular)
- Freiberg's disease (osteochondritis of second metatarsal head)
- Morton's metatarsalgia
- Verruca pedis
- Ligamentous strain/overuse injury.

Toes

- Hallux valgus
- Hallux rigidus

- Ingrowing toenail
- Lesser toe deformity, e.g. hammer toe, mallet toe, claw toe.

Other conditions

- Hypermobility
- Referral of symptoms from the lumbar spine, sacroiliac joint, hip or knee to the foot; or referral of foot structure and functional anomalies to more proximal structures in the locomotor system.

Further details of the questions asked during the subjective examination and the tests carried out in the physical examination can be found in Chapters 2 and 3 respectively.

The order of the subjective questioning and the physical tests described below can be altered as appropriate for the patient being examined.

Subjective examination

Body chart

The following information concerning the type and area of current symptoms can be recorded on a body chart (see Figure 2.3).

Area of current symptoms

Be exact when mapping out the area of the symptoms. Anatomical structures in the foot and ankle tend to produce local symptoms. Use this information to help you clinically reason underlying pain mechanisms. If the patient is able to tell you, ascertain the worst symptom and record both where the patient feels the symptoms are coming from and the patient's underlying thoughts as to the cause of these.

Areas relevant to the region being examined

All other relevant areas should be checked for symptoms as patients often forget to report relevant additional symptoms. Check for the presence of pain or even stiffness, as this may be relevant to the patient's main symptom, especially when considering referred pain. Mark unaffected areas with ticks (✓) on the body chart. Check for symptoms in the lumbar spine, hip joint and knee joint.

Quality of pain

Establish the quality of the pain.

Intensity of pain

The intensity of pain can be measured using, for example, a visual analogue scale, as shown in Chapter 2. This serves as one of a number of physical markers to monitor progress.

Depth of pain

Establish the depth of the pain. Does the patient feel it is on the surface or deep inside?

Abnormal sensation

Check for any altered sensation (such as paraesthesia or numbness) over the lower limb, ankle and foot. This may indicate a peripheral neurogenic contribution of reported symptoms.

Constant or intermittent symptoms

Ascertain the frequency of the symptoms, whether they are constant or intermittent. If symptoms are constant, check whether there is variation in the intensity of the symptoms, as constant symptoms, especially unremitting pain, require further investigation to exclude more serious pathology such as neoplastic disease.

Relationship of symptoms

Determine the relationship of the symptomatic areas to each other – do they come together or separately? For example, the patient could have ankle pain without back pain or the pains may always be present together. Such questioning will help you to build a pattern as to whether different symptoms share a common pain mechanism, e.g neurogenic pain, or a symptom is being referred.

Behaviour of symptoms

The following text will assume symptoms are due to a local nociceptive cause. The reader is encouraged to embrace current pain literature to help include the concepts of peripheral neurogenic pain, central sensitisation and supraspinal changes (van Griensven 2005). Ignoring this may cause the clinician to become confused by presenting symptoms that might not make sense without these considerations.

Aggravating factors

For each symptomatic area, discover what movements and/or positions aggravate the patient's symptoms, i.e. what brings them on (or makes them worse)? is the patient able to maintain this position or movement (severity)? what happens to other symptoms when this symptom is produced (or is made worse)? and how long does it take for symptoms to ease once the position or movement is stopped (irritability)? These questions help to confirm the relationship between the symptoms and serve as physical markers to gauge progress.

In addition, it is wise to question the patient about common aggravating factors for the anatomical structures within this region to implicate or exclude other structures which may form part of the clinical presentation. Common aggravating factors for the foot and ankle are weight-bearing activities such as stair climbing, squatting, walking and running, especially on uneven ground. Aggravating factors for other regions, which may need to be queried if they are suspected to be a source of the symptoms, are shown in Table 2.3.

The clinician ascertains how the symptoms affect function, such as: static and active postures, e.g. standing, walking (even and uneven ground), running, going up and down stairs, work, sport and social activities. Note details of sporting activities which the patient participates in, including surface, footwear and intensity. The clinician would be wise to question the patient on subtle variations in chosen sports to understand the stresses which the body is subjected to. It would be wise to check if the patient is left- or right-handed, especially in racket sports, as there may be different stresses which the foot and ankle are subjected to.

Detailed information on each of the above activities is useful in order to help determine the structure(s) contributing to symptoms and identify functional restrictions. This information can be used to explain symptoms and advise patients in understandable, non-threatening terms. In addition, it serves to determine both a treatment plan and the formulation of agreed goals. The most notable functional restrictions are highlighted with asterisks (*), explored in the physical examination and reassessed at subsequent treatment sessions to evaluate treatment intervention. It is best to clarify patients' understanding of symptoms and progress at subsequent points to ensure they have a clear and an accurate representation.

Easing factors

For each symptomatic area, the clinician asks what movements and/or positions ease the patient's symptoms, how long it takes to ease them and what happens to other symptoms when this symptom is relieved. These questions, along with a knowledge of relevant biomechanics and functional movement, help the clinician to reason why a movement might improve symptoms. For example, running may aggravate due to the increased range of dorsiflexion required, whereas walking may be symptom-free.

The clinician asks the patient about theoretically known easing factors for structures that could be a source of the symptoms. For example, symptoms from the foot and ankle may be relieved by weight-relieving positions, whereas symptoms from the lumbar spine may be relieved by lying prone or in crook-lying. The clinician can then analyse the positions or movements that ease symptoms to help determine the structure(s) contributing to the clinical presentation.

Twenty-four-hour behaviour of symptoms

The clinician determines the 24-hour behaviour of symptoms by asking questions about night, morning and evening symptoms.

Night symptoms. These are important to establish as they offer further insight as to the impact of symptoms on a patient's life as well helping to determine underlying pathology and pain mechanisms. Positions of comfort along with normal and current sleeping positions may help implicate or exclude certain anatomical structures. Symptoms which disturb or delay sleep and especially the way in which a patient manages them may help reasoning as to whether symptoms are nociceptive in nature or if more sinister causes might need to be considered. Recording the frequency of waking and time to return to sleep can serve as physical markers for reassessment.

Morning and evening symptoms. The clinician determines the pattern of the symptoms first thing in the morning, through the day and at the end of the day. This information may provide clues as to the pain mechanisms driving the condition and the type of pathology present. For example, early-morning pain and stiffness may indicate inflammatory-driven pain. Pain on the initial weight-bearing steps in the morning is commonly attributed to plantar fasciiosis; it should be noted that this is also reported with symptoms relating to tibialis posterior pathology (Patla & Abbot 2000). The pattern of symptoms may also be a helpful reassessment marker to establish the effectiveness of treatment and management.

Stage of the condition

In order to determine the stage of the condition, the clinician asks whether the symptoms are getting better, getting worse or remaining unchanged. Asking this allows one to question if symptoms are continuing beyond the expected time scale for recovery and, if so, to question possible factors to explain this.

Special questions

Special questions must always be asked, as they may identify certain precautions or contraindications to the physical examination and/or treatment (see Table 2.4). As mentioned in Chapter 2, the clinician must differentiate between conditions that are suitable for manual or manipulative therapy and systemic, neoplastic and other non-neuromusculoskeletal conditions, which are not suitable for such treatment and require referral to a medical practitioner.

The following information is routinely obtained from patients.

General health. The clinician ascertains the state of the patient's general health and finds out if the patient suffers from any malaise, fatigue, fever, nausea or vomiting, stress, anxiety or depression.

Weight loss. Has the patient noticed any recent unexplained weight loss?

Rheumatoid arthritis. Has the patient (or a member of his/her family) been diagnosed as having rheumatoid arthritis?

Drug therapy. What drugs are being taken by the patient? Has the patient been prescribed long-term (6 months or more) medication/steroids? Has the patient been taking anticoagulants recently?

Radiographs and medical imaging. Has the patient been radiographed or had any other medical tests? The medical tests may include blood tests, arthroscopy, magnetic resonance imaging, computed tomography scan, myelography or a bone scan.

Neuropathy secondary to the disorder. Has the patient any evidence of peripheral neuropathy – sensory, motor or autonomic – associated with a medical disorder such as diabetes (McLeod-Roberts 1995; Armstrong 1999)? Abnormality of skin and other structures will not necessarily be perceived or reported by the patient.

Neurological symptoms if a spinal lesion is suspected. Has the patient experienced symptoms of spinal cord compression (i.e. compression of the spinal cord to L1 level), which are bilateral tingling in hands or feet and/or disturbance of gait?

Has the patient experienced symptoms of cauda equina compression (i.e. compression below L1), which are saddle anaesthesia/paraesthesia and bladder and/or bowel sphincter disturbance (loss of control, retention, hesitancy, urgency or a sense of incomplete evacuation) (Grieve 1991)? These symptoms may be due to interference of S3 and S4 (Grieve 1981). Prompt surgical attention is required to prevent permanent sphincter paralysis.

History of the present condition

For each symptomatic area the clinician needs to know how long the symptom has been present, whether there was a sudden or slow onset and whether there was a known cause that provoked the onset of the symptom. If the patient is able to recall a traumatic onset, closer questioning as to the mechanism of injury may suggest structures which could have been injured and to what degree. Under the Ottawa ankle rules, determining whether a patient can weight-bear, in conjunction with the presence of specific bony tenderness after an injury, is highly sensitive (Bachmann et al. 2003) in determining if a fracture is present. If the onset was slow, the clinician finds out if there has been any change in the patient's lifestyle, e.g. a new job or hobby or a change in existing sporting activities, including alterations in footwear, equipment, surface or intensity. The goal here is simply to work out what has happened or to build a picture of what has changed so as to understand fully why a patient is presenting with symptoms. To confirm the relationship between the symptoms, the clinician asks what happened to other symptoms when each symptom began.

Past medical history

The following information is obtained from the patient and/or the medical notes:

- the details of any relevant medical history
- the history of any previous similar episodes: how many have there been? when were they? was a cause identifiable? what was the duration of each

episode? what did the patient think was happening? and did the patient fully recover between episodes? If there have been no previous attacks, has the patient had any episodes of any other symptoms in the lumbar spine, hip, knee, ankle, foot or any other relevant region? Check for a history of trauma or recurrent minor trauma

- ascertain the results of any investigations, past treatment and self-management strategies for the same problem or any others affecting the lower limb. Past treatment records may be obtained for further information. The clinician checks if orthotics have been prescribed. If so, check if the patient found them useful, which footwear they were recommended for and if the patient is still using them. It is wise to examine physically any prescribed orthotics or footwear to ensure it is adequate and is not defective or worn out.

Social and family history

Social and family history that is relevant to the onset and progression of the patient's problem is recorded. This includes the patient's perspectives, experience and expectations, age, employment, home situation, details of any leisure activities and how long the patient has participated in these. With sporting pursuits it can be helpful to check if the patient is planning to engage in any competitions or events to understand existing motivations towards continuing exercise programmes. Factors from this information may indicate direct and/or indirect mechanical influences on the foot and ankle and their frequency. It is helpful to have a working knowledge of these to equate them to tissue loading and the healing process for injuries in which this is a consideration for returning to activity. In order to treat the patient appropriately, it is important that the condition is managed within the context of the patient's social and work environment. This can serve as an area for both creativity on the part of the clinician and a helpful reminder for timing of completing home exercises for the patient. Taking the stairs instead of a lift and performing exercises when on a toilet break can be useful so that home programmes are less onerous.

The clinician may ask the following types of questions to elucidate psychosocial factors:

- Have you had time off work in the past with your pain?
- What do you understand to be the cause of your pain?

- What is your pain preventing you from currently doing?
- What are you expecting will help you?
- How is your employer/co-workers/family responding to your pain?
- What are you doing to cope with your pain?
- Do you think you will return to work? When?

Although these questions are described in relation to psychosocial risk factors for poor outcomes for patients with low-back pain (Waddell 2004), they can be highly relevant to other patients as they can be powerful factors in directing both response to treatment and overall recovery (Main & Spanswick 1999).

Plan of the physical examination

When all this information has been collected, the subjective examination is complete. It is useful at this stage to highlight with asterisks (*), for ease of reference, important findings and particularly one or more functional restrictions. These can then be re-examined at subsequent treatment sessions to evaluate treatment intervention. It is useful to communicate this to patients so they become proactive in monitoring progress.

In order to plan the physical examination, the following hypotheses need to be developed from the subjective examination:

- If pain is a feature of the presentation, what are the underlying pain mechanisms you suspect to be contributing to symptoms? It may be helpful to prioritise which of these is the most prevalent; this will help guide the depth and strength of your examination.
- The regions and structures that need to be examined as a possible cause of the symptoms, e.g. the lumbar spine, hip, knee, foot and ankle soft tissues, vascular and neural structures. Often it is not possible to examine fully at the first attendance and so examination of the structures must be prioritised over subsequent treatment sessions. Consider that a goal of the examination is to offer patients some explanation of their symptoms, and also, where possible, to eliminate more sinister causes of symptoms or facilitate further investigations for such if suspected.
- Other factors that need to be examined, e.g. working and everyday postures, leg length, associated footwear and orthotics.

- In what way should the physical tests be carried out? Will it be easy or hard to reproduce each symptom? Will it be necessary to use combined movements, repetitive movements and functional positions to reproduce the patient's symptoms? Are symptoms severe and/or irritable? If symptoms are severe, physical tests may be carried out to just before the onset of symptom production or just to the onset of symptom production; no overpressures will be carried out, as the patient would be unable to tolerate this. If symptoms are irritable, physical tests may be examined to just before symptom production or just to the onset of provocation with fewer physical tests being examined to allow for a rest period between tests.
- Are there any precautions and/or contraindications to elements of the physical examination that need to be explored further, such as neurological involvement, recent fracture, trauma, steroid therapy or rheumatoid arthritis; there may also be certain contraindications to further examination and treatment, e.g. symptoms of spinal cord or cauda equina compression.

A physical planning form can be useful for inexperienced clinicians to help guide them through the clinical reasoning process (see Figure 2.10).

Physical examination

The information from the subjective examination helps the clinician to plan an appropriate physical examination. Any underlying pain mechanisms, their severity and irritability and nature of the condition are the major factors that will influence the choice and priority of physical testing procedures. The first and overarching question the clinician might ask is: 'Is this patient's condition suitable for me to manage?' For example, a patient presenting with cauda equina compression symptoms may only need neurological integrity testing, prior to an urgent medical referral. The nature of the patient's condition has had a major impact on the physical examination. The second question the clinician might ask is: 'Does this patient have a neuromusculoskeletal dysfunction that I may be able to help and to what extent?' To answer that, the clinician needs to carry out a full physical examination; however, this may not be possible if the symptoms are severe and/or irritable. If the patient's symptoms are severe and/or irritable, the clinician aims to explore movements as much as possible, within a symptom-free range. If the patient has constant and severe and/or irritable symptoms, then the clinician aims to find physical tests that ease the symptoms. If the patient's symptoms are non-severe and non-irritable, then the clinician aims to find physical tests that reproduce each of the patient's symptoms. In conjunction with this the clinician would be wise to ask: 'Are there any psychosocial barriers that I need to consider/address prior to or within my physical examination, e.g. fear of movement, high level of distress?' Such things may heighten the patient's anxiety, which may increase existing pain.

Each significant physical test that either provokes or eases the patient's symptoms is highlighted in the patient's notes by an asterisk (*) for easy reference. The highlighted tests are often referred to as 'asterisks' or 'markers'. Throughout, a good working knowledge of possible mechanisms underpinning symptoms is vital to identify possible false positives when highlighting asterisks.

The order and detail of the physical tests described below need to be appropriate to the patient being examined; some tests will be irrelevant, some tests will be carried out briefly, while it will be necessary to investigate others fully. It is important that readers understand that the techniques shown in this chapter are some of many; the choice depends mainly on the relative size of the clinician and patient, as well as the clinician's preference. For this reason, novice clinicians may initially want to copy what is shown, but then quickly adapt to what is best for them.

Observation

Informal observation

The clinician needs to observe the patient in dynamic and static situations; the quality of movement is noted, as are the postural characteristics and facial expression. Informal observation will have begun from the moment the clinician begins the subjective examination and will continue to the end of the physical examination.

Formal observation

Observation of posture. The clinician examines the patient's posture in standing, noting the posture of the feet, lower limbs, pelvis and spine. Observation of the foot and ankle can also be carried out in a non-weight-bearing position. General lower-limb abnormalities include uneven weight-bearing through the legs and feet, internal femoral rotation and genu varum/valgum or recurvatum (hyperextension). It is worth noting the general foot posture and whether the foot has a particularly flattened or exaggerated medial longitudinal arch, as these may indicate pes planus or pes cavus respectively. The toes may be deformed – claw toes, hallux rigidus, hammer toes, mallet toe, hallux valgus, Morton's foot. It must be remembered that static observations are not strongly predictive of dynamic function (Cavanagh et al. 1997). Further details of these abnormalities can be found in a standard orthopaedic textbook (Magee 1997). Deviations observed in standing may be produced by a number of lower-limb factors, including tibial torsions and femoral anteversion or retroversion. Passive correction of observed deformity may give an idea of the ease by which this can be achieved and any associated impact on the lower limb and pelvis, but is not indicative of the cause of any deformity.

It is worth remembering that pure postural dysfunction rarely influences one region of the body in isolation and it may be necessary to carry out a full postural examination.

Observation of alignment of foot and calf alignment.

Leg–heel alignment. The patient lies prone with the foot over the end of the plinth and the clinician holds the foot with the subtalar joint in neutral. The clinician observes the position of the foot on the leg by using an imaginary line that bisects the calcaneus and the lower third of the leg (ignore the alignment of the tendocalcaneus). Normally, the calcaneus will be in slight varus (2–4°) (Roy & Irvin 1983). Excessive varus or presence of valgus alignment indicates hindfoot/rearfoot varus and valgus respectively; the latter is more likely to be observed following injury or disease process.

Forefoot–heel alignment. Test for forefoot varus and valgus with the patient in prone and the foot over the end of the plinth. The clinician holds the subtalar joint in neutral and the mid-tarsal joint in maximum eversion and observes the relationship between the vertical axis of the heel and the plane of the first to fifth metatarsal heads, which is normally perpendicular. The medial side of the foot will be raised if there is forefoot varus and the lateral side will be raised if there is forefoot valgus (Roy & Irvin 1983).

Tibial torsion. This test compares the alignment of the transverse axis of the knee with the ankle axis in the frontal plane. With the patient sitting, the clinician compares the ankle joint line (an imaginary line

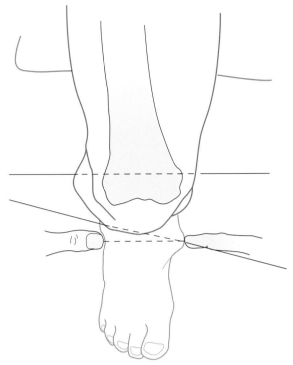

Figure 16.1 • Tibial torsion. The line of the ankle joint is compared with a visual estimation of the knee joint axis. (From Fromherz 1995, with permission.)

between the apex of the medial and lateral malleoli) and the knee joint line (Figure 16.1) (Fromherz 1995). The tibia normally lies in 15–20° of lateral rotation (Wadsworth 1988).

Pes planus and overpronation. Very high arched feet – pes cavus – may have a neurological or idiopathic aetiology and are invariably relatively rigid and have greater difficulty accommodating to uneven terrain, requiring other segments of the locomotor system to compensate for their relative lack of mobility. Feet that have an in-rolled appearance are termed over- or excessively pronated. On weight-bearing the calcaneus is usually in a valgus alignment and medial bulging of the navicular is evident. Those feet that appear flattened with no longitudinal arch, but without inrolling, are called pes planus. This latter condition is not very common.

Observation of muscle form. The clinician observes the muscle bulk and muscle tone of the patient, comparing left and right sides. It must be remembered that the level and frequency of physical activity as well as the dominant side may well produce differences in muscle bulk between sides. Some muscles are thought to shorten under stress while other muscles weaken, producing muscle imbalance (see Table 3.2).

Observation of soft tissues. The clinician observes the quality and colour of the patient's skin, any area of swelling, exostosis, callosities, joint effusion or presence of scarring, and takes cues for further examination.

Observation of balance. Balance is provided by vestibular, visual and proprioceptive information. This rather crude and non-specific test is conducted by asking the patient to stand on one leg with the eyes open; this can be timed until the patient needs to touch the other foot to the floor or hold on to restore balance. This can be repeated with the eyes closed and the times obtained used in the future to compare progress. If the patient's balance is as poor with the eyes open as with the eyes closed, this suggests a vestibular or proprioceptive dysfunction (rather than a visual dysfunction). The test is carried out on the affected and unaffected side; if there is greater difficulty maintaining balance on the affected side, this may indicate some proprioceptive dysfunction.

Observation of gait. Analyse gait (including walking backwards) on even/uneven ground and on toes, heels, and outer and inner borders of feet, as well as slopes, stairs and running. Always work in a logical manner from head to toe, or vice versa, observing each body segment for variations in the normal range. Look for asymmetries in each segment, e.g. head side flexion, arm swing, trunk rotation, uneven stride length from left to right, differences in weight-bearing. Each variation may indicate tight musculature, structural anomalies or functional movement patterns which may have altered through a habit, e.g. such as carrying a bag on one shoulder. Gait analysis serves as a physical measure which may assist in the identification of contributing factors in presenting symptoms. More detailed guidance on gait analysis can be found in Whittle (2007).

Whilst certain information can be gained from visual gait analysis, the use of a simple video camera and a treadmill offers the opportunity to view footage at a later stage. Depending on the software used, footage may be paused and viewed a number of times; software exists which allows for physical markers (angles, stride length) to be accurately measured, e.g. Dartfish, Quintic. This information may then be used to help direct treatment and evaluate the results of any intervention at future sessions.

The gait cycle is defined as 'the time interval between two successive occurrences of one of the repetitive events of walking' (Whittle 2007). It is often started at the point one foot touches the floor; this used to be referred to as heel strike but as it is not always the heel that strikes first it is now referred to as initial contact. The gait cycle consists of the following major events:

1. initial contact
2. opposite toe-off
3. heel rise
4. opposite initial contact
5. toe-off
6. feet adjacent
7. tibial vertical
8. initial contact – the gait cycle begins again.

The angle of heel contact with the ground is usually slightly varus. Marked variations from this will cause abnormal foot function, with compensation attained either in the foot across the mid-tarsal joint and first and fifth rays or more proximally in the ankle, knee (less often hip) and sacroiliac joints. Early heel lift may indicate tight posterior leg muscles which can be a cause of functional ankle equinus (Tollafield & Merriman 1995), where the range of dorsiflexion required for normal gait is lacking; this requires compensations throughout the foot, ankle and lower limb.

The degree of pronation of the foot during mid-stance is observed and noted. Pronation is a normal part of gait that allows the foot to become a shock absorber and mobile adapter. At heel lift the foot changes to a more rigid lever for toe-off. Limitation in range of motion of the metatarsophalangeal joints will affect gait also. Abnormality of function at any phase of gait may cause symptoms, varying from low-grade and cumulative to acute, in any structures of the locomotor system.

Summary of gait analysis:

• Systematically observe the alignment of each area from top to bottom during a number of gait cycles.
• Note any asymmetry from side to side.
• Note the point at which asymmetry occurs and consider why that might be.

Observation of the patient's attitudes and feelings. The age, gender and ethnicity of patients and their cultural, occupational and social backgrounds will all affect their attitudes and feelings towards themselves, their condition and the clinician. The clinician needs to be aware of and sensitive to these attitudes, and to empathise and communicate appropriately so as to develop a rapport with the patient and thereby enhance the patient's compliance with the treatment.

Joint integrity tests

Anterior drawer sign

The patient lies supine with the knee slightly flexed to relax gastrocnemius; this may be achieved by a pillow under the knee. The ankle needs to be relaxed in approximately 20° of plantarflexion. The clinician grasps the calcaneum and gently applies a postero-anterior force with the aim of drawing the calcaneum and talus forwards (Figure 16.2). Excessive anterior movement of the talus, with a loose end-feel, indicates a reduction in the passive stabilising function of the medial and lateral ligaments (Fujii et al. 2000).

Talar tilt

The patient lies supine with the knee slightly flexed to relax gastrocnemius; this may be achieved by a pillow under the knee. The ankle needs to be relaxed in approximately 20° of plantarflexion. The clinician grasps the calcaneum and slowly moves it into inversion; a small amount of traction can be applied (Figure 16.3). Monitor for range of movement, clicks or clunks. Excessive adduction movement, a reduced or absent end-feel and clicks/clunks suggest injury to the lateral ligament complex or that the calcaneo-fibular ligament is injured.

Some research suggests that these tests individually are not sufficient to differentiate which of the lateral ligaments has been compromised. It may therefore be wise to use these tests in combination with others to confirm an injury to the lateral ligaments (Fujii et al. 2000).

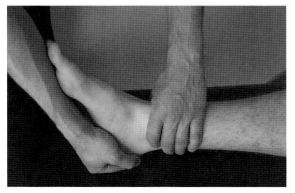

Figure 16.2 • Anterior drawer sign. The left hand stabilises the lower leg while the right hand applies a posteroanterior force to the talus.

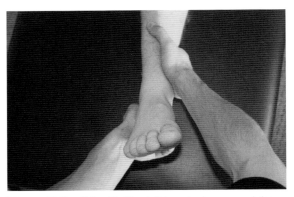

Figure 16.3 • Talar tilt. The left hand grips around the calcaneum and talus and moves it into adduction whilst the other hand stabilises the lower leg.

Active physiological movements

For active physiological movements, the clinician notes the following:

- quality of movement
- range of movement
- behaviour of pain through the range of movement
- resistance through the range of movement and at the end of the range of movement
- provocation of any protective muscle spasm.

A movement diagram can be used to depict this information. Active movements with overpressure to the foot and ankle are shown in Figure 16.4 and are tested with the patient lying either prone or supine. Depending on the size of the patient and the clinician's hands, it is often easier to perform inversion and eversion in supine and dorsiflexion and plantarflexion in prone. Movements are carried out on the left and right sides. Overpressure at the end of the range can be applied to the whole foot. For differentiation purposes, the foot may be considered in functional units: the rearfoot, midfoot and forefoot. These are described in Table 16.1. Using a knowledge of the joint lines the various regions may be individually examined with localised overpressure at the end of range. The clinician establishes the patient's symptoms at rest, prior to each movement, and notes the effect of passively correcting any movement deviation to determine its relevance to the patient's symptoms. Active physiological movements of the foot and ankle and possible modifications are shown in Table 16.2.

Numerous differentiation tests (Maitland 1991) can be performed; the choice depends on the patient's signs and symptoms. For example, when lateral ankle pain is reproduced on inversion, inversion consists of rearfoot, midfoot and forefoot movement along with a degree of adduction. The clinician takes the foot into inversion and, if symptomatic, the foot can be taken to a position short of symptoms and overpressure applied to each region and the effect on reproducing symptoms noted.

Other regions may need to be examined to determine their relevance to the patient's symptoms as they may be contributing to symptoms. The regions most likely are the lumbar spine, sacroiliac joint, hip and knee. The joints within these regions can be tested fully (see relevant chapter) or partially with the use of screening tests (see Chapter 3 for further information).

Some functional ability has already been tested by the general observation of the patient during the subjective and physical examination, e.g. the postures adopted during the subjective examination and the ease or difficulty of undressing and changing position prior to the examination. Any further functional testing can be carried out at this point in the examination and may involve further gait analysis over and above that carried out in the observation section earlier. Clues for appropriate tests can be obtained from the subjective examination findings, particularly aggravating factors.

Passive physiological movements

All of the active movements described above can be examined passively with the patient in prone with the knee at 90° flexion, or supine with the knee flexed over a pillow, comparing left and right sides. Comparison of the response of symptoms to the active and passive movements can help to determine whether the structures contributing to symptoms are non-contractile (articular) or contractile (extra-articular) (Cyriax 1982). If the lesion is non-contractile, such as ligament, then active and passive movements will be painful and/or restricted in the same direction. If the lesion is in a contractile tissue (i.e. muscle) then active and passive movements are painful and/or restricted in opposite directions. Metatarsophalangeal abduction and adduction can be tested (Figure 16.5).

It may be necessary to examine other regions to determine their relevance to the patient's symptoms; they may be the source of the symptoms, or they may

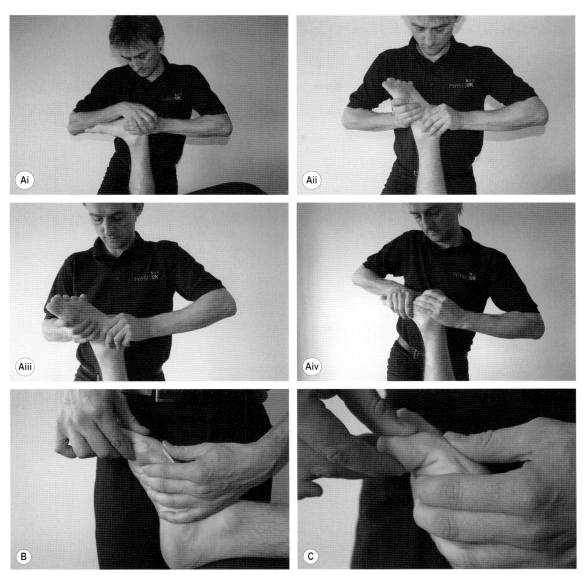

Figure 16.4 • Overpressures to the foot and ankle. **A (i)** Dorsiflexion. The left hand tips the calcaneus into dorsiflexion while the right hand and forearm apply overpressure to dorsiflexion through the length of the foot. **A (ii)** Plantarflexion. The right hand grips the forefoot and the left hand grips the calcaneus and together they move the foot into plantarflexion. **A (iii)** Inversion. The left hand adducts the calcaneus and reinforces the plantarflexion movement while the right hand plantarflexes the hindfoot and adducts, supinates and plantarflexes the midfoot and forefoot. **A (iv)** Eversion. The left hand abducts the calcaneus and reinforces the dorsiflexion while the right hand dorsiflexes the hindfoot and abducts, pronates and dorsiflexes the midfoot and forefoot. **B** Metatarsophalangeal joint flexion and extension. The left hand stabilises the metatarsal while the right hand flexes and extends the proximal phalanx. **C** Interphalangeal joint flexion and extension. The left hand stabilises the proximal phalanx while the right hand flexes and extends the distal phalanx.

Table 16.1 Functional units of the foot

Rearfoot	Midfoot	Forefoot
Talocrural joint	Talonavicular joint	Tarsometatarsal joints
Subtalar joint	Calcaneocuboid joint	Metatarsophalangeal joint Interphalangeal joints

Table 16.2 Active physiological movements and possible modifications

Active physiological movements	Modifications
Ankle dorsiflexion	Repeated
Ankle plantarflexion	Speed altered
Inversion	Combined, e.g.
Eversion	– inversion with plantarflexion
Metatarsophalangeal	– metatarsophalangeal joints: flexion and abduction
– flexion	Compression or distraction
– extension	Sustained
Interphalangeal joints:	Injuring movement
– flexion	Differentiation tests
– extension	Function
?Lumbar spine	
?Sacroiliac joint	
?Hip	
?Knee	

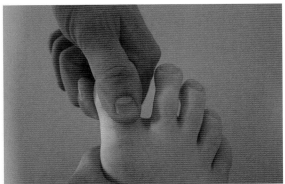

Figure 16.5 • Metatarsophalangeal joint abduction and adduction. The right hand stabilises the metatarsal while the left hand moves the proximal phalanx into abduction and adduction.

be contributing to the symptoms. The most likely regions are the lumbar spine, sacroiliac joint, hip and knee.

Muscle tests

Muscle tests include examining muscle strength, length, isometric muscle testing and some other muscle tests.

Muscle strength

The clinician tests the ankle dorsiflexors, plantarflexors, foot inverters, everters and toe flexors, extensors, abductors and adductors and any other relevant muscle groups. For details of these general tests readers are directed to Kendall et al. (2005), Cole et al. (1988) or Hislop & Montgomery (1995).

The strength of proximal muscles should be considered when deviations are observed during testing of functional movements which cannot be solely explained by the foot and ankle. Please refer to other relevant chapters and Kendall et al. (2005) for further details.

Muscle length

The clinician tests the length of muscles that may have an impact on lower-limb function, in particular those thought prone to shorten (Janda 1994, 2002); that is, piriformis, iliopsoas, rectus femoris, tensor fasciae latae, hamstrings, gastrocnemius and soleus (Jull & Janda 1987). Testing the length of these muscles is described in Chapter 3.

Isometric muscle testing

The clinician tests the ankle dorsiflexors and plantarflexors and any other relevant muscle group in resting position and, if indicated, in different parts of the physiological range. In addition the clinician observes the quality of the muscle contraction to hold this position (this can be done with the patient's eyes shut). The patient may, for example, be unable to prevent the joint from moving or may hold with excessive muscle activity; either of these circumstances would suggest a neuromuscular dysfunction.

Other muscle tests

Thompson's test for rupture of tendocalcaneus (Corrigan & Maitland 1994). With the patient prone and the feet over the end of the plinth or kneeling with the foot unsupported, the clinician squeezes the calf muscle; the absence of ankle plantarflexion indicates a positive test, suggesting rupture of tendocalcaneus.

Neurological tests

Neurological examination includes neurological integrity testing, neurodynamic tests and some other nerve tests.

Integrity of the nervous system

The integrity of the nervous system is tested if the clinician suspects that the symptoms are emanating from the spine or from a peripheral nerve.

Dermatomes/peripheral nerves. Light touch and pain sensation of the lower limb are tested using cotton wool and pinprick respectively, as described in Chapter 3. Knowledge of the cutaneous distribution of nerve roots (dermatomes) and peripheral nerves enables the clinician to distinguish the sensory loss due to a root lesion from that due to a peripheral nerve lesion. The cutaneous nerve distribution and dermatome areas are shown in Chapter 3.

Myotomes/peripheral nerves. The following myotomes are tested and are shown in Chapter 3:

- L2: hip flexion
- L3: knee extension
- L4: foot dorsiflexion and inversion
- L5: extension of the big toe
- S1: eversion of the foot, contract buttock, knee flexion
- S2: knee flexion, toe standing
- S3–S4: muscles of pelvic floor, bladder and genital function.

A working knowledge of the muscular distribution of nerve roots (myotomes) and peripheral nerves enables the clinician to distinguish the motor loss due to a root lesion from that due to a peripheral nerve lesion. The peripheral nerve distributions are shown in Chapter 3.

Reflex testing. The following deep tendon reflexes are tested and are shown in Chapter 3:

- L3/4: knee jerk
- S1: ankle jerk.

Neurodynamic tests

The following neurodynamic tests may be carried out in order to ascertain the degree to which neural tissue is responsible for the production of the patient's symptom(s):

- passive neck flexion
- straight-leg raise
- passive knee bend
- slump.

These tests are described in detail in Chapter 3.

Miscellaneous tests

Vascular tests

If it is suspected that the circulation is compromised, the clinician palpates the pulses of the dorsalis pedis artery. The state of the vascular system can also be determined by the response of symptoms to positions of dependence and elevation of the lower limbs.

Homans' sign for deep-vein thrombosis. The clinician passively dorsiflexes the ankle joint. If the patient feels pain in the calf, this may indicate deep-vein thrombosis. This needs to be integrated with other clinical findings suggestive of deep-vein thrombosis to confirm your diagnosis (van Beek et al. 2009).

Leg length

Leg length is measured if a difference in left and right sides is suspected (see Chapter 14 for details).

Palpation

The clinician palpates the foot and ankle and any other relevant areas. It is useful to record palpation findings on a body chart (see Figure 2.3) and/or palpation chart (see Figure 3.36).

The clinician notes the following:

- the temperature of the area
- localised increased skin moisture
- the presence of oedema or effusion. A tape measure can be used around the circumference of

the limb or joint and the left side compared with the right side

- mobility and feel of superficial tissues, e.g. ganglions, nodules, scar tissue
- the presence or elicitation of any muscle spasm
- tenderness of bone, ligament, muscle, tendon, tendon sheath, trigger points (shown in Figure 3.37) or nerve. Palpable nerves in the lower limb are as follows:
  - ○ The sciatic nerve can be palpated two-thirds of the way along an imaginary line between the greater trochanter and the ischial tuberosity with the patient in prone.
  - ○ The common peroneal nerve can be palpated medial to the tendon of biceps femoris and also around the head of the fibula.
  - ○ The tibial nerve can be palpated centrally over the posterior knee crease medial to the popliteal artery; it can also be felt behind the medial malleolus, which is more noticeable with the foot in dorsiflexion and eversion.
  - ○ The superficial peroneal nerve can be palpated on the dorsum of the foot along an imaginary line over the fourth metatarsal; it is more noticeable with the foot in plantarflexion and inversion.
  - ○ The deep peroneal nerve can be palpated between the first and second metatarsals, lateral to the extensor hallucis tendon.
  - ○ The sural nerve can be palpated on the lateral aspect of the foot behind the lateral malleolus, lateral to the tendocalcaneus.

- increased or decreased prominence of bones
- pain provoked or reduced on palpation.

Accessory movements

It is useful to use the palpation chart and movement diagrams (or joint pictures) to record findings. These are explained in detail in Chapter 3.

The clinician notes the:

- quality of movement
- range of movement
- resistance through the range and at the end of the range of movement
- behaviour of pain through the range
- provocation of any protective muscle spasm.

Accessory movements for the foot and ankle joints are shown in Figure 16.6 and listed in Table 16.3. Following accessory movements to the foot and ankle, the clinician reassesses all the physical asterisks (movements or tests that have been found to reproduce the patient's symptoms) in order to establish the effect of the accessory movements on the patient's signs and symptoms. Accessory movements can then be tested for other regions suspected to be a source of, or contributing to, the patient's symptoms. Again, following accessory movements to any one region, the clinician reassesses all the asterisks. Regions likely to be examined are the lumbar spine, sacroiliac joint, hip and knee (Table 16.3).

Mobilisations with movements (MWMs) are accessory movements applied during an active movement

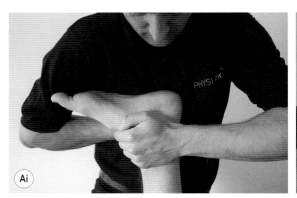 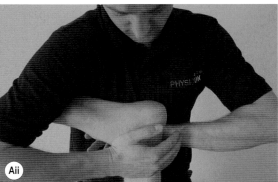

Figure 16.6 • Accessory movements for the foot and ankle joints. A Inferior tibiofibular joint. A (i) Anteroposterior. The heel of the left hand applies a posteroanterior force to the tibia while the right hand applies an anteroposterior force to the fibula. A (ii) Posteroanterior. The right hand applies an anteroposterior force to the tibia while the left hand applies a posteroanterior force to the fibula.

(Continued)

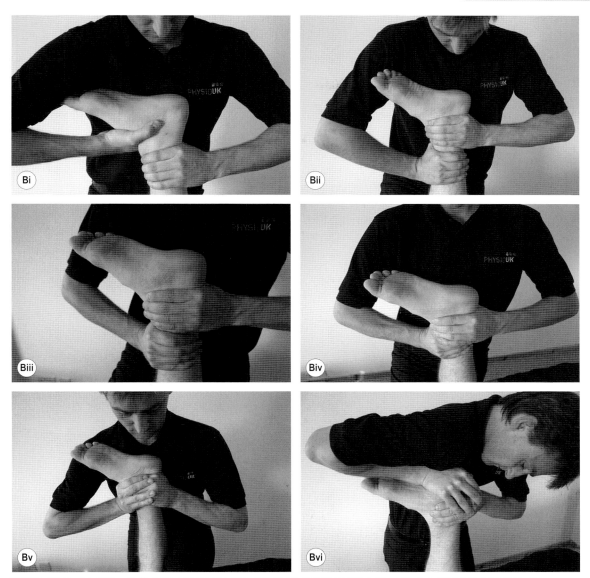

Figure 16.6—cont'd • B (i) Anteroposterior. The left hand stabilises the calf while the right hand applies an anteroposterior force to the anterior aspect of the talus. **B** (ii) Posteroanterior. The right hand stabilises the calf while the left hand applies a posteroanterior force to the posterior aspect of the talus. **B** (iii) Medial rotation. The right hand grasps the lower leg to stabilise the tibia while the left hand holds the talus posteriorly and rotates the talus medially. **B** (iv) Lateral rotation. The right hand grasps the lower leg to stabilise the tibia while the left hand holds the talus posteriorly and rotates the talus laterally. **B** (v) Longitudinal caudad. The clinician lightly rests the leg on the posterior aspect of the patient's thigh to stabilise and then grasps around the talus to pull upwards. **B** (vi) Longitudinal cephalad. The left hand supports the foot in dorsiflexion while the right hand applies a longitudinal cephalad force through the calcaneus.

(Continued)

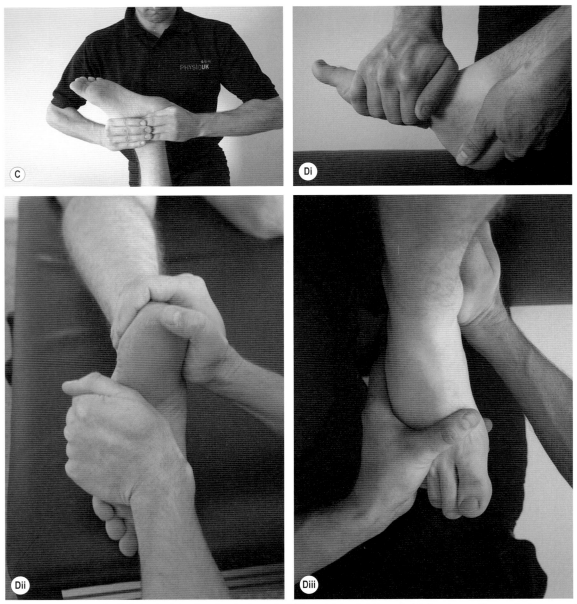

Figure 16.6—cont'd • C Subtalar joint, longitudinal caudad. The clinician lightly rests his/her leg on the posterior aspect of the patient's thigh to stabilise it and then grasps around the calcaneus with the left hand and the forefoot with the right hand, and pulls the foot upwards. **D** (i) Anteroposterior to the navicular. Pressure is applied to the anterior aspect of the navicular through the thenar eminence. The other hand stabilises the talus. **D** (ii) Posteroanterior to the cuboid. Pressure is applied to the posterior aspect of the cuboid through the thenar eminence whilst the other hand stabilises the calcaneum. **D** (iii) Adduction. The right hand grasps and stabilises the heel while the left hand grasps the forefoot. The left hand then applies an adduction force to the foot. The foot does not invert.

(Continued)

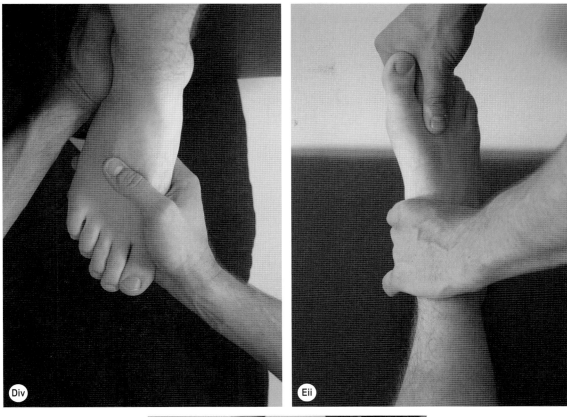

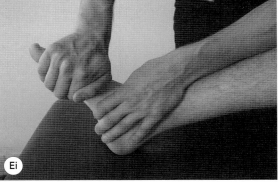

Figure 16.6—cont'd • D (iv) Abduction. The left hand grasps and stabilises the heel while the right hand grasps the forefoot. The right hand then applies an abduction force to the foot. The foot does not evert. **E (i)** Anteroposterior and posteroanterior movement of the first tarsometatarsal joint. The left hand stabilises the medial cuneiform while the right hand applies an anteroposterior and posteroanterior force to the base of the metatarsal. **E (ii)** Medial and lateral rotation of the second tarsometatarsal joint. The left hand stabilises the intermediate cuneiform while the right hand rotates the second metatarsal medially and laterally.

(Continued)

and developed by physiotherapist Brian Mulligan (1999). They can be used to assess changes in symptoms and, if they cause a noticeable change in symptoms or range, they may strengthen hypotheses relating to the structures moved contributing to symptoms and hence considered as treatment options.

Mobilisations with movement
(Mulligan 1999)

Inferior tibiofibular joint. The patient lies supine and is asked actively to invert the foot while the clinician applies an anteroposterior glide to the fibula (Figure 16.7). An increase in range and no pain or reduced pain are positive examination findings indicating a mechanical joint problem.

Plantarflexion of the ankle joint. The patient lies supine with the knee flexed and the foot over the end of the plinth. With one hand the clinician applies an anteroposterior glide to the lower end of the tibia and fibula and with the other hand rolls the talus anteriorly while the patient is asked actively to plantarflex the ankle (Figure 16.8A). An increase in range and no pain or reduced pain are positive examination findings indicating a mechanical joint problem.

Dorsiflexion of the ankle joint. The patient lies supine with the foot over the end of the plinth. The clinician applies an anteroposterior glide to the calcaneus and the talus while the patient is asked actively to dorsiflex the ankle (Figure 16.8B). Since the extensor tendons lift the examiner's hand away from the talus, the patient is asked to contract

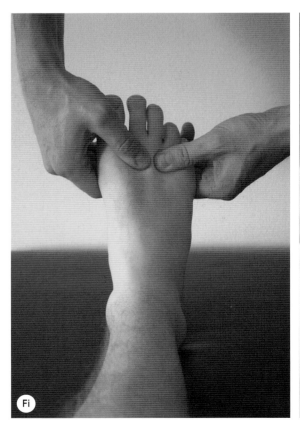

Fi

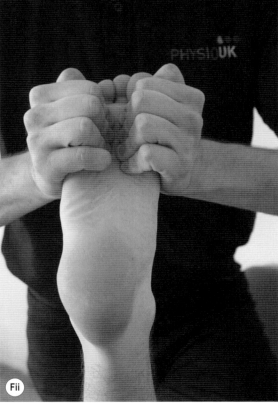

Fii

Figure 16.6—cont'd • F Proximal and distal intermetatarsal joints. Anteroposterior and posteroanterior movement. The hands grasp adjacent metatarsal heads and apply a force in opposite directions to produce an anteroposterior and a posteroanterior movement at the distal intermetatarsal joint. **F (ii)** Horizontal flexion. The fingers are placed in the centre of the foot at the level of the metatarsal heads. The metatarsal heads are then curved around the fingertips to produce horizontal flexion. You might think of folding the foot over.

(Continued)

repetitively and then relax. With relaxation, the clinician moves the ankle into the further range of dorsiflexion gained during the contraction.

Inversion of foot and ankle. This test is carried out on patients with pain over the medial border of the foot on inversion due to a 'positional' fault of the first metatarsophalangeal joint. The patient actively inverts the foot while the clinician applies a sustained anteroposterior glide to the base of the first metatarsal and a posteroanterior glide on the base of the second metatarsal (Figure 16.9). An increase in range and no pain or reduced pain are positive examination findings indicating a mechanical joint problem.

Metatarsophalangeal joints. This test is carried out if the patient has pain under the transverse arch

of the foot due to a positional fault of a metatarsal head. The patient actively flexes the toes while the clinician grasps the heads of adjacent metatarsals and applies a sustained posteroanterior glide to the head of the affected metatarsal (Figure 16.10). An increase in range and no pain or reduced pain are positive examination findings indicating a mechanical joint problem.

Completion of the examination

Having carried out the above tests, the basic examination of the foot and ankle is complete. Further testing may be carried out which considers the biomechanics of the foot and ankle complex but this

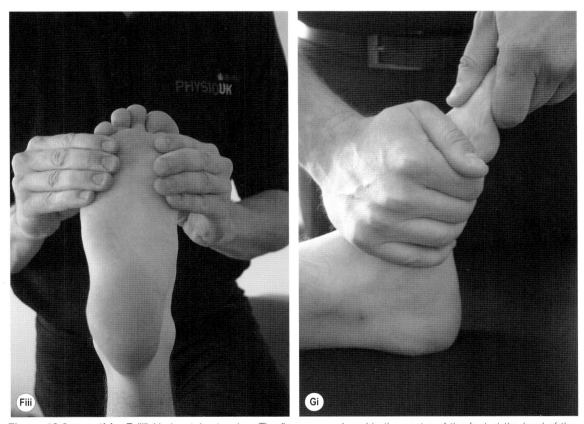

Figure 16.6—cont'd • F (iii) Horizontal extension. The fingers are placed in the centre of the foot at the level of the metatarsal heads. The metatarsal heads are then opened out, curving over the thumbs on the dorsum of the foot to produce horizontal extension. You might think of fanning the foot out. G First metatarsophalangeal joint. For all these movements, one hand stabilises the metatarsal head while the other hand moves the proximal phalanx. G (i) Anteroposterior and posteroanterior movement. The proximal phalanx is moved anteriorly and posteriorly.

(Continued)

is outside the scope of this text. Such information gained from further testing will enhance hypotheses regarding contributing factors.

The subjective and physical examinations produce a large amount of information, which should be recorded accurately and quickly. It is vital at this stage to highlight important findings from the examination with an asterisk (*). These findings must be reassessed at, and within, subsequent treatment sessions to evaluate the effects of treatment on the patient's condition.

The physical testing procedures which specifically examine joint, nerve or muscle tissues are summarised in Table 3.10. The strongest evidence that a joint is contributing to the patient's symptoms is that active and passive physiological movements, passive accessory movements and joint palpation all reproduce the patient's symptoms, and that, following a treatment dose, reassessment identifies an improvement

in the patient's signs and symptoms. Weaker evidence includes an alteration in range, resistance or quality of physiological and/or accessory movements and tenderness over the joint, with no alteration in signs and symptoms after treatment. One or more of these findings may indicate a dysfunction of a joint which may or may not be contributing to the patient's condition. A working knowledge of underpinning pain mechanisms should always be integrated into inferences drawn from physical testing to avoid false positives.

The strongest evidence that a muscle is contributing to a patient's symptoms is if active movements, an isometric contraction, passive lengthening and palpation of a muscle all reproduce the patient's symptoms, and that, following a treatment dose, reassessment identifies an improvement in the patient's signs and symptoms. Further evidence of muscle dysfunction may be suggested by reduced strength or poor quality during

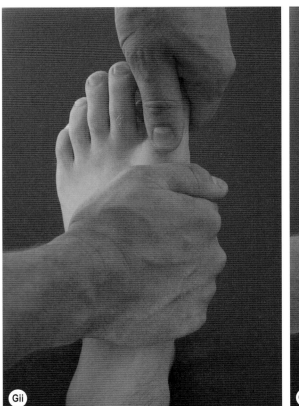

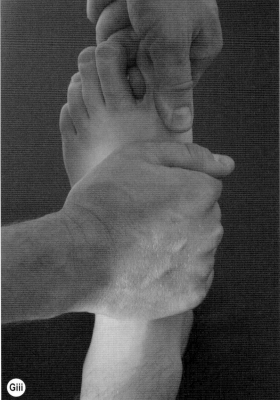

Figure 16.6—cont'd • G (ii) Medial and lateral transverse movement. The proximal phalanx is moved medially and laterally. **G** (iii) Medial and lateral rotation. The proximal phalanx is moved into medial and lateral rotation.

(Continued)

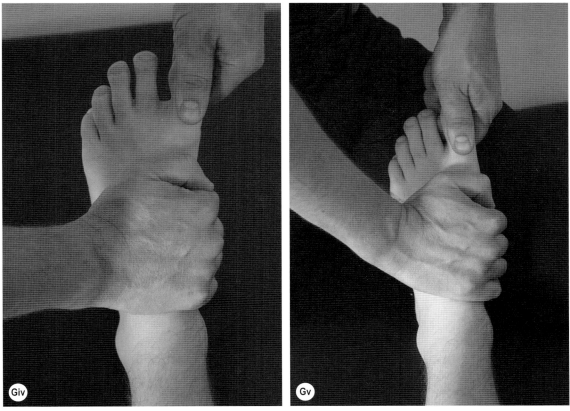

Figure 16.6—cont'd • G (iv) Abduction and adduction. The proximal phalanx is moved into abduction and adduction. G (v) Longitudinal caudad and cephalad. The proximal phalanx is moved in a cephalad and caudad direction.

Table 16.3 Accessory movements, choice of application and reassessment of the patient's asterisks

Accessory movements	Choice of application	Identify any effect of accessory movements on patient's signs and symptoms
Accessory movements for the foot and ankle joints	Start position, e.g.	Reassess all asterisks
Inferior tibiofibular joint ↕ Anteroposterior ↕ Posteroanterior ↕↕ Anteroposterior/posteroanterior glide	– in dorsiflexion – in plantarflexion – in inversion – in eversion	
Talocrural joint	Speed of force application	
↕ Anteroposterior ↕ Posteroanterior	Direction of applied force Point of application of applied force	

(Continued)

Table 16.3 Accessory movements, choice of application and reassessment of the patient's asterisks—cont'd

Accessory movements		Choice of application	Identify any effect of accessory movements on patient's signs and symptoms
Med	Medial rotation		
Lat	Lateral rotation		
Caud	Longitudinal caudad		
Ceph	Longitudinal cephalad		

Subtalar joint

Caud	Longitudinal caudad		

Intertarsal joints

	Anteroposterior		
	Posteroanterior		
	Anteroposterior/posteroanterior glide		
Abd	Abduction		
Add	Adduction		

Tarsometatarsal joints

	Anteroposterior		
	Posteroanterior		
	Anteroposterior/posteroanterior glide		
Med	Medial rotation		
Lat	Materal rotation		

Proximal and distal intermetatarsal joints

	Anteroposterior		
	Posteroanterior		
	Anteroposterior/posteroanterior glide		
HF	Horizontal flexion		
HE	Horizontal extension		

Metatarsophalangeal and interphalangeal joints

	Anteroposterior		
	Posteroanterior		
	Anteroposterior/posteroanterior glide		
Med	Medial transverse		
Lat	Lateral transverse		
Med	Medial rotation		
Lat	Lateral rotation		
Abd	Abduction		
Add	Adduction		
Caud	Longitudinal caudad		
Ceph	Longitudinal cephalad		

Ten accessory movements of the tarsal bones (Kaltenborn 2002)

Movements in the middle of the foot

– fix 2nd and 3rd cuneiform bones and mobilise 2nd metatarsal bone
– fix 2nd and 3rd cuneiform bones and mobilise 3rd metatarsal bone

(Continued)

Table 16.3 Accessory movements, choice of application and reassessment of the patient's asterisks—cont'd

Accessory movements	Choice of application	Identify any effect of accessory movements on patient's signs and symptoms
Movements on the medial side of the foot		
– fix 1st cuneiform bone and mobilise 1st metatarsal bone – fix the navicular bone and mobilise the 1st, 2nd and 3rd cuneiform bones – fix the talus and mobilise the navicular bone		
Movements on the lateral side of the foot		
– fix the cuboid bone and mobilise the 4th and 5th metatarsal bones – fix the navicular and 3rd cuneiform bones and mobilise the cuboid bone – fix the calcaneus and mobilise the cuboid bone		
Movement between talus and calcaneus		
– fix the talus and mobilise the calcaneus		
Movements in the ankle joint		
– fix the leg and move the talus or fix the talus and move the leg		
?Lumbar spine	As above	Reassess all asterisks
?Sacroiliac joint	As above	Reassess all asterisks
?Hip	As above	Reassess all asterisks
?Tibiofemoral joint	As above	Reassess all asterisks
?Patellofemoral joint	As above	Reassess all asterisks

the active physiological movement and the isometric contraction, reduced range and/or increased/decreased resistance, during the passive lengthening of the muscle, and tenderness on palpation, with no alteration in signs and symptoms after treatment. One or more of these

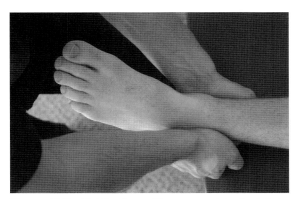

Figure 16.7 • Mobilisations with movement for the inferior tibiofibular joint. The left hand supports the ankle while the heel of the right hand applies an anteroposterior glide to the fibula as the patient inverts the foot.

findings may indicate a dysfunction of a muscle which may or may not be contributing to the patient's condition.

The strongest evidence that a nerve is contributing to the patient's symptoms is when active and/or passive physiological movements reproduce the patient's symptoms, which are then increased or decreased with the addition or removal of a sensitising movement respectively, at a distance from the patient's symptoms. In addition, there is reproduction of the patient's symptoms on palpation of the nerve and following neurodynamic testing, sufficient to be considered a treatment dose, results in an improvement in the above signs and symptoms. Further evidence of nerve dysfunction may be suggested by reduced range (compared with the asymptomatic side) and/or increased resistance to the various arm movements, and tenderness on nerve palpation.

On completion of the physical examination the clinician:

• warns the patient of possible exacerbation up to 24–48 hours following the examination

417

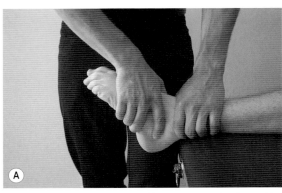

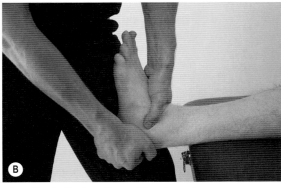

Figure 16.8 • Mobilisations with movement for the ankle joint. A Plantarflexion. The left hand applies an anteroposterior glide to the tibia and fibula while the other hand rolls the talus anteriorly as the patient actively plantarflexes. B Dorsiflexion. The right hand holds the posterior aspect of the calcaneus and the left hand grips the anterior aspect of the talus. Both hands apply an anteroposterior glide as the patient actively dorsiflexes.

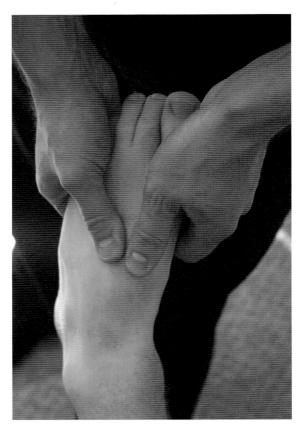

Figure 16.9 • Mobilisations with movement for inversion of the foot and ankle. The left hand applies an anteroposterior glide to the base of the first metatarsal and the right hand applies a posteroanterior glide to the base of the second metatarsal while the patient actively inverts.

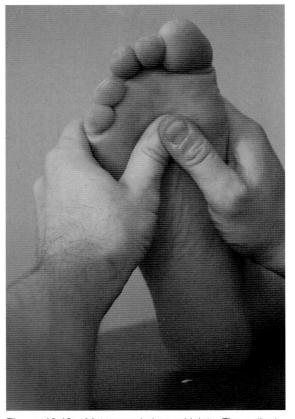

Figure 16.10 • Metatarsophalangeal joints. The patient actively flexes the toes while the clinician uses thumb pressure to apply a posteroanterior glide to the head of a metatarsal.

and reassures the patient this is normal. An explanation of things being moved in different ways may alleviate any anxiety associated with this. Explain, that, if it does occur, it will pass in a few days, much like the soreness felt after visiting a gym

- requests the patient to report details on the behaviour of the symptoms following examination at the next attendance
- explains the findings of the physical examination and how these findings relate to the subjective assessment. Any misconceptions patients may have regarding their illness or injury should be addressed
- evaluates the findings, formulates a clinical diagnosis and writes up a problem list
- determines the objectives of treatment
- devises an initial treatment plan.

In this way, the clinician will have developed the following hypotheses categories (adapted from Jones & Rivett 2004):

- function: abilities and restrictions

- patient's perspective on his/her experience
- source of symptoms. This includes the structure or tissue that is thought to be producing the patient's symptoms, the nature of the structure or tissues in relation to the healing process and the pain mechanisms
- contributing factors to the development and maintenance of the problem. There may be environmental, psychosocial, behavioural, physical or heredity factors
- precautions/contraindications to treatment and management. This includes the severity and irritability of the patient's symptoms and the nature of the patient's condition
- management strategy and treatment plan
- prognosis – this can be affected by factors such as the stage and extent of the injury as well as the patient's expectation, personality and lifestyle.

For guidance on treatment and management principles, the reader is directed to the companion textbook (Petty 2011).

References

Armstrong, D., 1999. Loss of protective sensation: a practical evidence based definition. J. Foot Ankle Surg. 38 (10), 79–80.

Bachmann, L.M., Kolb, E., Koller, M.T., et al., 2003. Accuracy of Ottawa ankle rules to exclude fractures of the ankle and mid-foot: systematic review. Br. Med. J. 326 (7386), 417.

Cavanagh, P.R., Morag, E., Boulton, A.J.M., et al., 1997. The relationship of static foot structure to dynamic foot function. J. Biomech. 30 (3), 243–250.

Christensen, J.C., Jennings, M.M., 2009. Normal and abnormal function of the first ray. Clin. Podiatr. Med. Surg. 26 (3), 355–371.

Cole, J.H., Furness, A.L., Twomey, L.T., 1988. Muscles in action, an approach to manual muscle testing. Churchill Livingstone, Edinburgh.

Corrigan, B., Maitland, G.D., 1994. Musculoskeletal and sports injuries. Butterworth-Heinemann, Oxford.

Cyriax, J., 1982. Textbook of orthopaedic medicine – diagnosis of soft tissue lesions, eighth ed. Baillière Tindall, London.

Fromherz, W.A., 1995. Examination. In: Hunt, G.C., McPoil, T.G. (Eds.), Physical therapy of the foot and ankle. Clinics in physical therapy, second ed. Churchill Livingstone, New York, p. 81.

Fujii, T., Luo, Z., Kitaoka, H.B., et al., 2000. The manual stress test may not be sufficient to differentiate ankle ligament injuries. Clin. Biomech. 15 (8), 619–623.

Grieve, G.P., 1981. Common vertebral joint problems. Churchill Livingstone, Edinburgh.

Grieve, G.P., 1991. Mobilisation of the spine, fifth ed. Churchill Livingstone, Edinburgh.

Hislop, H., Montgomery, J., 1995. Daniels and Worthingham's muscle testing, techniques of manual examination, seventh ed. W B Saunders, Philadelphia.

Janda, V., 1994. Muscles and motor control in cervicogenic disorders: assessment and management. In: Grant, R. (Ed.), Physical therapy of the cervical and thoracic spine, second ed. Churchill Livingstone, New York, p. 195.

Janda, V., 2002. Muscles and motor control in cervicogenic disorders. In: Grant, R. (Ed.), Physical therapy of the cervical and thoracic spine. third ed. Churchill Livingstone, New York, p. 182.

Jones, M.A., Rivett, D.A., 2004. Clinical reasoning for manual therapists. Butterworth-Heinemann, Edinburgh.

Jull, G.A., Janda, V., 1987. Muscles and motor control in low back pain: assessment and management. In: Twomey, L.T., Taylor, J.R. (Eds.), Physical therapy of the low back. Churchill Livingstone, New York, p. 253.

Kaltenborn, F.M., 2002. Manual mobilisation of the joints, vol I. The extremities, sixth ed. Norli, Oslo.

Kendall, F.P., McCreary, E.K., Provance, P.G., et al., 2005. Muscles: testing and function with posture and pain, fifth ed. Williams & Wilkins, Baltimore.

Magee, D.J., 1997. Orthopedic physical assessment, third ed. W B Saunders, Philadelphia.

Main, C.J., Spanswick, C.C., 1999. Pain management: an interdisciplinary approach. Churchill Livingstone, Edinburgh.

Maitland, G.D., 1991. Peripheral manipulation, third ed. Butterworths, London.

McLeod-Roberts, J., 1995. Neurological assessment. In: Merriman, L., Tollafield, D. (Eds.), Assessment of the lower limb. Churchill Livingstone, Edinburgh.

Mulligan, B.R., 1999. Manual therapy 'NAGs', 'SNAGs', 'MWMs' etc., fourth ed. Plane View Services, New Zealand.

Norkin, C.C., Levangie, P.K., 1992. Joint structure and function, a comprehensive analysis, second ed. F A Davis, Philadelphia.

Patla, C.E., Abbot, J.H., 2000. Tibialis posterior myofascial tightness as a source of heel pain: diagnosis and treatment. J. Orthop. Sports Phys. Ther. 30 (10), 624–632.

Petty, N.J., 2011. Principles of neuromusculoskeletal treatment and management: a guide for therapists, second ed. Churchill Livingstone, Edinburgh.

Roy, S., Irvin, R., 1983. Sports medicine: prevention, evaluation, management and rehabilitation. Prentice-Hall, Englewood Cliffs.

Tollafield, D., Merriman, L., 1995. Assessment of the locomotor system. In: Merriman, L., Tollafield, D. (Eds.), Assessment of the lower limb. Churchill Livingstone, Edinburgh.

van Beek, E.J.R., Büller, H.R., Oudkerk, M., 2009. Deep vein thrombosis and pulmonary embolism. Wiley Blackwell, Oxford.

van Griensven, H., 2005. Pain in practice. Butterworth Heinemann, Oxford.

Waddell, G., 2004. The back pain revolution, second ed. Churchill Livingstone, Edinburgh.

Wadsworth, C.T., 1988. Manual examination and treatment of the spine and extremities. Williams & Wilkins, Baltimore.

Whittle, M.W., 2007. Gait analysis: an introduction, fourth ed. Butterworth Heinemann, Oxford, p. 52.

Index

Note: Page numbers followed by 'b' indicate boxes, 'f' indicate figures and 't' indicate tables.

X

Y

Z